# REHAB
## SCIENCE

HOW TO OVERCOME PAIN AND HEAL FROM INJURY

## DR. TOM WALTERS

WITH GLEN CORDOZA

First published in 2023 by Victory Belt Publishing Inc.

ISBN-13: 978-1-628601-39-8

The information included in this book is for educational purposes only. It is not intended or implied to be a substitute for professional medical advice. The reader should always consult their healthcare provider to determine the appropriateness of the information for their own situation or if they have any questions regarding a medical condition or treatment plan. Reading the information in this book does not constitute a physician-patient relationship. The statements in this book have not been evaluated by the Food and Drug Administration, nor are they intended to diagnose, treat, cure, or prevent any disease. The author and publisher expressly disclaim responsibility for any adverse effects that may result from the use or application of the information contained in this book.

Cover design by Elita San Juan

Interior design by Yordan Terziev and Boryana Yordanova

Illustrations by Allan Santos, Elita San Juan, Crizalie Olimpo, Charisse Reyes, and Eugen and Arsim Loki of @Pheasyque

Printed in Canada

TC 0423

# contents

# BODY AREA MAP

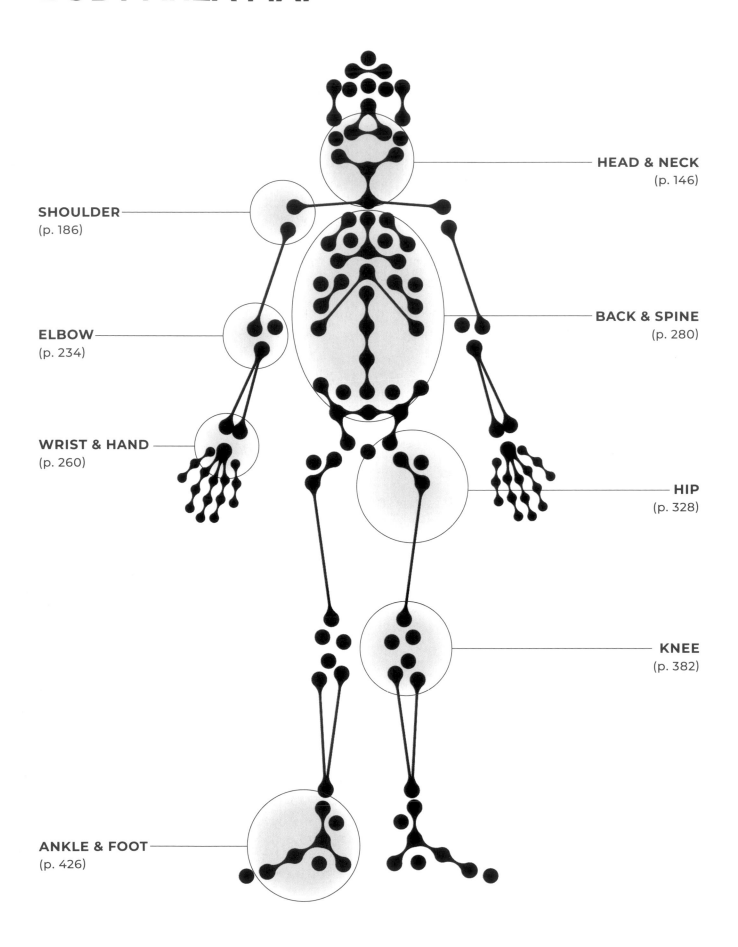

**HEAD & NECK**
(p. 146)

**SHOULDER**
(p. 186)

**BACK & SPINE**
(p. 280)

**ELBOW**
(p. 234)

**WRIST & HAND**
(p. 260)

**HIP**
(p. 328)

**KNEE**
(p. 382)

**ANKLE & FOOT**
(p. 426)

# INTRODUCTION

In many ways, the rehab model is broken.

It's not that the interventions practitioners provide aren't helpful or that rehab doesn't work—it's that the system is fundamentally flawed, and that has created a disconnect between the role of the practitioner, the goals of rehab, and the needs of the patient.

I became a physical therapist (PT) to help people. But when I started my first job in an orthopedic clinic nearly two decades ago, I was instantly hamstrung by the insurance-based model. I was expected to see a dozen patients a day, the sessions were kept too short, and return visits were spaced much too far apart. Before patients could make a full recovery, their insurance coverage would run out and treatments would end. Like many of my fellow PTs, I was overworked and frustrated knowing that I wasn't providing adequate care for those who were suffering.

I'm sorry to say that the same problems persist today. A patient might have insurance, but they have trouble finding a clinic that prioritizes their health. And when they finally manage to locate such a clinic, they have to wait months for an appointment. Worse still, there are many patients who don't have insurance, which can take even less-than-optimal treatment options off the table because they can't afford the out-of-pocket expenses.

These factors tend to leave people with just a few options:

- They can do nothing and hope that their pain goes away or their injury heals.
- They can seek alternative forms of treatment and pay out-of-pocket for in-person care.
- They can attempt to self-manage their condition.

Let's examine each option. Through that examination, I'll outline the solutions *Rehab Science* provides—and tell you what this book is about, who it's for, and how you can get the most out of it.

## OPTION 1: DO NOTHING

Some injuries and pain symptoms simply go away with time—you rest, avoid the behaviors and activities that led to problems, and get better. In this way, doing nothing can work, but only immediately following an injury that causes sudden or acute pain.

With most injuries, you need to implement techniques that reduce swelling, promote blood flow, and alleviate pain within a few days of getting hurt and then start rebuilding the tissue with movement and exercise. But most people do the opposite. The natural response is to protect the area, which is fine in the early phases of healing but can turn into a passive coping strategy that perpetuates a cycle of pain avoidance. When you move less, the area becomes deconditioned, and the likelihood of reinjury and developing chronic pain increases.

## OPTION 2: SEEK ALTERNATIVE IN-PERSON TREATMENTS

It's hard to beat in-person treatment from a skilled PT using science-based methods in a facility that prioritizes quality care. These PTs make assessments, design programs, select exercises, and use manual therapy techniques that are specific to the individual and the condition. If you have a catastrophic injury or need reconstructive surgery, it's the best option.

But let's assume you have pain or an injury that is less severe and not life-threatening—such as an overuse injury like a tendinopathy, muscle strain, joint sprain, sudden acute pain, or lingering pain. When in-person physical therapy is not optimal because the clinics in your area follow the broken model, you are left with complementary and alternative practices such as acupuncture, massage therapy, and chiropractic (to mention a few). Practitioners in these fields offer services that are typically not covered by insurance. You often pay out-of-pocket for treatment and, as a result, you may get more attention or receive a type of specialized care that can be helpful. But these modalities are not without flaws.

For starters, these services are out of reach for most people because they are too expensive or are not available locally. Even when complementary and alternative practices are an option, it can be difficult to find a practice that's geared toward mobility and resistance training, which have the best long-term evidence for resolving pain and rehabilitating injuries.

Even more concerning, many of these practices base their entire business model around the narrative that what they do is necessary for the patient to remain healthy. They stress the importance of return visits for tune-up treatments that might not really be needed. The role of a healthcare practitioner is to help patients find relief and heal—not to lock them into an endless cycle of follow-up. With this model, people can become dependent on the treatment and lose confidence in their ability to self-manage their condition.

## OPTION 3: SELF-MANAGE

Self-guided pain and injury management is the heart of *Rehab Science*. The goal is to confront the problem intelligently with active coping strategies—education, movement, and exercise. Through education, you can learn how to identify and address potential factors that influence the pain experience. Movement and exercise will break the pain cycle, improve tissue capacity, and boost confidence in the system, which ultimately encourages self-efficacy.

When you learn how to do something yourself and avoid becoming dependent on medication, surgery, or passive manipulations, you gain physical and psychological strength and resiliency. The problem is that most people have an incomplete picture of how their mind and body are connected to their symptoms and what steps they need to take to get better. It's difficult to know who to trust and how to filter through information to find the right treatment plan. People get stuck, or they jump from one program to another, never making progress.

I wrote this book to change that.

## BECOMING YOUR OWN PT

My intention with this book is to simplify the science so that it is accessible to everyone, and to provide stepwise strategies for dealing with the most common musculoskeletal conditions. I've done so with two groups in mind:

- People who want to better understand how to treat orthopedic pain and injuries on their own

- Medical and non-medical practitioners (doctors, physical therapists, personal trainers, and so on) who want to expand their knowledge, pass along evidence-based strategies to their patients or clients, and find concise methods and programs that they can reference and implement

To help you navigate this book, I've broken it into three parts.

Part I: Pain and Part II: Injury focus on education. Knowing what pain is, how it works, and what the different types are will give meaning and purpose to the strategies for alleviating and preventing both acute and chronic conditions. The same is true for injuries. There are many types, each of which has a different healing time frame and plays into how you should approach rehab. When you understand pain, you get better faster. When you understand what is injured and how long it should take to heal, you're less likely to make the injury worse, and you will recover more quickly. Understanding improves adherence, and adherence promotes consistency—both of which are necessary for getting better.

Parts I and II also explain how pain and injury are different, which is why I discuss them separately. They are often related because injuries can create acute pain, but you can have pain even when no tissue is damaged—as is the case with chronic pain. That's important to know because if you have pain that is not tied to an injury, you might need to address other aspects of your lifestyle that could be contributing factors, which I cover in Chapter 4.

Part III: Rehab provides comprehensive rehab protocols for the most common pains and injuries for all the main regions and joints of the body (see page 4 or 117 for the full body area map). Each protocol includes a movement and exercise program broken into three phases based on your pain symptoms, stage of healing, and functional abilities—similar to a program that a licensed PT would develop for you.

To address your particular pain or injury immediately, go to Part III, find the protocol that matches your symptoms or diagnosis, and then follow the rehab exercise program. Just be sure to review the introductory chapters in that part so you understand how the protocols are structured and how to get the most from the exercises.

I'd also like to point out that you do not need to be in pain or injured to benefit from the programs. Whether your goal is to address a weak link in your body, improve mobility with certain movements or ranges of motion, or strengthen a specific body region, the three-phase exercise programs will serve you well. Simply go to the body region that you want to improve or maintain and follow a program, or cherry-pick from the exercises to design your own program.

Remember, the exercises you do in rehab are the same exercises you use to maintain and improve the health of your body.

If you decide to go to Part III as your first stop, that is fine. You don't need to understand the science behind pain and injury to benefit from the programs. Although I believe the science is important to understand—the knowledge can expedite healing, prevent future occurrences, and help you approach rehab in a more efficient way—the protocols are the highlight of this book. When followed diligently, they are the quickest route to recovery. However, I've found that as patients go through them and experience the benefits, they often become more interested in the science, which is waiting for you in Parts I and II.

With a healthcare system designed to treat symptoms with medication and surgical interventions and a rehab model that doesn't always provide the best care, it's more important than ever to take control of your health—and that is exactly what *Rehab Science* will help you do. Through education and stepwise programs, it will empower you to self-manage common musculoskeletal issues and start resolving your pain and healing your injuries on your own terms.

# PART I
# PAIN

## CHAPTER 1

# WHAT IS PAIN?

"What is pain?" is probably not the first question you would ask when you are experiencing pain, but it's an important one to answer.

First, it's crucial to realize that pain is not only normal but also important to your overall health. **Pain is an unpleasant experience that helps keep you alive by alerting you to actual or potential bodily damage.**[1] It warns you that something might be wrong, and it gives you an opportunity to change or stop what you're doing to prevent further harm. But pain is a complex phenomenon, and many factors influence it.

In the coming chapters, I'll outline what's going on inside your body when you experience pain and equip you with the tools and knowledge to prevent and alleviate it. Because there are strategies that can help, even if you've been in pain for years and nothing has worked. By educating yourself, you can reshape how you think about pain and take the first steps toward healing.

But before you delve into the solutions and prescriptive protocols, it's helpful to understand why we approach pain the way we do. How did pain science get to where it is today? How do we know what pain is and how it works?

# THE CARTESIAN MODEL OF PAIN

Much of what we used to believe about pain was based on the Cartesian model established by philosopher, mathematician, and scientist René Descartes in his book *L'Homme,* published in 1644. He proposed that pain messages were detected by receptors in the body and sent along pathways to the brain. Those messages made us aware of a problem so that we could act in a way to reduce further harm.[2]

Back then, pain was thought to be a fairly simple sensory experience, as if the nervous system was merely detecting an external sensation—something that existed independent of the brain.

It would be wonderful if pain always worked that way. You could just stop doing the thing that was hurting you, and the pain would go away. Unfortunately, it's not that cut-and-dried.

The problem with the Cartesian model is that it separates the mind and body (a concept known as mind-body dualism) and doesn't explain the vast array of pain experiences that people report. As a result, researchers started to broaden their focus when studying mismatches between the physical stimulus and the person's pain experience. Ultimately, the research began to reflect a changing view of the brain's role in pain.

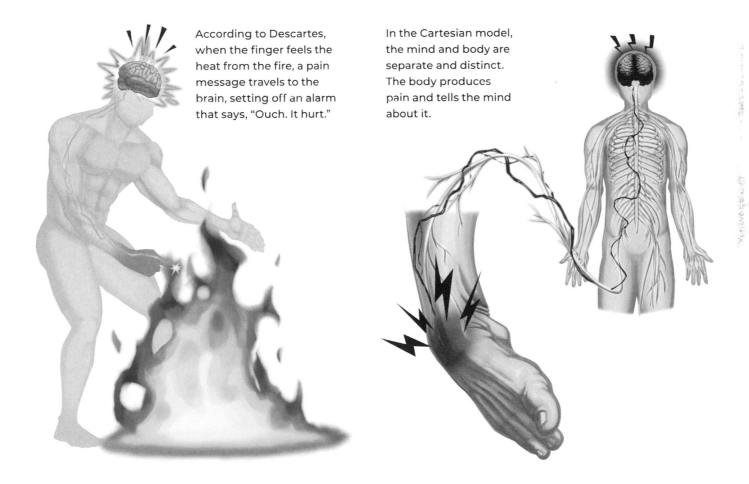

According to Descartes, when the finger feels the heat from the fire, a pain message travels to the brain, setting off an alarm that says, "Ouch. It hurt."

In the Cartesian model, the mind and body are separate and distinct. The body produces pain and tells the mind about it.

# MODERN PAIN SCIENCE

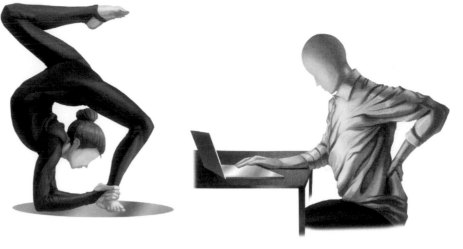

Pain is not always as simple as tissues being in danger. **Activities that should create pain—like a contortionist bending their body in unnatural ways—sometimes don't. And pain can exist when nothing dangerous is happening to the body, such as when sitting at a computer.**

This new understanding of pain stems from several types of studies, starting with phantom limb pain—a phenomenon in which up to 85 percent of people who have lost a limb complain about pain in the absent body part.[3-6] These studies show how complex pain can be and explain why pain is sometimes referred to as an illusion created by the brain. The fact that there are no messages traveling from the limb to the brain because the limb is gone demonstrates the role that the mind plays in the physical experience of pain.

Other studies have shown that people can feel pain even if their tissue isn't damaged or in danger. In these studies, subjects were made to believe through visual cues that harm was going to be done to their bodies, and their brains produced pain to protect them from potential tissue damage. In one study, subjects were shown a red or blue light just prior to being touched on the back of the hand with a metal rod. Even though the rod was always the same temperature, the subjects who saw a red light reported more pain because red signifies hot while blue means cold. Additionally, subjects who were allowed to watch the rod touch their hand reported more pain than those whose vision was blocked.[7]

PHANTOM LIMB PAIN

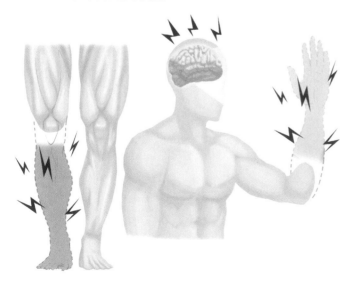

VISUAL CUES AND PAIN PERCEPTION

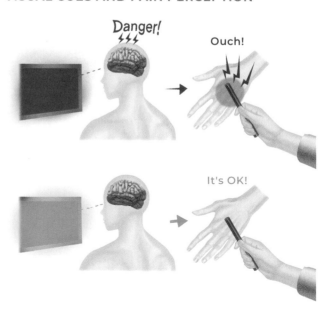

Danger!

Ouch!

It's OK!

There are also cases in which an MRI or X-ray shows evidence of injury, but the person feels no pain. Various studies on asymptomatic (pain-free) subjects found that 30 to 80 percent of them had a bulging disc,[8] 34 percent had a rotator cuff tear,[9-11] 30 percent had meniscus degeneration,[12,13] and the list goes on.

One such case study relayed the story of a soldier who had an X-ray for an unrelated reason and, despite experiencing no pain, was found to have a bullet lodged in his neck.[14] It's as if his brain decided, "This isn't dangerous. There's no need to create pain."

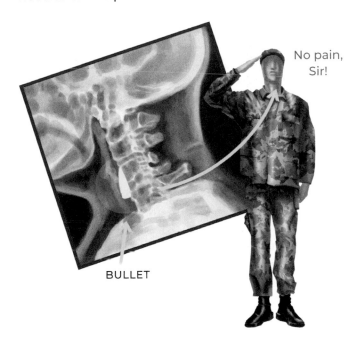

No pain, Sir!

BULLET

What these studies—and many more—illustrate is that pain comes exclusively from the brain, not from pain receptors or pathways in the body. With this new understanding, researchers started to consider a two-way model in which the brain receives stimuli and decides whether those stimuli warrant a pain response.

This model views the brain as a neuromatrix (network of neurons) with multiple inputs and outputs.[15] *Inputs* refers to sensations, but not only those things you touch, see, hear, or smell. You also have joint receptors called proprioceptors that tell you where you are in space, as well as emotional inputs that bring thoughts and feelings into the neuromatrix. Your brain constantly evaluates all these inputs (along with others) to determine whether your environment seems safe.

Touching a hot stove, for example, activates nociceptors—danger receptors that detect noxious stimuli. These stimuli can be thermal (such as something hot), chemical (such as a corrosive substance), or mechanical (such as a smashed finger).

When you touch something, a sensation called an afferent message travels from the tissue up through your spinal cord to a certain part of your brain, depending on the type of message it is. If the message is sensory, it usually goes to your sensory cortex. If it's dangerous, it's translated via a process called nociception. At that point, your brain makes decisions in the form of outputs, which fall into three categories:

- Pain (you hurt)
- Movement (you decide to move)
- A stress report (you feel anxiety)

The first type of output, pain, directly contradicts the Cartesian model, which presumes that pain comes *from* the body. Instead, sensations are constantly coming into the brain. The brain looks at all those inputs, weighs the situation, and chooses how best to protect you, possibly by outputting pain. Basically, it decides whether the circumstances you're in are dangerous and whether you need to alter your actions to avoid injury.

INPUT　　　　　　　　　　　　　　　OUTPUT
NEUROMATRIX

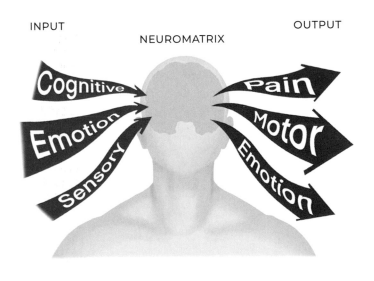

# PAIN COMES FROM THE BRAIN

With this new understanding of the brain's role, pain becomes a complex experience shaped by our thoughts, our emotions, our beliefs, our memories, our stress levels, the sensations we feel, the visual information we take in, and so on rather than simply being a message sent from the physical body.

Lots of people have pain that is largely due to high stress, poor mental health, lack of sleep, and other similar factors. But simply listing factors isn't helpful; you need to understand how these factors influence pain and, more importantly, how to treat it. In subsequent chapters, I'll dig deeper into the experiences and types of pain so that you can confidently evaluate your situation and choose the right rehab protocol to follow.

To sum up, **your brain produces 100 percent of the pain you feel.**[15,16] The brain is complex, thus so is pain. That said, the statement "pain comes from the brain" is often misinterpreted as "the pain is all in your head." That is not what I'm saying. While pain is created by the brain, it is not made up. Each person's pain experience is real and unique. To understand why, we must delve deeper into how pain works, which is the focus of the next chapter.

## THE BIOPSYCHOSOCIAL (BPS) MODEL: A COMPREHENSIVE APPROACH TO TREATING PAIN

It's natural to want to hunt for a direct cause of pain symptoms—a single variable that could be easily fixed. In most programs, practitioners and trainers are taught to think about pain as a tissue-driven biomechanical problem. We call it the postural-structural-biomechanical, or PSB, model. But over time, that model has been shown to be incomplete, especially in terms of fundamental takeaways from pain science research.[17] Certain people simply don't get better with that old-fashioned approach.

Yet this is the model that most physical therapists learn in school and most trainers and doctors base their treatments on—this idea that all pain and injuries stem from your structure, your posture, or your biomechanics (the way you move). Thinking about it from that limited perspective leaves out other factors that are often more closely tied to pain than anatomy is.

With the old PSB model, every problem has a mechanical answer. However, the mechanical treatment doesn't make every patient better. That's where modern pain science and neuroscience come in, analyzing the problem using the biopsychosocial, or BPS, model.[18]

To explain the word *biopsychosocial,* let's break it down into its three components:

- **BIO:** This component encompasses the traditional PSB model, which includes looking at structure, posture, biomechanics, and anatomy. These things are important because many people have pain issues that are driven by their tissues. We look at how force and load affect the body and whether certain postures or movements trigger a person's pain. "Bio" is necessary because we don't want to ignore the tissues of the body; in most cases, the problem really is mostly physical. It is what rehab explores first, trying to figure out if the pain is linked to a mechanical problem with a biological tissue. This is the acute pain phase—pain experienced immediately or soon after injury. Most people who have acute pain remain in "bio" territory, especially if they can point to some kind of physical trauma.

- **PSYCHO:** Thoughts, emotions, and beliefs are hugely important in how you evaluate the world and your own body. At the end of the day, pain is a protective mechanism—it helps you survive. This means your brain can create pain based on a perceived threat, even if there's no damage to your tissue. Pain can also be tied to stressful life events, making "psycho" an essential variable to consider when addressing chronic pain conditions that persist beyond the normal healing time frame.

- **SOCIAL:** The people you interact with are another huge element in pain. We are becoming more and more aware of how important social interaction is to overall health. Loneliness, for example, can be a significant factor for people with pain—lacking social engagement may predispose someone to depression, and that can lead to chronic pain disorders.

All these components are interrelated. And it's important to understand this, because once you realize how your mind, body, and environment (relationships) are connected to your symptoms, you can start to address all the potential factors that might be contributing to your pain.

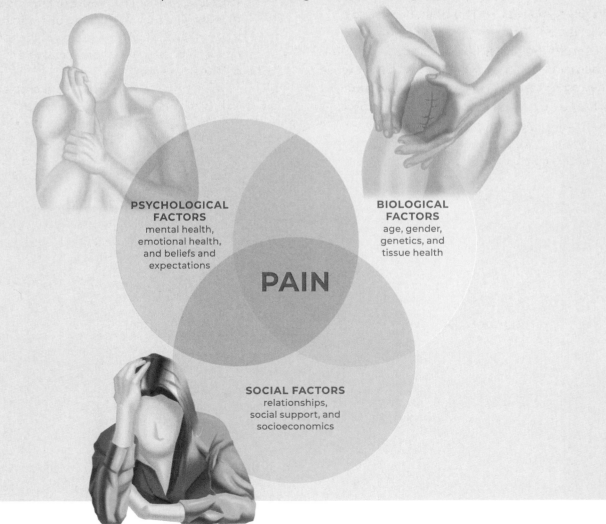

**PSYCHOLOGICAL FACTORS**
mental health, emotional health, and beliefs and expectations

**BIOLOGICAL FACTORS**
age, gender, genetics, and tissue health

**PAIN**

**SOCIAL FACTORS**
relationships, social support, and socioeconomics

## CHAPTER 2

# HOW
# PAIN WORKS

We know that pain is created by the brain and that everyone's pain is different.[1,2] But even though we understand pain better now than we used to, many people still struggle to manage pain on their own.

Pain is rarely hopeless, however. Once you know what it is and how it works, you can reshape how you think about pain and debunk myths that can influence your pain experience. For example, a common misconception is that nerves create pain, when in reality they are tied to pain but not directly responsible for it. Research shows that people who understand how their nerves function are less fearful and feel less threatened by pain, which can help reduce their symptoms.[3-8]

In this chapter, I dive deeper into how pain works and the role your nervous system plays in it. Let's start with the pain loop.

# SENSING THROUGH THE PAIN LOOP

The nervous system has pathways that begin with sensors in your skin, muscles, joints, and other tissues. These sensors, which comprise your peripheral nervous system, are always detecting sensations such as temperature, movement, and pressure and relaying that information to your central nervous system—your spinal cord and brain.

Put simply, nerves carry messages around the body, primarily to and from the brain. Information is constantly coming into the brain for analysis. As discussed in Chapter 1, you do not have pain sensors or pathways; you have receptors that detect sensations that could be dangerous, and those receptors send messages along the sensory pathways in your body.

Whether it's a light touch or contact with a sharp object, all information from the body—called ascending or afferent input—travels to the brain, which analyzes that sensory input to determine whether action is necessary. If it is, the brain sends information back down the system as descending or efferent output, producing a response, such as movement. That is the basic pain loop.

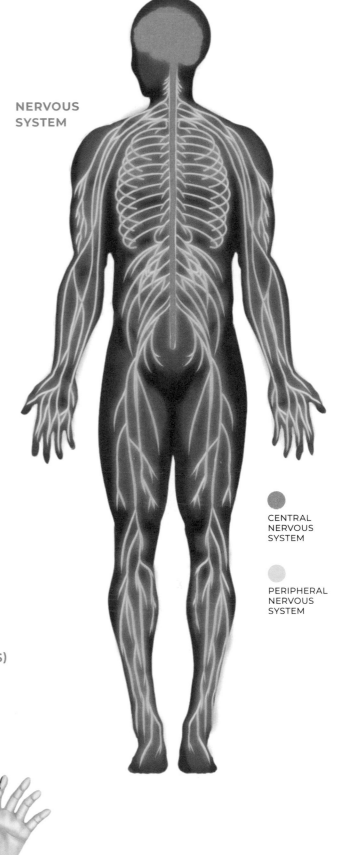

NERVOUS SYSTEM

● CENTRAL NERVOUS SYSTEM

● PERIPHERAL NERVOUS SYSTEM

## PAIN LOOP (AFFERENT AND EFFERENT PATHWAYS)

AFFERENT INPUT

EFFERENT OUTPUT

The sensors in your tissues work together all the time, and various factors can affect their sensitivity. You have sensors that detect the following information:

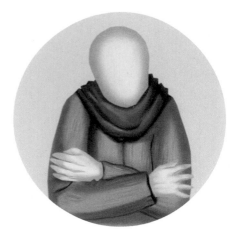

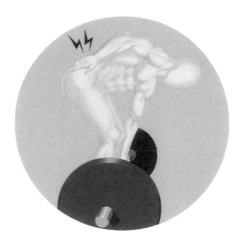

- TEMPERATURE. Some of our primary sensors detect heat and cold. When you hear someone say, "My pain gets worse when it's cold outside," it could mean their nervous system has assessed the situation and determined that cold weather is something to worry about, which can make their temperature sensors more sensitive.

- MOVEMENT. Mechanoreceptors and proprioceptors detect your position in space and how you are moving. Many people have pain that's triggered by certain movements or positions, so in physical therapy, we often try to reduce the sensitivity of these motion sensors. This is a primary area of emphasis in the rehab exercise protocols in this book.

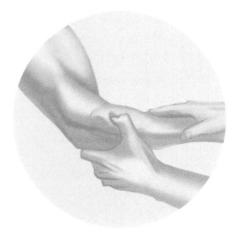

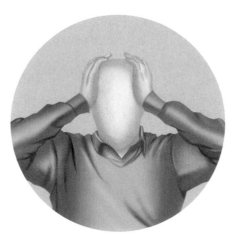

- PRESSURE. These sensors—most of which exist in the skin and muscles and have specific names, like Meissner's corpuscles and Pacinian corpuscles—grade how much pressure is being put on a tissue. When they become sensitized, pushing on the area or bumping into an object will cause pain. In the physical therapy world, this increased sensitivity helps us determine which structures might be contributing to a person's symptoms. We use a type of testing called palpation, which basically involves pushing on specific anatomical structures in an attempt to find the patient's familiar pain.

- STRESS. Elevated stress levels can activate the sensors that respond to stress hormones and make them more sensitive, which the nervous system may perceive as danger. As a result, some people experience pain simply from being stressed. They could be sitting still and experiencing no symptoms until they have a stressful thought, which increases the stress hormones in the bloodstream, activates their sensors, and relays a danger message to their brain, resulting in pain. Remember, thoughts and emotions affect your physical body.

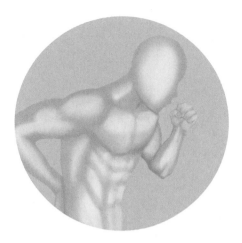

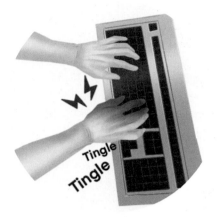

- IMMUNITY. These sensors detect immune system molecules. For example, some people report back pain when they're sick. This can happen because the nervous system has a sort of memory. If you've had previous back pain episodes, even if the pain was mechanical, you may experience that same pain when you're ill. The illness obviously didn't hurt your back, but the circulating immune system molecules may activate those sensors. Chronic inflammation can have the same effect. Normally, the immune system releases molecules to help repair injured tissue, which triggers inflammation, and the levels of these molecules return to baseline when the repair work is done. Sometimes, however, these levels stay elevated in chronic inflammatory states.

- BLOOD FLOW. One reason movement is thought to help pain is that it reduces ischemia, or a lack of blood flow to tissue. If blood flow is limited, oxygen and nutrient delivery decreases, which can activate nociceptors. It's natural for your body to detect low blood flow because it can be dangerous. You respond to these warnings subconsciously. For example, resting your wrist on the edge of your desk while typing for long periods slowly decreases blood flow to your median nerve, which runs through the carpal tunnel on the front of your wrist. These sensors detect the issue and signal you to change your position so that blood flow can return to normal.

Think of the lights on your car's dashboard. Oil pressure, engine temperature, tire pressure, and fuel level lights are there to warn you when something could stop working or be damaged if you don't act. Each light has a corresponding sensor in the car. Those same kinds of sensors are built into your nervous system.

# SENSORY SENSITIVITY

As a quick recap, stimulus starts at the tissue, where sensors pick it up. But your nervous system can dial up the sensitivity of those sensors to protect you, meaning that less stimulus is required to activate them.[9] This happens through neuroplasticity, and it can occur in two to three days if your nervous system considers your situation to be dangerous.[9-11]

Chronic or persistent pain that lasts beyond the normal healing time frame of three months is often the result of a sensor becoming so sensitive that it no longer accurately reflects the state of the tissue. But there's good news: you can use graded interventions (like the rehab exercise protocols in this book) to decrease the sensitivity of that sensor so it once again serves as a reliable indicator of what's happening in your body.

Say a man tries to lift the trailer off his truck, but he's cold, moves too quickly, and injures something. The injury starts as a physical one, but other stressors in his life might have been ramping up his nervous system, such as a strained relationship, bad job situation, or lack of sleep. The result is that six months to a year later, he still has pain when he bends down, even when he isn't lifting something heavy.

This person has moved from an acute pain state (short-term pain) to a chronic pain state (long-term pain). His current pain is likely not an accurate reflection of his physical body because the injured musculoskeletal tissues should have healed in that time. Instead, his nervous system may think it needs to protect him against the bending movement because that movement caused damage in the past. Now, when he bends over to tie his shoes or pick up a pencil, his nervous system recognizes the position as potentially dangerous. Because his brain senses a threat, the movement sensors in that area become more sensitive, and anytime he assumes that position—even though it's not damaging his tissues—he has a similar pain response.

This movement-based problem is called flexion sensitivity. To treat it, a professional develops an exercise program that exposes those sensors to graded amounts of stress. Instead of bending over and doing the exact movement that triggers his nervous system, the man might lie on his back and pull his knees to his chest, which creates flexion in a different context and helps gradually desensitize the sensors.

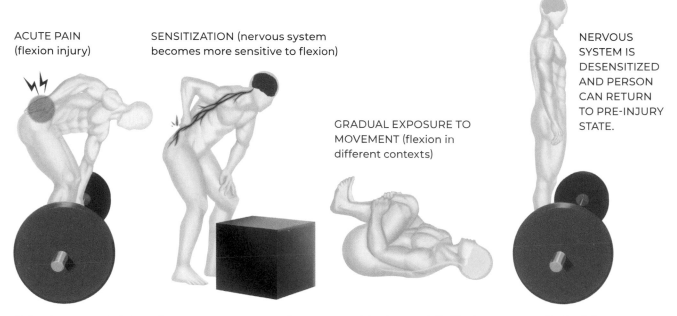

ACUTE PAIN
(flexion injury)

SENSITIZATION (nervous system becomes more sensitive to flexion)

GRADUAL EXPOSURE TO MOVEMENT (flexion in different contexts)

NERVOUS SYSTEM IS DESENSITIZED AND PERSON CAN RETURN TO PRE-INJURY STATE.

Following an acute injury, the nervous system can become sensitized, especially if other stressors (lack of sleep, work/relationship stress, poor nutrition, etc.) are present. The good news is that exposing the body to gradually increasing doses of movement stress can help desensitize the nervous system and promote recovery.

# HOW NEUROPLASTICITY WORKS TO REWIRE PAIN

Most people think neuroplasticity happens only in the brain, but your brain is part of your nervous system. Neuroplasticity rewires the nervous system in your brain, spinal cord, and peripheral nervous system, where nerves go all the way out into your fingers and toes.

The nervous system communicates using molecules called neurotransmitters. Along with other molecules like glucose and proteins, neurotransmitters enter and exit neurons (the long cells that make up nerves) via channels called receptors in the cells' protective membranes.

For example, you have movement sensors in your arms. To perform a movement, your brain releases neurotransmitter molecules into your bloodstream, and when those neurotransmitters approach the neuron, they try to match up with the appropriate membrane receptor. If a neurotransmitter matches the shape of the receptor, a cell "gate" opens, letting it enter and influence the cell.

Imagine a house with multiple sliding doors. If there are bugs outside and I open one sliding door, some bugs might get in. But the more doors I open, the more likely it becomes that I'm going to let bugs inside. Those sliding doors are like the receptors in your neurons, which open and close based on chemicals released by your nervous system.

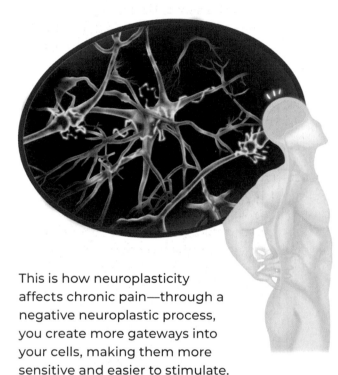

This is how neuroplasticity affects chronic pain—through a negative neuroplastic process, you create more gateways into your cells, making them more sensitive and easier to stimulate.

But neuroplasticity isn't a bad thing. If a movement sensor has become more sensitive, less of a particular movement will activate it and create a painful experience. If you reintroduce that threatening movement in graded steps, however, you can reduce the number of open gates in the cell, using neuroplasticity to your benefit. As you convince your nervous system that the movement is not dangerous, it will remove doors into the cell.

## HOW THE NERVOUS SYSTEM COMMUNICATES

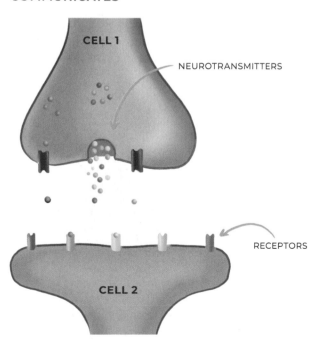

CELL 1

NEUROTRANSMITTERS

RECEPTORS

CELL 2

# ASCENDING (AFFERENT) PATHWAYS FOR PAIN

Your nervous system is like a network of highways. There are 400 nerves in the body totaling 45 miles of nerve pathways, which can be split into two types: ascending (afferent) and descending (efferent).

Your tissues are the starting point. You have sensors all over your body—in your skin, fascia, muscles, tendons, ligaments, and joints— and those nerves are always working in the background, monitoring your situation and environment. If a sensor is stimulated enough, it reaches a threshold and sends a message up to your brain—but to get to the brain, that message must travel through ascending pathways.

Nerves communicate by sending electrical impulses, and most run at a resting rate of about –70 millivolts. When a neurotransmitter activates a sensor, that resting millivolt level creeps up toward an activation threshold, which in most nerves is –55 millivolts. The activated sensor then sends a message to the central nervous system for analysis.

In this part of the pain loop, an ascending danger message is called nociception, or "danger reception." Your brain is constantly receiving information, including danger sensations from special nociceptors that only pick up potentially harmful stimuli. So, if something could damage your tissue, like too much pressure or heat, these higher-threshold nociceptors are activated, and a danger message is sent through an ascending pathway to your brain, where it is analyzed. But this does not always lead to pain.

For example, if you sit at a computer all day, nociceptors in your glutes may be activated because you're losing blood flow to that area. But when your brain receives the message from those sensors, instead of outputting pain, it sends down a movement program to get you to stand up or shift in your seat. Once you get blood flowing to the area again, those nociceptors turn off.

**SITTING ACTIVATES NOCICEPTORS**

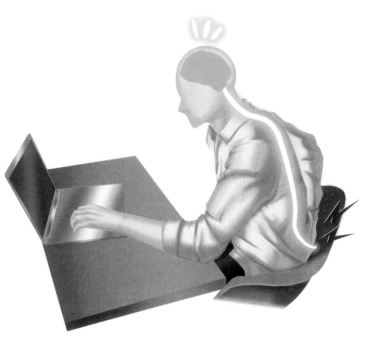

**BRAIN SENDS MOVEMENT PROGRAM**

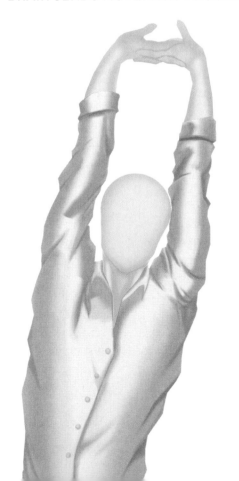

Think of nociceptors like little fingers—free nerve endings in your peripheral nervous system that are constantly on the lookout for danger. If you activate one of the standard sensors—say, by putting pressure on your finger—your brain will get sensory information about that pressure. But if the pressure becomes significant enough, the nociceptors will activate and relay a danger message.

Each sensation must hit a threshold to trigger such a message to the brain. You have the resting or "potential" state of the nerve, and the nociceptors in your nerves, tissues, and cells are always on, waiting for danger. When activated at a higher threshold, they send a message to the brain called an action potential. So, you're sitting at a certain resting voltage but then something stimulates a sensor, which changes the cell's voltage until it hits its threshold and sends an action potential up the spinal cord to the relevant areas of the brain.

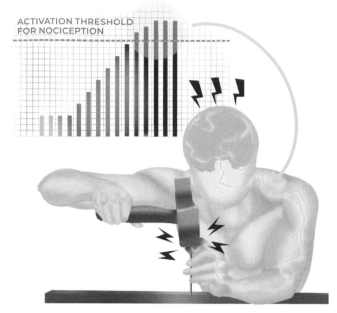

ACTION POTENTIAL

ACTIVATION THRESHOLD FOR NOCICEPTION

You have sensors all over your body. If a sensor is stimulated enough, higher-threshold nociceptors are activated, and a danger message is sent through an ascending pathway to your brain, where it's analyzed.

# HOW THE BRAIN CREATES UNIQUE PAIN

Many regions of the brain are involved in creating pain.[1,2,12] Because the ascending pathways mostly deal with sensory input, a message from an activated sensor will likely enter the somatosensory cortex first. Your brain will start analyzing that information, along with visual information in your occipital lobe, auditory information in your temporal lobe, and so on—every part of your current situation. All these pieces work together, which leads us back to the concept of the neuromatrix.

The brain has no single pain center, as people used to think.[13,14] Now, we recognize that when you feel pain, a certain pattern of brain structures has worked together to create an illusion of pain in your mind. That pattern is called a neurosignature.[1,2]

As the name implies, everyone's neurosignature is unique. You can take 100 people with similar back pain symptoms, and although their pain might involve many of the same regions of the brain, their neurosignatures will vary slightly because their brains are drawing on a variety of inputs to create unique patterns for pain.

These neuromatrix inputs fall into three categories: sensory, emotional, and psychological. Pain is different for everyone, and the brain must process a variety of information from these three inputs to produce it.

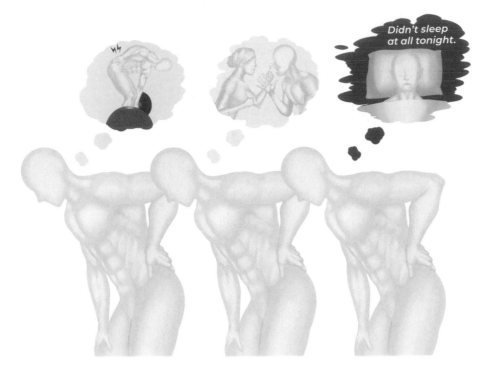

What all this means is that **you should approach pain as a process of rewiring your neurosignature through neuroplasticity—of pinpointing your own pain experience and retraining your nervous system to be less sensitive to those stimuli.** If you have chronic back pain that has lasted more than six months, for example, you shouldn't just unquestioningly follow the rehab protocol that matches your symptoms. You need to listen to your body, address other potential factors (like stress), and respect your pain symptoms by making any necessary modifications to the exercises. Otherwise, you may make your neurosignature even more sensitive and fall into the same loop that created the pain in the first place.

That's the power of the neuromatrix model. All these different brain structures are receiving, analyzing, and acting on information all the time, which creates a unique neurosignature when you have pain. And once that neurosignature exists, less stimulus is needed to trigger that pattern again and re-create the pain.

# DESCENDING (EFFERENT) PATHWAYS FOR PAIN

The descending, or efferent, pathway is the part of the pain loop that delivers a message to act. Although most messages that ascend through the afferent pathways are sensory, most that descend through the efferent pathways are motor, also called an action program.

An action program is usually a movement. Say you put your hand in a bucket of ice water. The temperature sensors in your fingers are switched on in response to the cold, and that stimulus is strong enough to activate a nociceptor, which causes an action potential to travel up your arm, into your spinal cord, and to the somatosensory cortex of your brain.

Using the different regions of the neuromatrix, your brain deems this input dangerous and then outputs not only pain but also an action program. The motor cortex transmits this action program down your spinal cord's corticospinal tract, sending it to the muscles that need to contract—in this case, your elbow flexors, which bend your elbow and draw your hand away from the cold water.

Most outputs from the neuromatrix are action programs or motor responses, but pain and emotions are other possible outputs. For example, if you step off a curb and sprain your ankle, a nociceptor is activated the moment the ligaments and other tissues in the region are stretched too far. After receiving this danger message, your brain decides to produce pain (to get you to protect the area), a new movement (to make you start limping), and fear (to get you to pay more attention the next time a similar situation presents itself).

**NEUROMATRIX OUTPUT**

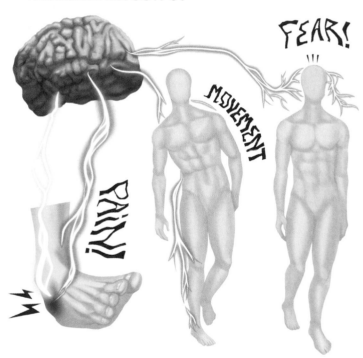

Remember when I said that your brain can inhibit danger messages? This happens in the brain and through descending tracts in the spinal cord. Your brain can produce endogenous opioids (naturally occurring morphine) and even flood your spinal cord with other powerful chemicals to block nociceptive messages so that sensory input doesn't make it to your brain and you don't feel any pain.

You see this process often in combat athletes. Mixed martial arts (MMA) fighters may incur significant tissue injuries during a fight but sometimes don't report pain until the fight is over and they are safe. Similarly, there are stories of soldiers getting shot or otherwise injured but not having pain until they get back to safety and can receive care for the injury.

There's a saying about the nervous system: neurons that fire together wire together.[15] Neurosignatures are unique patterns of neurons firing together, and the more you fire them together, the more they become wired together.

This is the same type of neuroplasticity that comes into play when you are developing a new motor skill. If you're learning to shoot a basketball, you're creating a neurosignature for that skill, and the more you practice, the better you get. It can work the same way for pain. When you have pain, you can use movement to desensitize the sensors and create a new neurosignature that doesn't involve pain. That's how neuroplasticity can play a positive role in the pain loop.

But the effectiveness of the rehab exercise protocols also depends on the type of pain you're experiencing, which is the focus of the next chapter.

## PAIN THAT FEELS GOOD

Sometimes pain feels good, such as a deep-tissue massage. The kneading activates sensors, but because you believe that the massage is helping you, your brain releases endorphins, blunting some of the danger messages traveling up your spinal cord. Just like with graded exposure, you can benefit from moving a sensitive body part in a novel way, which can change how your nervous system perceives that area.

## CHAPTER 3

# THE DIFFERENT
# TYPES OF PAIN

There are three main types of pain, and each has its own characteristics, signs, and symptoms:

- Mechanical (or nociceptive)

- Neuropathic (or nerve)

- Chronic (or persistent)

Figuring out which type you have can help you determine a strategy for treating it—a path forward for dealing with your unique pain experience. To do so, you combine your signs and symptoms with your history, such as how the pain started and what it feels like now. Using that information, you can choose the rehab protocol that most closely matches your condition, providing you with a framework to alleviate and treat your pain in an efficient way.

# ACUTE VS. CHRONIC PAIN: WHAT'S THE DIFFERENCE?

The terms *acute* and *chronic* typically describe the time frame of symptoms (how long the pain has been present).

- **ACUTE PAIN** is more predictable, usually begins suddenly, and goes away as the body heals (less than 12 weeks).

- **CHRONIC PAIN** is less predictable and persists beyond the typical healing time frame for most injuries (more than 12 weeks).[1-3]

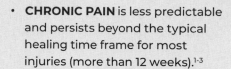
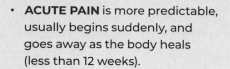
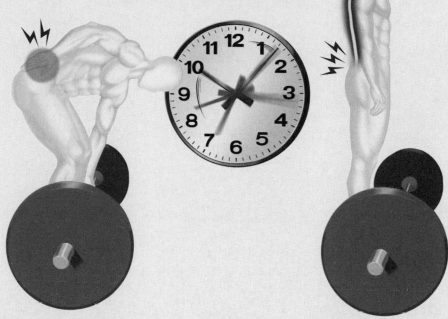

While these classifications are helpful, it's important to distinguish between them because the terms are often used interchangeably and in the wrong context, leading to confusion and misguided treatment strategies.

For instance, acute pain can last longer than 12 weeks if you keep aggravating the initial injury, such as with a repetitive overuse injury. The pain might start to go away but then come back if you engage in an activity that stresses the sensitive area before it has fully healed.

The problem is that reoccurring acute pain flare-ups are sometimes misclassified as a chronic condition when the pain lingers beyond the typical healing time for that tissue. And once the issue is labeled as chronic, your mindset and approach to rehab might change. The condition becomes more permanent and complex, and you may start to feel hopeless—like you will never get better.

But in most situations, reoccurring pain is acute pain rearing its ugly head over and over again. The pain system is healthy and accurately reflects what is happening with your body, which is good news. Simply avoid or modify aggravating factors (positions, movements, and activities that flare it up), follow the three-phase rehab exercise program, and you will get better.

If the pain doesn't get better, however, then it might develop into a chronic condition, which requires a slightly different approach. With chronic pain, the tissue has healed, but the nervous system continues to protect it. Maybe the brain remembers the movement that caused the injury and provides an exaggerated pain response even though the movement is not causing any damage. Or symptoms could be linked to your environment (such as unhealthy workplace conditions), lifestyle (poor sleep and diet), or psychology (excessive stress or depression).

To treat chronic pain—and keep it from coming back—you still follow the rehab exercise protocol, but you need to take a more comprehensive approach by addressing the factors covered in Chapter 4.

# MECHANICAL (OR NOCICEPTIVE) PAIN

The first type of pain involves non-nerve tissue, such as muscles, tendons, and ligaments. Mechanical pain is linked to the activation of nociceptors, the danger receptors described in Chapter 2. That is why mechanical pain is also called nociceptive pain.

A mechanical disruption of physical tissue is the most common cause of pain. During physical activity, you sustain some kind of injury—an ankle sprain, meniscus tear, or bone fracture, for example—and then you have pain associated with that injury.

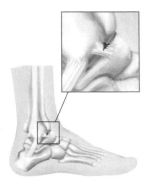

LIGAMENT SPRAIN

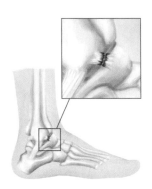

LIGAMENT TEAR

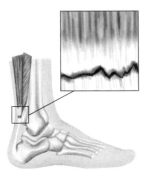

TENDON INJURY

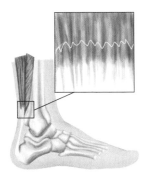

MUSCLE STRAIN

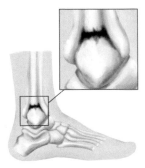

FRACTURE

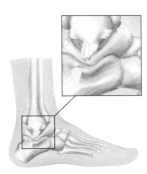

DISLOCATED JOINT

## mechanical pain: signs, symptoms, and characteristics

- This type of pain has clear on-off positions or activities. If you twist your body or move it in a certain way, the pain turns on. If you get out of that position, it turns off.

- If the pain is relatively new and you stress the area directly, it tends to be sharp. For instance, if you recently sprained your ankle and then twist it again in the same direction, you will probably feel a sharp pain.

- When the tissue is healing and is not being stressed directly, mechanical pain often presents as a dull ache.

- The pain usually has a clear border and stays localized to the site of injury. If you strain your hamstring, for example, it will hurt when you stretch, squeeze, or touch the injured area, but you won't feel pain in other areas that aren't mechanically associated with the hamstring muscles.

Most mechanical pain is acute—you suffer an injury, it heals within three months, and the pain goes away—but some tissues in the body heal more slowly than others, so mechanical pain can linger. The meniscus in your knee, for example, doesn't have great blood flow. If the injury is severe enough, it could produce pain beyond the average healing window for acute pain. Because that body part has a longer healing time frame, it may remain sensitive for longer than three months, but this doesn't mean it has turned into chronic pain. This is why you need to know what type of pain you're in before you decide how to treat it.

A low back injury initially produces acute pain, but if the pain keeps coming back, you need to ask yourself some questions: Did you re-aggravate it? Is it simply taking a long time to heal? Or did you sensitize those low back sensors? The answers depend on various factors, such as whether you followed a rehab exercise program to help you overcome the pain.

Most mechanical pain responds well to rehab, and your history can help determine whether you're experiencing lingering mechanical pain or if something is wrong with your pain system.

# NEUROPATHIC (OR NERVE) PAIN

Neuropathic or nerve pain occurs when there is irritation or damage to a portion of the nervous system. It can be related to both acute injuries and inflammation, or to systemic diseases that affect nerves, such as diabetes.

Nerves are like cords running through the body, and they have their own blood flow, their own microcirculation, and danger-detecting nociceptors. This is why hitting your funny bone hurts—you're striking the ulnar nerve and creating a high-threshold stimulus that activates nociceptors, but the pain is related to neural tissue. Nerve injuries result in neuropathic pain, which may create numb patches, tingling that radiates into specific regions, or sharp lightning-bolt pains.

Sciatica is one of the most common types of neuropathic pain. The sciatic nerve is composed of five small nerve roots coming from different parts of the low back. When these roots come together, they form a massive peripheral nerve that is roughly the diameter of a pencil.

Sciatica involves nerve irritation, which can be inflammatory or mechanical. It doesn't always mean something is touching or "pinching" the nerve. Maybe you strained your back and the resulting inflammation irritated the tiny branches of the larger sciatic nerve, which goes through your buttock, down your hamstring, and into your calf before branching into your shin, toes, and foot. In short, symptoms can develop if you have an irritation or injury to a nerve anywhere along its path.

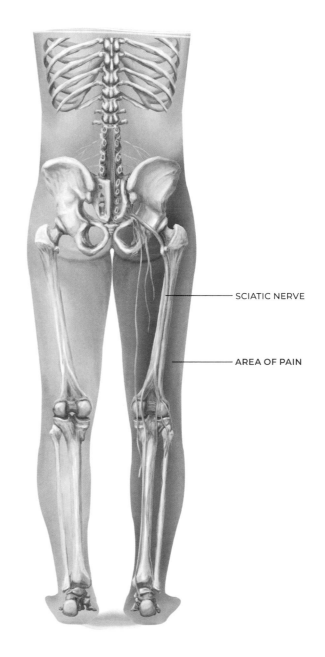

SCIATIC NERVE

AREA OF PAIN

# neuropathic pain: signs, symptoms, and characteristics

- For most people, the symptoms of neuropathic pain are numbness, burning, tingling, and traveling.

- Unlike nociceptive pain, which might spread only an inch or two into the surrounding area, neuropathic pain usually travels along a nerve's path. The worse it gets, the farther it travels. A mild irritation in the low back, for example, might travel only into the thigh and buttock, but as the nerve becomes more irritated, the pain will peripheralize and descend farther down the leg into the shin and foot.

Nerve pain that travels is called radicular pain. This differs from referred pain, which comes from non-neural structures—usually organs referring pain to the musculoskeletal system, like the heart referring pain to the left arm or a kidney stone referring pain to the low back.

Remember, pain without injury could be referred pain, and you should see your primary care physician to rule out serious medical conditions such as cancer. Referred pain differs from radicular pain because the cardinal symptoms are associated with an organ and don't improve with rehab. If you have a kidney infection, your back won't get better or worse with movement. It'll hurt whenever the organ is active, and the pain typically can't be reproduced mechanically.

Sciatica and carpal tunnel are examples of acute neuropathic pain, where you physically stress the nerve and make it hurt. But diseases and injuries of the nervous system such as cerebral vascular accidents (strokes), spinal cord injuries, and diabetic neuropathy can create chronic neuropathic pain along with numbness, tingling, and other sensations. Neuropathy usually refers to a systemic disease damaging the nervous system.

If you have numbness, tingling, or traveling pain influenced by body position or movement, the rehab exercise protocols in this book are applicable. If you have a disease that affects your brain or spinal cord, however, rehab exercises can help, but they may not change your neural symptoms that much. In those cases, medical treatment becomes the best option. For example, if you have diabetes and are experiencing pain, see a doctor to address the primary causes. This book addresses pain with roots in the musculoskeletal system. Anyone can benefit from the rehab protocols, but you shouldn't treat a neuropathy as if it were a mechanical issue.

Neuropathic pain can also occur within the central nervous system or peripheral nervous system. Sciatica causes neuropathic pain in the peripheral nervous system, but an injury to the spinal cord or brain can cause neuropathic pain in the central nervous system. This book primarily addresses issues of the peripheral nervous system because most central nervous system pains require medical management and the processes responsible for those pains are less responsive to exercise, movements, and physical interventions.

But that doesn't mean you should avoid exercise and movement. Rehab for a spinal cord injury might not change your pain symptoms much, but it can greatly influence your function—your ability to move safely and effectively through various ranges of motion. Although figuring out what type of pain you have can help determine how you move forward, you must not lose sight of the benefits of exercise for overall health and functional ability.

REFERRED PAIN    RADICULAR PAIN

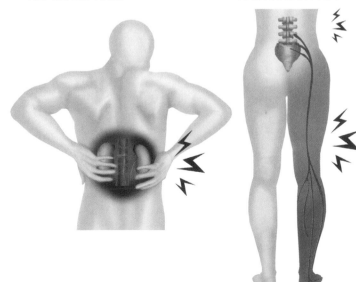

# CHRONIC (OR PERSISTENT) PAIN

Chronic pain indicates disease or malfunction in the pain portion of your nervous system, which is providing an overblown response that no longer reflects the state of your physical body. Because chronic pain is common, it is often perceived as normal.

Pain is normal and tells you about your body—but when it lasts too long and no longer reflects your physical well-being, it becomes abnormal and unhelpful. It represents a mismatch between what you're experiencing and what is happening with the tissues of your body.

With this kind of pain, everything might look normal on an MRI or X-ray, but you are still having pain symptoms, and sometimes they don't match the sensations coming from your body. For example, if you bend over to pick up a pencil and have a severe pain response that leaves you debilitated for days, that pain does not accurately reflect the health of your musculoskeletal system.

**TYPES OF CHRONIC PAIN**

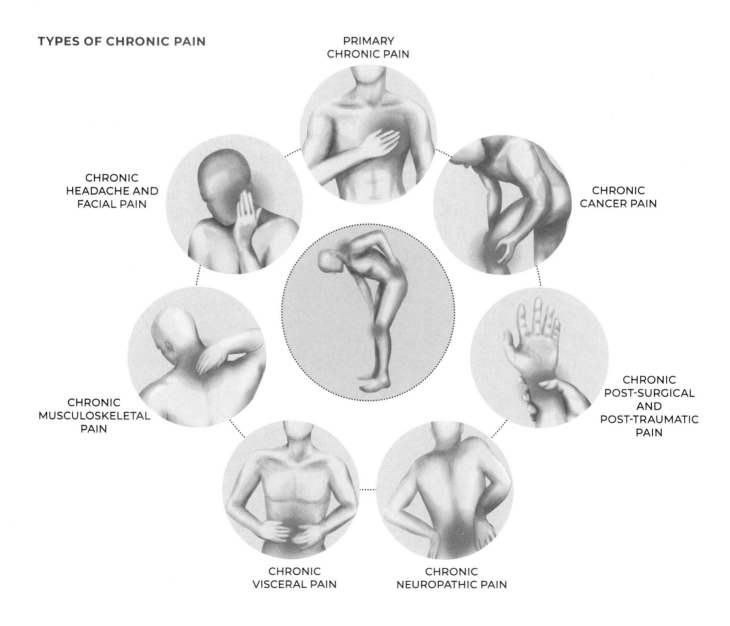

PRIMARY CHRONIC PAIN

CHRONIC CANCER PAIN

CHRONIC HEADACHE AND FACIAL PAIN

CHRONIC MUSCULOSKELETAL PAIN

CHRONIC POST-SURGICAL AND POST-TRAUMATIC PAIN

CHRONIC VISCERAL PAIN

CHRONIC NEUROPATHIC PAIN

# PATH TO CHRONIC PAIN AND RECOVERY (FEAR AVOIDANCE MODEL)

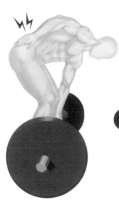

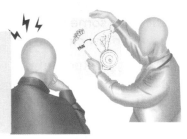

**(1)** **Painful experiences** can cause the brain to go into protective mode, making its "danger alarm" more sensitive.

**(2)** These experiences can force you to **create an ongoing state of tension and vigilance in the nervous system.**

*I have to perform the movement perfectly to avoid pain…*

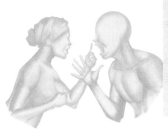

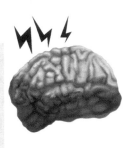

**(4)** **Everyday stress** combined with an overreactive nervous system will start producing physical symptoms, causing pain!

**(3)** **Incorrect diagnoses can also lead to pain catastrophizing,** making the pain experience worse and even more intense!

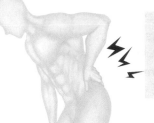

**(5)** These can create a **negative feedback loop** that begins every time the overreactive nervous system hits its tipping point.

**(6)** **The brain changes when pain becomes chronic** because the more the brain learns to act protectively, the better it becomes at doing it.

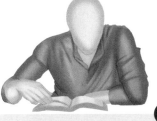

**(7)** **Painful responses are triggered even when no danger is present.** Activities become restricted and pain-related stress negatively impacts quality of life.

**(8)** **Education on the topic of pain science is the first step out of the negative feedback loop,** because it helps reduce fear around the symptoms.

**(9)** **Understanding how the nervous system reacts** during the "journey of pain" provides a clearer map of the way out.

*It's all right.*

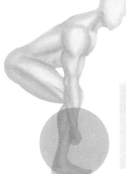

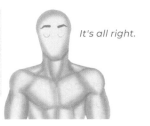

**(11)** Ultimately, the nervous system becomes less sensitive and pain symptoms abate, which leads to enhanced function and improved quality of life.

**(10)** New neural pathways are formed via education and graded exercise and when other factors (sleep, stress, nutrition, etc.) are addressed.

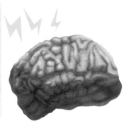

## chronic pain: signs, symptoms, and characteristics

- Symptoms are often hard to identify and may not be easy to reproduce mechanically (that is, by getting into a position that creates them).

- Chronic pain is often a vague sensation without a clear perimeter and can spread to different body regions. With mechanical pain and even some neuropathic pains, people can usually draw clear lines around the pain.

- An exaggerated, amplified pain response can occur with movement, physical touch, mental stress, or even ranges in temperature. Some people experience pain when they sit underneath an air-conditioning vent, for example, as if the cold air triggers their pain.

- The quality of chronic pain can change. Sometimes it's achy, sometimes it's sharp, and sometimes it burns or tingles.

Because chronic pain can mimic acute injuries and serious diseases (such as Lyme disease, which can cause physical pain), it's impossible to verify with a single test. So, the first step is to rule out autoimmune conditions, systemic diseases, or referred pain from an organ. If a medical professional determines through exclusion that your unrelenting pain is a chronic condition tied to your pain system, then you have to be your own advocate to figure out what triggers and eases it. You may notice that your pain can result from non-physical triggers, like worrying about an upcoming event. The fight-or-flight response can sensitize nerves, so if stress reproduces your pain, you might have a chronic pain system disorder, where pain in your musculoskeletal system is being activated by a different system.

In this scenario, you can implement a variety of strategies to reduce your symptoms, including not only movement and exercise but also sleep hygiene, diet, stress management, inflammation reduction, and so on. Although this book focuses primarily on resistance and mobility exercises, a great deal of evidence suggests that these other factors, which I'll discuss in the next chapter, are also important for alleviating chronic pain.

The key takeaway is that there is hope, even for chronic pain, because you can desensitize these systems through the protocols in this book and general awareness—knowing what the problem is so you can change your environment or alter your behavior in a way that puts your body's systems back into balance. Remember, the pain system is neuroplastic, and you can change it through gradual training.

# WHERE THE THREE TYPES OVERLAP

Mechanical. Neuropathic. Chronic. There is some overlap between these three types of pain because so many factors play a role.

Take low back pain. It can happen because you lifted something heavy and tweaked your back—that's a mechanical problem. You can also have low back pain as a result of sciatica, which is neuropathic pain. Then there's chronic pain, where we don't know exactly what's wrong but have ruled out everything else. This type of pain could be more closely correlated with your emotional state, your mindset, and other similar factors.

In the next chapter, I'm going to flesh out the factors that influence pain both positively and negatively—and explain how improving factors like sleep, diet, and stress can help with each type of pain.

## CHAPTER 4

# THE FACTORS THAT INFLUENCE PAIN

Pain is usually the number one symptom for people who come to a physical therapy clinic. As a rehabilitation practitioner, my main role is to resolve pain by addressing the needs of the physical body through movement and exercise. This is also the primary focus of this book. But other triggers may keep injuries from healing or cause prolonged pain. Thoughts, beliefs, stress, sleep, relationships, posture, exercise, anatomy, and environment are some of the factors that can influence your pain experience.

This is why education is incredibly beneficial—not only to understand how your pain works but also to help you get rid of it. If you address pain only from a mechanical standpoint (using movement and exercise), you may not get better because you're not addressing the other factors that can affect your physical system. What's more, if you overemphasize factors such as posture or biomechanics, you might miss other important factors contributing to your pain. Movement certainly plays a role and is important to address, but many of the biggest factors in prolonged pain are tied to lifestyle, beliefs, and environment. Appropriate steps might include seeking medical intervention or working with a psychologist or dietitian.

The rehab strategies in this book focus on the physical body, so I mainly discuss treating pain through movement and exercise. But other factors may be equally important. As such, this chapter includes the factors supported by the most evidence along with best practices and guidelines for addressing each of those factors. This will help you take a more comprehensive approach to addressing pain, whether you simply increase your awareness of the potential factors (both positive and negative), seek a more complete treatment plan, or pinpoint a factor that needs special attention.

# PAIN THRESHOLDS: PERCEPTION VS. TOLERANCE

When discussing the factors that influence pain and how those factors bias the pain experience, it's important to understand the two primary thresholds in pain science: pain perception and pain tolerance.

- **PERCEPTION:** As a potentially dangerous stimulus increases in intensity, your pain perception threshold describes the moment you first experience discomfort.

- **TOLERANCE:** After you start experiencing discomfort, your pain tolerance threshold is the point at which you are no longer willing or able to put up with that pain.

Imagine immersing your hand in ice water. The moment you register the cold as painful is your pain perception threshold.

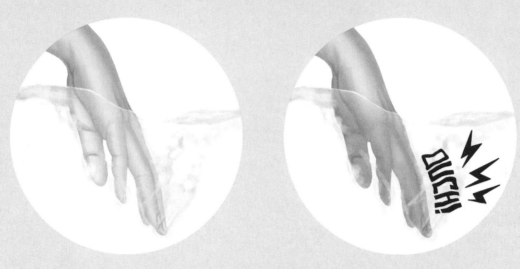

Your pain tolerance threshold is defined by how long you can keep your hand in the water after that.

Some individuals are more sensitive than others, but there is not much difference in "default" pain perception threshold from person to person.[1,2]

Tolerance is different because you can train your pain tolerance threshold. Endurance athletes and martial artists, for example, tend to have high pain tolerance thresholds because their training conditions teach them to endure physical suffering.[3-6] The significance of an event—such as childbirth—can also make a person willing to tolerate or endure great discomfort because of the good that results from their pain.[7,8]

# PHYSICAL INACTIVITY

The first factor that can influence pain is your physical activity level. The American College of Sports Medicine (ACSM) and U.S. Centers for Disease Control and Prevention (CDC) recommend that healthy adults engage in 150 minutes of moderate-intensity aerobic exercise each week (20 to 30 minutes per day) and implement resistance or strength training at least twice per week. While these recommendations have existed for some time, rates of physical inactivity and sedentary behaviors continue to climb across the globe.

Being physically inactive leads to detrimental changes in the nervous and immune systems and can increase the likelihood of developing chronic pain.[9-11] Human and animal studies have found that inactivity increases pain sensitivity (hyperalgesia), which is thought to be due to changes in the central nervous system that lessen its ability to inhibit nociceptive messages.[12-15] Furthermore, research shows that inactivity increases levels of inflammatory cytokines (immune system molecules) and decreases levels of anti-inflammatory cytokines. Inflammatory cytokines are known to activate receptors on nociceptors, making it more likely that you will experience pain, whereas anti-inflammatory cytokines help reduce nociceptor activity.[16-19]

The good news is that the type of exercise you engage in doesn't seem to matter as much as simply moving. Many forms of exercise, from aerobic training (walking, running, cycling, swimming) to resistance training to yoga, Pilates, and stretching, have been shown to help reduce pain sensitivity.[20-21]

The key is to pick something you enjoy doing and try to be consistent about getting in 20 to 30 minutes of that activity at a moderate intensity on most days of the week. Doing so will improve the health of your pain-related systems, which can reduce your current pain symptoms and your chances of developing chronic pain.

# MOVEMENT AND BIOMECHANICS

The study of biomechanics involves the intersection of the physics of movement and its effects on the biological systems, including the musculoskeletal system. In the context of pain, we look at how force (load) and mechanical stress impact tissues and whether that translates to pain.

Within the biopsychosocial, or BPS, model (see page 14), the "bio" component includes your physical body, the forces (pushes and pulls) you encounter, and the role your tissues play in the pain experience. With mechanical (nociceptive) and acute neuropathic pain, the physics of your movement (form and technique) helps explain why your pain is occurring. The musculoskeletal system is comprised of mechanical tissues (bones, muscles, tendon, ligaments, etc.), and when those tissues become sensitized following an injury or irritation, less force is required to activate your nociceptors and send danger messages to your brain—meaning you need to pay more attention to your form, technique, and training when you have acute pain.

Chronic pain is different, and the "bio," or tissue-driven, portion of the BPS model becomes less relevant. It still matters, but not as much as it would with a fresh injury or pain problem. In other words, you don't need to worry as much about the biomechanics of movement (how much force you put on the tissue) because it has already healed. Instead, you look at how movement is coupled with pain and think about how you can decrease your sensitivity to movement over time.

# THERE ARE NO "BAD" MOVEMENTS

Many people believe that pain is directly tied to form and technique as it relates to posture and biomechanics. In some cases, this might be true—certain positions or movements can create pain, and altering posture and form can reduce it.

But as with so many factors that influence pain, simply changing the way you move may not fix it. What's more, this way of thinking typically labels specific positions and movements as bad. Telling someone that they will have pain if they move a certain way or that they are "dysfunctional" can create anxiety and fear and make them feel as though their body is fragile, which can lead to an increase in pain and recovery time. That's why, as rehabilitation and fitness professionals, we have to be careful about the language we use when helping people navigate pain issues that are associated with movement and exercise.

Instead of labeling a movement as "bad," we need to point out that sensitivities to specific movements are common when pain is present. Say you have pain when rounding your back. That doesn't mean flexion is off-limits; it just means you are sensitive to flexion right now and you need to make modifications, such as keeping your back in the neutral zone or stabilizing your spine to avoid placing too much stress on the area.

For most people, it's not the position of their body or how they are moving that causes pain, but rather how long they remain in that position and how much they are moving. Put another way, it's less about the position and movement and more about the volume of that position and movement. Movement and exercise have a dosage just like medication. If you do too much for too long, or too much too soon, the dosage may be too high. When your tissues are not conditioned to handle the load and force being placed on them (it's "too much"), they become irritated or break, resulting in pain and injury.

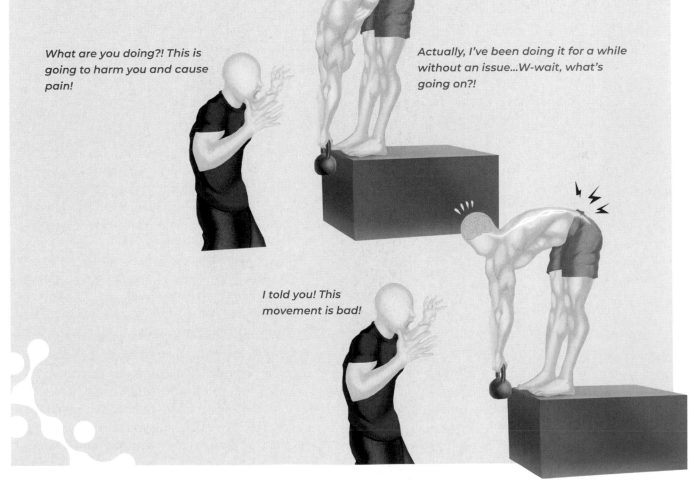

*What are you doing?! This is going to harm you and cause pain!*

*Actually, I've been doing it for a while without an issue...W-wait, what's going on?!*

*I told you! This movement is bad!*

This process can be confusing, but the key is that these differences don't necessarily change which exercises you use to relieve pain, but how you implement them.

For example, say two people have low back pain. The first person lifted something heavy a few days ago, and a mechanical muscle injury (a strain) occurred. This person should think about the mechanics of their movement as the injury heals so they don't reinjure the muscle. They also need to pay attention to the load they're placing on their body (and avoid lifting heavy things) for a few days to weeks, utilize exercises to reduce pain, and then rebuild the strength and integrity of their back muscles.

The second person has low back pain that has been coming and going over the last few years. They haven't sustained a recent injury, but they feel pain with certain activities or when sitting for long periods. In this case, movement and exercise can reduce pain, but this person should think about using movement more generally to reduce sensitivity. For instance, they might implement core exercises, not to build strength or stability but simply to move their low back and show their nervous system that everything is OK. They might also commit to regular walking because general movement

can achieve similar results in pain reduction compared to more specific core exercises in people with chronic low back pain.[21]

Whether you have an acute pain problem or a chronic pain issue, the rehab exercise protocols in this book can work. With acute pain, you typically pay more attention to how specific movements challenge certain tissues and work on calming those areas down and then using exercise to make them more resilient and mobile. With chronic pain, you think less about challenging certain tissues and more about moving the painful body region in a nonthreatening way that helps desensitize the pain system.

Movement and exercise stress your physical tissues, which helps them adapt. When you're in pain, movement that is dosed correctly can make you better; if it's dosed incorrectly, it can interfere with healing and cause pain to flare up. In short, rehab is all about using the right types of movement and exercise at the right time. That's why the process for addressing pain is to let the tissue calm down and move past acute pain (phase 1), gradually incorporate movement and mobility exercises to start rebuilding the tissue (phase 2), and then strengthen the body region with resistance training (phase 3).

# MENTAL HEALTH

Quite a bit of research links mental health issues, especially depression and anxiety, to the development of chronic pain.[22-25] For instance, people often report back pain while sitting, but that pain may occur only when they're at work or in a stressful environment—not when they're at home watching TV. Your mental health can be a huge factor in chronic symptoms, but treatment can be tricky when you start asking whether the depression caused the pain or the pain caused the depression.

If you are in pain and are experiencing anxiety or depression, please reach out to a mental health provider. These practitioners can help you sort through your thoughts and emotions and design a plan to help you cope with your situation. Addressing your mental health can have a profound impact on your ability to get your pain under control.

# THOUGHTS AND BELIEFS

I've already discussed the importance of thoughts and beliefs in terms of how pain works and how being educated about pain can shape our overall health and how we feel.

Most people are familiar with the placebo effect—how believing a treatment will have a positive effect can make it so. Many studies have demonstrated this effect, including sham surgery studies that randomly place patients with pain in either a real surgery group or a fake (sham) surgery group. A normal surgical procedure is performed on the first group, while the second group only has portal sites cut into their skin so it looks like they had the surgery. When the two groups are compared months later, they often report similar decreases in pain because both groups believed the surgery would positively influence their bodies.[26-28]

But many aren't as familiar with the nocebo effect, which occurs when a belief in something related to the body leads to negative outcomes and ultimately causes harm. Studies have shown, for example, that negative messages tied to doubt in the body can make pain worse and may make a person more likely to develop chronic pain.[29-32] If you're 35 years old and, after an MRI, a doctor says you have the spine of a 70-year-old, that message can harm you. Being told not to run or lift weights anymore can have a similarly negative impact on how you feel about your body and affect your trust in your system, possibly for life. You might have acute mechanical pain resulting from injury, but a message that triggers fear and anxiety can be harmful to your long-term health, too.

One of the most common examples of the nocebo effect is when someone with back or neck pain gets an MRI or X-ray and is told they have an injury or degeneration. Issues like disc bulges and arthritis are often a normal part of aging, but a medical professional telling you it's concerning can create a nocebic pattern, even if the "problem" identified in the image is not an issue for you at all. When a professional conveys a theory with confidence, most patients believe the explanation and feel that this new problem must be fixed in order for them to get better. Such a belief can negatively affect rehab outcomes. Fear and anxiety create stress, which can impede recovery and turn acute pain into chronic pain.[33,34]

Certain signs and symptoms do necessitate imaging, of course. If you have a severe loss of function, muscle weakness that has appeared suddenly, or a serious injury, then imaging can help you and your medical team formulate an appropriate treatment strategy. But imaging is just one piece of the puzzle.

Whether it's on the internet or from a practitioner, people will offer opinions about your pain. If you know the facts about what influences pain, you'll be able to navigate those opinions more effectively and create a buffer against how much a message can affect your experience. The more you understand your pain, the less threatening it is.

When working with a practitioner, speak up and ask questions. If the practitioner is unwilling to answer questions or can't communicate in a way that helps you understand the problem, get a second or even a third opinion, especially if something invasive like surgery is recommended.

# STRESS

Stress is a normal response to certain life events. Your sympathetic nervous system controls your fight-or-flight response, which is triggered by a perceived threat, either mental or physical. Sometimes, this response is helpful and normal; other times, it is harmful and abnormal. In this way, the stress response is similar to the pain response. When pain is acute, it helps keep you alive and avoid harm. When it is chronic, it provides an overreaction to a nonthreatening situation.

Many of us experience stress from things that aren't threatening to our immediate survival. Chronic stress, for example, is often tied to psychological fear rather than physical threats. This could include having an upcoming speech to give at work, an argument with your spouse, or a sudden loss. The event or the fear of the event activates your sympathetic nervous system and prepares you for action by releasing hormones like cortisol so that you can either confront the threat or flee from it. But when the fight-or-flight system remains activated for prolonged periods, it becomes more and more sensitive to stressful events and the anxiety associated with those events. This can have negative effects on immune function and the nervous system and make you more sensitive to pain.[35-37]

Reducing stress and the associated pain starts with understanding your triggers and changing your behaviors to avoid those stressors. This might involve improving your mindset and relationships by strengthening healthy social connections and removing toxic ones and taking control over your health by improving your sleep, diet, and exercise habits. Breathing exercises and meditative practices can help, too. Deep breathing activates the parasympathetic nervous system and returns the body and mind to a calm and relaxed state, while mindfulness meditation can break the conditioning of anxiety-inducing thought patterns. See page 52 for more on these practices.

# SLEEP

Numerous pain disorders, such as neck pain, low back pain, and headaches, are associated with insufficient sleep.[38] You might experience pain and not sleep well, and then the poor sleep exacerbates the pain, creating a loop.

During sleep, your musculoskeletal and nervous systems remodel themselves, healing physical injuries, regenerating neurons, and changing through neuroplasticity. If your sleep is interrupted or you have poor sleep habits (such as drinking caffeine or alcohol too close to bedtime), your body will have a hard time regenerating, which may influence or exaggerate your pain symptoms.

While sleep requirements vary from person to person, medical professionals recommend that most adults get seven to nine hours per night.[39] But data from the CDC show that approximately 35 percent of Americans average less than seven hours of sleep.[40] If you have chronic pain, improving your sleep could help considerably. Develop a routine that helps you wind down before bed, sleep in a completely dark room, keep the temperature at around 70 degrees, and do not look at your phone or do things that might cause stress. Other strategies that encourage a parasympathetic state, like deep breathing or light stretching (the phase 1 exercises included in the rehab protocols are good examples), can help you build a routine that encourages better rest.

# DIET

Some studies show that inflammatory foods—which include highly processed products that contain refined carbohydrates, trans fats, and excessive amounts of sugar—may sensitize nerve fibers, potentially causing throbbing, aching, or dull pain, making food a factor in the development and severity of chronic pain.[41-44] The less healthy you are, the more susceptible you are to pain, especially if you're in a chronic pain state or have an autoimmune condition.

But we aren't always sure what causes pain. Unhealthy eating can be tied to many other factors (stress, sleep, etc.), which also affect pain. Another source of uncertainty is that dietary needs are unique to the individual, so you may want to seek out a nutritionist or dietitian to determine what's right for you. Still, it's good to highlight that diet can be a factor in chronic pain, and you may benefit from eliminating or cutting back on potentially inflammatory foods. Working toward a healthier diet that focuses on whole foods and energy balance (weight management) is a good move in general.

As previously mentioned, all these factors are interconnected. If you sleep poorly, you might wake up groggy. When you're tired, you're more likely to make poor food choices and move less, which can cascade into familiar pain symptoms.

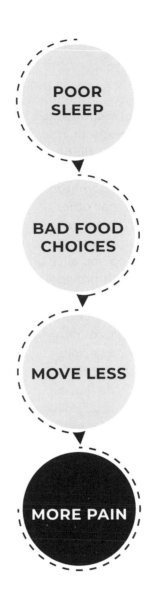

# GENETICS, ENVIRONMENT, AND HISTORY (TRAUMA)

Chronic pain often begins with inflammation or a traumatic injury, but it doesn't develop for everyone. Of the people who get whiplash in motor vehicle accidents, only 30 to 50 percent develop chronic whiplash symptoms.[45,46] So, what makes that injury grow into chronic pain?

Some research suggests an interaction between genetics and environment to explain why some people heal and others develop chronic symptoms.[47] Most studies show that both factors play a role in pain, but since you don't have control over your genetics, let's dig into the factor you do have some influence over: your environment. This may include family, history, and associated social pressures. For example, social pressure often pushes people who participate in contact sports to have a greater pain tolerance.

On the flip side, a parent who overreacts to their child's small scrapes and bruises may be more likely to raise a sensitive kid with a lower pain tolerance threshold.[48] Kids who end up in the NICU and undergo invasive procedures (such as injections and IVs) also tend to have more sensitivities than children who haven't experienced such things.[49] But these sensitivities can be modified through environmental changes later in life. By choosing to pursue activities that challenge your mind and body in appropriate doses, you can push your pain tolerance higher, making you less likely to experience pain while doing everyday tasks.

So, your genes and environment may work for or against you, but there's a great deal of variability. It's a delicate balance. The key is to make decisions and lifestyle changes based on what you can control. If you have genes linked to autoimmune diseases such as celiac disease—you are allergic to gluten—eliminating certain foods will dramatically improve your health and pain symptoms.

Both physical trauma following surgery or an accidental injury (car accident, sports injury, fall, act of violence, etc.) and psychological trauma (PTSD) are associated with the development of chronic pain states. If you have endured a trauma in the past that activates a pain response, you need to confront it so that you can remove those triggers and heal. This might mean combining movements and exercises, like those found in this book, and working with a psychologist who can help you work through any negative thoughts and emotions tied to the trauma you experienced.

# CULTURE AND MEANING

Culture is one of the most fascinating factors that can influence pain.[50] Consider the Sateré-Mawé, an Amazon tribe that requires boys to be stung by bullet ants as a rite of passage. When people do painful things as a cultural practice, they often report less pain.

Pain science shows that meaning can modulate the pain experience. If you find a practice like sticking your hand in bullet ants meaningful, you may be less fearful and experience less pain from it.[51,52] But if the act had no cultural significance to you, the threat would be different.

I saw this factor at play firsthand while working with Cirque du Soleil. There were three Russian contortionists who never wanted to come to PT. One of them was always in pain, but she would never talk about it; she considered it a sign of weakness. It took a lot of persuading to get her to let me work on her. Some people ignore pain as a sign of cultural strength. It's good to be aware of these differences. Pain is not weakness, and neither is acknowledging it. The attitude that pain should be ignored can lead to serious injury.

On the other hand, if someone has learned to exaggerate pain—maybe doing so got them attention from their parents—they may have developed a high sensitivity to pain that doesn't indicate an actual injury.

I grew up doing Judo, and I've always thought that people who are extra sensitive to pain should try martial arts. You choose to do it, which makes it meaningful, and you pursue goals, which can desensitize your system and make you more resilient.

This goes for other forms of movement, too. If you have musculoskeletal pain and a certain type of movement or exercise that you want to engage in triggers it, the best strategy is to implement small doses of that activity and try to increase the dose over time. Doing so will help decrease the sensitivity of your nervous system not only because the physical activity is graded but also because you are participating in an activity you value.

# SOCIAL INTERACTION AND HUMOR

This factor is part of the psychosocial dynamic of pain. Regular and healthy social interaction is important for boosting the immune system and overcoming pain.[53]

People with chronic pain often withdraw from social interaction because they're uncomfortable and don't want to risk flaring up their symptoms. Another reason often cited in the research is that they become so fixated on their pain that they talk about it all the time. They pick up on reactions from friends and family who grow tired of hearing about it, and that makes them feel like their pain is not being validated, pushing them toward isolation. They start to pattern an association between social interaction and pain. It's a downward spiral where they become anxious about engaging in social situations, so they go out less. Then they get lonely and slip further into depression, which makes their pain worse and harder to treat.

The goal is to deny the urge to pull away and try to integrate yourself into positive social situations. Identifying supportive relationships is a good place to start. Empathetic individuals, whether they're friends, family members, or practitioners, can validate your symptoms. People who put you in a negative frame of mind can affect your pain, too. You might feel dismissed, especially by medical providers. Try to identify positive relationships that make you feel better about yourself—and avoid people who exacerbate your pain.

Humor is tied to immune system health as well, so you'll often see recommendations to watch something funny or engage in an activity that makes you laugh, both of which can provide a positive experience when you're dealing with pain.[53] Even smiling can improve how you feel.

It's all connected. Making an effort to smile and laugh can have a positive effect—not only on how you think and feel but also on the people around you, improving your relationships.

# ANATOMY

Anatomy is your physical structure—the architecture of your body that you're born with. Although the organization and orientation of our skeletons and soft tissue structures tend to fall within a certain range, some people have deviations that predispose them to certain injuries and pain issues. For example, hypermobile joints can make you more susceptible to injuries like joint subluxations or dislocations. Similarly, a variation in the orientation of the hip socket can increase your likelihood of developing a labral tear, hip impingement, and/or osteoarthritis later in life.

A common misconception is that anatomical deviations predispose you to pain and injury, but the musculoskeletal system is incredibly adaptive; as you develop from a child into an adult, you expose it to gradual stress that helps it grow stronger.

Many people have musculoskeletal issues that might be categorized as dysfunctional, but they operate without pain because their system has adapted to that stress. Take the example of Paralympic and adaptive athletes, who do amazing things, often without pain. Anatomy is just one of many factors.

If you do have an anatomical finding that could be related to your pain, identify movement modifications to work around the anomaly so you can continue participating in the activities you enjoy without increasing your risk of injury and pain. For instance, people with femoracetabular hip impingement (FAI) demonstrate a deviation in either their hip socket bone (acetabulum) or the top of their thigh bone (femur) that leads to premature contact between bones and pain when they move their hips into extreme positions, like the bottom of a squat. To relieve this discomfort, these individuals often adopt a wider stance or a toes-out position when squatting.

If rehab and behavior modification can't help an anatomical anomaly much, surgery is sometimes an option. With a hip impingement, for example, surgeons can remove the bony buildup on the acetabulum or femur, allowing for better movement and less pain. Get an opinion from a trusted practitioner (or several) who is up-to-date on these principles and options.

# POSTURE

Posture refers to the alignment and orientation of the entire body and all its segments, not just the spine. As with biomechanics and movement, posture influences pain in that certain positions may trigger symptoms. For example, if you have sustained a recent injury such as a ligament sprain, certain postures might stress the healing tissue and cause pain. This doesn't mean the posture that triggers your pain is bad; it just means that your body isn't ready for it yet.

In other cases, different body positions can trigger pain even though you haven't suffered an injury to the area. When you adopt a position, you apply low levels of stress to the tissues that allow you to maintain that position. If you look down at something (maybe to read an article on your laptop), for instance, your neck extensor muscles must contract isometrically to hold your head in position. If you hold this position for an extended period day after day (such as at a desk job) and exceed the capacity of your tissues, you could develop a type of postural sensitivity where you have neck pain.

But posture doesn't play as big a role in pain as you might think.[54-56] Temporarily modifying your posture can help you desensitize and recover, but research shows that body segments have considerable variability and that posture doesn't correlate well with the development of pain. In short, we can't blame "bad" posture for most pain symptoms because what is considered "good" varies from person to person.

What's typically more important is your dynamic posture or form, especially when you're putting load on your system, like when lifting weight. Many people get hung up on their posture while standing or sitting at a desk, but posture at rest for short periods of time is not that stressful, so it rarely correlates to pain.

When a position does become painful, it's usually because you've been in it for too long. Spending prolonged periods in one position can lead to ischemia (reduced blood flow), which causes chemicals to build up and activate sensors in the body, creating a danger signal. You may feel the urge to move, but it doesn't matter what position you're in—being static is the problem. There's a common ergonomist saying: "Your next posture is the best posture."

"Dysfunctional" posture isn't what causes pain. Even exercise, whether it's stretching or resistance training, doesn't permanently alter your default posture. People with "bad" posture may feel better than those with "ideal" posture. And if you're forced to maintain a "good" postural position for too long, you will eventually report discomfort. Essentially, if you hold any position long enough, it'll start to hurt. Posture should be dynamic, so listen to your nervous system and move when it tells you to.

# TOUCH

For many people, being touched helps with pain by causing the body to release the hormone oxytocin, which aids in social bonding and may reduce fear and anxiety.[57] Not being touched is associated with social withdrawal and depression, which can sensitize the body. Even a practitioner's touch can help by building a therapeutic alliance. Whether it's the endocrine system or the nervous system itself, touch seems to positively influence pain.

That said, there are conditions like hyperalgesia and allodynia where the body becomes overly sensitive. For people with these conditions, being touched—a stimulus that's normally not painful—creates pain. But being sensitized to touch doesn't mean that touch is bad. You can use touch to desensitize the body, but you have to be thoughtful in figuring out the problem and navigating those conditions.

# BREAKING THE LOOP

All the factors outlined in this chapter can influence pain.

The world's best centers for pain management are integrative facilities that address the entire biopsychosocial continuum, employing specialists such as social workers, psychologists, physical therapists, yoga instructors, and more. There is always hope, but you need to consider all the variables that contribute to pain.

The best way to approach pain is to address as many factors as possible. Take an active approach to addressing these influences and implement the strategies that work best for you and your situation—all these steps can help alleviate your symptoms.

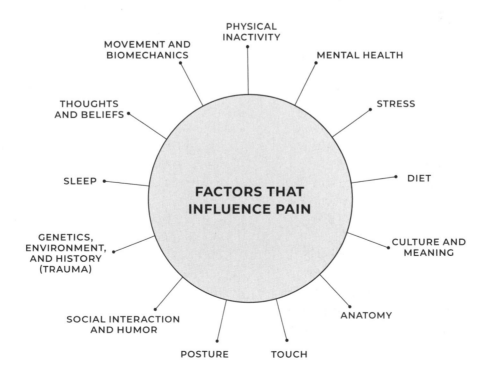

CHAPTER 5

# HOW TO
# OVERCOME PAIN

Whether you have sudden acute pain from an injury, pain that appeared for unknown reasons, or persistent chronic pain, the strategies to manage and resolve your symptoms—and the general order in which you will approach those strategies—are the same.

**PHASE 1: Reduce pain symptoms.**

Pain makes it difficult to do the things you enjoy, so the first step is getting it under control. To address your current pain, you must avoid or modify activities that flare it up (I call these aggravating factors) and implement strategies that will alleviate your symptoms. Soft tissue mobilization (self-massage), aerobic exercise, and flexibility/mobility strategies are perfect for that. They will reduce pain and prepare your body for the next phase.

**PHASE 2: Address impairments or deficits caused by pain (such as muscle weakness and range of motion limitations).**

Pain inhibits muscle activation and can impair your ability to move. As your pain symptoms improve, you need to implement more mobility, movement, and isometric and eccentric resistance exercises to eliminate impairments in your system and improve your functional ability. You might still have mild to moderate pain, but you can move and do certain things without making it worse. That's how you know you are getting better and are ready to move to the final phase.

**PHASE 3: Build capacity and prevent flare-ups by strengthening your body.**

Once you've regained some functional ability, the next step is to load your system with full range of motion resistance training. This type of exercise changes ligaments and spinal discs, enhances muscle strength, and increases bone density, muscle fiber diameter, and tendon size—all positive adaptations within the musculoskeletal system that make your body more resilient.

| REDUCE PAIN SYMPTOMS | ADDRESS IMPAIRMENTS | BUILD CAPACITY |
|---|---|---|
| • Soft tissue mobilizations<br>• Aerobic exercise<br>• Flexibility and mobility exercises | • Flexibility and mobility exercises (continued)<br>• Isometric and eccentric resistance training exercises | • Full range of motion resistance training exercises |

This three-phase approach to alleviating and resolving pain is similar to the three-phase approach you would take when rehabbing an injury (see Chapter 10). That's why the protocols in Part III can be used to address both pain and injury—and why the strategies in this chapter are the same strategies used in rehab.

But in some cases, we must separate pain from injury when progressing through the phases because not all injuries cause pain, and not all pain is caused by injury. With an injury, you must consider not only your pain symptoms and functional ability but also the tissue that is injured and the typical healing time. With a purely pain-based problem, you're not worried about the tissue because you might not have an injury, or the tissue has already healed. Instead, you're thinking about the type of pain you're feeling, how long you've had it, and your sensitivity to movement. Keep that in mind as you implement the strategies in this chapter, review the injury management phases in Chapter 10, and navigate the protocols in Part III.

## ACTIVE VS. PASSIVE STRATEGIES: WHAT'S THE DIFFERENCE?

In physical therapy, "active strategies" refers to movements generated by an internal force, whereas "passive strategies" refers to movements influenced by an external force. Lifting weights and walking are active strategies because the movement comes from an internal source—you're contracting your muscles to move your body. Using a band to stretch your hamstring, moving on a foam roller, and applying heat or ice to a body region are passive strategies because the movement or stimulus is facilitated by an external object or force rather than your own working muscles.

Active strategies like mobility, aerobic exercise, and resistance training have the best evidence for creating lasting change.[1-3] Passive strategies like soft tissue mobilizations and flexibility exercises have their place but are mainly used to alleviate symptoms and address range of motion impairments. The idea is to use passive strategies to get pain under control (phase 1) and then implement active strategies to prevent pain, address impairments, and stay healthy (phases 2 and 3).

In Part III of this book, I provide specific pain and injury rehab protocols and help you navigate the exercises in those protocols with information about acceptable pain levels. In general, it's OK to feel mild discomfort when doing both active and passive exercises; it's important to work through a certain level of discomfort to desensitize your system and break the persistent pain cycle. Rehab drills are safe if your baseline symptoms aren't flared up a few hours after performing them.

However, not every exercise will help you, and some might make your pain worse. If your symptoms worsen after performing the exercises, take some time off and eliminate the movement that flared up your pain. Movement is medicine and dosage is important, so be sure to follow the protocol and review the exercise guidelines in Chapter 12.

# SOFT TISSUE MOBILIZATIONS

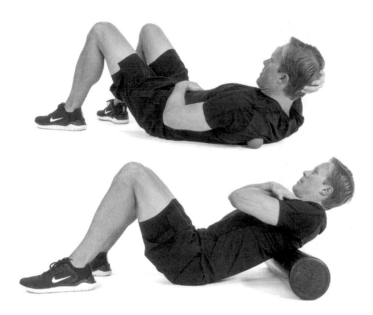

Soft tissue mobilizations (also known as myofascial release techniques) are primarily used during the first phase of rehab to alleviate pain symptoms. They include foam rolling and massage.

Soft tissue mobilizations are often combined with other mobilizations to improve range of motion impairments faster and more comfortably—you're loosening up the soft tissue (muscles, tendons, and fascia) and getting it ready for the mobility exercises to come. You can also implement them to address tender spots in muscles or joints and relieve tension in any area that feels stiff—if raising your arm overhead (shoulder flexion) feels restricted, for example, rolling out your thoracic spine and lats might temporarily increase your mobility.

There are many tools you can use to perform self-guided myofascial release, such as foam rollers, massage balls (lacrosse ball, peanut tool, etc.), and even a percussion massage gun. Each tool has its pros and cons. In general, foam rollers are good for large muscles like the quads and lats, while smaller balls are more precise and good for targeting areas around joints and insertion points (attachments in a muscle where movement occurs). Massage guns offer the best of both worlds but may be too intense for some people, and they are difficult to use in hard-to-reach areas, like the back. The best approach is to experiment and figure out which tools you prefer for specific areas and situations.

Soft tissue mobilizations are thought to work in two main ways, regardless of the tool you use:[4,5]

- Moving or massaging tissues can create vasodilation (the widening of blood vessels) to improve blood flow to the area, which can reduce pain symptoms. If you have a swollen injury, increased blood flow improves nutrient delivery and clears out the chemical irritants causing swelling and inflammation.

- Soft tissue mobilizations modulate pain by introducing a novel stimulus, as if you're distracting your nervous system. They do not seem to mechanically alter tissue; it's more likely that a neurological mechanism changes the pain experience. Say you have pain in your low back, and you use a ball to massage the muscles. You're introducing a new stimulus to the low back sensors and increasing blood flow to the area, and that's what helps reduce pain symptoms temporarily—not breaking up knots or adhesions in the muscle as many people think.

The pressure you use should feel like a "good hurt," meaning it feels therapeutic and doesn't make your pain worse. Applying too much pressure could flare up pain symptoms, cause spasms, or tighten the muscle. Stop if you feel sharp or traveling pain, tingling, or numbness. If your pain is worse after you finish, wait until it calms down before doing any more soft tissue work.

You can massage along the length of a muscle or across it, whichever feels better. Stop on sensitive areas and spend one to two minutes massaging the tender point. (Anything more probably won't offer additional benefits.) Working adjacent joints and muscles (above, below, and around the area) can be helpful, too.

When you find a tender point, play around with these three methods to help desensitize and relax the area:

- Take a big breath in and then, as you exhale, try to relax and sink deeper into the tissue (apply more pressure) with the tool you are using.

- Contract the muscle you are massaging for a few seconds and then relax (also referred to as proprioceptive neuromuscular facilitation, or PNF).

- Add movement while staying on a specific spot—if you're foam rolling your quads, for example, bend and straighten your knee.

People tend to overcomplicate soft tissue mobilization and put way too much emphasis on it as an intervention. It is a temporary strategy that does not last long—maybe 20 to 30 minutes. Even though it can feel good, the evidence (at least for now) doesn't support the idea of "prehab" soft tissue work to prevent injuries and pain. You're better off following the injury prevention and management strategies covered in Chapters 9 and 10 and sticking to a mobility and resistance training program if you're healthy and pain-free.

However, you can do these mobilizations as often as you like if they help your symptoms. If foam rolling on a specific spot every couple of hours reduces your pain, relieves stiffness, and helps you move better, that's great. But this should be a temporary behavior modification to desensitize your system, not a mandatory routine that replaces active strategies like mobility, aerobic exercise, and resistance training.

## TRIGGER POINTS AND MUSCLE KNOTS

You're probably familiar with the terms "trigger points" and "muscle knots." Both refer to sensitive or hyper-irritable spots in soft tissue that are often found in close proximity to areas of pain or injury.

These terms—and the treatment strategies used to address them—have led to a lot of misinformation and debate among practitioners and therapists. Some argue that you need to address trigger points and release muscle knots to alleviate pain and optimize function. While addressing tender points can relieve pain, release tension, and potentially promote healing, it's not an end-all-be-all treatment strategy. As with many treatments, the science doesn't support the most commonly given advice. Myofascial release techniques should be viewed as complementary and temporary, meaning you use them in conjunction with other resistance and mobility training strategies and mainly for short-term relief of pain, tension, and other symptoms.

We all have trigger points that are sensitive to pressure. People spend way too much money and time trying to "fix" trigger points that will always be present. If you have a spot that is tender when you are at rest or with movement (referred to as an active trigger point), you should address it with soft tissue mobilizations. But if it doesn't hurt at rest, and you feel only mild discomfort when you press on it (known as a latent trigger point), you don't need to worry because it's not affecting your functional ability or influencing your pain symptoms.

The same is true with so-called muscle knots. There are a lot of spots in your body that have a ropy feel. As with trigger points, these are usually natural components of your anatomy. A lot of people feel a tight knot in the trapezius or levator scapulae muscles at the top of their shoulder blades and think, "Oh, I have a big knot," and then spend a ton of time trying to reduce the size of it. But it's not a knot; it's just the anatomy of the muscle, and all that massaging won't change anything structurally. If you had surgery or some kind of trauma to your skin, muscle, or fascia, however, scar tissue and adhesions often form that can influence how the fascia and muscles move. In that case, spending time on the area to alleviate symptoms and restore function might be helpful.

With trigger points and muscle knots, it's largely about perception and nervous system sensitivity. If there were adhesions or inflammation in the structure of the soft tissue, you would be able to see them with imaging, and that is not the case. These issues are not visible on an MRI or with a real-time ultrasound, which is why some theorize that they are related to increased activity in free nerve endings rather than actual bunching up or tightening of a muscle.[6,7]

The key takeaway is this: If an area feels tight or tender, spend a little bit of extra time there until you feel the muscle relax or the pain dissipate, and then move on. Don't worry about trying to make a bump or "knot" go away, as it is likely a part of your normal anatomy and not something you want to try to permanently alter.

# AEROBIC EXERCISE

Aerobic exercise is not included in the rehab protocols, but it's an important element for managing pain and recovering from injury.[8] Increasing blood flow can alleviate pain and improve healing by transporting nutrients and oxygen throughout the body and clearing inflammatory chemicals that may be increasing nerve sensitivity. Sustained aerobic exercise also increases blood flow to the brain, promoting the growth of new neurons (a process called neurogenesis). Given the brain's role in pain, more blood flow is certainly not a bad thing.[9]

If you have pain—whether it's chronic or from a recent injury—doing 20 to 30 minutes of aerobic exercise like walking, swimming, cycling, or hiking can reduce symptoms. But you must be careful about choosing the right kind of aerobic exercise when you have acute, injury-related pain. If you sprained your ankle recently and then go for an hour-long walk, you risk a flare-up and might extend the healing time.

While the research supports mobility and resistance training for chronic pain conditions, aerobic exercise has better evidence for reducing many persistent symptoms.[2,10] I recommend that you use resistance exercises to desensitize your system and boost strength and function, but make sure to prioritize aerobic exercise if chronic pain is your main problem.

## JUST MOVE: THE SCIENCE OF EXERCISE AND PAIN

Whether it's aerobic exercise, therapeutic movements designed to target a particular joint or muscle group, or whole-body options like yoga or Pilates, research shows that regular, sustained movement decreases pain sensitivity and positively alters the pain experience.[11] For instance, exercise increases blood flow to the brain and promotes neuroplasticity, which can alter pain processing. It helps prevent hyperalgesia (increased sensitivity to stimuli) by decreasing excitability within the central nervous system and by improving your ability to inhibit incoming nociceptive signals.[12] It also positively affects the immune system by increasing levels of anti-inflammatory cytokines and decreasing levels of inflammatory cytokines. These molecules are highly relevant to pain because inflammatory cytokines activate nociceptors, while anti-inflammatory cytokines reduce nociceptor activity and can prevent pain from occurring.[12]

Outside of effects on the physical body, people who exercise regularly demonstrate improved mental health and psychological well-being as compared to their sedentary counterparts. When you exercise—whether it's going to the gym or playing a sport—you're likely in a social situation, and that might make you feel less stressed. You're doing something that makes you feel better about yourself and more confident in your body, and that may help with other factors, such as depression.

As I've said, all the factors that influence pain are interrelated. Addressing one helps the rest. Exercise is possibly the most important factor of all. Getting 20 to 30 minutes of exercise— regardless of what type it is—has a positive effect on your health and just might help with your pain, too. It has an important place in pain management because it affects so many factors that are interwoven with both acute and chronic pain.

# FLEXIBILITY (STRETCHING) EXERCISES

Flexibility exercises are what we think of as classic stretches. As with mobility exercises (see the next section), you mainly see flexibility training in phases 1 and 2 of the protocols.

Holding a static stretch improves not only the flexibility of your soft tissues (muscle, tendon, fascia, etc.) but also your stretch tolerance.[13-15] In other words, you're conditioning your nerves to be less sensitive to positions of increased stretch. This is a major element in techniques like nerve mobilizations and nerve flossing.

For example, stretching your hamstrings to temporarily relieve pain in your low back may affect your stretch tolerance at the nervous system level. Since your sciatic nerve is located in your hamstrings and low back, you're stretching the muscles and tendons as well as the sciatic nerve and its branches. Similar to the soft tissue mobilizations, this improves blood flow to the sciatic nerve, which enhances nerve health and helps with pain.

To perform flexibility exercises correctly, experiment with these two methods:

- Move as far into the stretch position as you can without pain and hold it there. Focus on your breath. As you exhale, try to relax into the stretch and move a little bit farther until you reach end range.

- Contract and relax a muscle (PNF) at the point of restriction to improve your stretch tolerance. Many people gain more range of motion faster with this technique compared to static holds. To do it, contract the muscle that is being stretched for five to seven seconds, relax and hold for 10 to 15 seconds, and then repeat two to four times.

When holding a stretch, it's important not to push into pain. When your stretch receptors detect a threat, your body responds by contracting muscles or producing pain to prevent you from stretching too far. Pay attention to these signals. Stop at the point of restriction, hold, and breathe into the stretch until your stretch receptors no longer detect the threat, and then let go.

In general, two to three sets with 15- to 30-second holds are enough for people in pain. Anything more and you risk flaring up your symptoms. Once you are asymptomatic, longer holds—30 seconds all the way up to several minutes—are great for improving flexibility.

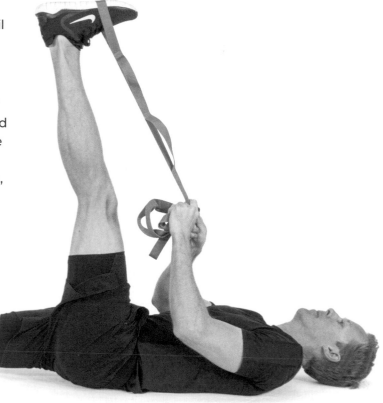

# RELAXATION AND MEDITATION

Breathing can be a huge piece of pain management because it affects your whole system.[16,17] It ties directly to stress, which is why I count it among active treatments even if it isn't as exercise or movement heavy. You're still doing something to confront your pain, and research proves that meditation and breathwork can help reduce sympathetic nervous system activity and improve all areas of health.[18,19]

Your diaphragm is your primary ventilatory muscle, assisted by the intercostal muscles between your ribs. When people get stressed or feel threatened, they often switch from stomach or diaphragmatic breathing to "chest breathing," which incorporates accessory muscles in the neck and shoulder blades and increases tension throughout the upper body, dumping adrenaline into the bloodstream and making pain worse.

Incorporating diaphragmatic breathing—such as the "in and out through the nose" or "in through the nose, out through the mouth" method—can help you slow down, become more in-tune with your body, and realize where you're holding tension. Box breathing is another popular exercise for reducing stress. It involves breathing in through your nose while slowly counting to four, holding your breath while slowly counting to four, exhaling while slowly counting to four, and then holding your breath again while slowly counting to four. Repeat these steps at least three times or until you feel calm.

Whether it's due to the increased oxygen, decreased sympathetic nervous system activity, or boosted awareness of the state of your body, this meditative process can reduce stress and help with chronic musculoskeletal pain. Worrying about pain, however, can put you in a sympathetic fight-or-flight response state, and breathing can ramp the system up or slow it down. The more threatened you feel, the more likely you are to breathe rapidly—igniting pain or making it worse. But slower breathing can help reduce that response by telling your brain and nervous system that you're OK, potentially reducing symptoms and connecting you with your body.

Meditation, which is essentially time set aside to focus on breathing, can dramatically improve your mindset and reduce pain symptoms. This mindfulness practice is all about observing your thoughts as they come rather than engaging with them, which ties into reducing stress and addressing the other factors that influence pain discussed in Chapter 4.

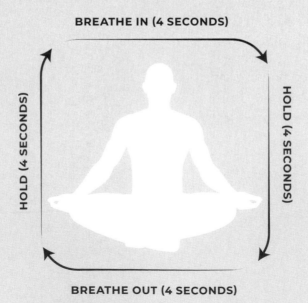

**BREATHE IN (4 SECONDS)**

**HOLD (4 SECONDS)**

**HOLD (4 SECONDS)**

**BREATHE OUT (4 SECONDS)**

# MOBILITY EXERCISES

Mobility exercises are similar to flexibility exercises in that they appear in phases 1 and 2 of the rehab protocols and primarily address range of motion impairments. But instead of targeting soft tissue with stretching (flexibility), you're targeting your joints with movement (mobility). Mobility exercises take a joint to end range (a position of maximum resistance) or through a full range of motion (the full movement potential of the joint) to desensitize the system through movement, improve stretch tolerance, and decrease pain in the affected joint.

Because flexibility and mobility exercises are similar, they complement each other—stretching can help with soft tissue limitations, and mobility can improve joint restrictions. But the focus and methods differ slightly.

In the protocols, you will encounter three mobility methods: passive, active assisted, and active range of motion. They are typically performed as a stepwise progression based on the severity of pain and functional ability.

- **PASSIVE RANGE OF MOTION (PROM)** mobility exercises require a tool such as a dowel, stretch strap, or band to move a painful or injured joint. Say you have a torn rotator cuff tendon or you're unable to move your shoulder due to pain. In that scenario, you would hold a dowel or similar object (like a broomstick or golf club) with your healthy arm and then use it to move your hurt shoulder into positions that challenge the mobility of the joint. Start with PROM when pain is limiting your ability to move or when moving without assistance makes your pain worse. The idea is to reduce stress on the injured or painful joint and surrounding tissues to keep pain at a minimum. Progress to the next method as your pain decreases and function improves.

- **ACTIVE ASSISTED RANGE OF MOTION (AAROM)** mobility exercises also involve the use of an external object like a dowel or strap to assist with the movement, but instead of completely relaxing the painful joint and surrounding soft tissue, you start to actively move the joint. With the shoulder example, you would use a dowel to facilitate the movement, but you would actively move your painful or injured shoulder to end range—splitting the effort between both arms. As your functional ability improves and you're able to move more freely without making your pain worse, progress to the next method.

- **ACTIVE RANGE OF MOTION (AROM)** mobility exercises are performed without external assistance. These are the exercises most people think of when they see or hear the term "active mobility." You use your muscles to actively move the painful or injured joint through a full range of motion.

### PROM AND AAROM SHOULDER FLEXION

PROM: Use the dowel to perform 90–100% of the movement.

AAROM: Use the dowel to perform about 50% of the movement.

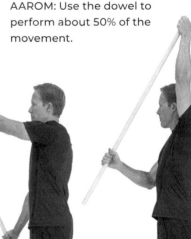

## AROM SHOULDER FLEXION

AROM: Use your muscles to perform 100% of the movement.

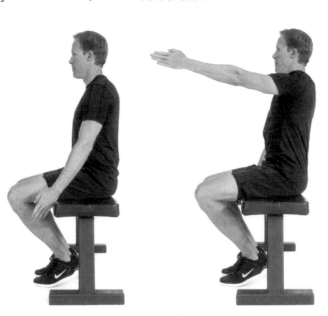
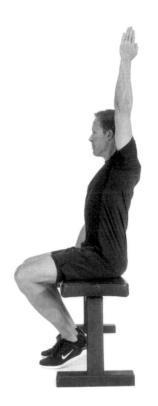

With all three methods, the goal is to slowly move the joint through a full range of motion and hold end-range positions for a few seconds. The exercise photos in the protocols show you what those positions look like.

As with flexibility exercises, you're not pushing into pain. Mobility exercises might be mildly uncomfortable, but you can move in and out of the demonstrated range without making your pain worse. Once you can perform the AROM exercises with control and relatively free of pain, you're ready to start loading the joint with resistance training exercises.

If you have a contracture (see below) or a joint-based restriction that is preventing you from moving into certain ranges, you need to isolate that position and perform a low-load, long-duration (LLLD) stretch.[20-22] For instance, say you have a shoulder flexion restriction—you try to move your arm overhead and it feels blocked. Go to the point where you can't move any farther and then apply a low-load external force to hold the position. "Low-load" means

## ADDRESSING CONTRACTURES AND JOINT RESTRICTIONS

Positions or ranges of restriction where movement feels stiff or blocked often relate to changes in the tissues surrounding the joint due to a prolonged lack of activity. Maybe you were immobilized after a severe injury or major surgery, or you stopped moving due to chronic pain.

Your body adapts to your movements and positions or lack thereof. When you routinely express the full movement potential of your joints, your tissues remain elastic and mobile. If you don't, they become inelastic and restricted. Left unchecked, structural shortening can start to occur in the skin, muscles, tendons, or ligaments (known as a contracture), which limit or prevent movement. That's why you perform mobility exercises early on in the rehab process—because minor impairments can turn into permanent restrictions.

Most contractures improve with LLLD stretches performed three to five times a day, consistently for several weeks or months. But if you aren't seeing any improvements after a few weeks of consistent work, you might consider seeking out a practitioner who specializes in manual therapy and joint mobilizations.

it's a stretch with a low magnitude of force that is tolerable and can be sustained for a long duration. This can be done using a dowel or by placing your arm against a wall at the point of restriction.

Space the LLLD stretches out throughout the day (three to five times each day) and hold for two to 10 minutes (referred to as total end range time, or TERT). Joints have denser connective tissue and require longer hold times and sessions to get the desired results. The goal is to maximize TERT as long as it doesn't cause flare-ups or make you too sore.

## JOINT MOBILIZATION AND MANIPULATION

A joint mobilization or manipulation is a technique in which a practitioner—usually a physical therapist or chiropractor—moves your joint in a way that you can't achieve on your own, typically in an oscillation or push, to reduce pain or increase mobility.

Joint mobilizations and manipulations involve moving two bones that come together to form a joint. So, if your shoulder is being mobilized, that ball-and-socket joint, where the glenoid (socket) and humeral head (ball) of your humerus bone come together, is being moved. The joint capsule that goes around it, with ligaments and other structures that affect range of motion, stability, and mobility, is also being moved. There are mechanical receptors in your joints, and oscillating those joints can stimulate those receptors, which can change how your brain perceives the area.

As with other forms of manual therapy, joint mobilizations and manipulations work well in many cases to temporarily reduce pain and improve mobility.[23-26] If you have a stubborn issue that seems to be related to a joint and isn't fully improving with exercise alone, you might consider working with a physical therapist or chiropractor who specializes in manual therapy while continuing with your exercise program to further reduce symptoms and keep your system healthy for the long term.

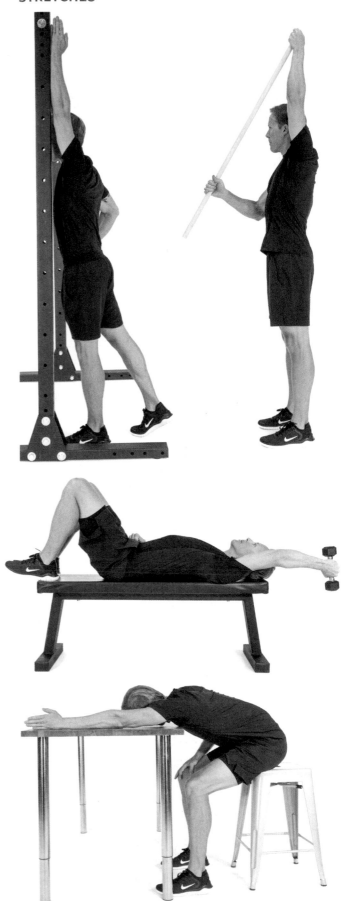

# RESISTANCE EXERCISES

Resistance training encompasses exercises that include a static or dynamic muscle contraction that is resisted by an external load or force.

When you're in the early acute pain phase of rehab, you will primarily use isometric and eccentric resistance exercises. Isometric exercises contract a muscle with no movement. Imagine you're doing a biceps curl and you stop halfway up and hold it there. The muscle isn't changing length, but it is contracting. In rehab and after surgery, people with pain usually start with isometric exercises to create a hypoalgesic response (alleviate pain), especially in tendons.[27] I often tell patients that this process is like a natural ibuprofen. You typically do four or five repetitions and hold them for 30 to 45 seconds. Isometric contractions are often used in exercises like pause squats to increase strength in a portion of the range of motion where you are weak, which is important in the early phases of injury or pain.

Eccentric contractions involve a muscle contracting and lengthening. In the biceps curl example, this is the lowering phase; your elbow is moving into extension, so your elbow flexors are contracting and lengthening. Eccentrics are a great way to reduce pain symptoms while also addressing range of motion and strength impairments associated with pain and injury.[28] In terms of movement and injury prevention, eccentrics make muscles longer, help with flexibility, and reduce the likelihood of future strains (because strains often happen during eccentric contractions).

The protocols often start with isometrics (phases 1 and 2), then go to eccentrics (phase 2), and add full-range movements (phase 3) that include the concentric contractions. This is the "up" portion of the biceps curl, where the muscle is contracting and shortening. It's usually the most difficult and causes the most discomfort, which is why it's in phase 3, after your pain is mostly gone.

There are two main reasons why resistance exercise is so effective at treating many types of pain.

## ISOMETRIC CONTRACTION
MUSCLE CONTRACTS BUT DOES NOT SHORTEN

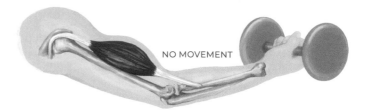

NO MOVEMENT

## CONCENTRIC CONTRACTION
MUSCLE CONTRACTS WHILE SHORTENING

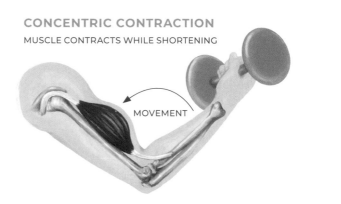

MOVEMENT

## ECCENTRIC CONTRACTION
MUSCLE CONTRACTS WHILE LENGTHENING

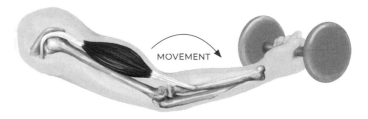

MOVEMENT

**First, improving strength and control within the neuromuscular system makes your active subsystem elements (muscles and nerves) more efficient and resilient.**

To alleviate issues like tendinopathy (tendon pain and dysfunction), muscle strains, and myofascial pain problems associated with prolonged postures and repetitive tasks, resistance exercises that apply gradually increasing loads to the body should be your primary focus in rehab. These exercises not only reduce pain but also improve function and reduce the odds that the issue will reoccur in the future.

Take myofascial neck and shoulder pain associated with workplace ergonomics. Research in this area shows that regular short doses of resistance training that target the neck and shoulder muscles—such as the upper trapezius and levator scapulae—can alleviate pain by helping overactive muscles relax. Research on the benefits of resistance training for painful tendon conditions demonstrates that loading painful tendons, like the Achilles and patellar tendons, is probably the best thing you can do to overcome this type of issue.[29,30] Resistance training in the correct dosage leads to significant reductions in tendon pain and, when implemented a few times a week, helps prevent the issue from coming back.

When it comes to the benefits of resistance training for painful passive subsystem structures, individuals with knee pain associated with osteoarthritis are a good group to consider. In these cases, knee pain can partially be explained by the deterioration of the protective cartilage that covers the ends of bones. When this cartilage breaks down, the underlying bones, which have numerous nerve endings, touch and create pain. However, individuals with this issue who participate in resistance training a few times each week have less pain and better functional ability.[31,32] While there are likely several mechanisms at play here, improving neuromuscular efficiency and strength may translate to less stress on the bones as the muscles become better at accepting load. This is a great example of how sensitive passive subsystem structures can be desensitized via training of the active subsystem.

**Second, by placing gradual doses of load on your system—and keeping them below the level that causes your pain to flare up—resistance exercise can help desensitize your nervous system and improve your tolerance to load.**

Graded exposure starts with finding the movements that exacerbate pain and then gradually building up doses to desensitize your system. Your goal is to continually "poke the bear" and beat your previous best by progressively confronting the threat. You take whatever movement or position you're sensitive to, break it into pieces, and gradually expose yourself to it. But remember, chronic pain is not an accurate indicator of the state of your physical body. If a movement flares up your pain, it's probably not because you've damaged something; it's because your system has become hypersensitive. You're trying to find your tolerance level and move your flare-up line. If you do have a flare-up, reduce the load or go back to the previous phase of the rehab protocol you are following.

Due to the individual variability of the pain experience, the process is different for everyone. You need to determine the training frequency and volume you can handle, which is another reason why education is so important. Once you understand the categories, principles, and phases along with your type and base level of pain, you can tweak the rehab exercises to your needs, using the appropriate protocol to gradually expose your system to more physical stress and create your own graded exposure program.

## THERAPEUTIC, NOT CORRECTIVE

I don't usually use the term "corrective exercise" with patients—and if I do, it always comes with an educational message: if these exercises help with your pain, it's not because they're correcting a biomechanical fault or postural issue in your system.

The problem with the term "corrective" is that it makes people think of pain as a mechanical problem requiring mechanical fixes, as if you're replacing a part in your car. Even when pain is mechanical, that word often leads people to look for a linear relationship between their pain and their body—the idea being that if you fix one physical factor, your pain will get better. Yet many people "correct" their physical problems—if they even have one—and their pain doesn't improve. As such, "therapeutic exercise" is a more appropriate term because the movement has a therapeutic effect, meaning it reduces pain and improves function.

# PART II
# INJURY

## CHAPTER 6

# WHAT IS AN INJURY?

In simple terms, an injury is an identifiable physical disruption of musculoskeletal tissue, such as a ruptured tendon, torn ligament, strained muscle, or fractured bone.

There are many types of injuries, and the time frames for healing vary widely. Diagnosing an injury provides a framework for the treatment strategies you should follow to address it. Knowing which tissues are involved, how those tissues typically heal, the factors that aggravate the injury (or may have caused it), and how to best address them are all part of designing an effective rehabilitation program—one that not only optimizes recovery but also strengthens the tissue so that you can return to the activities you enjoy and prevent the injury from reoccurring.

Possessing this knowledge, you can actively confront injuries—like pain—with confidence and purpose. Suffering an injury, whether minor or severe, is often scary and can lead to despair. The associated pain can compromise your physical regimen and distract you from your daily routine. The little things that you took for granted, like picking up your child, playing sports, or just moving and feeling good, are put on hold, and that can take a heavy toll on your mindset. Left unchecked, it can cause you to spiral into a pattern of worry, imagining the worst possible outcomes and wondering if you will ever get back to your pre-injury self.

Those thoughts and feelings are perfectly natural, but they may contribute to more pain—the kind that is directly linked to chronic pain states. Just as you need to actively confront pain, you need to realize that injuries—and the symptoms associated with them—are temporary, and there is a lot you can do to manage and prevent them.

# THE INSIGHT INJURY PROVIDES

Injuries are unfortunate, but they are wake-up calls that expose weaknesses in your lifestyle and training. Maybe you got injured because you are deconditioned, and through the rehab process you realize that you need to be more physically active, follow a consistent resistance and mobility training program, or address one of the many other factors covered in Chapters 4 and 9.

Or perhaps an injury highlights that you need to modify some aspect of your training, such as your program design, training frequency and/or volume, recovery time, or exercise variations. These changes, though seemingly small, can have a huge impact on how you feel and perform as you transition back to normal activity.

Whether they are lifestyle issues or issues related to training, addressing the factors that contribute to pain and injury will help you come back stronger and more resilient while developing habits that improve your performance and overall health. It may even prevent another injury.

Say you have pain associated with a tendon injury that is disrupting your ability to move. This type of injury is usually brought on by doing an activity too fast or at too high a volume and is typically labeled a repetitive use injury. If you pay attention to the signals your body is sending you—the pain you feel when you move or perform the irritating activity—you can pinpoint the factors that aggravate and potentially caused it and follow the appropriate rehab protocol to get better. You can then apply what you learned and make the necessary adjustments to your lifestyle and training to not only prevent tendinopathy in other areas but also keep the condition from turning into something worse, like a full tear or rupture.

Or, say you strained your back while lifting something heavy, and you realize that you didn't warm up properly, moved with poor form, or made some other error. It's unfortunate that it took an injury to make you aware of those missteps, but the information highlights strategies that you can apply to your future practice. If you implement those strategies during rehab, they can become habits, and you'll be much less likely to sustain the same injury (or related ones) when you return to the activity that caused it. What's more, having successfully rehabilitated the injury, you're less fearful and can move with confidence knowing that you are equipped with the tools to prevent problems and treat them as they arise.

Obviously, not all injuries have an identifiable cause or factors that you can pinpoint and work on to prevent the injury from getting worse or reoccurring. Sometimes an injury is sudden, traumatic, and outside of your control—like a car accident, a fall off your bike, or a hit while playing a sport. But even in the most unfortunate circumstances, you can adopt an active coping strategy that is optimistic and purposeful. You might discover that training around an injury opens your eyes to modalities and exercise variations that you hadn't tried before but enjoy and find helpful—which you can then incorporate into your post-injury routine. The habits you form through rehab can make you healthier overall—you gain knowledge, and that knowledge leads to positive change.

Viewing injuries with this active coping perspective is essential because you will get injured at some point in your life. Regular exercise, movement, and training—especially resistance, mobility, flexibility, and proprioceptive training—can greatly reduce your risk.[1] However, you can never ensure 100 percent prevention, so you need to know how to think about injury—and your own abilities—to avoid negative outcomes. Before you jump into the protocols, it's important to learn the types of injuries, the contributing factors, what you can do to prevent and manage them, and how long they take to heal, all of which is covered in this part of the book. These chapters explain the why behind the rehab strategies you will implement for specific injuries and give you the autonomy to make adjustments to suit your unique situation.

Then, in Part III, I provide the how in the form of rehab exercise protocols for specific injuries. But the protocols are not just for addressing injuries; they are also for addressing pain symptoms. Now, you might be thinking, aren't pain and injury one and the same? They are certainly related, but it's important to distinguish between them.

# SEPARATING PAIN FROM INJURY

Most people who have pain assume it comes from injury. And sometimes that is the case—there's an obvious mechanical insult that is creating pain. In this way, injury and pain are connected. But the relationship is not always clear-cut.

Remember, pain is a neurogenic phenomenon that the brain produces to protect the body from actual or potential damage.[2] Pain is an important survival mechanism, but sometimes your brain creates it even though no physical damage to your body has occurred. Conversely, you can have an injury without experiencing pain if your nervous system doesn't find that injury threatening. That means you can have an injury and feel pain, have an injury and feel no pain, or feel pain but have no injury.

So, if injury is not always directly tied to pain, how should we think about the association between them? To answer this question, we must examine how the scientific community arrived at this injury–pain paradox.

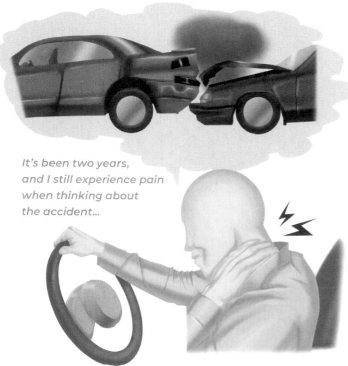

*It's been two years, and I still experience pain when thinking about the accident...*

At one point, it was thought that if a person was in pain, they had an injury to their physical body. And if a person had an injury, it would always lead to pain—it was a cause-and-effect relationship. But that all changed with advancements in medical imaging and studies of people who have injuries but not pain. Researchers started to put people who were asymptomatic—they had no pain symptoms—through MRIs and realized that a significant percentage of them had identifiable disruptions to their musculoskeletal tissue. Around 40 to 50 percent of the population experiences no symptoms despite having labral tears, meniscus tears, disc herniations, tendon problems, arthritis, and so on.[3-8]

As researchers started to pull apart injury from pain, they also realized that there are people who have pain but don't have identifiable injuries. A huge percentage (90 to 95 percent) of low back pain diagnoses are nonspecific, meaning a specific underlying cause or problem cannot be linked to the person's pain.[9] Lots of people who experience pain latch onto this idea of finding a physical problem—something to blame the pain on. But a clean or inconclusive MRI doesn't mean that a person's pain is not valid or real. It just means that injury and pain are different.

You could be in pain, and an MRI could show an injury, but because pain and injury are not always directly linked, there's no way to prove that the injury is the cause of your pain. That "injury" could be benign—a normal part of the aging process, like developing wrinkles.

Take someone who has back pain and goes to the doctor for spinal imaging. The radiology report comes back saying there are small disc herniations, facet joint arthritis, and stenosis. If that person fixates on these diagnoses and believes their pain will get better only when there are no visible signs of injury, they may never again feel confident in their body—even if their pain symptoms and function improve with rehab.

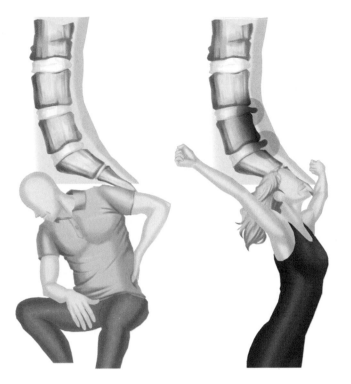

PAIN WITH NO "INJURY"          NO PAIN WITH "INJURY"

This is the main problem with imaging: the results provoke anxiety, which impedes recovery.[10-11] The injured person starts to worry about making the injury worse and stops stressing the area in any way. As a result, the area becomes deconditioned and the body atrophies, and then they're even more likely to get injured when they try that activity again.

You need to respect an injury by not putting too much physical stress on it, but becoming inactive and fearful has equally negative effects. That could be how you got injured in the first place.

Decoupling pain from injury is important because if all you're thinking about is the injured tissue, you might miss the bigger picture—the other factors that could be contributing to or causing your pain. Your symptoms and how well you are functioning are a much better gauge of your progress. You'll know you're getting better because you can feel and see the improvement, whether or not the injury is still present. All this gives you a greater sense of confidence in and awareness of what is happening with your body. Once you tune in to your pain symptoms and functional ability—and let go of the idea that pain always means injury—you'll be less fearful when something flares up. You'll recognize it not as an injury that you need to worry about, but as a temporary sensitivity that you can easily address.

Bring this concept with you into this part of the book, because as we transition into the core of this injury section, I'm going to talk about injury separate from the component of pain. To wrap your head around these concepts, you must shake the mindset that pain means injury and injury means pain. This is not always true, and it factors into how both are approached in the protocols.

That said, when an injury is associated with pain or leads to a functional problem, knowing which tissue is injured can help you determine how to move forward with the rehab process. This includes treatments such as movement and exercise protocols, and it provides an expected timeline for healing, as different tissues heal at different rates. Whether or not pain is a factor, when you're navigating an injury, you must respect the injured tissue and how long it takes to heal, which I cover in the coming chapters.

## CHAPTER 7

# THE TYPES
# OF INJURIES

When it comes to injury, relating pain and other symptoms to a specific tissue is not only reassuring but also helps you navigate the path forward.

Knowing whether you have a strained muscle, torn ligament, nerve irritation, or tendinopathy is important because it tells you which of the rehab protocols you should follow to get the best results. Although many of the exercises are similar from one protocol to the next, each injury has impairments associated with it, along with its own aggravating factors (behaviors you need to modify to prevent flare-ups) and treatment strategy based on the tissue that is most involved in your symptoms. The closer you get to identifying the type of injury, the more precise the treatment plan will be.

# MUSCLES—STRAINS

A lot of people have pain related to muscles, and it mostly comes in the form of strains.

Muscle has fibers that form a sort of "belly," and on either end, tendons attach the muscle to bone. The muscle is the meaty, fibrous portion in the middle. So, in essence, a muscle injury is a physical disruption of that muscle fiber structure.

**MUSCLE BELLY AND TENDON**

— MUSCLE

— TENDON

## MECHANISM OF INJURY (HOW IT HAPPENS)

Muscle strains typically occur when a muscle is performing an eccentric contraction—that is, squeezing and stretching forcefully at the same time. Imagine lifting a heavy backpack off the ground. This is a concentric contraction; when you lift the pack, the elbow flexor muscles are squeezing and shortening. When you lower the pack back down, however, the muscles are squeezing but the fibers are lengthening. This is an eccentric contraction.

For example, sprinters are more likely to strain their hamstrings when the knee is kicking out straight to make the foot touch the ground for the next step. As the knee flies forward, the hamstrings contract to act like a brake and slow it down. That's what eccentric contractions do—serve as brakes. And that braking motion is where strains usually happen.

Strains most commonly occur at the musculotendinous junction, where the muscle belly turns into a tendon (it's not a separate structure; it literally becomes a different type of tissue). We think of muscles as one big unit, but inside there are fascicles, which are like little ropes running in parallel. A strain tears those fascicles, and the severity of the strain depends on how many fascicles are torn.

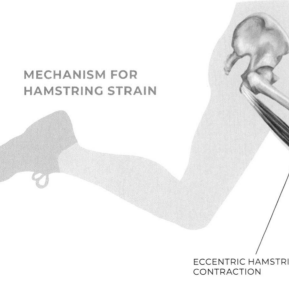

**MECHANISM FOR HAMSTRING STRAIN**

ECCENTRIC HAMSTRING CONTRACTION

# INJURY GRADES (GAUGING SEVERITY)

Muscle strains are graded based on the severity of the damage and how much they affect function:

- A grade I strain indicates damage to the muscle that causes pain but has a minimal impact on function. The strength of the muscle and its ability to stretch and contract aren't severely impaired.

- A grade II strain causes pain that affects function by limiting range of motion and the ability to forcefully contract the injured muscle. You have swelling and minor weakness, and stretching the muscle is painful.

- A grade III strain is a major muscle tear that is evident on medical imaging. These strains share the same pain symptoms and functional impairments as grade II but are more severe and take longer to heal. Increased swelling and a complete loss of muscle function are common with grade III strains.

**RECTUS FEMORIS MUSCLE STRAIN INJURY GRADES**

GRADE I      GRADE II      GRADE III

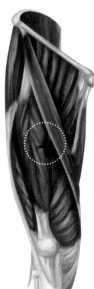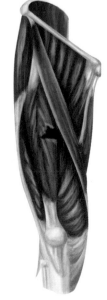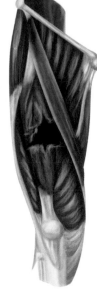

# SIGNS AND SYMPTOMS

Strains feel similar as you go up the scale, just more intense. You may notice bruising and bleeding in the surrounding tissues with a grade II or III strain, whereas a grade I strain might hurt, but you won't see any discoloration in the limb.

A grade II or III strain can cause bruising and bleeding because blood leaks into the surrounding tissues. (This happens with muscle tears but not with most other types of injuries.) Because muscles and tendons are connected, major strains or ruptures in either can also cause a divot or discontinuation in the muscle—a spot where the muscle doesn't feel connected anymore that you can feel with your hand.

When you stress a fresh muscle injury, the pain is sharp. At rest, the pain is achy, throbbing, or pulsating. But what's unique about muscles is that contracting or squeezing an injured muscle can reproduce the pain because you've damaged a contractile structure. Those fibers have to grab each other and squeeze, and if you pull on a tear, it hurts.

If you strain your hamstring, for example, you may feel pain when you're walking and swinging your leg forward—when you're performing that eccentric contraction. As your knee straightens, you swing your foot to take the next step, and when the hamstring starts braking to slow the leg down, you feel soreness and pain in that muscle.

Strains also usually hurt when the muscle is stretched. Lying on your back so that somebody can push your leg toward your chest to stretch your strained hamstring usually reproduces pain because you're putting tension on a tear.

# IMPAIRMENTS ASSOCIATED WITH MUSCLE INJURIES

Because muscles are contractile units, the most noticeable impairment related to strains is weakness or a reduction in power when actively engaging the muscle. This weakness can be due to pain inhibition or physical damage—a torn muscle has damaged connections, so it cannot generate as much force, especially if the strain is a grade II or III.

Flexibility impairments are also common. Putting the muscle in a lengthened position pulls on the injured tissue and triggers pain, so you will naturally protect yourself by limiting how far you are willing to stretch.

# WHEN TO SEEK PROFESSIONAL HELP

Grade III muscle strains tend to be fairly obvious. If you have bruising and bleeding in the area along with weakness and difficulty moving (loss of function and impaired range of motion), consult with a physical therapist or doctor. A lot of severe strains can be managed with rehab, and the body may be able to recover on its own, but sometimes—depending on the muscle group—strains need to be repaired with reconstructive surgery to get the muscle back to normal function.

In the protocols in Part III, I provide some basic guidance regarding surgery. But you'll want an answer for your specific situation, especially if your injury is a grade II or III. That's why I'm teaching you how to identify what the injury is—so you can figure out the best course of action for your situation.

In some cases, especially for competitive athletes, reconstructive surgery may be necessary to correct functional impairments and return performance to the pre-injury level. For people who train recreationally, getting the injury checked can't hurt. But most strains respond well to rehab and heal to a point where the injury doesn't significantly impair function.

There's so much redundancy in your muscles that if you strain one, and you're active, you can probably get by using the surrounding muscles. It depends on how badly the muscle is injured—if it's a full tear, the muscle could become nonfunctional. But in some cases, a tear won't greatly impair function because the muscles underneath and around it can carry the load. Still, for grade II and III tears, it's good to visit a specialist to determine the appropriate treatment.

## OTHER CONNECTIVE TISSUES—FASCIA

Fascia is a band or sheet of connective tissue under the skin that attaches, stabilizes, and encloses muscles and organs. It plays an important role in pain, injury, and movement.

Fascia runs parallel to muscles, tendons, ligaments, and bones. It's like a sleeve that envelops a muscle and helps transmit force. Think of a sausage casing, only way more useful. Fascia stores energy when you're moving, just like muscle. This is partly why you are stronger when doing eccentric contractions—not only because the muscle is creating torque but also because the fascia is storing energy and allowing you to handle more load. So, when you strain a muscle, it is possible to injure the fascia as well.

This interconnectedness makes it hard to differentiate muscle and fascia injuries because they often feel the same and happen simultaneously. Luckily, rehab for fascial structures is very similar to muscle rehab. If you suspect you have a fascial injury, follow the protocol that targets and strengthens the muscles in that area.

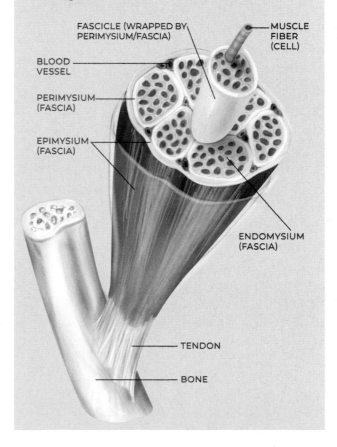

FASCICLE (WRAPPED BY PERIMYSIUM/FASCIA)

MUSCLE FIBER (CELL)

BLOOD VESSEL

PERIMYSIUM (FASCIA)

EPIMYSIUM (FASCIA)

ENDOMYSIUM (FASCIA)

TENDON

BONE

# TENDONS— TENDINOPATHY AND RUPTURE

As I mentioned earlier, tendons connect muscle to bone. The three types of tissue lie in a series like train cars on a track. Tendons help transmit force so that your muscles can contract to move your bones and joints—the muscle connects to the bone via the tendon, and that tendon pulls on the bone and rotates your joint. That's how you move.

## MECHANISM OF INJURY (HOW IT HAPPENS)

The vast majority of tendon problems are associated with "overuse" or repetitive stress injuries and involve low-magnitude forces being applied in high volumes—running or walking long distances, for example. You essentially do too much of an activity and exceed your tissue capacity. It could be a brand-new activity or an activity you are used to but do way more of than normal, and as a result, the tendon gets irritated.

Tendons can also be injured when exposed to high-magnitude forces, which often happens suddenly rather than gradually like repetitive use issues. In these situations, the muscles that attach to the tendon are typically contracting forcefully and end up pulling hard enough to rip the tendon off the bone.

## INJURY GRADES (GAUGING SEVERITY)

Tendon injuries tend to come in two types. At the less severe end of the spectrum is tendinopathy, which is one of the most common injuries and is thought to account for more than 30 percent of all musculoskeletal consultations.[1] Tendinopathy used to be called tendinitis, but that term isn't accurate because it's not a true inflammatory state. Rather, tendinopathy is an irritation that causes structural changes in the tendon—if you keep irritating it, the tendon can become enlarged (referred to as tendinosis).[2]

On the more severe end of the tendon injury spectrum are ruptures or avulsions, where the tendon tears away from the bone. An Achilles rupture fits into this category and involves a strong calf muscle contraction paired with the ankle moving rapidly into dorsiflexion, stretching and tearing the tendon from the calcaneus bone. Many people who tear their Achilles report making a quick, explosive movement (landing from a jump and trying to jump again, or stepping back with one leg and trying to push off) and then feeling a pop on the back of the ankle. Many don't experience significant pain but have difficulty using their calf muscles; they are unable to do a calf raise, for example.

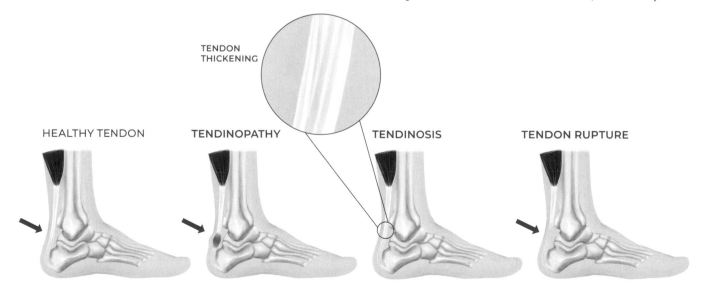

TENDON THICKENING

HEALTHY TENDON     TENDINOPATHY     TENDINOSIS     TENDON RUPTURE

When the tendon pulls away from the bone, the entire muscle-tendon unit shortens and balls up, causing a deformity in the affected limb. A great example is a biceps rupture where the tendon tears either near the elbow or near the shoulder at the attachment point. In either case, the biceps retracts and pulls closer to the side where it is still attached, creating an unusual-looking ball of tissue in the arm. When a tendon is fully torn, you can sometimes feel a gap or discontinuation in the area.

## SIGNS AND SYMPTOMS

Tendon injury pain isn't in the muscle; it's in the cord connecting muscle to bone, so it is closer to the joint. In some cases, such as Achilles tendon injuries, it's obvious which tendon is hurt. That tendon attaches to your calf muscles, but it doesn't hurt in the muscle; tendinopathy hurts right on the tendon when it is stressed, usually when you're squeezing the attached muscle. If you had an Achilles tendon problem, doing a calf raise would probably cause pain because you're squeezing your calf muscle, which pulls on the tendon and reproduces the pain.

When a tendon flares up, you may feel achy, dull pain at rest and sharper pain when you stress it, usually when squeezing the muscle that connects to it. Once they're flared up, injured tendons can take days to calm down. But you can distinguish a tendon injury from a muscle strain because you don't get bruising or bleeding with a tendinopathy. It also hurts only at the tendon, close to the bone, not in the muscle belly. For instance, tennis elbow is a tendinopathy. It hurts right where the wrist extensor tendon attaches to the bone on the outside of the elbow, but not in the middle of the forearm where the wrist extensor muscles are located.

A tendon injury (such as a rotator cuff injury) can feel sharp when you stress it, but the pain can linger and might throb afterward. You will probably also notice a cycle of pain in that the tendon will hurt more when you are cold and feel better after you warm up. This occurs often in runners who have Achilles tendinopathy. They notice more pain at the start of their run and less pain later in the run as the tissue warms up.

Pain can also occur when the tendon is stretched. If you stretch your calf while your Achilles tendon is injured, it will hurt right at the tendon. Many tendons get irritated when they are compressed as well. The hamstring tendons that attach to your pelvis under the sit bones are known to remain aggravated with prolonged sitting because they are compressed between your pelvis and the chair.

## IMPAIRMENTS ASSOCIATED WITH TENDON INJURIES

Impairments associated with tendon injuries are similar to those for muscle injuries because the tendon is a part of the muscle-tendon contractile unit. With tendinopathies, pain usually occurs when you place load on the tendon or contract the muscle to which the injured tendon connects. This pain causes weakness or inhibition—your nervous system shuts down the muscle connected to the irritated tendon to prevent further damage.

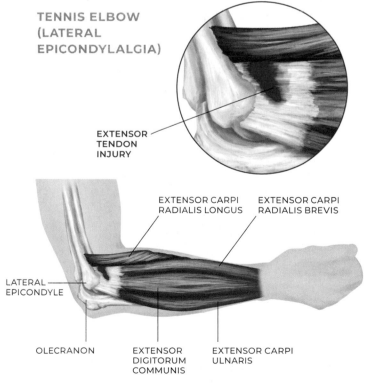

TENNIS ELBOW
(LATERAL
EPICONDYLALGIA)

EXTENSOR
TENDON
INJURY

EXTENSOR CARPI
RADIALIS LONGUS

EXTENSOR CARPI
RADIALIS BREVIS

LATERAL
EPICONDYLE

OLECRANON

EXTENSOR
DIGITORUM
COMMUNIS

EXTENSOR CARPI
ULNARIS

With partial and full tendon ruptures, weakness is significant because the tendon is physically damaged and can no longer transfer force as it normally would.

As with muscle pain, tendinopathy-related pain limits flexibility. Stretching a muscle and its tendon applies load to the tendon and exacerbates pain, limiting how far you are willing to stretch.

## WHEN TO SEEK PROFESSIONAL HELP

Tendinopathy and tendinosis usually don't require specialized care; they respond well to rehab when you eliminate or modify aggravating factors. However, if you suspect you have a tear, it's a good idea to consult with a doctor or physical therapist. If the tendon is ruptured, you may need to undergo reconstructive surgery in order to regain full function.

# LIGAMENTS— SPRAINS AND RUPTURES

Ligaments are connective tissues like tendons, except they connect bone to bone. Unlike tendons, you don't have voluntary control over them. You can't squeeze a ligament such as your anterior cruciate ligament (ACL); it simply guides and restrains your movement, holding your bones and joints tightly together so they don't move or slip against one another and harm other structures. An injury to a ligament is called a sprain and can range from a minor stretch injury to a full rupture or tear. An ankle sprain, for example, is a ligament injury.

## MECHANISM OF INJURY (HOW IT HAPPENS)

Ligament injuries often occur under high force when a joint is twisted or a ligament is stretched too far. Imagine a soccer player tearing their ACL while sprinting and pivoting to cut across the field. Their foot is planted when their body changes direction, which twists the knee bones and sprains the ACL inside the joint.

Stress buildup over time also can cause repetitive use ligament injuries. For example, baseball pitchers usually tear their ulnar collateral ligament in one moment, but many microtraumas occur before the ligament snaps.

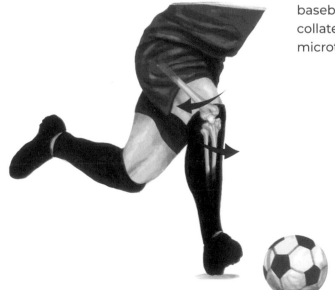

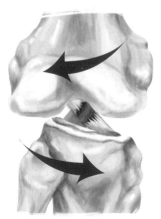

# INJURY GRADES (GAUGING SEVERITY)

Ligament injuries, like muscle strains, are graded on a three-point scale that indicates increasing severity:

- With a grade I ligament sprain, there's pain near the ligament but no instability in the joint. You may experience discomfort when moving in a way that stresses the ligament (such as turning your foot inward after an ankle sprain), but the pain is not debilitating, and the joint doesn't feel like it's going to give out when you're using it.

- A grade II sprain causes more intense pain and swelling (rather than bleeding or bruising as in the case of muscle strains) because ligaments are usually inside joints. So, you get balloon-like swelling inside the joint and some instability. With certain movements, you may notice that the bones slip and move apart a bit because the joint has lost some of its integrity.

- A grade III sprain is a full ligament tear or rupture. In this case, joint instability is much more obvious, and it feels like the bones move apart easily or the joint doesn't want to stay connected. If you have a full ACL tear, for example, your tibia and femur bones will slide apart and your knee will buckle.

You can almost think of a grade I ligament sprain as a "stretch injury." The ligament is usually stretched and swollen but isn't torn, and the change isn't permanent. With grades II and III, however, the change usually becomes permanent. A grade II sprain can heal somewhat, and people sometimes regain stability in the joint. When you get to grade III, though, some amount of instability usually remains, and reconstructive surgery is often advised.

# SIGNS AND SYMPTOMS

Similar to muscle and tendon injuries, a ligament sprain comes with sharp and achy pains. As such, identification is chiefly about what provokes it (I refer to these as aggravating factors). With a ligament injury, you're less likely to be able to turn on the pain by squeezing a muscle. You'll usually feel it only when you move the joint in a specific direction. Say you sprain your ankle by rolling it inward. If you turn your ankle in that same direction, you will stretch the injured ligament(s) and reproduce the pain.

Ligament pain is easy to differentiate from muscle pain because all ligament injuries occur close to a joint. Ligament and tendon injuries can be harder to tell apart because tendon injuries can also cause pain near a bone and some instability (if a muscle is inhibited, you might feel unstable). The difference is that with a ligament injury, the joint will have lost some structural stability, whereas with a tendon injury, the joint won't shift apart if you grab it and try to move it.

ANKLE LIGAMENT GRADES OF INJURY

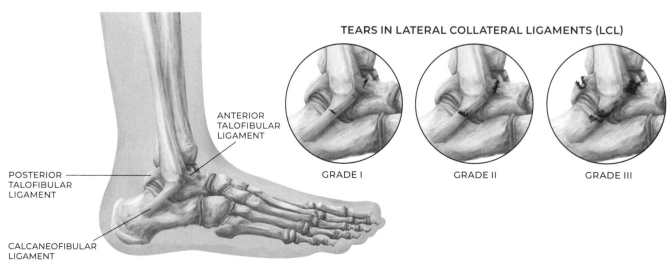

ANTERIOR TALOFIBULAR LIGAMENT

POSTERIOR TALOFIBULAR LIGAMENT

CALCANEOFIBULAR LIGAMENT

TEARS IN LATERAL COLLATERAL LIGAMENTS (LCL)

GRADE I          GRADE II          GRADE III

What's more, when a ligament experiences a more severe tear, you often hear a pop. This can happen with tendon ruptures as well, so you have to look closely at the site of injury to determine whether a tendon or a ligament was involved.

# IMPAIRMENTS ASSOCIATED WITH LIGAMENT INJURIES

The hallmark impairment associated with ligament injuries, especially grades II and III, is joint instability. Ligaments are passive stabilizers designed to protect joints by holding bones together. If they are damaged, the bones that make up the associated joint will be able to slide farther away from each other than normal. For instance, if you tear your ACL, your femur and tibia will not be held as tightly to one another and will slide apart. When you perform standing tasks that require knee stability (e.g., stand and pivot), the joint may feel like it is going to shift out of place and buckle.

In addition to instability, ligament injuries often lead to joint range of motion impairments, especially when moving the joint into a position that stretches the injured ligament. For example, if you fall down and sprain your wrist by trying to catch yourself, you are likely to experience discomfort when the wrist moves into extension, which stretches the healing ligaments. Other motions of the wrist might also be painful, but extension will probably be the worst.

# WHEN TO SEEK PROFESSIONAL HELP

With a full ligament tear (grade III), most people need surgery. Some can use their neuromuscular system to cope and avoid surgery; for example, the quadriceps and hamstring muscles can make up for instability due to an injured MCL or LCL in the knee. But with most severe ligament injuries, surgery is needed to restore full function to the joint. If you have pain, especially if you're also noticing instability, I recommend seeking professional help.

## OTHER CONNECTIVE TISSUES—JOINT CAPSULES

A joint capsule is a balloon-shaped connective tissue that surrounds a joint and holds the joint fluid, called synovial fluid. When something inside the joint is injured, the swelling stays in the joint because the capsule is holding it in. So, your joint balloons, but you don't get a lot of swelling in the surrounding muscles.

The capsule is made of a similar tissue to a ligament, so it almost fits into the same category. Like a ligament, it holds the joint together and protects the bones from slipping around too much. Twisting the joint under high force can result in a severe tear to the joint capsule, but the ligaments and cartilage usually tear at the same time. For example, if you dislocate your shoulder, you're probably going to tear your labrum (a type of cartilage) as well. And if it's a severe dislocation, the shoulder capsule could also tear. As a result, some people need to have the shoulder capsule repaired along with the ligaments and labrum. Joint capsules are so far on the periphery that you usually need to tear ligaments and cartilage to make the bones slip far enough to injure them.

**SHOULDER JOINT CAPSULE**

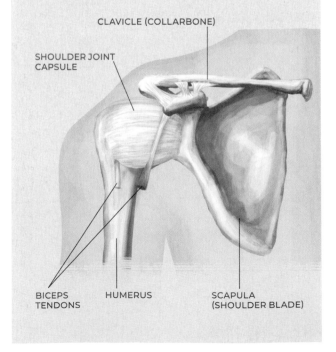

CLAVICLE (COLLARBONE)

SHOULDER JOINT CAPSULE

BICEPS TENDONS

HUMERUS

SCAPULA (SHOULDER BLADE)

# CARTILAGE—TRAUMATIC AND DEGENERATIVE INJURIES

The musculoskeletal system contains skin, nerves, muscle, and connective tissues. The four types of connective tissue are tendons, ligaments, bones, and cartilage. Cartilage helps absorb force, reduces friction in joints, and—like ligaments—provides stability.

There are different types of cartilage. Fibrocartilage is one type—that's your meniscus, the labra in your hip and shoulder, and the discs in your spine. The other important type is articular or hyaline cartilage, which covers the ends of bones and joints to reduce friction. Without hyaline cartilage, your joints would grind together, as in osteoarthritis. (A third type of cartilage is elastin, which is in your ears and nose, but it doesn't really apply to the musculoskeletal system.)

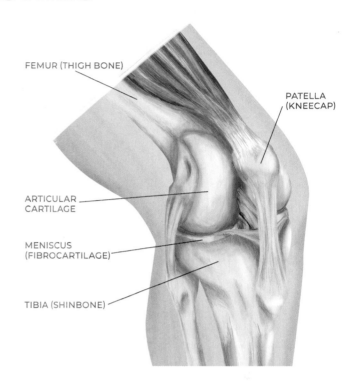

FEMUR (THIGH BONE)

PATELLA (KNEECAP)

ARTICULAR CARTILAGE

MENISCUS (FIBROCARTILAGE)

TIBIA (SHINBONE)

## MECHANISM OF INJURY (HOW IT HAPPENS)/ INJURY GRADES (GAUGING SEVERITY)

Cartilage injuries can be broken into two categories: traumatic and degenerative.

Traumatic cartilage injuries occur in a single moment and involve putting increased force or load on the tissue in a compromising position. For instance, you might injure the labrum in your shoulder when you are reaching overhead, your arm goes behind your body, and the head of the humerus pops forward out of the socket, dislocating your shoulder and tearing the labrum. Or you might bend your spine under heavy load—maybe you're new to deadlifting and trying to lift more weight than you've trained for. That might cause a disc bulge or a tear in the disc wall, which is also classified as a cartilage injury.

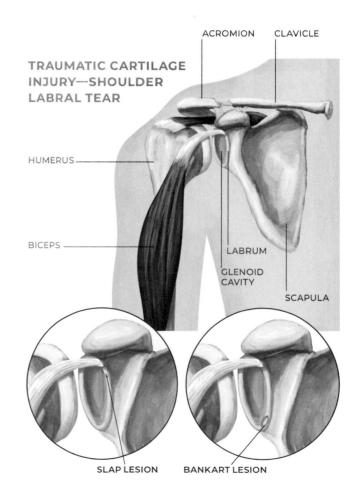

**TRAUMATIC CARTILAGE INJURY—SHOULDER LABRAL TEAR**

ACROMION    CLAVICLE

HUMERUS

BICEPS

LABRUM

GLENOID CAVITY

SCAPULA

SLAP LESION    BANKART LESION

Degenerative cartilage injuries—small tears and disruptions in the shape of the tissue—are also common and are now considered a normal part of aging. Many meniscus and spinal disc injuries are categorized as degenerative because changes to the tissue can be seen on an MRI, but they occur over many years rather than in one instant.

Most articular or hyaline cartilage injuries fall into the degenerative category as osteoarthritis. As the cartilage breaks down, the articulating bones, which have tons of nerve endings, come into contact and create severe pain.

**DEGENERATIVE CARTILAGE INJURY—KNEE**

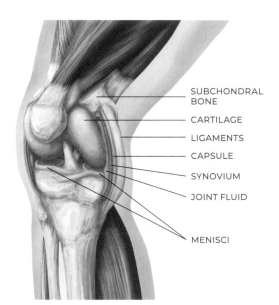

- SUBCHONDRAL BONE
- CARTILAGE
- LIGAMENTS
- CAPSULE
- SYNOVIUM
- JOINT FLUID
- MENISCI

NORMAL KNEE

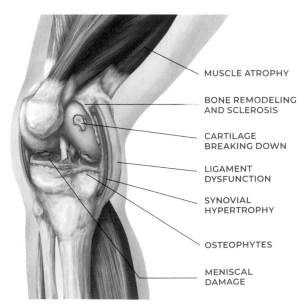

- MUSCLE ATROPHY
- BONE REMODELING AND SCLEROSIS
- CARTILAGE BREAKING DOWN
- LIGAMENT DYSFUNCTION
- SYNOVIAL HYPERTROPHY
- OSTEOPHYTES
- MENISCAL DAMAGE

OSTEOARTHRITIC KNEE

Interestingly, the way to keep hyaline cartilage healthy is to subject it to moderate stress over your lifetime. It can deteriorate if you repetitively stress it too much or don't stress it enough. For example, a moderate dosage of running has been shown to protect the hyaline cartilage in the knee and hip. But both sedentariness and high-volume running are associated with quicker deterioration of hyaline cartilage.[3]

## SIGNS AND SYMPTOMS

Many degenerative cartilage injuries produce no pain or other symptoms, but those that do create swelling and deep pain at different points in the joint (front, back, or side), which can affect function.

Traumatic cartilage injuries like labral and meniscus tears also create pain and swelling but may lead to joint instability as well, similar to ligament injuries. The labrum in your shoulder or hip, for example, goes around the rim of the socket, creating a tight fit around the adjoining bone. If you tear that rim, the ball can slip out easier, making you lose stability and increasing your chances of future dislocations. With a meniscus injury, the knee can get stuck, catch, or feel unstable when bent or straightened. If you put weight on it, it may hurt or start to buckle.

## IMPAIRMENTS ASSOCIATED WITH CARTILAGE INJURIES

Cartilage injuries can cause joint mobility impairments and weakness due to pain but are mostly associated with joint instability, especially in traumatic cases. If you dislocate your shoulder and tear your labrum, your shoulder joint will lose some stability. Your neuromuscular system may be able to make up for the problem, but you may continue to feel like your shoulder is going to slip out of the socket again.

With an injury like a meniscus tear, joint instability is common, and you are likely to experience joint mobility impairments due to pain or a piece of the meniscus getting in the way and preventing the joint from moving normally.

## WHEN TO SEEK PROFESSIONAL HELP

If you have pain from a cartilage injury that doesn't resolve after six to 12 months, or you notice ongoing joint instability and/or joint restriction in certain movements and positions, you should seek professional help. For instance, with shoulder labral tears, some people experience recurrent shoulder dislocations even after going through rehab. In these cases, surgical repair of the labrum may be the best path forward to prevent future dislocations. With a more severe meniscus tear, you may feel like your knee is going to give way or buckle and notice that it gets stuck, meaning you have difficulty bending and straightening your leg. In this scenario, especially if you are a young athlete, surgical repair of the meniscus might be the best option.

With degenerative tears, on the other hand, evidence suggests that you should avoid surgery when possible. In fact, several studies show that degenerative meniscus tears improve equally well when comparing physical therapy to arthroscopic surgery.[4-5] Surgery might be the faster option, but it comes with much more risk, such as developing arthritis or infections. For this reason, I almost always recommend that people with degenerative cartilage injuries—where pain is the chief symptom—choose rehab as their primary treatment as opposed to surgery.

# NERVES—TENSION AND COMPRESSION

Nerves transmit electrical signals throughout your body, providing sensory feedback and allowing you to detect sensations, contract your muscles, and move. Injuries to nerves are more straightforward than other injury types because they produce unique symptoms.

## MECHANISM OF INJURY (HOW IT HAPPENS)

Nerves can be injured through tension, compression, or laceration—a nerve is stretched too much, compressed for too long, or cut. Injuries can also result from trauma or overuse.

Traumatic nerve injuries usually fall into the stretching or tension category. In a traumatic injury like whiplash, a nerve gets stretched too hard. All the nerves exiting the neck are stretched quickly, which can cause nerve palsies, tingling, numbness, and weakness everywhere those nerves enter the arm.

Traumatic compression injuries can occur in situations like motor vehicle or contact sport–related accidents. If you are rear-ended and suffer whiplash, your neck first stretches forward into flexion and then whips back into extension, which slams the joints together and compresses the nerves where they exit the neck.

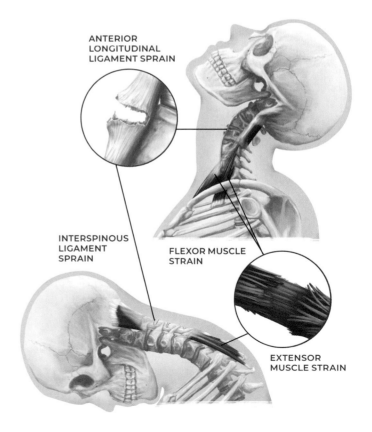

ANTERIOR LONGITUDINAL LIGAMENT SPRAIN

INTERSPINOUS LIGAMENT SPRAIN

FLEXOR MUSCLE STRAIN

EXTENSOR MUSCLE STRAIN

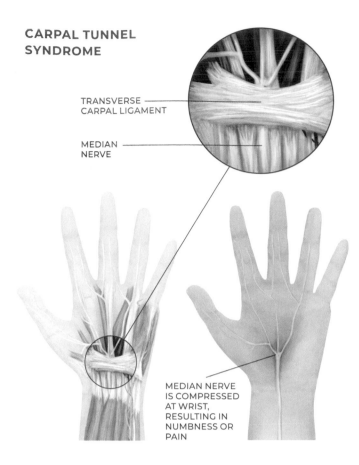

## CARPAL TUNNEL SYNDROME

TRANSVERSE CARPAL LIGAMENT

MEDIAN NERVE

MEDIAN NERVE IS COMPRESSED AT WRIST, RESULTING IN NUMBNESS OR PAIN

The protocols in Part III mainly address overuse compression injuries, which are more common than the other types. Carpal tunnel syndrome, for example, is an overuse compression nerve disorder where the desk hits or rubs against your carpal tunnel as you type at your keyboard, compressing and irritating the nerve.

# INJURY GRADES (GAUGING SEVERITY)

Peripheral nerve injuries are classified based on how severely the nerve is damaged. They range from mild injuries where the structure of the nerve is not damaged to severe injuries where a nerve is completely transected, or separated into two segments. However, most people who come to physical therapy with nerve-related issues are experiencing less severe nerve problems where pain, numbness, tingling, and maybe weakness are their primary complaints.

In rehab, we gauge the degree of nerve irritation based on how far the symptoms travel and whether there is weakness. If a nerve in the neck or low back is irritated and symptoms travel only partway down the arm or leg, we consider the injury to be less severe than if the symptoms went all the way to the hand or foot.

Nerve symptoms that move farther down the arm or leg (referred to as peripheralization) typically signal that things are getting worse. On the flip side, nerve pain that moves up toward the spine and leaves the arm or leg is referred to as centralization and usually indicates that the nerve is healing. So, the goals when rehabbing nerve-related issues are to get the nerve to calm down and for the symptoms to leave the limb.

## PINCHED NERVES

I'd like to clear up some misconceptions about nerve injuries. A pinched nerve, for example, is not usually the result of a mechanical pinch. It can feel like a pinch when you move your neck and pain shoots down your arm, but in most cases, medical imaging reveals that nothing is touching or pinching the nerve. This pinching feeling is more often caused by inflammation around the nerve.

This concept comes up most often with disc bulges in the neck or low back. Most people who have these injuries think that they have nerve symptoms because the disc bulge is pushing on the nerve. In reality, most disc bulges aren't large enough to touch the nerve, and the pain is due to inflammation in the area. Once the inflammation goes away, the nerve desensitizes and the pinching feeling disappears, even though the disc bulge may still be visible on a follow-up MRI.

# SIGNS AND SYMPTOMS

Nerves are unique in that they create pain along their path, and the pain might manifest as tingling, numbness, or burning sensations—it can even shoot down an arm or leg like lightning bolts. As a result, nerve injuries are typically easy to diagnose because they feel a lot different from injuries to other tissues.

Nerve pain also tends to get worse the longer you hold a position or touch the nerve. (With light pressure, you have to hold it longer to create an effect.) That's why a lot of people wake up with nerve pain. You may have twisted your neck in your sleep, and holding that position for hours irritated the nerves.

Numbness and tingling are common, but you might also feel heaviness, weakness, and other symptoms. Nerves allow you to squeeze your muscles, so if you have a more severe nerve problem, you may notice weakness in the muscle through which the nerve travels. For instance, if you had a severe C5–C6 nerve injury in your neck, your biceps could weaken.

## IMPAIRMENTS ASSOCIATED WITH NERVE INJURIES

Nerves supply muscles with electrical current and allow you to sense the world around you. When they are injured, altered sensation (numbness, tingling, etc.) and pain are the primary issues. These symptoms may cause mobility and flexibility impairments as you alter your movement patterns to avoid stressing the sensitive nerve. If nerve irritation increases, weakness impairments will begin to appear as the muscles no longer generate their normal levels of force and power.

## WHEN TO SEEK PROFESSIONAL HELP

Most nerve pain cases respond well to rehab. However, if you have a persistent nerve problem like carpal tunnel syndrome or sciatica that is not improving with rehab and you notice progressive weakness and/or atrophy in the related muscles, immediately consult with a physical therapist or orthopedic doctor, as other interventions may be necessary. Certain physicians can perform nerve conduction velocity (NCV) tests, which can be used to determine the severity of the nerve issue and the best treatment strategy.

As nerves become more compromised (due to either injury or inflammation), they produce pain, numbness, and tingling, and you will begin to lose strength in the muscles the nerve supplies. For instance, if you have severe inflammation in your low back near the L4 nerve root, you might feel pain, numbness, and tingling down your leg along with weakness in the ankle dorsiflexor muscles on the front of your shin. Left untreated, the nerve can become permanently damaged.

## OTHER CONNECTIVE TISSUES—BONE

It may seem odd, but bone is a type of connective tissue. Ligaments, tendons, and cartilage are soft connective tissues that hold your skeleton together, whereas bones make up the hard structure of your skeleton.

When we think of bone injuries, we tend to think of fractures, but a bone injury is any kind of fatigue or break. Bones can bend and break in different ways: there are bending fractures, which most people are familiar with; compression fractures, where bones break under pressure; distraction fractures, where bones pull apart; spiral fractures, where bones get twisted; and stress fractures, where the bone is repeatedly loaded to the point of breaking.

Bone fractures usually heal back to almost full strength because most bones have great blood supply. But fractures are extremely painful because bones also have a ton of nerves. It's usually obvious when you sustain a major fracture: you hear a loud snap, the limb looks distorted, and it hurts a lot. There is also a lot of swelling, and movement of the limb is limited. If the pain is so intense that you can't even try to move, you should seek medical help right away.

Because bone has so many nerve endings, injuries produce sharp pain right on the bone. If you are a runner and are developing a stress fracture in your shin or one of the bones of your foot, for example, a specific spot will hurt, and pushing on that spot will re-create pain. If the bone is fatigued or failing, you'll also feel pain when the bone is loaded—when you put stress on it. If you have pain on a bone that's not getting better, schedule an appointment with a doctor. Most of the time, an X-ray will find the problem.

## CHAPTER 8

# HOW LONG
## INJURIES TAKE TO HEAL

Once you know what type of injury you have, the next question to ask is, "How long will it take to heal?"

The answer to this question involves many variables. Injuries to muscles, tendons, ligaments, cartilage, or bones take different amounts of time to heal, and your healing time will depend on the severity of your injury, your lifestyle (among other factors that influence injury), and how you approach rehab.

After you've used the information in Chapter 7 to figure out what you've injured (or a medical professional has issued a diagnosis), you can determine roughly how long the injury will take to heal.

# FACTORS THAT INFLUENCE HEALING TIME

As you know, injuries are graded based on severity, and the severity of your injury will play a role in how long it takes to heal. For example, a grade III ligament injury such as a full tear will take longer to heal than a grade I. Put simply, the more damage done to the tissue, the longer the healing time.

The type of tissue also matters. A grade I muscle strain is different from a grade I ligament sprain. Blood flow to the tissue brings oxygen and other nutrients that serve as building blocks for tissue repair. A tissue that receives less blood flow, such as cartilage, will take longer to heal than one that receives more blood flow, such as muscle. Even within the same tissue type, blood flow matters. Similarly, a tendon in one part of your body may have better blood flow than a tendon in another part, and the one with better blood flow will heal faster.

The rehab exercise protocols offered in Part III are designed to increase blood flow, and following the appropriate protocol can help you avoid reinjury because you're stressing the tissue in the right dosage. What's more, the aggravating factors listed in the protocols will help you avoid activities that might make the problem worse, giving the damaged tissue time to heal while maintaining a level of movement that doesn't cause further irritation.

Sometimes medical professionals suggest that when you're injured, you should only rest. Resting temporarily lets injured tissues calm down, but it will not help you address impairments or deficits—whether they're related to mobility, strength, or neuromuscular control (movement control through coordinated muscle activity). If you don't address those impairments, your likelihood of reinjury goes up. That's what the protocols are designed to do: take you through a progression that helps you get out of the acute pain phase by allowing the tissue to calm down and then addressing major deficits and impairments. That way, you recover faster and are less likely to experience reinjury.

## SMOKING AND ALCOHOL CONSUMPTION

Many of the factors covered in Chapters 4 and 9 can negatively influence healing time, but smoking and alcohol consumption are also worth mentioning.

Smoking significantly impairs healing.[1-5] Tobacco, whether it is smoked or chewed, harms the vascular system, impeding blood flow to the point where tissue heals much slower. As a result, some surgeons will not perform surgery on smokers.

Alcohol consumption inhibits protein synthesis, which can negatively affect muscle adaptations and slow recovery.[6-7] If you have an identifiable tissue injury, drinking alcohol can delay the rebuilding process. It can also negatively affect your sleep and might exacerbate other factors that affect healing time, like stress.

# THE PHASES OF HEALING

There are three main phases of healing: inflammation, maturation, and remodeling, which correlate with the three-phase rehab exercise protocols in Part III. As you go through the protocols, you progressively apply more stress to the injured tissue, just as you would in strength training, to build up its capacity. Later in this chapter, I will discuss how long you can expect to spend in each of these phases depending on the type of injury you have.

INFLAMMATORY
PHASE

CELLS REPAIRING
TISSUE

TISSUE ALMOST
HEALED

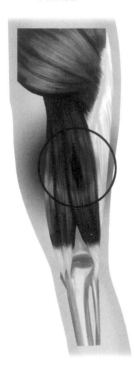 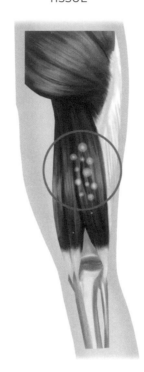 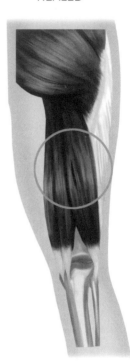

## PHASE 1: INFLAMMATION

When you first sustain an injury, there is an inflammatory phase, which usually lasts for about 72 hours. However, it can be longer if the injury is severe or you keep aggravating it. If you have an ankle sprain, for example, you still need to walk around. The more you irritate the injury, the longer you will have pain, and the slower your recovery will be. But if you implement the right amount of rest and get your pain under control, the inflammatory phase typically lasts about three days.

During this first phase of healing, your immune system is actively repairing the injured tissue, which makes the region more sensitive. Keeping with the ankle sprain example, you wouldn't start rehab by doing calf raises, because loading the ankle would slow the healing process. Instead, you should do general unloaded movements, which increase blood flow and clear out the swelling and fluid that tend to accumulate. Think of this as the "pain management and general movement" phase.

## PHASE 2: MATURATION

After about 72 hours, you enter what is sometimes called the fibroblastic or maturation phase, which typically lasts up to three weeks. This phase comprises the initial steps of rebuilding the integrity of the tissue. You may still have pain and other symptoms during this stage.

In these three weeks, you should start to incorporate more movements and methods for addressing mobility, strength, and stability. If you have mobility deficits, you want to get those under control early on so that the tissue doesn't get stiff or stuck.

## PHASE 3: REMODELING

After about three weeks, you enter the third phase: remodeling. This stage could be as short as four to six weeks for minor injuries (grade I and II tears, and tendinopathies) or as long as a year for more severe injuries (ligament or tendon ruptures). Your body is constantly remodeling tissue, but with an injury to a tissue like a ligament—to which blood flow is not great—studies have shown evidence of remodeling up to a year or two later. That's why you shouldn't return to sports any sooner than nine months after an injury like an ACL tear.

Certain ligament, tendon, and cartilage injuries take a long time to heal, even if you no longer have pain. If you try to push the tissue before it's ready, your likelihood of reinjury increases. That's why, in phase 3, you work on rebuilding tissue capacity through resistance training and a slow reintegration into the physical activities and sports that you have been avoiding since your injury.

# TYPICAL TIME FRAMES FOR HEALING

It's important to understand that the length of time associated with each phase of healing is a general estimate and could change depending on the severity of the injury. For instance, if you have a grade I ankle sprain, you will likely spend minimal time in all the phases of healing, which is why the anticipated total healing time for a grade I ligament injury is only one to three weeks. However, a grade III ankle sprain can take two to 12 months to heal, so you would spend much more time in each phase, especially the remodeling phase.

The time frames listed for each injury type are averages. Keep these durations in the back of your mind when going through the protocols, but also remember to focus on your symptoms and functional capacity as the primary clues for how you are healing and when you should progress to the next phase of rehab.

You'll also notice that the recommended time for performing the rehab protocol often extends past the healing time frame listed for that grade of injury. These discrepancies are purposeful. Even though the injury may be mostly healed, you want to continue strengthening the surrounding muscle groups to ensure the area is protected and less likely to be reinjured. If you've suffered a major (grade III) injury, you may need to continue with the phase 3 exercises for much longer than is listed in the protocol. For example, if you have a grade III ligament or tendon injury, you don't stop doing the phase 3 exercises after four to six weeks, because those tissues could be remodeling for up to a year. Rather, you should do the phase 3 exercises for six to nine months to ensure that tissue integrity and joint stability return to full capacity. Stopping shy of this mark translates to a much higher risk of reinjury.

# MUSCLE INJURIES

| GRADE I:<br>1–3 weeks | GRADE II:<br>4–12 weeks | GRADE III:<br>3–6 months |
| --- | --- | --- |

A grade I muscle strain has a relatively fast healing time range of one to three weeks because muscles have good blood flow. With a less severe muscle injury, you will move through the protocol phases fairly quickly and might spend only a few days in phase 1, another week in phase 2, and four to six weeks in phase 3. Even though your injury is mild, muscle tissues need this amount of training time to return to full function and strength.

Recovering from a grade II strain can take four to 12 weeks. These strains are more than just uncomfortable; they impair strength and/or mobility. You can't stretch or load the muscle in the early phases of healing. Sometimes there's even damage that's identifiable on an MRI—some inconsistency or tear in the muscle. With this grade of strain, you will spend more time in each phase of rehab. Phase 1, which focuses on reducing pain, might last two weeks. Phase 2 begins looking at flexibility and mobility exercises, which are usually somewhat impaired in people with grade II strains, so make sure you don't leave phase 2 until you can perform all the exercises with full range of motion and no more than mild pain, which will probably take another two weeks. Considering that grade II strains can take up to 12 weeks to heal, I recommend performing the phase 3 resistance training exercises three or four times per week for another six to eight weeks to ensure that the tissue heals with maximum strength.

If you have a grade III strain, you might need surgery to repair it, and then you're looking at three to six months of recovery time. Because severe strains often require surgery, you should seek the guidance of a physical therapist who can work with you personally and design a rehab program that is specific to your individual needs. The protocols in this book can complement your care, but working with a professional who can assess your injury and make specific recommendations will help you recover optimally.

# TENDON INJURIES

| TENDINOPATHY:<br>2–12 weeks | TENDINOSIS:<br>3–6 months | RUPTURE:<br>3–12 months |
| --- | --- | --- |

In terms of severity, tendon injuries range from tendinopathy to a rupture. Recovery from tendinopathy takes two to 12 weeks according to most studies.[8-11] In the case of tendinosis, which involves recurrent bouts (you get pain, it calms down, and then you get it again)—the tendon can change shape and even look thicker on an MRI.[12] Those injuries can take three to six months to heal, but you can dramatically reduce that time by following the rehab protocol and modifying or avoiding aggravating factors when symptoms start to appear.

With tendinopathy, the severity of your pain symptoms will guide your rate of progress through the phases. Mild tendon pain during the prescribed exercises is usually fine unless your symptoms flare up after the training session. If you can perform all the exercises with no more than mild pain, then you are probably ready for the next phase. In general, you can expect to spend one to two weeks in phase 1, two weeks in phase 2, and four to six weeks in phase 3 of the rehab protocol.

Even after your injury has healed, make sure to perform the phase 3 exercises two or three times per week to reduce the likelihood of a recurrence. This is especially important if you are returning to a high-volume activity that led to the tendinopathy. For instance, if you are a runner and developed Achilles or patellar tendinopathy after increasing your mileage, you should continue with the phase 3 strengthening exercises as you ease back into your regular running program to keep your tendons strong and healthy.

Tendinosis results from repeated bouts of tendinopathy, meaning it's an overuse injury that never fully heals due to persistent flare-ups. Over a long period—say, six months to a year—the tendon starts to thicken. When that occurs, the healing time extends to three to six months, so you should consider spending an extra week or two in phases 1 and 2 and eight to 12 weeks in phase 3 before gradually returning to your sport.

Finally, a tendon rupture can take anywhere from three months to a year to heal, depending on the severity and whether reconstruction is needed. The Achilles tendon, for example, can take up to a year to return to normal. Tendon ruptures, like grade III muscle injuries, typically require more personalized care. Whether or not you have surgery, I highly recommend that you work with a skilled orthopedic or sports physical therapist and use the protocol in this book as a secondary resource.

# LIGAMENT INJURIES

| GRADE I:<br>1–3 weeks | GRADE II:<br>4–6 weeks | GRADE III:<br>2–12 months |
| --- | --- | --- |

With a grade I ligament sprain, where you have pain and swelling but not much loss in the integrity of the ligament—if you tweak your ankle and it gets a little swollen, for example—recovery time is between one and three weeks, similar to a muscle strain. With this level of injury, let your symptoms guide you through phases 1 and 2 of the protocol. You use the phase 1 exercises to get pain and swelling under control, which will probably take one to two weeks. Then you add phase 2 and keep performing those movements until you can complete all the mobility exercises with minimal to no pain and full range of motion, which will take approximately one to two weeks. Lastly, even though the joint is stable, you should perform the phase 3 resistance training exercises for at least four to six weeks to improve strength, motor control, and proprioception.

A grade II sprain involves stretching of the ligament, and you're looking at four to six weeks to heal. The process for grade II sprains is similar to what was outlined for grade I injuries, but you are likely to spend more time in each phase of rehab. It will probably take a bit longer to get your swelling and pain under control, which means more time in phase 1 (an additional one to two weeks). The phase 2 exercises, especially the sensorimotor control drills, will require more focus and practice because your joint may feel somewhat

unstable, so you may need to spend an extra two to three weeks in that phase. Make sure the joint feels stable before jumping into the phase 3 exercises. Once your pain is minimal when doing everyday tasks and the phase 2 exercises, you can move to phase 3. Again, I recommend performing the phase 3 exercises three or four times per week for at least four to six weeks, or until you don't have any pain or notice any feelings of instability, before returning to more complex sport-related activities.

If you have a grade III ligament injury—a full rupture—you're looking at eight weeks to a year of recovery time. For example, with a full ACL tear, most people are not back to full function until nine months to a year later. Again, grade III injuries often require surgery and an individually tailored rehab program, so working with a licensed PT is ideal. Not all grade III ligament injuries require surgery, but it's best to consult with an orthopedic doctor or physical therapist to determine the best path forward.

# CARTILAGE INJURIES

| GENERAL TIMELINE:<br>3 months to 2 years |
| --- |

Blood flow to cartilage is not great; a lot of cartilage is aneural and avascular, meaning it lacks both nerve endings and blood flow. Cartilage is meant to reduce friction and serve as a shock absorber, so this is a good thing; it would not feel good to have nerve endings in the cartilage between bones and joints, letting you feel every impact.

Thanks to its low vascularity, cartilage doesn't heal well, and it can take a long time—anywhere from three months to two years. A disc herniation, for example, sometimes reabsorbs and goes away, but the process can take several months or more. Still, many people who have cartilage injuries like meniscus, labrum, and disc tears don't have pain symptoms or impaired function.

In some cases, a cartilage injury doesn't heal at all—but don't let that concern you too much, because you can get better. Again, it's important to differentiate between injury and pain. The injury might be present, but that doesn't mean there's pain or function is compromised.

I once experienced a meniscus tear that resulted in some loss of function and instability for several months, but I followed the Knee Instability protocol on page 400 and stayed active, and eventually my symptoms went away. If you did an MRI of my knee today, however, you would probably still see evidence of the tear.

So, if cartilage injuries don't always heal, what do the protocols do? They improve the performance of the rest of the neuromuscular chain—everything you have control over. Immediately following a knee injury, for example, the muscles around it are inhibited, especially the quads. As the pain and swelling dissipate and the tissue begins to heal, those other neuromuscular elements will come back online and reduce your instability.

For cartilage injuries, as with most other injuries, let your pain level guide the rehab process while also factoring in typical healing times and other symptoms like joint instability.

For example, a disc herniation, a labral tear in the hip, or arthritis primarily limits people due to pain. You need to pay close attention to your symptoms and move through the rehab phases in accordance with how your body is responding to the exercises. In the beginning, you may have pain at rest, and you will use the phase 1 exercises to reduce pain for around one to two weeks. When your resting pain has dissipated, you move to phase 2, where you should plan to spend two to three weeks. Once you can complete the phase 2 exercises with minimal pain and with good control and range of motion, you can progress to phase 3. Perform the phase 3 exercises until your symptoms have resolved with daily tasks and then for several months afterward to strengthen the surrounding muscles and protect the cartilaginous structure from reinjury.

With other cartilage injuries, especially traumatic ones like certain meniscus tears and shoulder labral tears following a dislocation, you also need to pay attention to how stable the joint feels as you progress through the protocol. In phase 2, for instance, you begin

working on motor control and stability. Practice these exercises until you feel confident and stable using the joint before moving to phase 3 and adding more challenge or load to the system. Also, keep in mind that traumatic injuries take longer to heal, so you will need to practice the phase 2 control exercises and the phase 3 strengthening exercises for four to six months to ensure that the surrounding muscles are capable of protecting the area and the tissue has had time to complete most of the healing process before you return to full-force sport-related activities.

# NERVE INJURIES

| IRRITATION: 4–6 weeks | LACERATION: 3–12 months |
| --- | --- |

The most common nerve injuries include sciatica and other mild irritations like carpal tunnel syndrome. Severe nerve injuries like lacerations are rare and typically occur in patients who've had surgery where the peripheral nerves are cut or who have experienced traumatic insults, such as car accidents or falls.

Surgeons say that once those sensory nerve endings are cut, they're unlikely to recover fully, and the patient may have numb patches forever. What's interesting about the nervous system, however, is that these peripheral nerves, which are like long spaghetti strands that go from your spine out to the ends of your fingers and toes, do have the capacity to heal. The rate at which a peripheral nerve heals depends on the severity of the injury, but, in many cases, nerve function does return. Though the healing process can take a long time, nerve regeneration can occur at a rate of a millimeter per day, or about an inch per month.[13-14]

A nerve irritation like sciatica tends to get better in four to six weeks, whereas a more severe nerve injury from surgery can take from three months to a year to heal. Other issues like radicular pain (see page 30) usually heal within a month or two because they have more to do with inflammation or irritation than actual injury.

For nerve issues, you generally spend about two weeks in each phase of the rehab protocol, but the timing may vary depending on how fast your symptoms dissipate. Also, it's not uncommon for people to experience flare-ups in nerve pain, which means you may need to spend more time in a particular phase or move back to the previous phase to get your pain under control. If you have a more severe nerve issue that is causing weakness in the muscle it travels to, rehab can take longer (several months), and you need to pay attention to whether the weakness is getting worse. If you notice a progressive loss of strength associated with other nerve symptoms, it is important to consult with your doctor immediately.

Nerve issues that get progressively worse can turn into permanent problems, so you need to stay ahead of them. Rehab is not the answer here. You might need surgery, an injection, or some other intervention. For example, if you have carpal tunnel syndrome and you have weakness and atrophy in your hand muscles, you may need surgery to release pressure on the nerve. Another common example is neck and low back disc herniations, which cause weakness in an arm or leg. You may need an epidural to reduce inflammation or a discectomy to remove the disc bulge. Early detection is key, so don't hesitate to make an appointment with a specialist if you have nerve-related issues.

# BONE FRACTURES

| SIMPLE: 6–8 weeks | COMPLEX: 3–6 months |
|---|---|

Bone is a surprisingly resilient tissue because it has the next best blood flow after muscle. But the healing time depends on the complexity of the fracture. If you have a stress fracture or a simple fracture that's not displaced and just needs to be stuck back together, it is likely to heal back to 95 to 100 percent in six to eight weeks.

Even complex fractures rarely take beyond six months to heal. If the bone comes apart, the treatment team might use plates, rods, and screws to restabilize it, and the bone should heal relatively well. It may even end up stronger than before. The potential caveat is that these kinds of fractures—especially compound fractures that poke out of the skin—can cause nerve damage because the sharp ends of the bone can cut through nerves.

Whether you have been placed in a cast or had surgery for a bone injury, you will probably have some impairments in range of motion and strength after the bone has healed, so it's good to work with a physical therapist once your doctor has cleared you—especially if you sustained a fracture close to a joint, which can lead to permanent mobility limitations if it isn't addressed with the appropriate interventions and exercises.

I don't cover bone fracture rehab in this book, but the protocols in Part III can serve as a great supplement while you are in physical therapy. They can also help you continue to gain strength, control, and mobility once you have been discharged from PT so that you can lessen your injury risk when returning to activities such as sports.

It's important to reiterate that all these healing timelines are just estimates. They vary based on a number of factors, including the effort you put into recovery and rehab. The next chapter looks at factors that influence injury, which you can use to not only reduce your risk of injury but also speed up healing if you are currently injured.

## CHAPTER 9

# FACTORS THAT INFLUENCE INJURY

Nobody wants to get injured, but it's a reality we all have to deal with from time to time. Some injuries are outside our control, while others occur because of poor planning and training practices.

Although you cannot eliminate risk entirely, knowing the variables that increase your risk of injury can reduce your vulnerability because you're more likely to take an active approach to mitigating them. This chapter focuses on those factors, some of which are covered in Chapter 4 as factors that also influence pain, including sleep hygiene, nutrition, diet, stress, and mental health. It is important to study both chapters and learn how to address these factors in each context.

To help you navigate this chapter, I've categorized the factors into four groups: training variables, physical variables, mental variables, and external variables. They are presented in hierarchal order, meaning that training variables are the most influential. The same is true for the factors listed within each category. This system is not perfect—some factors may have more influence than others depending on your unique circumstances—but it gives you a framework for approaching and prioritizing factors that can decrease your risk of injury.

THE INJURY PREVENTION VARIABLES HIERARCHY

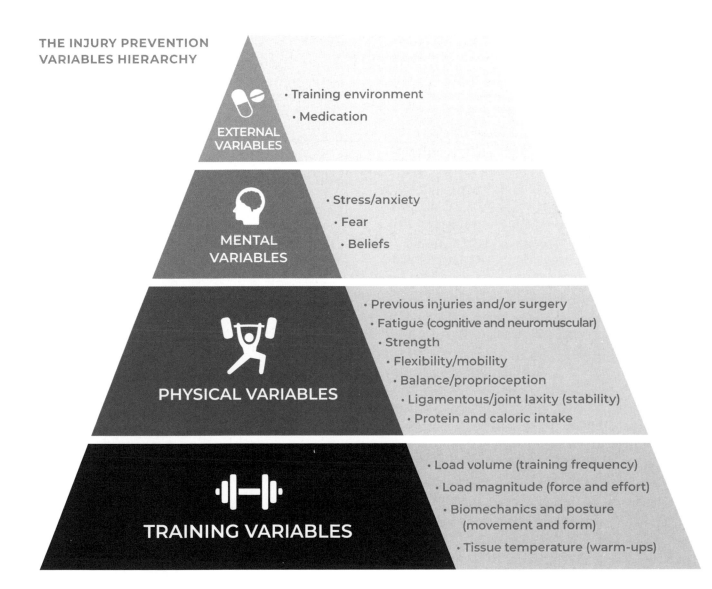

EXTERNAL VARIABLES
• Training environment
• Medication

MENTAL VARIABLES
• Stress/anxiety
• Fear
• Beliefs

PHYSICAL VARIABLES
• Previous injuries and/or surgery
• Fatigue (cognitive and neuromuscular)
• Strength
• Flexibility/mobility
• Balance/proprioception
• Ligamentous/joint laxity (stability)
• Protein and caloric intake

TRAINING VARIABLES
• Load volume (training frequency)
• Load magnitude (force and effort)
• Biomechanics and posture (movement and form)
• Tissue temperature (warm-ups)

# ·|I—|I· TRAINING VARIABLES

Training variables include the type of training you're doing, the length of time you're active, the force you're putting on your tissues, the speed of your movement, and the positions you're in. They're at the top of the list because they are the most common cause of injuries.

## LOAD VOLUME (TRAINING FREQUENCY)

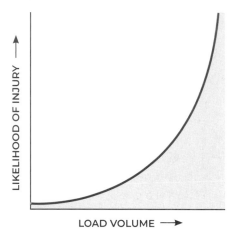

Load volume refers to your training frequency, or how often you work out, the number of sets and reps you do, and the time you spend performing a specific exercise or activity. Doing too much too fast—either in a single workout or over a series of workouts—places a volume of loading on your tissues that they're not conditioned to handle.

Most people with pain problems have repetitive use injuries, which typically occur when the musculoskeletal system does not possess the capacity to handle the total load volume. It's not that the load is too forceful or heavy; instead, you've performed a movement so many times that the tissue fatigues, which can result in injuries like stress fractures and tendinopathies.

A common example is plantar fasciitis. Say you rarely walk more than a mile at home, but then you take a vacation in a new city and walk five miles every day. The load isn't super heavy, but the higher volume surpasses the capacity of your tissue.

To prevent this type of injury, you must condition your tissues to handle that load volume. If you're going to engage in a high-volume activity—such as a long hike or a marathon—you need to train for it. Specificity in training is important, but you don't want to jump in too fast and risk an injury during conditioning. Start with less load volume than you think you can handle and see how your body responds. Use muscle soreness as an indicator that you did too much too soon and need to dial back your training. Take a few days off to recover and then try again at a lower volume. If you feel good after doing less, you have a benchmark, and you should let yourself adapt to that before adding more. This is the progressive overload (more over time) model.

Keep in mind that taking time off from an activity wipes the slate clean. Jumping back in at the same load volume increases your injury risk because some deconditioning may have occurred (unless you lifted weights or did something else to keep your tissues strong during your hiatus). If your activity is an endurance sport, it's extra important to come back at a lower load volume and build it up gradually. This is true regardless of your reason for stopping, but especially if you sustained an injury. Take it slow and test your body before a repetitive use injury starts to develop.

# LOAD MAGNITUDE (FORCE AND EFFORT)

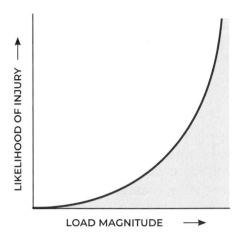

Load magnitude relates to the force on a tissue—specifically a heavy or quickly increasing force. This category is most applicable to traumatic injuries. When a tendon pops or a bone fractures, it's usually because the magnitude of force that was applied was greater than what the tissues were conditioned to handle.

Both moving faster and increasing the load amplify force on the musculoskeletal system. As with load volume, you can exceed the capacity of your tissue, just in a different way. Take someone who used to play volleyball but now works at a desk and has gained 20 pounds. He joins a weekend beach volleyball game with friends, having not played in a while, and fatigues quickly. Yet he's still playing and jumping with the same enthusiasm and force as his younger, fitter, and lighter self. He attempts an explosive, high-magnitude movement, and the extra weight on his system increases the force, resulting in an Achilles tendon tear.

# BIOMECHANICS AND POSTURE (MOVEMENT AND FORM)

*Biomechanics* refers to your form during movement, and posture relates not only to your physical position when in a static posture such as sitting or standing but also to the alignment of your body segments during dynamic tasks like landing from a jump and running.

Some trainers and PTs put a lot of emphasis on biomechanics and posture being a direct cause of pain and injuries. But form and pain/injury are not as closely correlated as many are led to believe.

I'm not saying the quality of your movement isn't important. Maximizing joint stability and improving movement efficiency is generally a good thing. Biomechanics and posture influence the muscles you use to hold a position or perform a movement—and you want to train your muscles to provide stability for your joints in a wide range of postures.

The problem is when movements and postures are labeled as "dysfunctional" or "bad" and people adopt the belief that they will get injured or develop pain if they move in a certain way. While moving from an unstable position can contribute to pain and injury, other factors play a much bigger role.

**Pain and injury prevention is less about how you are moving and more about what your joints and tissues are conditioned to handle.** This goes back to the load volume and magnitude factors. If you do too much too soon, do too much over time, or add more load than your body is capable of controlling—whether you're moving with "good" or "bad" form—then your likelihood of injury goes up.

To be clear, form and technique are important. In general, when you practice using your muscles in ways that maximize stability, you will experience fewer injuries. Functional stability helps you avoid injury, whether it is related to acute loading or repetitive use and whether it's in a passive subsystem like bone or an active subsystem like muscle.

However, it's also important to realize that labeling a movement or posture as "dysfunctional" or "bad" can negatively influence how a person perceives and approaches movement in daily life and sport. Instead, we should encourage others to listen to their bodies and move in ways that feel right to them.

# TISSUE TEMPERATURE (WARM-UPS)

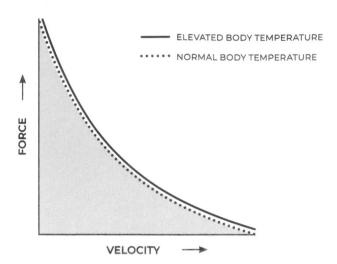

Legend:
— ELEVATED BODY TEMPERATURE
····· NORMAL BODY TEMPERATURE

FORCE (vertical axis) / VELOCITY (horizontal axis)

Warming up allows you to move with greater velocity and generate more force, which can help reduce injury risk and boost performance.

Warm-ups can be helpful for boosting performance and reducing the risk of injury.[1-3] That's why the exercise community has largely shifted from long-duration static stretching to dynamic warm-ups, which involve going through the movements you're about to engage in at a lower intensity. You're raising your heart rate and getting your blood pumping, which elevates your tissue temperature and primes your muscles for more strenuous movement.

Research shows that when you elevate tissue temperature, the tissue becomes more elastic, which changes the influence of the load volume and magnitude factors, allowing you to accept more load and complete faster contractions before getting injured.[4-6] Even better, it changes the contractile features of the tissue, altering muscle conduction so that the recruitment of muscle fibers happens faster after a warm-up.[7,8]

In general, your warm-up should mimic the movements you're going to perform. For example, if you're about to do heavy squats, start with bodyweight squats and then incrementally increase the weight. If you're going to run sprints or play pickup basketball, do a dynamic warm-up that primes your body for explosive, high-magnitude movement (see the sidebar "Dynamic vs. Static Stretching," opposite, for a sample dynamic warm-up).

Warm-ups are also a good time for active mobility drills, which look like stretches or poses but are not static or do not involve holding a position for extended periods. Instead, you're moving in and out of end-range positions with the intention of expressing the full movement potential of the joint. The goal here is to not only increase tissue temperature but also improve position, range of motion, and stability, resulting in more efficient movement and performance. These types of warm-ups are often done—typically in conjunction with dynamic stretching—before weightlifting and other high-intensity training.

# DYNAMIC VS. STATIC STRETCHING

You can stretch before explosive exercise, but make it dynamic stretching rather than static stretching to avoid injury and increase muscle output.

Dynamic stretches take your tissues through length changes, just like playing a sport. For example, in sprinting—where hamstring strains are common—you want to warm up with high-knee marching, Frankenstein walks, and dynamic leg swings. These stretches require the tissue to change length rapidly, replicating the activity you're going to do. This is important because, in an explosive sport like sprinting, power is all about generating force rapidly. Static stretching, on the other hand, has been shown to reduce maximal muscle power and strength, which will not only impair performance but could also increase the chances of injury.[9-10]

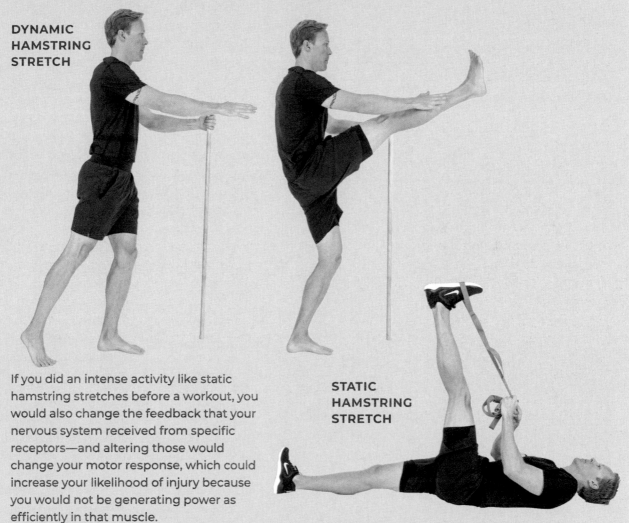

**DYNAMIC HAMSTRING STRETCH**

**STATIC HAMSTRING STRETCH**

If you did an intense activity like static hamstring stretches before a workout, you would also change the feedback that your nervous system received from specific receptors—and altering those would change your motor response, which could increase your likelihood of injury because you would not be generating power as efficiently in that muscle.

If you're not going to be applying explosive force to your tissues—if you're doing an activity like yoga, for example—then warming up with static stretching is probably fine. If you are involved in explosive sports, however, do static stretching afterward. You can even mix these styles for sports like jiu-jitsu, where you might adopt both dynamic and static positions. Perform both active and passive mobility exercises so that you can get into the positions the activity requires.

But in general, the end of a workout is the best time for static stretching. You're already warmed up, so it's a good time to improve your flexibility. Long-duration static stretches can be a nice cool-down so that you're not going from explosive activity to nothing at all. Some people even believe it can help with delayed onset muscle soreness (DOMS).

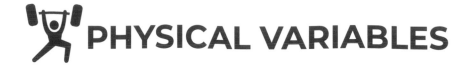

# PHYSICAL VARIABLES

This section is closely tied to mental variables (the next category), but it comes second in the hierarchy because physical variables tend to be simpler to control than mental and external variables.

## PREVIOUS INJURIES AND/OR SURGERY

If you've injured a specific area, your likelihood of reinjuring that area is much higher than it would be if you'd never had an injury.[11-13] For example, if you tore your meniscus—and your knee is a little loose or the tissues are still sensitive when you return to training—you are more likely to sustain another injury because the tissue is already compromised. The ligaments may be a little stretched, or perhaps the joint has lost some of its structural integrity and stability.

The same goes for surgeries, especially reconstructive surgeries. If you return to a movement or activity before going through the appropriate stages of healing or regaining full function, your likelihood of injury goes up.

Step one in reducing your risk of injury is being more conscious about the previously injured area. Think about the other factors discussed in this chapter and take appropriate steps to reduce your susceptibility to reinjury.

With some injuries, such as ACL tears, you are more likely to not only reinjure the same area but also sustain an injury to the opposite side.[14-16] It may be because you're compensating and bearing more weight on the uninjured side, which relates to load magnitude and volume; you're changing the force on those tissues. This is why I recommend performing the rehab exercises on both sides. For instance, if you tore your Achilles tendon and are going through rehab, it would be wise to perform the phase 3 exercises on your uninjured side to make sure you are doing everything you can to strengthen and protect the healthy tendon.

## FATIGUE (COGNITIVE AND NEUROMUSCULAR)

This factor can be broken down into two subcategories, cognitive and neuromuscular fatigue, but the two are interconnected, and sleep is a huge factor in both. Most research on the link between sleep and physical performance shows that impaired sleep leads to decreased performance, which increases injury risk.[17-19]

Sleep deprivation obviously affects both cognitive and neuromuscular fatigue, but it has a more profound impact on cognition. Another factor that exacerbates cognitive fatigue is stress. If you're mentally exhausted and you try to engage in an activity that requires focus, the increased demand on your attention creates anxiety about being a step off or behind, and you're more likely to make a mistake and suffer an injury.

Neuromuscular fatigue, or fatigue of the physical body due to activity, is also important.[20-22] Most people experience it as muscle fatigue—you play a sport until your body starts to tire. What many don't realize is that nervous system fatigue also exists, and it can affect the peripheral or the central nervous system.

Peripheral nervous system fatigue is what most people experience as burning tiredness in a muscle group. But central nervous system fatigue is a bit different. Remember, the central nervous system is your brain and spinal cord, which also can tire from activity. This type of fatigue often results in systemic symptoms, such as deep tiredness throughout the body.

Whether you're playing a sport or lifting weights, listen to your body and pay attention to the other factors. Did you get enough rest the night before? Are you tired or feeling off? Is a stressful event compromising your focus? How you answer these questions should play a role in how you approach the activity. You may need to take the day off, slow down, or rest more frequently.

Many experienced athletes who get injured say that they knew something was off before they got hurt—they weren't focused, or they were tired, and that played a role in the injury that occurred.

# STRENGTH

To some degree, the next four factors boil down to impairments. Physical deficits are closely related to training variables like load volume and magnitude. If you have a strength deficit, for example, you are more likely to injure yourself when you place your system under high force.

When I talk about strength, I don't mean just muscle strength, but tendon, bone, and other tissue strength as well. It's the integrity of all your tissues and how they adapt to loading.

Research suggests that resistance training strengthens and thickens the discs in your spine, bones, tendons, and ligaments.[23-26] This is known as Wolff's law, which outlines the idea that tissue will adapt and get stronger when progressively loaded.

So, strength is one of the physical factors associated with injury risk, and it has been shown to be more important than flexibility, mobility, balance, or proprioception.[27] The strength of a tissue determines how much force it can take before failing. A stronger tissue will be able to accept greater loads without becoming injured. This is why physical therapists focus so much on resistance training after most musculoskeletal injuries.

It's important to follow a resistance training program, not just for rehab but for general health and longevity. Increasing the strength of your musculoskeletal tissues by increasing the loads on your system and learning how to move your body with control can significantly decrease your susceptibility to injury.

# FLEXIBILITY/MOBILITY

Flexibility and mobility are other areas where you could have deficits. Flexibility refers to a muscle's capacity to passively stretch or lengthen, and mobility refers to the ability to move your joints both actively and passively through their available range of motion.

There are different flexibility and mobility tests for different muscles and joints, but generally, we ask whether a person has the range of motion to carry out the tasks they want to do. This relates to injury only if you lack the mobility to perform an activity you want to take on, or if an action you don't normally engage in happens suddenly, such as you slip and bend your leg in an unusual way.

Flexibility is often tougher to control than strength, but again, the best way to avoid injury is to do full range of motion resistance training exercises (often referred to as compound or functional movements) that increase your range of motion, like squats, deadlifts, push-ups, and pull-ups. These exercises will improve your mobility and neuromuscular control. Mobility is just another tool in your arsenal for avoiding injury. Whether it's passive stretching or full range of motion resistance training, you should put yourself in the positions required by the tasks you want to perform. That way, when you assume those positions, your tissues will be better prepared to handle them.

Ask yourself, what activities do I want to do? Can I perform the necessary movements and get into the positions those activities require? If you can't, your risk of injury is higher, and you should implement both active and passive mobility and flexibility training to increase your joint and tissue range of motion.

# BALANCE/ PROPRIOCEPTION

As you age, balance, which describes your ability to maintain and move your center of mass over your available base of support without falling, can become a significant factor.

Most young people don't think much about balance because it comes naturally. But for older people, especially those who do not engage in sports or other regular physical activity, balance plays a much larger role in injury risk.[28] Many people suffer from falls; some even become sedentary because they develop a fear of falling again. And sedentary behavior leads to deconditioning, which increases the risk of all sorts of health problems in addition to injury.

The ankle is the primary joint involved in static balance, so having strength and control over your calf and shin muscles should be a focal point if you are an older person who is vulnerable to falling. The tibialis anterior and calf (soleus and gastrocnemius) are muscles that fire in a near-constant alternating pattern, co-contracting to maintain ankle stability so that you don't fall. Your vision, inner ear, and joint receptors all play roles in maintaining balance as well, with vision being the primary contributor. That's why you sway when you close your eyes.

When testing young, healthy people in physical therapy, we ask them to balance on one leg for 30 seconds to a minute. But if you've sustained an injury—say, you sprained an ankle or tore your ACL—or if you're older, you may have a balance impairment. Training can help improve your proprioception and kinesthesia, which refers to knowing how your body is moving through space. Having a better sense of where you are in space will sharpen the sensory information entering your nervous system, allowing it to make better action programs and recruit your muscles in more efficient ways. In many of the lower body protocols, you will encounter exercises such as the clock, skater squat, and step-up/down movements that will not only improve strength and motor control but also challenge your balance and proprioception.

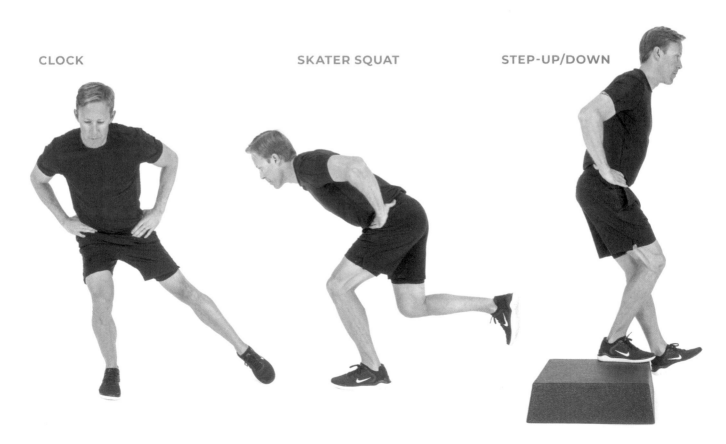

CLOCK

SKATER SQUAT

STEP-UP/DOWN

## LIGAMENTOUS/JOINT LAXITY (STABILITY)

Certain collagen disorders are more prevalent than was once thought. People with these disorders display changes in the collagen makeup of their tissues, which can affect connective tissues such as ligaments and joint capsules. Some of these disorders can even cause joint hypermobility, which is often congenital (present at birth). As a result, these passive subsystems often provide less stability overall.

If you have a hypermobility issue, you will need to work harder to maintain stability throughout your neuromuscular system. But all of us exist along a continuum. Some are stiff and must work harder on mobility and flexibility, while others are hypermobile and should do more stability-focused training.

The rehab protocols show you what a healthy range of motion looks like. If one or more of your joints falls outside that range, you may be congenitally hypermobile, or you may have had an injury that provided extra mobility. Losing integrity in one of these passive subsystems increases your likelihood of injury because the joint becomes less stable. For example, if you dislocate your shoulder, permanent joint instability is common, and you may need to be more conscious of recruiting your neuromuscular system to avoid reinjury.

If you do resistance training and pay attention to technique, biomechanics, and posture, you can train the stability of your joints by recruiting your muscles to maintain good positions. Doing resistance training "correctly" is a form of stability training.

Although we all exist on a spectrum of mobility, there are ideal "zones" for positions during an activity, and a zone may be larger or smaller depending on the individual and the activity. You can usually feel whether your muscles are working correctly or your joints are unstable.

## PROTEIN AND CALORIC INTAKE

Some research suggests that protein and caloric intake may influence injury, but most of it focuses on expediting healing in a person who is already injured.[29-30] Being able to build your tissue back up to full strength is an important part of not getting reinjured. And that's where calories and protein play a role.

When most people think about protein and caloric "needs," they think about muscle maintenance or growth. Your caloric needs depend on your goals. If you want to be in a caloric deficit in order to lose weight, you must recognize that a caloric deficit can hinder your athletic performance. Cognitive and physical fatigue will set in more quickly, too.

When you're injured, meeting your caloric needs is hugely important. Even if you stop working out while you recover, your body still requires energy (calories) to go through the inflammatory response and repair the damaged tissue. And most of your tissues are made of protein, so adequate protein levels are particularly critical. Researchers recommend consuming 1.6 to 2.5 grams of protein per kilogram of body weight to heal faster after an injury, but protein needs can vary from person to person based on their goals and individual biology.[31] I suggest consulting with a dietitian or nutrition expert to determine your caloric and protein requirements.

# MENTAL VARIABLES: STRESS, FEAR, ANXIETY, AND BELIEFS

Mental variables include stress, fear, anxiety, and beliefs, which I covered in Chapter 4. For this reason, I've lumped them into one group here, but it's important to revisit them because they do play a role in injury prevention and healing.

Any outside stressor—such as a divorce or an illness in the family—can be a distraction during physical activity. And when you are paying less attention to the activity you're performing, your injury risk increases. If you can't be 100 percent present, participating in that activity may not be a good call.

Another variable is the fear of reinjury, which can change the way you move. The irony is that you are more likely to get injured when you're fearful of injury because the fear changes your movement patterns and makes you less confident.[12,32-36] In that situation, you need to take steps to rebuild your confidence in your movement system, which you can do by using the appropriate rehab protocol for your injury. This means using graded steps to perform activities that replicate your sport without fully engaging the injured area.

Beliefs—especially negative ones—are another factor in injury risk. If you have a negative belief about something, it may be more likely to come true. If you believe an activity will injure you, that belief could end up being harmful in that it changes how you move or engage with that activity.

These factors are often unique to the individual. We all have different beliefs and stressors. So, it comes back to awareness. Stress, fear, or negative thoughts can affect your ability to be present in the moment, which may influence your ability to react and move in a way that helps you avoid injury.

The protocols in Part III are designed to take you through steps that gradually increase the stress on your tissues, and as you move through the phases, you should start feeling better. Progressing through the phases will also boost your confidence in your musculoskeletal system, which should decrease your injury risk.

# EXTERNAL VARIABLES

You may have some control over these external variables, but they are mostly outside influences. For example, if you go on a hike and there is only one trail, you can't control the terrain, but you can control the shoes you wear. Your decisions based on outside variables can increase or decrease your injury risk.

## TRAINING ENVIRONMENT

Training environment includes things like weather, training surfaces, and equipment.

For example, heat and humidity make you sweat more, decreasing hydration and causing fatigue.[37] If you're a runner, there are different risks associated with concrete versus sand. These factors change the stresses on your tissues, and if you're not prepared for them, they can result in injury.

Shoes are probably the biggest external factor for the musculoskeletal system. And there is considerable debate about them. Should you go barefoot? Should you wear minimalist shoes? Should you wear supportive shoes? Research suggests you should pick a shoe that feels comfortable rather than one that matches your foot type (high vs. low arch).[38,39] Injury risk is lowest, especially for running-related injuries, when you wear comfortable shoes.[40] If a shoe is uncomfortable or you develop pain symptoms quickly when wearing them, it may be time to change footwear.

Weight room equipment can play a role as well. If you're always working out on machines and then you try free weights—which have radically different stability demands—that abrupt change could increase your injury risk. You might need to reduce the load and/or volume, pay more attention to your form, and so on to prevent injury.

Regarding your training environment, it all comes back to awareness and making smart decisions based on the circumstances. You can't control the weather or other environmental factors, but you can plan accordingly and make choices that reduce your risk of injury.

## MEDICATION

As mentioned elsewhere in this book, anti-inflammatory medications can be helpful for getting through the acute pain and inflammation phase after an injury. A cortisone injection might allow you to return to your sport, but it will also weaken your tissues to some degree, which might factor into your injury risk.

Research into the effects of various medications on wound healing shows that steroids, which include cortisone injections, and nonsteroidal anti-inflammatory drugs (NSAIDs), such as ibuprofen, cause the biggest delays in healing.[41-43] Antibiotics are another type of drug to be wary of. The warning labels say to avoid strenuous exercise because antibiotics can weaken tissue integrity and potentially increase your susceptibility to injury.[44,45]

Get a cortisone injection for pain management only if the pain is not getting better with any other treatment, and try not to get more than one shot. The same goes for NSAIDs; if you decide to take them, the usual recommendation is to do so temporarily. Long-term use of anti-inflammatory medications can cause a host of negative side effects. They're a short-term solution to get you through the acute phase.

If you're taking any of these medications, it's because you're recovering, so you shouldn't be doing resistance training or any other activity that stresses the injured tissues. These meds are not designed to help you push through a workout. Don't use medication to mask pain so you can participate. Doing so only increases your risk of injury and delays healing. In fact, if you have to play a sport while injured, it's better to feel the pain so you can listen to your body and avoid making the injury worse.

If you're in phase 2 or 3 of a rehab protocol, you shouldn't be taking these meds anymore because your pain should have diminished—unless you have a flare-up, in which case you should go back to phase 1.

## CHAPTER 10

# HOW TO HEAL
## FROM INJURY

Regardless of the severity or type of injury, there's a basic rehab progression that is universally helpful. This chapter explains the three phases you will go through and will help you connect the dots between injury, the phases of healing, and the stepwise rehab exercise protocols you will follow in Part III.

If you've read Chapter 5, you'll notice that the three phases outlined here—and the exercise strategies—overlap with the phases and strategies for overcoming pain. This is where pain and injury intersect. The phases of treatment follow a similar framework, which is why the protocols in Part III can be used to treat injuries or general or specific pain from unknown causes.

But knowing you have an injury gives you additional information to work with and should be factored into rehab. You will still use the severity of your pain symptoms and your functional ability to guide you through the phases, but you also need to consider the type of injury you have, how long it typically takes to heal, and the impairments it can cause.

# MOVING THROUGH THE PHASES

Say you sprained your ankle. The first thing to think about is where you are in the healing process. If the injury is fresh, then your first objective is to calm the tissues and reduce inflammation so you can assess the damage.

Most ankle sprains involve one or more of the four ligaments running along the outside of the ankle. A mild sprain (grade I) could take about three weeks to heal. A more severe sprain (grade II) could take up to six weeks. Without a doctor's assessment, it's difficult to know exactly how bad the injury is, but you can use pain, swelling, and bruising (covered in Chapter 7) as a guide.

If you feel sharp and throbbing pain with small movements and have significant swelling and bruising after 72 hours, then it could be a grade II. In that case, you should remain in phase 1 until your symptoms calm down—maybe one to two weeks. Knowing that this kind of sprain takes six weeks to heal, you might remain in phase 2 for another three to four weeks to address mobility, strength, and stability impairments caused by the injury. As your range of motion and strength improve and your pain becomes more manageable, you can move to phase 3 and focus on resistance training exercises that rebuild tissue capacity. The idea is to perform the phase 3 exercises until your pain is gone and all impairments have been resolved, which may take four to six weeks.

Remember, pain is not always a good indicator of tissue health. With ligament injuries such as ACL tears, pain starts to go away, but the tissue is still in an early phase of healing, so you need to be careful about how hard you exercise and how quickly you advance through the phases.

This is also true with many post-surgery protocols, including ligament, tendon, meniscus, and labral reconstructions. You may experience reduced pain, but you don't want to load the repaired tissue too soon. Because you feel better, you may think it's OK to start pushing harder with exercise, but if you don't understand the tissue that's injured and how long it takes to heal, you could reinjure it.

All this means that you might need to spend more time in phases 1 and 2 and then remain in phase 3 for several months before returning to explosive activities, especially for ligament and cartilage injuries.

In the rest of this chapter, I discuss each phase and provide general progression guidelines and time frames. But remember, the protocols are meant to be modified based on your unique circumstances. Again—and I can't emphasize this enough—you must use your signs and symptoms, functional ability, and knowledge of injury to progress safely and effectively through the phases.

While the exercise strategies and the time you spend in each phase might depend on the type of injury you have, the end goal is always the same: to get you out of pain, return you to full function, and reduce your susceptibility to future injuries.

# PHASE 1: PAIN MANAGEMENT (INFLAMMATORY PHASE)

When you're in the beginning stages of injury, the first step is to reduce pain. Phase 1 of every protocol incorporates general movement strategies—ranging from soft tissue mobilizations to mobility and stretching drills and, in some cases, low-load resistance training exercises like isometrics—that decrease inflammation, boost blood flow, and get pain under control.

Another big part of the pain management phase is temporarily changing your behavior so that you don't put stress on the injured tissue and make the pain worse. (I'll cover that in more detail in the aggravating factors portion of the protocols.) This is difficult for a lot of people because it requires modifying deeply ingrained habits. If you have a rotator cuff injury, for example, sleeping on the injured side or moving in certain ways can cause pain. Or say you injured your low back and your pain flares up every time you sit at your workstation for too long. Whether it is a normally benign task or an activity you enjoy, stressing the tissue during the initial phase of healing can slow your recovery. So, you must be aware of the aggravating factors and modify your behavior to give the injured tissue time to calm down.

Complementary and alternative medicine interventions (CAMs), which I discuss in Chapter 14, can also reduce pain and decrease inflammation. These modalities include electrical stimulation, ice and heat, compression, and more—any treatment strategy that helps get pain under control and enhances healing is a good option during this phase. Just make sure to prioritize the exercises; don't substitute a CAM intervention for a rehab protocol. CAM treatments are supplemental, meaning you do them in addition to the exercises.

The general timeline for phase 1 ranges from a couple of days to weeks. Again, you have to listen to your body and assess the severity of your injury. My general recommendation is to progress to phase 2 when you no longer have pain at rest and can perform the phase 1 exercises with no more than mild pain.

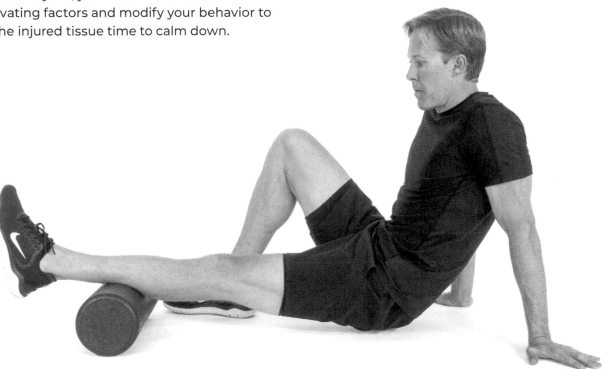

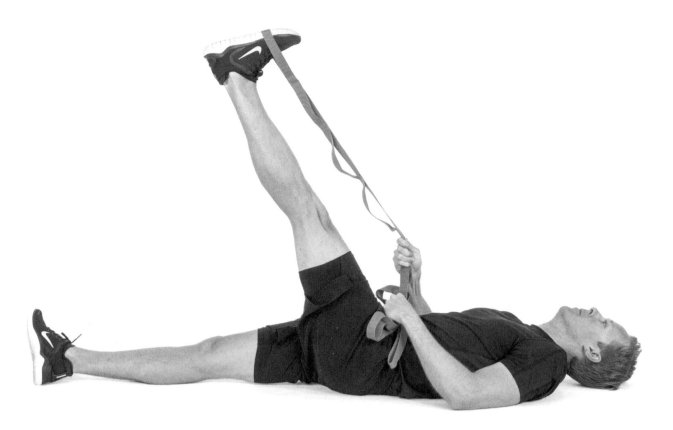

# PHASE 2: RANGE OF MOTION AND SENSORIMOTOR CONTROL (MATURATION PHASE)

Once you're out of the acute pain phase, you enter the maturation or repair phase. This is where you start to address range of motion, sensorimotor control, and in some cases strength impairments caused by your injury.

In rehab, you must tackle mobility impairments within the first few weeks of the injury. If you don't, the injured joint (depending on the location and severity of the injury) can stiffen, develop contractures (structural changes in non-bony tissue), and even become stuck. For example, if you have a meniscus injury and stop moving your knee for a couple of months, you could develop a joint contracture that restricts your ability to fully straighten or bend your knee. Or, if you have a rotator cuff injury and avoid full-range movements for an extended period, you could develop frozen shoulder. This would set you back, as getting past either of those more severe issues takes extensive work.

In addition to performing mobility and flexibility exercises to address range of motion impairments, you will tackle sensorimotor control deficits in phase 2. This refers to your nervous system and the way it turns on your muscles to control your kinetic chain. With sensorimotor exercises, you're looking to improve control and coordination by moving slowly and focusing on the quality of your movement. By doing so, you refine the communication between the sensors in your muscles and joints and your central nervous system (brain and spinal cord), which leads to better form and technique and reduced stress on healing tissues.

The link between the muscle and joint sensors and the nervous system is known as the sensorimotor control system because it's a loop: your sensory neurons detect inputs, and your motor neurons react to those inputs. This loop refines your control over the system. If you tore your meniscus and only rested to recover, healing might take a long time. But if you train your sensorimotor system to control your body without putting too much stress on the injured area, you will recover much more quickly. For example, with a meniscus injury, you might use the lateral step-down exercise to improve how your gluteal and quadriceps muscles control your knee joint. As your nervous system gets better at recruiting these muscles, your form with the exercise—as well as any activity that involves standing on the injured leg—will improve. This positive change in movement quality means that the muscles are more capable of acting as shock absorbers so that too much force isn't applied to the healing meniscus. You're increasing functional stability in the region and limiting stress on the injured tissue so that it can heal.

Phase 2 also includes isometric and eccentric exercises, which are an early form of resistance training that is mainly used to further reduce pain and improve tissue strength. As I covered in Chapter 5, concentric muscle contractions, which you will do in phase 3, produce tension in the muscle as it shortens and often create pain in the early phases of healing. That's why you start with isometric and eccentric contractions because you can start to put small doses of stress on your system and rebuild the tissue without interfering with the healing process or making your pain worse.

Once you can easily perform the phase 2 exercises—that is, complete the full range of motion with control and with mild to no pain—you can move to phase 3. If a movement from phase 2 provokes symptoms—you experience acute pain in the area, you're unable to perform the full range of motion, or you have poor motor control (coordination and stability)—do not progress to phase 3. Again, you have to listen to your body and respect the healing time for the injury you're rehabbing.

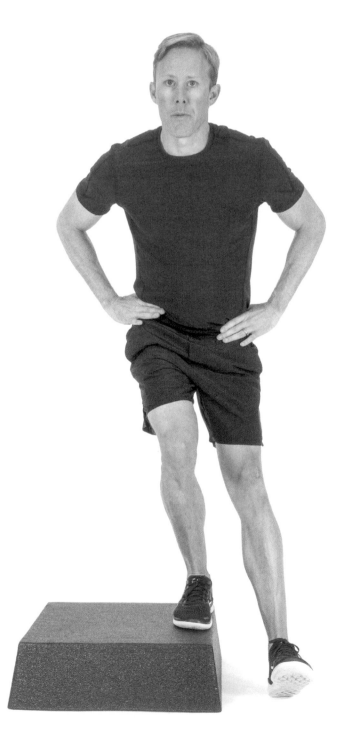

# PHASE 3: RESISTANCE TRAINING (REMODELING PHASE)

When you sustain an injury to any type of tissue, you're unable to do some of the activities that you did before. As a result, the muscles in the region will weaken and atrophy, which reduces tissue integrity and compromises the capacity of your musculoskeletal system.

Even though the body is complex, it's also mechanical. And you want a mechanical structure to have the highest capacity possible. A bridge that's weak in one spot is more likely to collapse. The same goes for your body. If you have a tendon or ligament that's been weakened by injury, you need to rebuild that tissue so you don't injure it again.

This is accomplished primarily through resistance training. In the remodeling phase, you incorporate bodyweight exercises (such as push-ups and squats) and loaded movements that involve external resistance, such as dumbbells, kettlebells, and bands. Your effort revolves around improving the integrity and capacity of your body through full-range muscle contractions (concentric and eccentric), which strengthens the injured and surrounding tissue.

People often don't have much pain when they get to phase 3, so it's all about incrementally challenging your body to do more over time—otherwise known as progressive overload. That means increasing range of motion, load, volume (training frequency, sets, or reps), and effort (movement speed) as your injury continues to heal.

In phase 3, I provide specific resistance training exercises to rehab common injuries with general recommendations for sets and reps. However, everyone has a unique starting point and experience level, and that might determine how you approach the program.

## BACK TO SPORT AND PLAY

Phase 3 is when most people reintroduce activities they were limiting. If you are a runner, for example, you'll start reintegrating running. But this is a tricky phase because you're beginning to combine a lot of variables, and increasing the volume of activity can flare up many musculoskeletal issues. That doesn't necessarily mean the activity is bad, but adding too much stress too quickly could knock you back into the inflammatory phase, and then you would have to go through the phases again, letting the area calm down again before you can build it back up. Although you'll probably move through the protocol faster the second time, you can avoid this cycle by closely monitoring the total stress your preferred activities and rehab exercises are putting on your healing tissue.

In terms of time spent doing rehab exercises as opposed to your normal sports or other physical activities, you can implement a progressive overload approach. With most musculoskeletal conditions, you should not stop doing your regular activities or you could become deconditioned, but you should significantly dial back any aggravating activities for two to four weeks while you're focusing on rehab. Maybe you can swim instead of run while you're letting the running tissues calm down. After that two-to-four-week window, you can start to slowly ramp up running—do a little at a time and see how your body responds.

Regardless of the activity, don't try to jump into the same volume of training that you did prior to your injury. Treat that activity like an aggravating factor. If your pain flares up, reduce the dosage and then build it back up over time by doing a little more every week.

If you are a beginner who is new to resistance training, stick to the prescribed exercises, focus on your form, and listen to your body. If something feels off—a certain movement causes pain, for example—you may need to modify the exercise. The guidelines in Chapter 12 answer common troubleshooting questions that might not be addressed in the exercise descriptions and will help you adapt the exercises to suit your individual needs.

If you are a more advanced athlete or lifter, use the programs and exercise selections as a general guide. Depending on the severity of your injury, you might need to add more load, modify the set and rep scheme, or swap one exercise variation for another that you prefer. Just remember, I picked those exercises because they work!

While some movements might seem basic or easy, I carefully selected them to address the specific impairments associated with the injury. If you decide to swap one exercise for another, pick a variation that shares the same movement pattern and plane of motion. That way, you work the same muscle groups and target the tissue in a precise way.

It's also important to keep the phase 3 exercises in your toolbox even after you've completed rehab and are pain-free. Again, these strengthening exercises are the best way to prevent pain from coming back or reinjuring the area, especially for tendinopathies. Say you have a history of tennis elbow or jumper's knee, and you're going to engage in an activity that could flare it up. Using the phase 3 exercises in the relevant protocol to condition and strengthen the area prior to the activity will dramatically reduce the likelihood of a flare-up.

Most importantly, I want you to create a habit around resistance training. The work is not done once you've completed a protocol, your injury has healed, and your pain is gone. Resistance training—as well as aerobic, mobility, and flexibility exercises—is crucial to maintaining physical resilience and long-term health. The idea is to develop a routine you enjoy so that you can stick with it for the rest of your life and continue to reap the countless benefits that regular exercise offers.

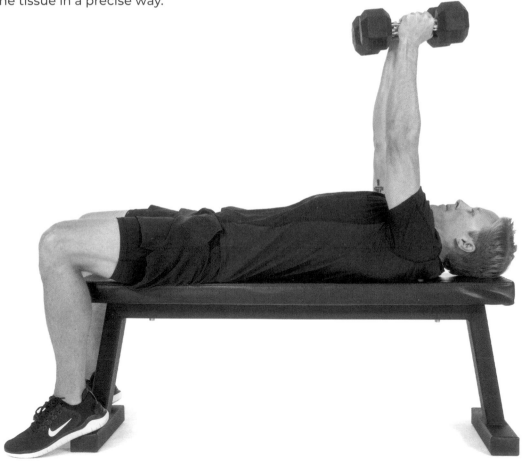

# SAME FRAMEWORK, DIFFERENT EXERCISE STRATEGIES

While the three-phase framework is the same for all injuries, the exercise strategies and the order in which they appear vary based on the type of injury, the affected body region, and the associated impairments and pain symptoms.

For example, the rehab protocols that address low back pain, neck pain, and other general pain typically start with soft tissue mobilizations and stretching and then progress to mobility and resistance training. This is a great template for treating minor pain impairments because soft tissue mobilizations and stretching can alleviate symptoms and prime your body to tackle the mobility and resistance exercises in later phases. But it is by no means a universal blueprint.

With muscle and tendon injuries, you might need to skip or be careful with soft tissue mobilizations and stretches because they can flare up symptoms. Stretching into a muscle strain or compressing an injured tendon with a soft tissue mobilization is generally a bad idea, as it can make pain worse and slow healing. Instead, you might incorporate isometric and eccentric exercises in phase 1 or 2—even though they are technically resistance training exercises—because they can reduce muscle and tendon pain and address weakness, which is the primary impairment associated with those types of injuries.

The order of exercise strategies also differs for ligament and cartilage injuries. Soft tissue mobilizations and stretching are not likely to help and may not have a place in the program. With these injuries, the primary impairment is joint instability, so active mobility and neuromuscular control (low-load resistance exercises) become the primary strategies and show up much earlier than in the protocols that address muscle and tendon injuries and general pain.

I wish there were a clear-cut, one-size-fits-all exercise blueprint that I could provide for all pain and injuries. Unfortunately, that is not how rehab works. There is a lot of nuance and individual variability when it comes to programming exercises, which is why some programs differ from others and some exercise strategies appear earlier or later in the phases.

If this is confusing, don't worry. I have designed the rehab protocols to take the guesswork out of it. Find the protocol that matches your injury, do the exercises, and trust that they will reduce pain, correct impairments, and get you back to normal function.

In Part III, I provide guidelines for progressing through the programs and modifying the exercises as needed. Without a practitioner to guide you through rehab, it's important to understand how to choose the right protocol and adapt it to your unique circumstances and symptoms. The chapters in Part III will get you moving in the right direction and help you gain the most benefit from the protocols.

# PART III

# REHAB

## CHAPTER 11

# PROTOCOLS
## OVERVIEW

You may have arrived at this part of the book as your first stop. You have pain, an injury, or both, and you want to know what to do about it. That's where rehab comes into play. In this part, I provide rehab exercise protocols (programs of treatment) for the most common musculoskeletal conditions. Consider each protocol a step-by-step strategy for addressing pain symptoms, improving movement and recovery, and rehabilitating and preventing injuries.

This chapter explains the organization and structure of the protocols—and how to navigate them to get the most from them.

# SELECTING A PROTOCOL

The protocols are organized by body region: head and neck, shoulder, elbow, wrist and hand, back and spine, hip, knee, and ankle and foot. (See page 4 or 117 for a full body area map.)

At the beginning of each body region chapter are illustrations that represent the protocols in that section. If you have pain in your shoulder, for example, go to the shoulder chapter, look at the illustrations, and choose the protocol that best matches your symptoms. Or, if you already have a diagnosis from a healthcare provider or otherwise have a general idea of what is causing your pain, you can flip to that protocol by injury name.

Note that many of the protocols capture more than one condition because the rehab exercise program for those conditions is the same. For instance, the Hip Pain protocol that begins on page 329 includes hip impingements, labral tears, osteoarthritis, gluteal tendinopathy, and trochanteric bursitis.

If I've included more than one protocol for the same body region and you don't know which one to follow, or you have a general idea of what your problem is but want confirmation, read the descriptions and other categories to match your symptoms to the condition. Most body region protocols are similar and include many of the same exercises, but there are some overlapping protocols targeting a common area that may require different treatment strategies. Shoulder labral tears and biceps tendinopathy both create pain in the front of the shoulder, for example, but the programs of treatment are different, and it's important to pick the right one. That's what the descriptions and other categories are for—to help you determine which protocol to follow.

## REHAB IS PREHAB

A lot of people mistakenly think that rehab exercises are only useful in the case of injury. That may be true for certain exercises, but not all of them. Although the protocols are designed to address pain symptoms and injuries, the exercises—which are primarily resistance exercises that improve movement, coordination, mobility, and strength—are just as good for preventing pain and injuries as they are for healing them.

Here's the deal: strengthening your joints and tissues through all ranges of motion makes your body more resilient. Resistance training has the best evidence for reducing the long-term likelihood of reinjury. You must keep your musculoskeletal tissues (bones, joints, muscles, tendons, ligaments, and soft tissue) strong even after you're better to prevent a problem from coming back. Everyone, regardless of athletic background, should do some form of resistance training a few days a week to ensure optimal physical health.

When it comes to prehab—whether you are preparing for surgery or simply looking for an injury prevention program—you can cherry-pick from the exercises in the protocols and design a program that suits your needs. This also applies to general fitness training. Maybe there are soft tissue mobilizations that are helpful for reducing reoccurring pain and stiffness, or perhaps you have a range of motion impairment that needs constant maintenance. The idea is to select mobility and resistance training exercises from the protocols that are helpful and continue doing them—and that can serve as your prehab or mobility and body region–specific strength training program.

# REHAB PROTOCOL OVERVIEW

Each protocol includes a description, a list of signs and symptoms, aggravating factors, a prognosis, a treatment strategy, and a rehab exercise program broken into three phases. When taken together, these categories provide a comprehensive framework for identifying, treating, and preventing the pain and injury associated with that protocol. Learn what is covered in the categories and you will have a better grasp of how to use the information to guide your rehab.

## DESCRIPTION

The first part of the protocol describes which tissues are affected and how commonly the condition or injury occurs. In essence, it's a quick overview of what the pain or injury is, who it commonly affects, what activities cause it, and what potential vulnerabilities it creates.

This is an important section to read, not only to identify the problem but also to pinpoint the potential mechanism of injury and pain. Reinjury and recurrence of pain (flare-ups) are frustrating and common. But you can safeguard yourself and reduce your susceptibility to reinjury by understanding what may have caused the issue and making the necessary adjustments—such as reducing your training volume, giving yourself ample time to recover, adjusting your technique or form, or addressing lifestyle factors that contribute to inflammation and pain.

## SIGNS AND SYMPTOMS

Common signs and symptoms include where the pain is located and what it typically feels like (numbness, aching, tingling, stiffness, weakness, and so on). Do a symptom check to determine whether the protocol is the appropriate match.

## AGGRAVATING FACTORS

During physical therapy evaluations, I ask patients what activities, tasks, and movements trigger their pain or make it worse. These are called aggravating factors. I use them in the clinic as a part of my differential diagnosis process, and you can use them in the same way.

Put simply, you can use the aggravating factors section as a screening tool. It lets you know what movements and activities you should avoid or modify to promote healing and prevent flare-ups, and it can help confirm that you are following the most appropriate protocol.

I don't recommend putting yourself in pain on purpose, but pay attention to what you're doing when you do feel pain. Also note that with a lot of conditions, aggravating factors can change throughout the phases of healing.

The protocols teach you how to calm the tissue before building it back up so that the aggravating factors no longer cause you pain. Because aggravating factors are often functional tasks, you can't avoid them forever, but your tissues may be sensitized to them or not ready for them right now. For example, a lot of knee problems are aggravated by stair climbing, but you will need to climb stairs at some point. Each protocol has exercises meant to help rebuild capacity so that when you go back and retest a functional task, it's easier to do.

# RED FLAG SYMPTOMS:
# READ THIS BEFORE YOU START A PROTOCOL

If you have pain and visit a doctor, the first thing they are going to do is rule out what are called "red flags." These are potential signs of a more serious underlying condition—the kind that rehab exercises won't fix. If you are experiencing any of these symptoms, speak with your doctor before beginning any of the protocols in this book.

## RED FLAGS INCLUDE[1,2]

- **RECENT TRAUMA.** *Incidents like car accidents and serious falls can cause fractures or other injuries that may require medical attention.*

- **RESTING/NIGHT PAIN.** *Unrelenting pain that is present at rest and at night may be associated with more serious medical conditions.*

- **SADDLE ANESTHESIA.** *Absence of sensation in the saddle (perianal) region can be related to a serious compromise of low back nerves and may require immediate surgical intervention.*

- **LOWER EXTREMITY NEUROLOGICAL DEFICIT.** *Progressive weakness and loss of function of the legs, like saddle anesthesia, can point to a serious compromise of low back nerves.*

- **BLADDER DYSFUNCTION.** *Changes in bladder function (such as incontinence, blood in urine, or pain) can be related to infection or nerve compromise and can produce back pain.*

- **HISTORY OF CANCER.** *Having had cancer increases your risk of developing the types of cancers that cause musculoskeletal pain.*

- **UNEXPLAINED WEIGHT LOSS.** *Weight loss of over 10 pounds in three months that is not related to a change in diet or activity may be associated with an infection or cancer.*

- **FEVER, CHILLS, OR NIGHT SWEATS.** *These types of constitutional symptoms can point toward infection or cancer.*

- **RECENT INFECTION.** *A recent infection increases your risk of developing another infection, which may cause musculoskeletal pain.*

- **AGE OVER 50.** *Being over 50 comes with an increased risk of infection, fracture, cancer, and aortic aneurysm.*

These symptoms aren't always cause for alarm. Night pain, for example, is a symptom of arthritis for some people. Only around 1 percent of musculoskeletal issues are due to serious pathology, so the likelihood is low, but you don't want to miss a life-threatening condition.[3-5] If you combine several of these red flags—night pain plus a history of cancer and you're over 50—then you should talk with your doctor to make sure nothing else is wrong before starting any of these protocols.

If you don't have any red flags, most doctors will have you try physical therapy. That's why there's no real downside to working through the rehab exercises on your own (assuming you have ruled out obvious red flags). Then you can screen yourself and get close to what an actual PT would do. But keep in mind that, while the protocols in this book address most musculoskeletal conditions, they are not a substitute for direct medical care.

# PROGNOSIS

This category lays out the typical recovery time—that is, how long you can expect something to take to get better. Remember that your prognosis is based mainly on the type and severity of the injury and the type of tissue that was damaged (tendon versus muscle versus ligament and so on). In Chapter 7, I cover the different grades of injury, and in Chapter 8, I cover the different tissue types and how they relate to pain and healing.

Prognoses often range from weeks to months. That range might seem broad, but every person and every injury is different, and it may take you longer to progress than someone else. That's OK.

The prognosis section also offers recommendations about when you might want to seek professional care. For example, you should start noticing small positive changes in about two weeks. If you've modified or eliminated the aggravating factors and followed the rehab exercise program for at least six weeks but you're not getting better, it's usually a good time to have an in-person evaluation.

# TREATMENT STRATEGY

The treatment strategy explains how the condition or injury is typically treated to facilitate healing. Think of it as a general summary of treatment and rehab exercise options—and how to approach those options.

Within this category, there are three important factors to be aware of: medication, the potential for surgery, and the exercises you will perform during rehab.

In some cases, I recommend anti-inflammatory medication, but I don't advise taking medication for a long time because it can have negative side effects.[6] However, in short bursts, it can help calm irritated musculoskeletal tissues. So, in phase 1, you might use it temporarily.

Certain injuries may not respond well to rehab exercises—specifically, injuries that compromise the stability of a joint (for example, a knee that wants to give way). In this case, you might be a candidate for surgery. Or you may need to avoid certain exercises if you've had a previous surgery. I provide guidelines for approaching these situations in the treatment strategy sections. I also unpack the rehab exercise programs by explaining why I picked certain exercises and how they fit into the framework of the phases. This is the core of your treatment strategy because it details the rationale and methodology used to construct the programs, and the role the exercises play during rehab.

As I said, some programs encompass more than one condition. With these protocols, it's important to pay attention to the treatment strategy because there might be certain exercises that are great for one condition but must be approached with caution for other conditions. For example, the Neck Pain protocol can be used to treat non-specific neck pain or an injury like whiplash. If you have non-specific neck pain, the stretches included in the program are probably fine. But if you have a strain (whiplash), you need to be extra careful because stretching a strained muscle can flare-up symptoms and slow healing. That doesn't mean that stretching is bad. It all depends on the severity of the injury and where you are at in the healing process. You might be fine stretching, or you may need to modify the exercise (such as by reducing the load or range of motion), or skip it and add it to the next phase.

My biggest fear is that you will blindly follow the program, perform an exercise that makes your symptoms worse, and then give up on rehab. Remember, the rehab programs include exercises that have the best evidence both in the literature and in my practice for specific pain symptoms, body regions, and conditions. But they are general programs, meaning they are not specific to individuals with unique circumstances. Without a PT there to make modifications, it's up to you to read the treatment strategies, guidelines, and captions, and then make informed decisions based on how you feel and perform.

## ARE YOU A CANDIDATE FOR SURGERY?

If you have pain and your doctor spots an irregularity on an MRI, they may recommend surgical intervention. But it's not always that simple. Something showing up on an MRI doesn't automatically make you a candidate for surgery. There are other factors you must consider.

For example, maybe you've been in chronic pain, and nothing has helped. Or maybe you've followed the appropriate protocol for eight to 12 weeks, and you haven't gotten better. Or maybe you have some of the red flag symptoms covered earlier. If any of those apply to you, surgery might be an option worth exploring. I recommend you talk with a doctor—and seek a second opinion if that is an option for you—before deciding.

I chose the musculoskeletal problems listed in this book because they respond well to rehab-based interventions that revolve around mobility and resistance training. But other interventions—mainly medication or surgery prescribed by non-rehab medical providers—should become options if you have gone through the rehab protocols but aren't seeing the desired results after eight to 12 weeks—the typical length of time you would spend with a physical therapist.

It's also important to realize that certain conditions can flare up, prolonging the healing process and making a problem seem worse than it is. I've had injuries that caused me pain for over a year, not because rehab didn't work but because I did something that aggravated the area and set me back. If I hadn't known better, I might have thought I was a candidate for surgery. It's easy to think, "Something is really wrong here; surgery might be the best course of action," when in reality, you should be thinking, "This is just a flare-up; I need to let the tissue calm down and then build it back up so that it can get better."

Here's the truth: surgery for degenerative tears and most minor injuries is not a guaranteed fix, and it comes with risks. There are better options, such as following a rehab program and avoiding aggravating factors—even some of the CAM interventions offered in Chapter 13 are worth exploring first. If those efforts don't help, then it might be time to consider more invasive options.

# REHAB EXERCISES

Finally, you'll find stepwise programs for dealing with your pain or injury. For every protocol, there are three rehab exercise phases. As I covered in Chapters 5 and 10, how you progress through those phases is based on your symptoms—how much pain you're in and how much functional ability you have—as well as the type of injury and typical healing time.

The protocols list the exercises you need to do in each phase and how to do them. Keep in mind that the time you spend in each phase will depend on your injury and how quickly you are able to resolve the associated impairments.

Here's a summary of the phases and how to progress through them:

- **PHASE 1** is for getting pain under control and mainly includes soft tissue mobilizations (self-guided massage). These can be done after an injury or anytime you experience a flare-up—when you're not injured but you have minor pain due to an aggravating factor. Once pain is no longer present at rest, move to phase 2.

- **PHASE 2** addresses range of motion, sensorimotor control, and strength impairments using mobility, flexibility, isometric, and eccentric exercises. Once you can perform the movements in phase 2 with mild to no pain, move to phase 3.

- **PHASE 3** is all about rebuilding capacity and tissue integrity through full-range resistance training exercises. Continue following the phase 3 program until your pain is resolved or your injury is fully healed.

Each phase includes a set of exercises with instructions on how to perform them, along with the training frequency (how often to do the workout) and the number of sets and repetitions (reps) for each exercise. The reps are the number of times you perform the exercise, and the sets are the number of cycles you complete for each exercise.

Here are some general guidelines:

- Perform the exercises in sequence. In other words, perform all the sets and reps of each exercise before moving on to the next one.

- Rest for 30 seconds to a minute between sets.

- I typically give a range of reps and hold times. Perform the number of reps or hold for a period that is challenging for you.

- Gradually increase your range of motion and effort (the number of reps or the hold time) week by week.

- If a movement causes pain, shorten the range of motion and/or reduce the load, reps, or hold time. If the issue gets worse, consider a different exercise variation that shares the same movement pattern or skip it and add it to the next phase.

See Chapter 12 for more about the training variables and modifying exercises to address common issues.

## POST- OR PRE-SURGERY PROTOCOLS

Some of the protocols feature post-surgery movements and exercises. Maybe you've just gone through a procedure, or you have one coming up. Perhaps you've been told you need surgery and you're considering your options. Whatever your prognosis, you might be wondering what comes next.

No matter which phase you are in, these protocols can help you recover after surgery. Working through them before surgery can help, too; going in strong with better neuromuscular control will help you recover faster. But keep in mind that surgeons often assign specific protocols, and the ones listed in this book should not supersede or replace those.

If you are a post-op patient, I recommend that you use this book to supplement the rehab you're doing with your physical therapist. After surgery, it's important to have a program that's tailored to your needs and work with a professional who can guide you through the process with easier exercises and more specific tests. But the education found herein can be an awesome complement. It can help you understand what's going on with your body and ask your PT the right questions. It can provide context and accountability for whatever recommendation the PT is making and enable you to make suggestions of your own. It gives you power when you're feeling powerless.

# WHERE TO START AND HOW TO IMPLEMENT THE PHASES

As I've said, your pain symptoms can help you decide where to start and when to move from one phase to the next. In some of the protocols, I provide general guidance and timelines based on the injury. In other cases, I generally use the visual analog scale (VAS). Zero is no pain, and 10 is the worst pain you can imagine. If your pain is greater than a three out of 10, start with phase 1. If your pain is less than a three out of 10, move to phase 2. If your symptoms don't flare up and you can complete all the exercises easily (full range of motion with control), advance to phase 3.

People often have a hard time putting an exact number on their pain, so you can also think about it as mild, moderate, or severe. Mild pain is in the one to three range. Moderate pain is four to seven, and severe pain is eight and above.

Even if you are not in pain, I recommend progressing through the phases sequentially. You might feel fine starting with phase 3, but the phase 1 and 2 exercises will provide some benefit—they serve as a warm-up, improve range of motion, prep your body for loaded movements, and help you identify and address potential impairments.

Even within the phases, the path to getting better is rarely linear. When you go through rehab, occasional setbacks and flare-ups are inevitable. If you experience them, give the tissue time to calm down, often by going back to the previous phase.

# WHAT IF I HAVE PAIN IN MULTIPLE AREAS?

You might be wondering what to do if you have pain in more than one area, or if more than one protocol fits what you're feeling. (This applies more to generalized pain; an injury is usually quite specific.)

Within a protocol, all the rehab exercises are designed to address a particular issue. You can expect that your pain will decrease over time as you move through the phases of healing. But pain in more than one area—either in one body region or two different body regions—changes things a bit.

If you have two different pains in one body region—your shoulder, for example—I recommend picking the protocol that addresses the more painful area or the pain that limits your function more. Performing all the exercises from two protocols in one region is too much exercise volume and could make the problem worse, seeding doubt that rehab may not be the best path forward.

In some ways, having pain in two different body regions is easier than having two pains in the same region because the movements are different; the tricky part is ensuring that exercises for one region don't aggravate your other injury.

If you have more than one injured body part, you can approach the protocols in various ways. You can combine exercises from both protocols into a single training session or focus on one area one day and then the other area the next day. You'll notice some overlap between exercises, especially if you have different pains in adjacent regions—your neck and shoulder, for example. If an exercise appears in both protocols, don't do it twice; just do it once to cover both areas.

# TRAINING BOTH SIDES OF YOUR BODY

Pain and injury typically affect one joint, limb, or side of the body. Even so, I encourage you to do the rehab exercises in this book with a "both sides" mentality. This specifically applies to single-joint or unilateral exercises.

Say you've got plantar fasciitis in your right foot. Should you do the exercises on the other side, too? Yes. It certainly can't hurt, and chances are it will safeguard your left foot from pain and injury down the road. Furthermore, performing the exercises on the uninjured side helps inform your neuromuscular system as to how the movement should be completed when you shift to the injured side, which is called cross-transfer education (see page 134). I often have my patients start on the uninjured side so that they can get an idea of how the movement should feel, which typically leads to better movement performance on the injured side.

# LET YOUR BODY BE THE GUIDE

As you go through the protocols, pay attention to how your body responds to the movements. Because I'm not evaluating you in person, these protocols aren't specific to you—they're generalized for everyone. In the clinic, I would test you to see how your body and symptoms responded to physical stresses. Since I can't do that in this book, you need to be aware of your own body, test them on yourself, and see how your body responds.

The protocols are set up so that you can simply follow them and see results, but to get the most out of them, you need to make modifications that suit your unique circumstances, functional ability, and symptoms. For example, say a movement triggers your pain or makes it worse. You need to know how to modify the training and programming plan based on how your body responds, which you will learn how to do in the next chapter.

# BODY AREA MAP

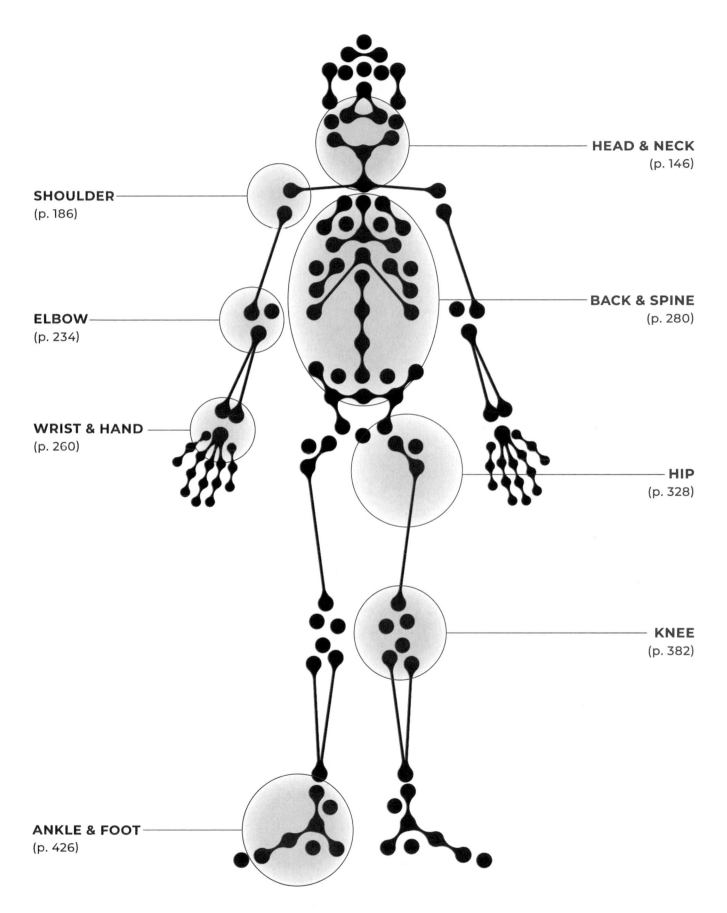

HEAD & NECK
(p. 146)

SHOULDER
(p. 186)

BACK & SPINE
(p. 280)

ELBOW
(p. 234)

WRIST & HAND
(p. 260)

HIP
(p. 328)

KNEE
(p. 382)

ANKLE & FOOT
(p. 426)

## CHAPTER 12

# TRAINING & PROGRAMMING GUIDELINES

This chapter provides training and programming guidelines that apply to all the rehab protocols in this book. Look to the training and exercise guidelines for solutions to the most common problems and questions associated with the exercises—pain, load (weight), range of motion, and tempo (movement speed), and look to the programming guidelines for clarification on the program structure—sets and reps, rest periods, and training frequency.

I recommend reading through these guidelines before you start any of the protocols. Doing so will help you get the most from the training routines and give you direction when making modifications to the exercises and programs.

# TRAINING AND EXERCISE GUIDELINES

When you start a rehab protocol, you're bound to encounter problems with certain exercises that will raise questions. What should you do if an exercise causes you pain? What if your pain is worse the next day? How do you determine the right load for an exercise?

These guidelines show you the best ways to modify an exercise if you experience pain or compromised quality of movement. They address load, range of motion, neuromuscular control (stability), tempo, stance/posture, and variations (with the mind-muscle connection as a bonus). Don't just throw out an exercise because it is giving you problems. There are many ways to adapt an exercise to suit your ability, but removing it entirely might interfere with your recovery because every exercise in a protocol is important. If you struggle with any of the movements, refer to these guidelines, and hopefully you can find a solution that allows you to stick with the program.

## What should I do if an exercise causes pain?

**Mild discomfort is generally OK. Stick with the exercise if you experience no more than a three out of 10 on the pain scale; modify the exercise if it's too painful or causes a flare-up.**

Pain is usually the first big problem people experience. You do an exercise, it causes pain, and your movement quality goes down—you can't perform the full range of motion, you lose neuromuscular control, or you compensate by performing the exercise incorrectly. Remember, in rehab, we use the visual analog scale for pain, which goes from zero to 10. Zero is no pain, five is moderate pain, and 10 is the worst pain you can imagine.

A little discomfort is acceptable when doing the exercises; it means you're applying enough stress to challenge the tissue. If the exercise is super easy and you feel nothing, you might not be creating enough stress to cause adaptation in the musculoskeletal system. But if you hit four out of 10 or above, you're probably putting too much stress on the tissue, which can interfere with the healing process. In that case, you should modify the exercise by following the subsequent guidelines—reduce the load, range of motion, or volume (sets and reps); skip it and add it to the next phase; or switch the variation.

By "mild discomfort," I don't mean normal exercise fatigue or muscle burn; I mean your unique, familiar pain—the pain you came to rehab to address. You want to lightly trigger that pain. For many conditions, just starting to activate symptoms means you're applying the right amount of stress to facilitate positive adaptation and desensitize your system. But pushing into pain—beyond a three out of 10—can risk injuring tissue or cause a flare-up, which may lead to setbacks.

As you go through the phases and your system becomes less sensitive, you'll be able to handle more load before triggering a pain response. By the time you reach phase 3, your pain should be dying down, and you'll be feeling more muscle challenge and fatigue. But regardless of phase, be aware of your unique pain experience and try not to push past mild discomfort—and that applies to soft tissue mobilizations, isometrics, stretching, mobility, and resistance exercises.

## My pain is worse the day after a training session. What should I do?

**If your pain is worse the next day, you need to modify the exercise that is giving you problems, or skip it and add it to the next phase.**

Think about pain in a 24-hour window. If your resting pain is worse the day after working out, you may need to modify the exercise. If you exercised on a Monday morning and felt a bit of discomfort while doing the exercise, that's OK. But if you were at two out of 10 at rest on Monday, and on Tuesday morning your baseline pain level has increased to a four, you may have stirred things up too much. In that case, you need to modify the exercise during the next training session—by decreasing the load, number of reps, or range of motion, for example.

If your resting pain is worse, think about what you did the day before. Did a certain exercise cause more pain than others? How many sets and reps did you do? How much weight did you use? Keep a log that you can review to determine what might've caused the flare-up.

If your resting pain has increased, let your body recover and return to baseline—only then can you determine how to modify the exercises so you do not trigger your pain again. This involves some trial and error. You're constantly adapting.

Reducing your baseline pain level is the goal; staying at or under that baseline indicates that the dosage is right and you don't need to modify the exercise. But if it does flare up, it's not a big deal. Just give yourself a few days to rest without doing whatever movements triggered the area. A lot of people worry about taking time off, but it's important for getting your pain back to baseline. Once you resume training, pay attention to how you feel during the exercise. If certain exercises make your pain worse, you can either modify the load and range of motion, or skip the exercise and add it to the next phase.

## I feel pain or a loss of control with a specific range of motion. How should I modify the exercise?

**Reduce range of motion or perform partial reps to work around pain restrictions or a loss of neuromuscular control/stability.**

If you have reduced the load for an exercise and your pain is still higher than a three, and/or you have a loss of neuromuscular control with an exercise, the next step is to temporarily reduce the range of motion or perform partial reps.

People often have pain or a loss of control—muscles feel weak or a joint feels less stable—at a specific point in an exercise, typically as the joint moves toward end range. So, if you need to modify the exercise, go right up to the point where your pain starts to hit a three out of 10 and/or you start to lose control, and stop there. Just work that range from no pain to mild pain, or from total control to a drop in control. As your system desensitizes and you work through the healing phases, your range of motion will gradually increase, and your control will improve. For example, if you're doing squats and going too deep hurts your knee, do partial-range squats and see if you can increase that range over time.

This applies mainly to the resistance and mobility exercises in phases 2 and 3 of the rehab protocols. Even if you're just stretching, go to the point where pain starts and don't push past it. Pushing too far into pain can aggravate many conditions. At the same time, you have to gently challenge your pain threshold to improve your flexibility and mobility. To do so, you use the familiar progressive overload (more over time) model, just with range of motion instead of load. If you're at your baseline pain level and you no longer feel mild discomfort, take the movement closer to end range until you can perform the full range of motion for the exercise.

If you are at a three out of 10—and you can maintain control—prioritize full range of motion, particularly for the start and finish positions for each exercise. Using full range of motion during resistance exercise maximizes strength and hypertrophy (muscle growth). When you're injured, you want to work toward maximizing tension in the muscle-tendon unit to promote muscle strength, and that's best achieved by performing the full range of motion.

Prioritizing full range of motion also helps with active mobility. If you want to rehabilitate a body region and reduce your risk of future injury, you need to train that region through all its available ranges of motion. This also ensures you have neuromuscular control. If you have a joint that moves 180 degrees but you can only control it through 150, you have a 30-degree range in which you are at higher risk of injury.

## How do I determine the right load for a resistance exercise?

**Choose a load (weight, band, etc.) that is challenging and fatiguing by the end of each set but doesn't create more than mild discomfort or cause you to sacrifice movement quality.**

Once you're back to baseline pain level or better, the first factor to adjust is load. If a load is easier than it was the previous week and doesn't cause you more than mild discomfort, then you can add load or reps.

Here's how to approach it: First, respect your pain, keeping it at a three out of 10 and trying not to flare it up. But, especially with resistance training, choose a load that leaves only a few reps in reserve—meaning that by the end of the set, you would be able to perform only two or three more reps. With progressive overload, you need to increase the load to keep the muscle-tendon unit continuously adapting, but you still need to consider your pain. If your pain will allow it, continue to increase the load so that you maintain the challenge that triggers positive adaptation.

For example, if the prescribed movement is a bodyweight squat and that is too easy for you, increase the load by performing a goblet squat or barbell back squat. Or modify the exercise by switching it from a bilateral (both limbs) to a unilateral (single-limb) variation—for example, bodyweight squat to single-leg squat.

If an exercise is too hard, then reduce the range of motion, slow down the movement, or stick with the phase 2 exercise that shares the same movement pattern and works the same muscles. Using the bodyweight squat example, you might choose to perform a chair squat or wall sit.

Whether you're modifying exercises to make them harder or easier, it's a balance between choosing a load that challenges your muscle-tendon unit and one that challenges the pain system. If you increase the load too fast, you may not be able to control the movement. That's why I put movement quality up there with pain as the top priorities; ensure you have those dialed in before you start increasing load.

## At what tempo should I perform the exercises?

**When it comes to movement speed (tempo), start slow, and move at a rate that allows you to maintain stability and control.**

People who are new to training or lack neuromuscular control often try to move too fast. Doing so can produce more pain because a faster tempo places more force on your tissues and makes the movement harder to control. This can increase your injury risk, especially with a load on your system.

So, if an exercise is still causing you pain after you've reduced the load and range of motion, slow it down. Slowing down improves the interaction between the sensory and motor divisions of your nervous system, which helps optimize neuromuscular control and stability. This gives you time to improve your movement quality, which often helps with pain and reduces injury risk.

Similarly, if you notice that you're losing stability or control, you're probably going too fast and need to slow down. This is especially important for people who are used to doing resistance training with heavier loads. In rehab, you need to wait until the final stages of the healing process before doing the exercise with the same speed or force you applied before getting injured.

## Can I modify an exercise, or do I need to perform it exactly as shown in the photos?

**Stance and posture are highly individualized. Choose a position that feels comfortable, doesn't cause you pain, and allows you to express your full movement potential.**

By stance, I mean your foot and hand position, such as foot flare or hand placement on the floor. By posture, I'm referring to your body position. It could be your torso angle, spinal position, or how your body changes positions during the movement.

This book provides standard starting positions, but if you need to tweak them slightly—maybe you need to turn your feet out for a squat—that's OK. Find a position that's comfortable for you while allowing you to maintain good form.

The same is true for your posture. For standing movements like squats, hip hinges, and upper body dumbbell and band exercises, try to keep your spine in neutral—the zone where you feel stable without excessively rounding or hyperextending (arching) your back. For horizontal movements where you're lying on the ground or on a bench, try to maintain the natural curvature of your spine throughout the exercise.

In other words, you can change your stance and posture slightly, even if it doesn't perfectly match the exercise images. If a certain starting position produces pain, adjust it. If a certain posture doesn't feel right, modify it. The positions shown are close to ideal, but they aren't always the best for everyone. If you need to modify something slightly based on what your body is telling you, do it—as long as you don't change the form so completely that you alter the effect of the exercise.

It might take a bit of experimentation to find the best stance and posture for you. That's the case with every exercise, whether you're doing it as a part of a rehab protocol or as a part of your normal training routine.

## The exercise doesn't feel right—it causes more than mild discomfort—even after I modify the load, range of motion, tempo, and stance. What should I do?

**If an exercise is giving you problems and making the previously suggested modifications doesn't alleviate your symptoms, skip it and add it to the next phase, or choose a different variation that shares the same movement pattern.**

If reducing the range of motion, load, and tempo and adjusting your stance and posture haven't alleviated your symptoms, temporarily remove the exercise from the program by shifting it to the next phase, or choose a different variation that shares the same movement pattern. Remember, I chose the exercises in the protocols for a reason, so try to work through the other variables first before switching an exercise.

If you do switch variations, pick one that has a similar movement pattern and trains the same muscle groups. For example, you wouldn't want to replace a quad exercise with one that works your hamstrings. If you have knee pain and a forward lunge triggers your symptoms, for example, you can try replacing the forward lunge with a reverse lunge or split squat, which changes the stress a bit. The movement pattern is similar, but it might not flare up your pain as much.

I provide variations for certain exercises in the protocols. In those cases, experiment with both versions and stick with the one that you prefer.

## Where should I direct my focus during an exercise?

**In the beginning, think about the working muscle (mind-muscle connection).**

A lot of people doing rehab for pain and injuries are thinking about other things. But the mind and body are interconnected. Research shows that when people look at and think about a muscle while it contracts, they perform better than people who are distracted.[1,2] So, in the beginning, think about the muscle and the area you're working as you perform each exercise. In rehab, we often have people look in a mirror so they can see what's going on with their body, which helps improve that mind-body connection.

As you learn to move better, however, you should start shifting your focus outward, thinking less about what's happening in a specific body region and more about the movement as a whole. For example, if you're bench-pressing to heal a pec strain or tear, you should adopt an internal focus to start, thinking about what your muscles are doing to move the bar. You're focusing on how to rehab that muscle, and you want to learn how to squeeze it and improve neuromuscular control. But as time goes on, you should develop an external focus. With a bench press, that means thinking more about moving the bar up and down.

Stated differently, thinking about the body region will help you improve your mind-muscle connection and neuromuscular control. But as you get into phase 3, you should be thinking less about the specific muscles that are contracting and more about performing each movement with good form and control. Focus on your technique and movement quality throughout the entire range of motion.

# PROGRAMMING GUIDELINES

In the rehab protocols, I include the recommended number of sets and reps and other details. Stick to these recommendations, as they are specific to the injury, pain symptoms, and prescribed exercises. The programming guidelines offered here provide a basic framework and explanation for those recommendations.

## How often should I perform the exercises?

**Perform the soft tissue mobilizations, stretching, isometric, and mobility exercises every day. Perform the resistance exercises at least three times per week with a day off between training sessions.**

Your training frequency, or how many days you perform exercises during the week, will vary based on the type of exercise. I include the training frequency for each phase of exercises within the protocols, but it's important to modify them if you experience a flare-up of symptoms.

Mobilizations and exercises that are designed to treat pain (phases 1 and 2) are typically performed every day until pain resolves and mobility improves—unless you have delayed onset muscle soreness (DOMS) or your symptoms flare up, in which case a day or two of rest between training sessions is recommended.

Do the resistance training exercises (phase 3, and sometimes in phase 2) three times per week with at least one day of rest between sessions. You can add a fourth day if you have zero pain and aren't sore after your workouts. As with the mobilizations, training frequency with resistance training will depend on whether or not the movements provoke your symptoms and how much DOMS you experience. If your pain is worse or you have more than mild muscle soreness, take another day or two off and consider implementing phase 1 exercises such as soft tissue mobilizations or a non-exercise physical activity, like walking, to help reduce soreness.

## How many sets and reps should I do?

**Stick to the recommended number of sets and reps listed in the rehab protocols.**

"Reps" refers to how many times you perform the exercise, and "sets" refers to how many times you repeat that number of repetitions. For example, say the program includes three sets of 10 reps of bodyweight squats. That means you perform 30 squats in total, resting after each round of 10.

Sets and reps vary and are listed in the protocols. However, here are the general recommendations:

- For soft tissue mobilizations (myofascial release and self-guided massage), spend one to two minutes covering an entire muscle or region, stopping for five to 10 seconds on sensitive areas.

- For nerve mobilizations and mobility exercises (PROM, AAROM, and AROM), perform three sets of 10 to 15 repetitions.

- For stretching exercises (muscle and tendon flexibility), perform two to four reps with 30- to 60-second holds.

- For isometric exercises, do four or five reps with 30- to 45-second resisted holds.

## How long should I rest between sets?

**In general, rest for 30 seconds to 1 minute between sets (or reps with stretching and isometrics).**

Rest intervals are most important with resistance exercises, as your muscles require a bit of time to recover between sets in order to maximize recruitment potential. For resistance training exercises and mobility exercises, 30 seconds to a minute is good for most people. If you're performing a stretch or an isometric hold, 15 to 30 seconds of rest is usually sufficient.

However, recovery times vary from person to person and depend on the exercise—some people need longer to recover, and some exercises require longer rest periods because they are harder. Just don't rest so long that you get cold between sets. You also don't need to be overly concerned with timing your rest periods. If you like to do it because it keeps you on track or you're susceptible to distraction, then do it. But in many cases, going by feel leads to the best results. If you listen to your body and pay attention to your pain symptoms and form, you'll know when you're recovered and ready for the next set.

It's also important to realize that you're not lifting a lot of weight when doing rehab exercises. As you progress through phase 3 and start lifting heavier weight, moving more explosively, or performing more reps, you may need longer recovery times—say, two to three minutes.

## The phase 3 exercise program is too easy or too hard. What should I do?

**Adjust the total training volume to match your fitness and experience level.**

If the exercise program is too easy—and you've already increased load, range of motion, etc.—then consider adding another training day, increasing the number of reps, or adding exercise variations that work similar muscle groups. Assuming the tissue is already healed and you are no longer in pain, you might also consider transitioning to a more comprehensive resistance training program that is specific to your goals and preferences.

If the exercise program is too hard, consider reducing the sets or reps. Instead of performing three sets of 15, you might do two sets of 10. Or continue performing the phase 2 exercises and perform only the phase 3 exercises that you feel comfortable doing. As your fitness and strength improve, add the phase 3 exercises one at a time, week by week, until you are able to complete all the exercises in phase 3.

# How do I modify a program to make it more specific to my sport?

**Once you finish or are in the late stages of rehab, modify your sets and reps to match your training focus and goals.**

In rehab, most people should stick to three sets of 10 to 15 reps. However, as you progress through phase 3, you may require more specificity, and the breakdown of sets and reps may change. For example, you might incorporate more strength, power, or endurance interventions depending on what you need to get back to full function and what impairments you have.

If you're an endurance athlete or you have an impairment associated with fatigue—meaning your muscles can't perform repeated contractions to complete a task—then you can increase your reps. For example, hamstring endurance deficits have been linked to increased muscle strain injury risk in athletes who sprint and change direction rapidly while fatigued, such as soccer players.[3] Doing more repetitions can increase endurance and make muscles more resistant to fatigue.

- **ENDURANCE:** 3–5 sets, 12–20+ reps, <65% one-rep max, 30–60 seconds of rest, 2–4 times per week

Power refers to rapid force generation, which is required in sports that involve sprinting, lifting, and other explosive movements. But it also affects non-athletes, especially those who are at risk of falling—if an 80-year-old cannot generate power in their glutes and quads quickly enough to catch themselves when they trip, they are more likely to sustain a serious injury. Some neuromuscular disorders can cause deficits in the connection between the nervous system and muscles, which also reduces power. Most power-focused exercises are normal resistance training exercises with decreased weight and increased speed. Stop the set once the tempo or movement speed slows down.

- **POWER:** 3–5 sets, 1–3 reps, 80–85% one-rep max, 2–4 minutes of rest, 2–4 times per week

Strength relates to the ability to generate maximum force. A strength impairment means you can't generate enough force to complete a task. It differs from power in that you're not moving explosively—you're just moving the heaviest weight you can by performing slow, grinding reps.

- **STRENGTH:** 3–5 sets, 1–5 reps, >85% one-rep max, 2–5 minutes of rest, 2–4 times per week

## CHAPTER 13

# TOOLS & EQUIPMENT FOR THE REHAB EXERCISES

Although most of the exercises in this book use body weight for resistance and don't require equipment, you should consider acquiring a few essential and condition-specific tools to complete the programs.

# ESSENTIAL TOOLS

At least one of these essential tools is used in every protocol. They should be available at most public gyms. That said, every exercise in the book can be done from the comfort of home—the essential tools are relatively inexpensive, easy to acquire, and don't take up a lot of space. My goal is to make rehab easy and accessible. These tools provide everything you need to complete the rehab exercises.

Some of the tools can be swapped out for household replacements. I provide equipment recommendations, alternatives, and uses.

## bench

- **RECOMMENDATION:** weight bench with a firm cushion
- **ALTERNATIVES:** table bench or sturdy chair
- **USES:** seated and supine exercises

## dowel

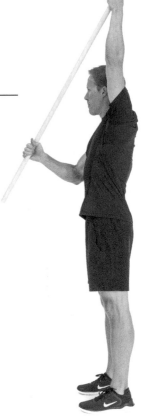

- **RECOMMENDATION:** 1-inch by 48-inch dowel
- **ALTERNATIVES:** PVC pipe, broomstick, or golf club
- **USES:** passive and active assisted range of motion exercises

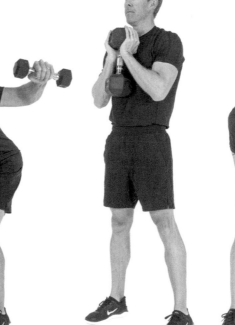

## dumbbells

- **RECOMMENDATION:** two light dumbbells (5–10 pounds) and one heavy dumbbell (25–45 pounds)—choose the brand and weight you prefer and that suits your fitness level
- **ALTERNATIVES:** kettlebell in place of a heavy dumbbell (in most cases)
- **USES:** resistance exercises

## foam roller

- **RECOMMENDATION:** long (36-inch), firm (black high-density foam), smooth roller
- **ALTERNATIVES:** soft (white) foam roller or studded roller
- **USES:** soft tissue mobilizations for large muscle groups and shoulder mobility exercises (such as angels)

## massage balls

- **RECOMMENDATION:** small massage ball (the size of a tennis or lacrosse ball) and large massage ball (the size of a softball)
- **ALTERNATIVES:** there are several brand-specific options for self-guided massage, such as Trigger Point Therapy and Yoga Tune Up—choose the brand, firmness, and texture you prefer
- **USES:** soft tissue mobilizations that target small muscle groups and insertion points

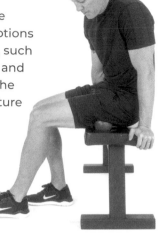

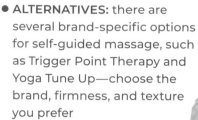

## peanut tool

- **RECOMMENDATION:** peanut massage ball roller
- **ALTERNATIVES:** tape two lacrosse balls together
- **USES:** soft tissue mobilizations for the spine (neck and back)

## physio (exercise) ball

- **RECOMMENDATION:** 55-centimeter ball—choose the brand you prefer
- **USES:** hamstring curls and core (back and abdominal) exercises

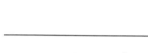

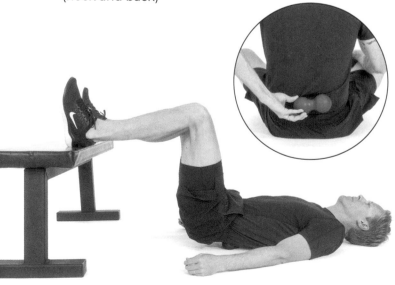

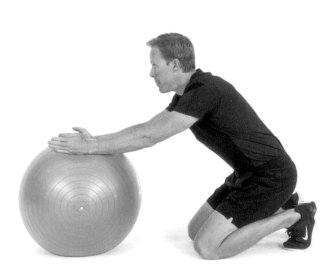

# resistance band (roll)

- **RECOMMENDATION:** Thera-Band, medium resistance (red); a 6-yard roll provides enough length to cut the needed sizes
- **ALTERNATIVES:** choose the brand, length, and resistance level you prefer
- **USES:** resistance exercises

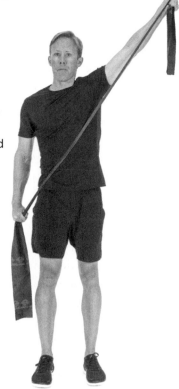

# resistance loops

- **RECOMMENDATION:** variety pack with multiple resistance levels
- **ALTERNATIVES:** thin rubber/latex (easier) or thick elastic fabric (harder)
- **USES:** hip and shoulder training exercises

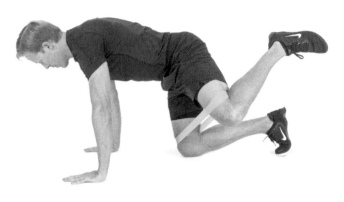

# resistance tube bands

- **RECOMMENDATION:** variety pack of resistance bands with handles in multiple resistance levels and a door anchor (if you don't have sturdy/stable attachments like a squat rack)—choose the brand you prefer
- **ALTERNATIVES:** cable machine
- **USES:** resistance exercises

# stretch strap

- **RECOMMENDATION:** nonelastic stretch strap with end loops
- **ALTERNATIVES:** belt or strap that won't break or stretch
- **USES:** stretching exercises

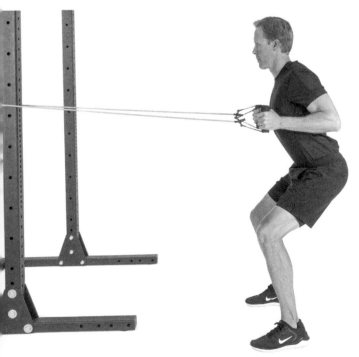

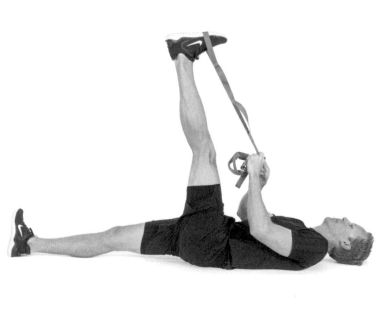

# CONDITION-SPECIFIC TOOLS

Some programs require specialized equipment to treat specific injuries. You can perform most of the programs without this equipment or swap in a household substitute.

## balance pad

- **RECOMMENDATION:** AIREX Balance-pad
- **ALTERNATIVES:** any balance pad or a thin, firm pillow or cushion
- **USES:** protecting the knees when kneeling on the floor; increasing elevation for adduction exercises

## fasciitis fighter

- **RECOMMENDATION:** Fasciitis Fighter
- **ALTERNATIVES:** rolled-up towel
- **USES:** stretching and strengthening the plantar fascia and big toe

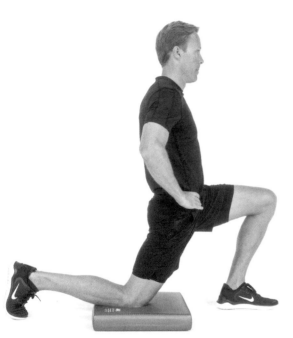

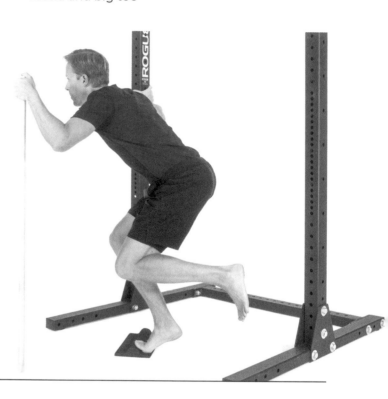

## grip strengtheners

- **RECOMMENDATION:** hand gripper for closing strength and finger extensor resistance exerciser for opening strength—choose the brand and style you prefer
- **ALTERNATIVES:** any tool or exercise that challenges the grip when opening and closing the hand
- **USES:** treating tennis elbow, golfer's elbow, and carpal tunnel syndrome; hand and finger strengthening

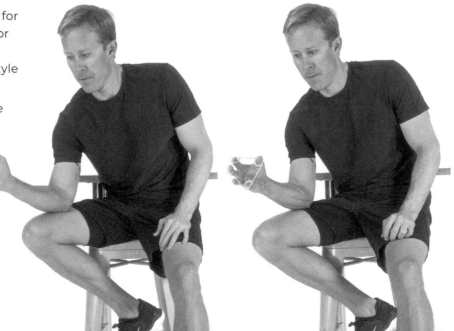

## plyometric (plyo) boxes

- **RECOMMENDATION:** two boxes that are 6 to 8 inches and 16 to 18 inches tall
- **ALTERNATIVES:** chair, step, or any stable raised surface
- **USES:** step-ups and step-downs

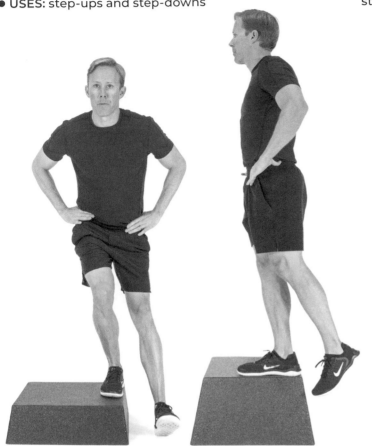

## slant board

- **RECOMMENDATION:** adjustable slant board with a nonslip surface
- **ALTERNATIVES:** any raised (3- to 6-inch) step
- **USES:** calf stretching and patellar tendon strengthening

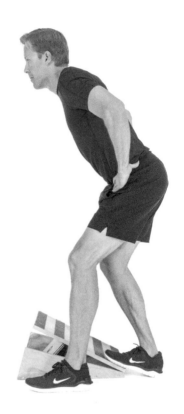

## sports ball

- **RECOMMENDATION:** soccer ball, volleyball, or basketball
- **ALTERNATIVES:** any ball that is firm and can resist inward pressure
- **USES:** adduction bridges

## yoga block

- **RECOMMENDATION:** square yoga block—choose the brand and style you prefer
- **USES:** neck soft tissue mobilizations

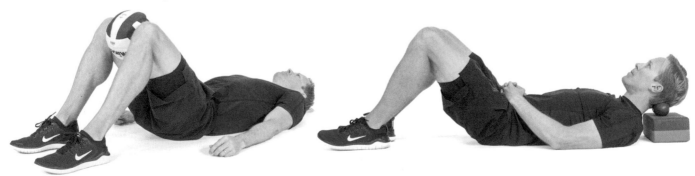

CHAPTER 14

# COMPLEMENTARY & ALTERNATIVE MEDICINE (CAM) INTERVENTIONS

Whether you're suffering from chronic pain, you were recently injured, or you're a practitioner working with somebody who is struggling with pain, you'll probably want to explore all the options available.

When it comes to the most effective treatments for pain and injury, look no further than education, graded movement, and manual therapy. However, I realize that you might want something more—something you can do in conjunction with the rehab protocols outlined in this book. Sauna, cryotherapy, acupuncture, and neuromuscular electrical stimulation, to list a few examples, are all considered complementary or alternative medicine (CAM) treatments, and they may be used to supplement the protocols.

Perhaps you have a resistant pain problem or an injury that hasn't responded well to traditional care. Or maybe you're the type of person who is willing to do anything (within reason) to stimulate healing. That's why I'm including these CAM treatments—to give you options.

I want to be clear: many of these treatments have low to moderate evidence to support their efficacy, or the research is inconclusive. Perhaps we don't know why they work, but many do seem to produce positive outcomes. And questions about these interventions come up often in my clinical practice, so I would hate to leave something out that you might be curious about.

What's more, the power of belief is real and should never be underestimated. How you think about a treatment matters. If you believe it will work—whether there's evidence to support it or not—and it isn't extremely invasive, doesn't have adverse side effects, and isn't going to drain your wallet, then I say sure, try it. If it helps you, that's great!

Now I will summarize some of the most popular CAM treatments based on what I know about them and the research that is available. It's important to realize, though, that I am not an expert in these fields. Some of them, such as acupuncture, require years of specialized education. Entire books have been written on many of these treatments. What's more, the degree of effectiveness might depend on how much you believe the treatment will work. While some interventions have some science to support them, how much they can help is still based on the individual and many other variables.

My intention is not to convince you that one is better than another or even to provide a detailed overview, but rather to help you determine what each treatment is good for, when to consider using it, and what evidence (if any) supports its efficacy.

I've broken them into three categories and listed them in a hierarchical order that I believe is logical and approachable. You or your practitioner may value one over another or have a better experience with an intervention listed lower or in another category, and that is perfectly fine. Do what's best for you and your unique circumstances. If a CAM treatment is presented here, then chances are it can be helpful in some way.

# TRY THESE TREATMENTS FIRST

Interventions from this category include treatments that I have found to be helpful for my patients, are fairly easy to access and generally affordable, and have some research support behind them.

## CROSS-TRANSFER

Cross-transfer is a unique phenomenon by which, when training one limb, transfer occurs through neural connections in the brain and spinal cord, resulting in changes in the untrained opposite limb.[1-5] This fascinating effect can be used to reduce strength deficits in an injured extremity or after surgery.

For people who have injuries or pain—especially in the acute window when they can't move very well—I almost always recommend not only to keep training the whole body, but also to train the opposite limb because it will influence the side that can't currently be used. Say your right arm is immobilized in a cast or brace. Continuing to do curls, presses, rows, and so on with your left arm will help reduce the severity of the strength deficits that occur on the immobilized side.

A lot of people who get injured simply stop moving, which is not ideal. But cross-transfer primes your nervous system for when you do that exercise with the injured side. The nervous system "informs" the other side and gives you a feel for the activity, which makes it easier to recruit the affected limb.

This doesn't mean you want to ignore the injured side. You want to get to a point where you can do equal weight on both sides. That's why I encourage everyone to go through the protocols with a "both sides" mentality. There's no downside and probably a major upside thanks to cross-transfer. Whatever rehab protocol you're using and whatever phase you're in, you can use the uninvolved side to inform your involved limb. It will help the whole protocol, and it also helps with both the mental and the physical sides of the healing process.

## MENTAL IMAGERY

Visualization in rehab typically involves thinking about moving an injured or painful body region either when it cannot be moved (such as after surgery) or when actual movement induces severe pain. Imagining movement activates similar neural networks to those used when actually moving and can be a helpful complement to the rehab process when movement isn't possible. Humans are visual beings, and studies have shown that mental imagery exercises can reduce injury-related anxiety and the amount of strength that is lost in individuals who are injured and immobilized.[6-11]

Especially if you're in phase 1, you should spend time imagining using the injured or painful limb or joint in the complex ways you would've before your injury, just to fire up those mental circuits. This will help when you're doing a workout, too. There is value in imagining using that area in its normal ways to enhance your recovery.

Say your right knee is injured and you can't bend it fully. Just sitting and bending the left side for a few reps, and then thinking about doing so on your right side, will fire up the neuromuscular circuits that get that joint moving. It incorporates cross-transfer to create a positive experience that makes it easier to form that mind-body connection.

## BLOOD FLOW RESTRICTION

This treatment is becoming more popular in rehab, and it can be useful for people who are injured, especially in the acute pain window when you can't fully load the tissue.[12-16] I see it a lot with ACL tears when patients start quad strengthening.

Blood flow restriction (BFR) occludes mainly venous blood flow, which causes blood to pool in the limb. That pooling creates a buildup of metabolites, which means you can lower the load of the exercise—it could be a resistance-type exercise or even an aerobic exercise that works the muscles in that region—and induce the same changes in strength and hypertrophy. That's awesome because you often can't add much weight during the initial healing phases.

Basically, a strap is fastened around either an arm or a leg, usually close to the top of the limb—up by the armpit or high on the thigh. That way, it will provide benefits farther downstream. It might not help something like a rotator cuff tear, which is above where the strap would go, but it can help an injury farther down.

Say you had an ACL reconstruction and haven't been cleared to do bodyweight squats yet. You could put on a BFR strap while you're doing easy bodyweight leg extensions. The exercise will feel much more challenging because of the pooling blood and metabolites that come from working the area. That, in turn, stimulates muscle growth and increases strength while putting less mechanical strain on your body. This is most helpful in phase 1 or maybe at the end of phase 2, depending on the diagnosis.

Remember, you need to position the strap correctly and get the pressure right; it can be dangerous if you occlude an artery. So, it's best to visit an experienced practitioner who can show you how to do blood flow restriction properly.

# HEAT

Heat is thought to increase circulation and reduce pain, which may speed healing.[17-20] Research suggests that localized heat such as from a heating pad activates heat-sensitive calcium channels, and when those are activated, they inhibit peripheral receptors, which are involved in nociception, or the process by which danger messages travel up the spinal cord to the brain.[21,22] Other heat sources like saunas (which I'll discuss next) may have similar effects.

Heat also makes tissue more elastic. Like with a good warm-up prior to an exercise session, increasing tissue temperature and elasticity may reduce injury risk when performing mobility and resistance training drills. This can be especially useful when working through the early phases of a protocol.

Many studies suggest that sauna use can reduce muscle atrophy.[23-26] This can help in the acute phase if, for example, you are post-surgery and have doctor approval that you're not at risk for infection. Even if you can't do resistance training, sauna can potentially help you hang on to muscle longer.

There's also an inflammation management strategy involving ancient stressors, or stressors our hunter-gatherer ancestors used to encounter often but don't come up as much now. Extreme temperature is one of them. Exposing yourself to extreme heat, whether it's a hot yoga studio or a sauna, may provide the right dosage of stress to activate protective mechanisms in your body. Supposedly, it activates genetic pathways related to longevity and health that reduce inflammation. (Extreme cold can do it, too.) And reducing inflammation can improve lots of health factors, including cardiovascular health.[27-30]

Remember, acute inflammation is a normal immune response—when you sprain your ankle, for example, inflammation occurs and the injured area gets warm, which helps you heal. Sauna use is more beneficial for chronic inflammatory states, where the immune system remains active and continues to produce inflammation past that acute window. That's when we start to see diseases that have a chronic inflammatory component, which is why sauna can be useful for people who have had longer, persistent, chronic pain.

This book is largely focused on mechanical, nociceptive-type pains, but a lot of chronic pain disorders are thought to have a chronic inflammatory component. So, if sauna or extreme heat exposure does help reduce pain, it's worth trying. Even if it doesn't, it certainly can't hurt. You get all the health benefits—specifically reducing muscle atrophy and inflammation while improving cardiovascular health—and you're not having to move if you're in that early window when you're building yourself back up.

If you have chronic pain or you're in the early phases of an injury, sauna is one of the few interventions that's easy for most people. Plus, it has a variety of health benefits even if you're not injured and is relatively low cost and low risk (assuming you don't have an open wound and are cleared by a doctor).

# NEUROMUSCULAR ELECTRICAL STIMULATION (NMES)

Neuromuscular electrical stimulation, aka e-stim, is often used to control pain and swelling with recent injuries. Basically, a machine delivers electrical currents to a patient's tissues as a means of increasing muscle strength and reducing pain.

The e-stim unit used to treat acute pain and swelling is called a TENS unit, which stands for transcutaneous electrical nerve stimulation. These units can provide temporary relief but are not typically effective from a long-term standpoint.[31-33]

To use e-stim, you stick pads onto your skin, usually around the region that's injured, and follow the instructions provided with the unit. It's thought to help with pain by temporarily distracting the nervous system from nociception. This new sensory input travels

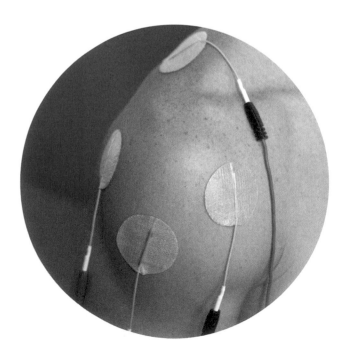

through myelinated neurons, which have faster conduction velocities than nociceptors. As a result, e-stim for pain is only going to help while you have it on or for up to 15 minutes afterward.

Electrical stimulation for strengthening and neuromuscular recruitment, however, shows better results. Research has indicated that when e-stim is combined with traditional physical therapy, strength gains can be greater following some orthopedic surgeries compared to physical therapy without e-stim.[34-36] Say you've had an injury that caused your nervous system to inhibit your quads, meaning you're having a hard time recruiting them for movement—in that case, e-stim is like an external brain. If your brain won't turn those muscles on, you can use the machine to help activate your quads by using certain currents.

We typically use Russian or high-voltage currents for strengthening. You turn them up until the person's muscle contracts on its own. And then you have them do the exercise so they're doing something active when the e-stim turns on, and it helps them the same way cross-transfer does. You're hijacking the nervous system to improve activation and recruitment, which enables greater improvements during rehab.

In either of these scenarios, e-stim alone will not solve your problem. But there's very little harm in trying it, especially for strengthening and improving neuromuscular recruitment after surgery.

# COMPRESSION GARMENTS

Although more research on compression garments is needed, much of the research that does exist follows strenuous bouts of exercise and has found that compression garments can reduce an individual's perception of the severity of delayed onset muscle soreness (DOMS).[37-39] Some studies have even found that, after strenuous exercise, these garments accelerated functional muscle recovery (measured by power and maximum force output) and reduced concentrations of creatine kinase (which is produced with muscle breakdown). This is likely due to the fact that these garments help with venous return, meaning they get blood pumping back to the heart instead of pooling in the tissue. This is especially true of graduated compression, where it's squeezing more distally and forcing blood proximally toward the heart.

To be clear, most of these studies used high-tech compression systems, which are expensive devices that fill up with air—the kind you usually see in a physical therapy or sports performance clinic. Not all compression garments are created equal. Again, these studies also examined subjects following strenuous exercise and looked at how compression affects muscle soreness and recovery.

When it comes to injury and pain rehabilitation, the application of compression can be quite helpful. After a traumatic injury, most orthopedic healthcare practitioners recommend limb elevation and compression.[40] Compression for the acute phase of an injury is traditionally thought to reduce swelling and restore movement. We're all familiar with the ACE bandage, for example. Another example is the post-injury compression sleeve, which people often wear to improve circulation, proprioception, and joint stability. If you have an ankle or knee sprain, or even an irritated meniscus or arthritis flare-up in a joint—anything with swelling—compression does seem to help push fluid out of the area and allow for greater joint mobility.

There are best practices for how to wrap, too. Generally, start tighter. If you sprained your ankle, for example, begin near your toes, where the wrap should be a little tighter, and slowly loosen it so that it becomes less tight as it goes up your ankle. You're trying to move fluid through your veins back toward your heart.

Remember, you don't want to see discoloration, bruising, or redness below the compression site. If you see that, it's probably too tight where you started. After an injury, you may want to leave the compression device on for an extended period, and there's no real danger in doing so if it's not wrapped too tightly. You should be able to press on your skin and watch it lighten before blood returns. If you see discoloration, you're likely blocking blood flow, which means it's too tight for extended use.

If you're worried about doing it wrong, buy a graduated compression sock or sleeve. But keep in mind that a wrap gives you more control over the degree of compression, and you can do a more aggressive, moderate, or slight compression for different periods of time. Also, be aware that most compression sleeves are not strong enough to stabilize a joint. They're not going to hold your bones together if you've had a ligament injury, which is why implementing the strengthening exercises in the protocols is so important. Our muscles are our internal stabilizers!

# ACUPUNCTURE AND DRY NEEDLING

Acupuncture comes from traditional Chinese medicine and involves the use of needles, meaning it's a little more invasive than some other CAMs. This makes some people shy away from it, while others believe it's more likely to have a positive effect.

Acupuncture and dry needling are similar in a lot of ways, but acupuncture is an Eastern medicine technique that uses meridians and energy (rather than muscle and nerve anatomy) to determine where the needles are placed. This means, in terms of the research, acupuncture is a bit more controversial.

For example, there are studies showing that real and simulated acupuncture produce similar results.[41-43] Still, some people believe it helps them. And some studies show that, for problems like low back pain, neck pain, osteoarthritis of the knee, and certain types of headaches, acupuncture can be a good complement to physical therapy.[44-46] Again, if the potential for adverse side effects is low and the intervention isn't horribly expensive, it might be worth a try.

Dry needling is essentially the same thing; it just follows a different school of thought for implementation—dry needling is targeted and deeper and mainly for muscles. Needles are inserted into the muscle belly, the surrounding fascia, or in proximity to nerves to treat musculoskeletal pain and improve function. Some studies suggest that dry needling is not more effective than sham treatment and should not be considered as a first line of defense, and others have found it to be superior to sham.[47-49]

# THINK ABOUT THESE TREATMENTS NEXT

The interventions in this section have less research support, tend to cost more, and only help people occasionally (and are highly tied to placebo).

## TAPE

Tape is primarily used in rehab to enhance joint stability, reduce pain, and serve as a tactile cue to maintain a particular postural position, such as sitting up straight.

Although the use of tape to treat various pain conditions is controversial, the skin is an organ with millions of nerve endings, and so many interventions involve touching the skin because doing so can modulate the pain experience. Tape provides sensory feedback to your skin, which might change pain, and that could alter your motor response by introducing novel sensory information.[50] As with other CAM interventions such as compression sleeves, the psychological side is important to consider. Some people feel more secure in their body when wearing tape, and the fact is, placebo likely explains much of the effects we see.[51]

Also, there are different types of tape. Leukotape is a strong product that can be used on your kneecap to help ease patellofemoral pain. In this case, you push the kneecap, glide it into a slightly different position, and tape it, and there is evidence that the tape can help reduce pain for some people.[52] Then you have stretchy tapes like Kinesio tape, where it's probably more of a tactile sensory feedback effect, like posture taping.

Posture taping really seems to help some people. You might have them sit up straight and then apply tape down their back in two lines. Every time they slouch or move into a position that was previously painful, the tape pulls on their skin. They can still adopt the painful posture; the tape is not going to hold them up. But it can be helpful as a sensory feedback reminder.

## INSTRUMENT-ASSISTED SOFT TISSUE MOBILIZATION (IASTM)

Coming from traditional Chinese medicine, IASTM is a soft tissue mobilization technique in which specially designed instruments are used to treat myofascial restrictions (scar tissue, adhesions, and so on) with the goal of reducing pain, improving range of motion, and improving overall function. Evidence is still emerging, but some studies suggest that IASTM may be useful for improving short-term joint range of motion.[53-55]

Say you had surgery and have a large scar. IASTM would involve scraping around the perimeter of that scar to help treat the pain. Keep in mind, it does not penetrate deeply like a deep tissue massage. It really is just scraping the surface, the idea being to clear underlying adhesions so the skin "slides" against the fascia and other tissues more easily. Although there isn't much evidence to support these claims, IASTM is relatively low cost and is not going to cause much damage. Some people with conditions like plantar fasciitis have found it helpful. And pushing on areas that are sore can feel good.

If you have pain that's resistant to other interventions, and you feel as if you've tried everything else without improvement, you can give something like IASTM a try. But again, remember to approach it like an experiment: add one new variable at a time and see if it changes anything.

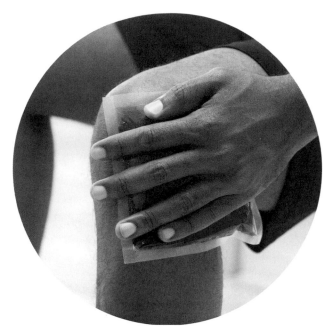

## ICE

While applying an ice pack used to be a staple part of an injury treatment plan, this strategy is no longer recommended as new research has shown that ice blunts the inflammatory phase of healing and may slow a person's return to full function. When ice is applied to an injury, it slows the infiltration of immune cells such as macrophages, which clean up damaged tissue and start the healing process.[56,57]

This change seems to be most appropriate for less severe soft tissue injuries (think grade I). When it comes to more severe strains and tears (grades II and III) and after surgery, ice may still be useful to control swelling and reduce pain. In fact, several studies have shown that applying ice after ACL reconstruction surgery leads to a significant reduction in knee pain and the use of pain medications.[58,59] Other research has shown that using ice to slow the inflammatory response after a muscle injury can help reduce secondary injuries.[60]

Full disclosure: I haven't used ice on myself in a long time. If I get injured, I'm more apt to rest the area for a few days and then gradually start adding movement; that's just my personal preference. That said, to throw out ice completely based on a few recent studies may not be appropriate. A large body of research suggests that ice does reduce pain and can help keep swelling from getting out of control and causing secondary problems.[61]

As with all treatments, there's a continuum of possible ways to use ice. If you have a grade I injury, you may not want to ice it. Maybe the inflammation is appropriate for what's happening and will be helpful. But if you have a grade III injury with a torn ligament, applying ice for a few days might help stop the inflammatory process from going overboard.

## COLD WATER IMMERSION AND CRYOTHERAPY

Many people believe that whole-body cryotherapy is better than localized icing for reducing systemic inflammation, swelling, and pain and boosting recovery. Whole-body cryo with cold, dry air has less research behind it, which is partly due to the fact that it is newer. Cold water immersion has better support, especially when looking at athletic recovery and strategies that can reduce fatigue and soreness.[62]

In these studies, people are taken through a strenuous workout and then are either exposed to whole-body cryo or cold water immersion. When the results are compared, cold water immersion comes out on top with those people showing a decreased perception of fatigue and soreness and lower inflammatory markers.[62-64]

That said, for conditions like arthritis, whole-body cryo isn't usually found to be better than traditional rehab movements such as strengthening and stretching. But I've worked with osteoarthritis patients who believe it is helpful, and, as with a lot of these treatments, there might be benefits beyond the scope of injury and pain. Some people even claim it can be used to treat depression because it provides a shock to the nervous system.

This is a treatment that is relatively easy to access and doesn't cost much, so it might be worth trying. Keep in mind, though, that it probably won't dramatically accelerate healing or eliminate pain permanently.

# MEDICATION

Many different medications can help with injury, many of which are available over the counter. But keep in mind that almost all of them have negative side effects, and I don't recommend using them without first consulting a doctor.

Most of the time, when I refer to over-the-counter medications, it's either pain medication or anti-inflammatory medication. Ibuprofen is one of the more common anti-inflammatory medications and often works well in terms of reducing pain-related symptoms. Most people are aware that ibuprofen typically comes in 200-milligram tablets, and physicians usually prescribe three of those or provide a prescription for stronger ibuprofen at 600 milligrams per tablet.

Tylenol is another popular pain medication, but many people don't realize it is not an anti-inflammatory; it simply helps with pain. There are also prescription-strength medications, like muscle relaxants. Some people need muscle relaxants for specific conditions, but those are prescribed by a physician.

The medications that are most often used in the musculoskeletal world are nonsteroidal anti-inflammatory drugs, or NSAIDs, which include ibuprofen and naproxen. When I say "medication" in a treatment strategy, I'm talking about NSAIDs.

So, specific anti-inflammatory medications seem to be helpful in certain cases—say you tweaked your back and have sciatica pain radiating into your leg, or you spent the day walking more than normal and your plantar fascia or Achilles tendon is irritated. In these situations, limited ibuprofen use might be appropriate.

However, in rehab, we generally try to stay away from these meds because even the mildest anti-inflammatory drugs have negative side effects when they're taken chronically. Ibuprofen, for example, can lower testosterone, impair healing, and cause stomach issues.[65-69] You don't want to be on anti-inflammatory meds for a long time, but if you need to use them to calm things down, it's generally OK to do so. Just make sure it's temporary in the acute phase to manage the early pain and inflammation so that you can start doing some of the phase 1 exercises.

But—and I can't emphasize this enough—it's important to talk to a doctor before taking any medication. There are lots of medications available, and even over-the-counter medications or supplements can have unpredictable interactions.

As with every part of this CAM section, I'm simply listing the pieces that are common in a treatment strategy (inside or outside of a doctor's care), but I can't tell you if taking a medication is right for you. I recommend doing the rehab exercises (unless they make the problem worse or a red flag shows up, in which case you should seek medical care immediately) because that is the best way to bounce back from an injury and alleviate pain. I'm simply saying that medication might be part of the treatment strategy under a doctor's care. Always check with your physician first.

# STEROID INJECTIONS

You may hear these called cortisone injections, corticosteroid injections, and so on, but they're all steroid injections. A physician—often an orthopedic surgeon or someone who specializes in pain medicine, like an anesthesiologist—injects a steroid into a localized area to reduce pain and inflammation. And such injections do have strong evidence to support their use in certain phases of healing and for specific issues.

Frozen shoulder is a good example. If it's caught early, in the acute phase 1, research suggests that cortisone injections can help keep frozen shoulder from progressing into the later stages or becoming more severe.[70] With most other issues, it's generally recommended that you go through six to eight weeks of physical therapy before seeking an injection.

For instance, say you tear your meniscus or rotator cuff and the pain is related to inflammation. If it doesn't improve to an acceptable degree after six to eight weeks of physical therapy, then a steroid injection might be the first medical intervention recommended before surgery.

One problem with steroid injections is the highly varied durations of effectiveness, which may have to do with how many shots a person has had and the nature of the injury. With some people, the problem never comes back. With others, relief may last only for a week or two.

Steroid injections are like a bandage—it's helping, but if the issue keeps getting aggravated, it's not going to heal. And then the inflammation will come back. But for a lot of people, a shot knocks the inflammation down enough that they can continue physical therapy, do mobility and strength training, and implement behavior modification—whatever they need to do to let that tissue calm down so they can build it back up.

This is a truly complementary treatment, as it can be done during or after several weeks of therapy. If the area is still painful—it's gotten better, but not enough—you can get a cortisone injection and then see if it calms the pain enough to get you past that hurdle so you can enter a true buildup phase.

But what happens if you do a cortisone injection and the pain comes back? Is it OK to get another one knowing that it worked the first time and then try to identify some aggravating factors and see if it works again? How many cycles will be recommended before surgery becomes a more effective option?

You don't want to get too many steroid injections because they can weaken connective tissue, possibly to the point of contributing to a tendon tear in extreme cases.[71,72] If you have an injury that's appropriate for this treatment, start with one injection. Deciding whether to get a second shot will depend on how long the first one helped. If it helped you for only a week, it probably doesn't make sense to get another one. In fact, many medical professionals won't give you another shot for a while; most orthopedic surgeons will let you do a maximum of three in a year because of the negative side effects. Some athletes want injections so that they can return to play, but due to the risk to the connective tissue, I do not recommend this practice.

So, if you had a steroid shot, and it helped for three months but the pain came back, maybe a second injection would be reasonable. But you would need to base it on how you responded to that first one and consult your doctor.

# SHOCKWAVE THERAPY

Shockwave is like ultrasound, but it's a much higher-energy acoustic wave—some studies have shown it to be a thousand times stronger.[73] You can direct those acoustic waves into musculoskeletal tissue, which is thought to induce a microtrauma and stimulate the healing response.

It's hard to say whether shockwave therapy promotes healing, but it supposedly reduces pain and has been used for plantar fasciitis, tennis elbow, Achilles and patellar tendinopathy, accumulated calcium deposits on tendons, and bone injuries. There are numerous studies supporting its use, but for painful conditions such as tennis elbow, other studies show that shockwave therapy is no more effective than a placebo.[73-77]

# PLATELET-RICH PLASMA (PRP) INJECTION

With a PRP injection, a doctor draws your blood, pulls out the platelets or thrombocytes, which are cells involved in growth and healing, and then injects this platelet concentration back into an area to theoretically help reduce pain and encourage tissue regeneration.

PRP is said to help a number of conditions, including tennis elbow (lateral epicondylitis), rotator cuff tears, Achilles tendon injuries, and knee osteoarthritis.[78-80] But this is another intervention that, if it worked as well as advertised, we'd hear a lot more people talking about having it done. In reality, evidence supporting it is limited.

But PRP may work better than we know, especially for resistant injuries that aren't responding well to traditional rehab. I know a couple of physicians who really believe in PRP, but researchers haven't been able to reproduce studies because the preparation protocols weren't documented thoroughly enough.[81]

So, PRP could be useful for conditions that aren't healing well. I would certainly try PRP before surgery. If you've done eight to twelve weeks of rehab consistently, and the only option left is surgery, options like PRP and stem cell (discussed later in this chapter) are less invasive and could help with pain. Just keep in mind there is not much hard evidence suggesting that it accelerates injury recovery.

## BRACES

Braces have a specific use, and they can be used incorrectly. The problem is that some people wear them habitually to reduce or prevent pain and end up developing disuse atrophy and deconditioning problems because the musculotendinous system, which is our natural bracing system, is no longer being challenged. Your muscles, tendons, and ligaments are your built-in braces. Most of the time, you shouldn't use an external brace, and if you do need to, you should use it only temporarily.

If you're relying on back braces, elbow braces, patella or tendon braces, or solid metal knee braces, you are probably going to create some deconditioning in your neuromuscular system. If you need to use a brace temporarily after surgery, immediately after an injury, or for

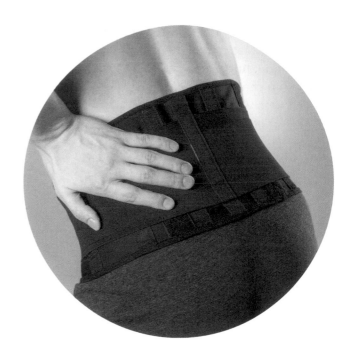

some activity where injury risk is higher, that's fine. But most of the time, your focus should be on building the capacity of your system so that you don't have to wear a brace. This book has programs that will help you enhance your tissues so that you don't have to rely on an external brace for stability or control.

# CONSIDER THESE TREATMENTS LAST

The interventions in this section have either poor clinical efficacy or minimal research support to date and, in some cases, are very expensive and difficult to access.

## STEM CELL THERAPY

Stem cells are specialized cells that have the ability to transform into other cell types, such as bone, muscle, or nerve cells. Because of this capability, researchers and clinicians are hopeful that stem cells will be able to be used to regenerate and repair injured or diseased tissues. When it comes to orthopedic injuries, stem cell therapy involves using a syringe to remove bone marrow from the pelvic bone. Stem cells are then

harvested from the bone marrow and injected into an area where an injury has occurred. This therapy can be used on numerous joints and tissues, including shoulders, knees, hips, muscles, ligaments, and bones.

I know physicians who have spent their lives studying regenerative medicine and believe in stem cell therapy for certain conditions. But when you look at the research, it typically says, "Largely safe. Tends to create positive outcomes, but the quality of the current research is poor."[82,83]

The main problem is that a lot of the studies don't incorporate a control group using a sham intervention. And if you don't have a control group, you can't really prove anything. That's the problem with pain: if people think they're getting an effective intervention, they usually feel better. The best research, which provides the best evidence, always includes a control group.

Most of the stem cell therapies offered in the US are orthopedic injections using mesenchymal stem cells pulled from adult fat, bone marrow, muscle, and other tissue. And drawing these cells, especially from bone marrow, can be extremely painful. Stem cell IV treatment is another option, but it is only available outside the US at the time of this publishing.

Is stem cell therapy worth trying? Maybe. You hear stories of people who claim it really helped or even cured their pain. There could be a group that has a great way of doing it or a concentration that's super effective, but it hasn't been studied enough to nail down the ideal preparation and method.

# PEPTIDE THERAPY

This type of therapy is even more controversial than stem cell treatment. Most of the studies are still done on rats, and when you buy peptides, the label usually says, "Not for human use." But there are a ton of studies on rats, especially regarding the stomach and GI system.

Basically, a peptide chain is extracted from a protective protein in the stomach and then injected into your body. When administered to rats, peptide therapy seems to help the gut-brain axis with healing, angiogenesis (sprouting new blood vessels), and a lot of issues related to the stomach and intestinal tract. There are some rat studies that show ligament and tendon regeneration and healing too—specifically, the peptide known as BPC-157 may have this effect.[84-86]

Peptide therapy is so controversial because there are thousands of peptides, and anybody can make them. Who knows what will happen when you start to play with the switches and mechanisms in the human body? This is a new field of study, and the FDA is not likely to approve peptides anytime soon because they're not proprietary. Anybody can do peptide therapy, and that has produced some slightly sketchy results.

Even so, a lot of regenerative medicine doctors prescribe peptides from compounding pharmacies—labs that test the compounds for purity—and many people are willing to accept the potential risks.

If testing improves and studies on human subjects begin, peptide therapy could be the future of regenerative medicine. We just don't know yet.

# ULTRASOUND

Ultrasound has what is referred to as a piezoelectric effect, where crystals inside the ultrasound head vibrate and create an acoustic wave that's directed into tissue. And obviously it works because it's used for medical imaging. Not just for pregnancy either; ultrasound is used often in musculoskeletal medicine because it lets you see certain injuries without having an MRI.

Some clinicians use ultrasound in practice to help reduce pain. It's thought to create a deeper heating of the tissue, depending on which frequency is used. There are two frequencies to which the machine can be set, and that setting determines how many centimeters the wave supposedly penetrates the tissue.

But in tests against a sham ultrasound, actual ultrasound usually scores about the same as the control group—meaning it doesn't hold up as an evidence-based treatment, and any benefits are likely attributable to the placebo effect.[87-92]

# CUPPING

Full disclosure: I haven't tried cupping myself, but it is mostly used for muscles and myofascial issues. Much of the higher-quality research (randomized, placebo-controlled trials) shows that cupping isn't more effective than sham cupping, which suggests that placebo plays a major role in this intervention.[93,94]

Put simply, a practitioner attaches suction cups that pull the skin up into the cup. Some cups are heat-based while others are connected to an air chamber to create suction. Cupping is thought to help with pain, inflammation, blood flow, and relaxation. It's an old technique and can be done using different types of suction cups and wet and dry methods.

To further explain how it works, let me use a firsthand example. A patient of mine had a wrist fracture—she fell off a bike and broke the bone, then had it surgically repaired using internal fixation with hardware. Like many people who injure their joints, she was having a hard time regaining range of motion, with only about 50 percent of her usual wrist mobility eight weeks after surgery.

When she tried cupping for the first time, it was with a practitioner who used a needle to go into the joint capsule and then applied a suction cup. As the cup came off, it pulled up a disc of blood. Then he wiped it away, claiming it was wiping away inflammation. And she was left with the telltale circle on her wrist.

From a pain standpoint, cupping does not have a lot of research to support it, but many people believe it helps. Like a lot of these interventions, it may interact with the skin and deeper tissues, where there are lots of free nerve endings and receptors that can influence pain, which is highly subjective. Studies on cupping aren't common, but many people in the pain science world believe it's probably the placebo effect at work.

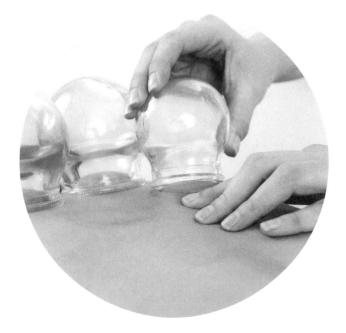

But what's interesting is that in my example—which was related not to pain but to mobility—the patient saw a significant improvement in her range of motion after cupping. She gained 10 degrees in her wrist flexion and extension. Now, that's just one person, but I think it'd be an interesting intervention to study for people who have mobility restrictions after surgery.

In the end, if you want to add cupping to your exercise routine, go ahead. It's probably just influencing sensory receptors in the skin, but if it helps, it helps.

# HYPERBARIC OXYGEN

With this intervention, you are put in a chamber where you breathe 100 percent oxygen, which leads to a higher saturation of oxygen in your blood. There's a lot of research into hyperbaric oxygen (HBO) as a treatment for wounds such as burns, nervous system injuries like stroke, traumatic brain injury, and other major tissue damage.[95-98] In the musculoskeletal system, HBO has been used with peripheral nerve injuries, exercise-induced muscle damage, and various other injuries, such as ankle sprains and medial collateral ligament (MCL) tears in the knee. The results of these studies are mixed, with some showing positive results and others showing no difference between HBO and sham treatment.[99-102]

The theory is sound. Hyperbaric oxygen works because blood flow is hugely important to healing. Nutrient delivery is one factor, but the other is how much oxygen is getting to the tissue and cells. And that's where hyperbaric oxygen helps.

Your cells rely on oxygen, and a lack of oxygen for too long—called hypoxia—leads to cell death. So, boosting oxygen is going to help that tissue stay aerobic, which is going to benefit you as a whole.

However, in most cases, you need extended and continued treatments to reap the benefits. And it's unclear if hyperbaric oxygen (HBO) dramatically improves healing following a musculoskeletal injury. Plus, you have to go to a treatment center that has an HBO chamber; it takes time, and it's definitely not cheap.

# TRY IT...WITHIN REASON

Some people want to try every intervention under the sun. So, is it OK to try as many CAM treatments as possible to see what works, or is it better to stick with one at a time? Well, it depends.

One of the best things about CAM treatments is that they can usually be integrated into a rehab program without compromising the protocol. This is especially true with at-home treatments like cross-transfer training, mental imagery, icing, and compression. But whatever you do, stick with the protocols first—continue the therapy and interventions that we know will work.

I encourage you to think of your rehab strategy as an experiment in getting rid of pain and recovering. As with any experiment, if you add too many variables, you won't know what may be effecting a change. Not knowing which treatment was the most effective makes it harder to self-manage pain if it comes up again. Also, interventions can sometimes cause pain flare-ups, and if you add a bunch right before a flare-up, you'll have a hard time pinpointing what caused it.

As a general guideline, for any treatment that requires outside help (think dry needling,

cryotherapy, platelet-rich plasma injections, and so on), add one intervention at a time and track your symptoms. That way, you know which treatment was the most useful for you (or which one caused pain). However, you may choose to combine the CAM treatments that are accessible and easy to do on your own.

For example, maybe you're in that acute pain window—the inflammatory phase 1. Perhaps you sprained your ankle and have severe swelling, and you're planning to rest and then do the necessary movements to help it heal. But you also read that e-stim and compression can help, so you want to try those things to manage the swelling. You have time on your hands, so you decide to do some cross-transfer and mental imagery practice as well. That's OK. These interventions won't hurt and might even help alleviate pain and accelerate healing.

But remember that most musculoskeletal issues get better with time and movement. Don't assume that simply sticking with the protocols will slow the healing process. Even if you don't do these extra CAM activities, you will heal.

# CONCLUDING THOUGHTS: SIMPLE COMPLEMENTS FOR COMPLICATED PAIN

It probably sounds as though I'm dismissing a lot of these interventions, but that's not my intention. I think anything that helps and doesn't hurt is worthwhile, even if the clinical evidence doesn't currently support it. I just want you to have all the facts before trying something.

Again, your beliefs play a huge role in pain. If you like doing something and it helps you—and doesn't carry the risk of causing harm—keep doing it. Just bear in mind that the rehab protocol should be your primary focus, and you don't want to overdo it with too many CAM interventions at once. As with the protocols, I recommend that you consult with a specialist before you implement any CAM treatment, especially after a traumatic injury or surgery.

## CHAPTER 15

# HEAD & NECK PROTOCOLS

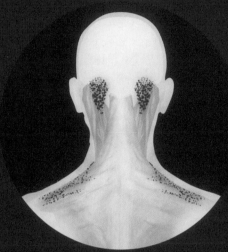

**NECK PAIN**
(p. 147)

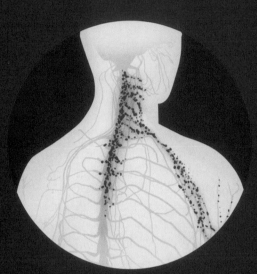

**NERVE PAIN**
(p. 161)

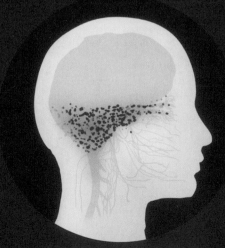

**HEADACHE PAIN**
(p. 172)

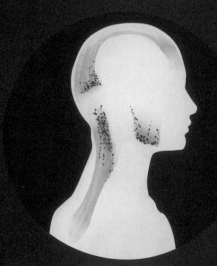

**JAW PAIN**
(p. 180)

# NECK PAIN

**Follow this program to treat:**

- General neck pain and stiffness (back and side)
- Neck strains and sprains (whiplash)
- Cervical spondylosis (arthritis)

## GENERAL (NON-SPECIFIC) NECK PAIN

**DESCRIPTION:** Approximately 22 to 70 percent of people will experience neck pain at some point in their lives.[1] In most cases, a specific nociceptive source of the pain (disc, muscle, joint, etc.) cannot be determined. Medical and rehab providers chose the term *non-specific* to describe general pain that exists when an obvious source cannot be linked to a person's symptoms. More than one-third of individuals with non-specific neck pain have lingering or recurring symptoms after one year, and in some cases, the pain becomes chronic.[2,3]

**SIGNS AND SYMPTOMS:** Typically, non-specific neck pain is dull, achy pain along the sides or back of the neck or in the shoulder or upper back region, but the location of symptoms varies. Symptoms may become sharp with certain movements and limit range of motion.

**AGGRAVATING FACTORS:** Non-specific neck pain is often unrelated to injuries (strains, disc herniations, etc.). It may be influenced by other factors, such as stress, sleep, and general physical activity level,[4] so pay attention not only to the physical movements and positions that make your pain worse, but also to the less obvious factors that can influence pain (see Chapter 4).

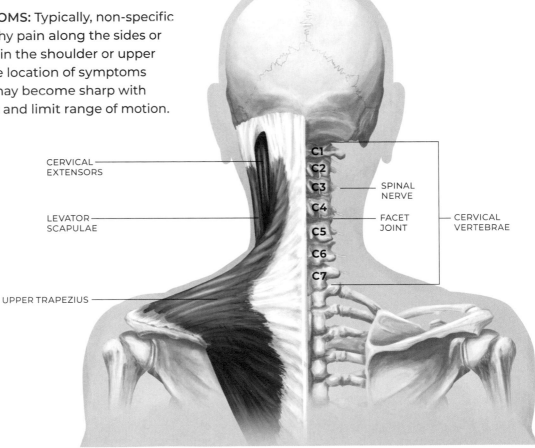

CERVICAL EXTENSORS

LEVATOR SCAPULAE

UPPER TRAPEZIUS

C1
C2
C3
C4
C5
C6
C7

SPINAL NERVE

FACET JOINT

CERVICAL VERTEBRAE

**PROGNOSIS:** Most general neck pain cases resolve within four to six weeks after starting rehab, which combines massage, range of motion work, and gradual strengthening. If left untreated (meaning without doing rehab or modifying aggravating factors), the pain can last much longer.

**TREATMENT STRATEGY:** A rehab program to treat non-specific neck pain—whether acute or chronic—combines passive strategies (self-guided soft tissue mobilizations and joint mobilizations) with mobility, sensorimotor control, and resistance training exercises.

In phase 1, you start with soft tissue mobilization techniques that reduce pain and tension in the muscles that control, support, and connect to the neck: the cervical extensors, upper trapezius, levator scapulae, rhomboids, and thoracic spine.

In phase 2, you start stretching some of the primary neck muscles (levator scapulae and upper trapezius) and the pectoral muscles, which are associated with tension and pain through the shoulder blade and neck regions. In this phase, you will also perform cervical mobility drills, which take the neck through all ranges of motion (flexion, extension, lateral flexion, and rotation). Pain can reduce neck mobility, so target these movements to prevent lasting range-of-motion impairments. Lastly, you implement cervical isometrics as an early strengthening exercise and to gradually improve stress tolerance and capacity. Push on your head in each of the directions demonstrated in the protocol, but use only as much force as your neck muscles can tolerate. Modify the resistance of your arm so that it provides some challenge but does not cause more than mild discomfort (three out of 10 on the pain scale).

In phase 3, you focus on sensorimotor control and resistance training exercises that build neck control and strength in all planes of motion (sagittal, frontal, and transverse). Sensorimotor control and strength changes can occur in individuals with neck pain, but this may be because the development of chronic neck pain is linked to unaddressed impairments in sensorimotor control and strength. The neck curl exercises use gravity and the weight of the head to strengthen the neck muscles. Banded cervical retractions also strengthen the neck extensors and the muscles that help maintain a neutral neck posture (rather than the forward head position many of us find ourselves in).

The other resistance training exercises focus on the scapular muscles that attach to the neck. Evidence shows that loading these muscles can reduce neck tightness and pain.[5,6] The lateral raise and shrug, for instance, can alleviate occupational neck pain when implemented periodically throughout the workday.

If an exercise causes more than mild discomfort, modify it by reducing the range of motion or temporarily remove it from your program. You can test the exercise again in one to two weeks to see if your body can tolerate the stress without flaring up your pain symptoms. With non-specific pain, we are concerned less about reinjury and more about desensitizing the neck through graded doses of stress. Phases 2 and 3 provide exercises that progressively put more stress on the neck, so pay attention to your symptoms and modify the program to match your current capacity.

# NECK STRAINS AND SPRAINS (WHIPLASH)

**DESCRIPTION:** Neck strains and sprains involve the muscles that run along the posterior (back side) and/or the anterior (front side) of the neck and the small facet joints that connect one vertebra to the next. Both are typically associated with traumatic injuries in which high forces stretch the neck muscles or push the joints past their available range of motion. Traumatic neck strains and sprains are common in car accidents (think whiplash) and in contact sports, such as American football, grappling, and rugby. With whiplash, the injury occurs when the body moves forward, typically from a rear impact—the head is forced into extension and then whips forward into flexion as it catches up with the body, causing muscle strains, facet joint sprains, or both.

**SIGNS AND SYMPTOMS:** Strains and sprains typically cause dull, achy pain along the side or back of the neck, in the shoulders, or in the upper back region, which can become sharp with certain neck or shoulder movements (see Aggravating Factors). You may also experience pain in the front of your neck or limited range of motion, especially when turning your head to one side.

**AGGRAVATING FACTORS:** For strains, stretching or contracting the muscles along the side or back of the neck usually produces pain. If you strain the right side of your neck, for example, it will often hurt to stretch (by tilting your neck to the left) or contract (by tilting your neck to the right).

If you have a sprain, compressing the tissues to end range (by rotating the head, tilting the head toward the injured side, or looking up) typically reproduces pain symptoms.

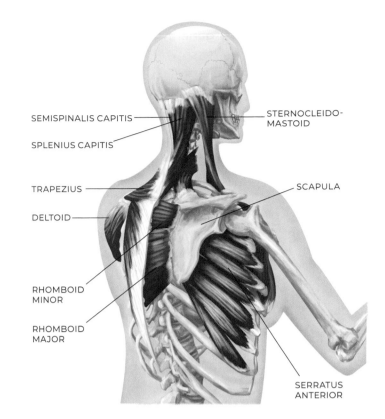

SEMISPINALIS CAPITIS
SPLENIUS CAPITIS
TRAPEZIUS
DELTOID
RHOMBOID MINOR
RHOMBOID MAJOR
STERNOCLEIDO-MASTOID
SCAPULA
SERRATUS ANTERIOR

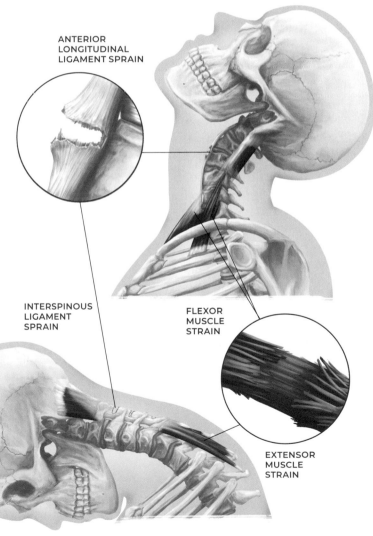

ANTERIOR LONGITUDINAL LIGAMENT SPRAIN
INTERSPINOUS LIGAMENT SPRAIN
FLEXOR MUSCLE STRAIN
EXTENSOR MUSCLE STRAIN

**PROGNOSIS:** Most strains and sprains resolve within four to six weeks of starting the appropriate recovery and treatment regimen, which includes a combination of massage, range of motion work, and gradual strengthening.

**TREATMENT STRATEGY:** Most strains and sprains are treated conservatively with a combination of soft tissue mobilizations (phase 1), mobility exercises (phase 2), resistance training (phase 3). Whether you have a sprain or a strain, you approach the phases in the same manner.

In phase 1, the exercises are designed to reduce pain and improve mobility, but be careful with soft tissue mobilizations that target injured tissues (cervical extensor mobilization) because applying too much pressure to a muscle strain can delay healing. The key is to apply just enough pressure to relieve tension and pain without making your symptoms worse after the exercise.

It's also important to mobilize the thoracic spine and surrounding soft tissues (such as the rhomboids) because research shows that mobilizing the thoracic spine (especially with thoracic extension) can reduce neck pain.[7] The thoracic spine is adjacent to the neck or cervical spine, meaning it influences how the neck moves and hurts, especially when the region is stiff or hypomobile.

In phase 2, you start stretching some of the primary neck muscles (levator scapulae and upper trapezius) and pectoral muscles. If you have a more severe neck strain, do not apply too much force when performing the levator scapulae and upper trapezius stretches, as these exercises can make your symptoms worse and delay healing. The process is different for everyone. Some people feel fine when stretching; it may even reduce symptoms because adjacent uninjured muscles can get tight and spasm. If you feel worse when stretching, skip those exercises and add them to phase 3.

Phase 2 also includes cervical mobility drills, which take the neck through all available ranges of motion (flexion, extension, lateral flexion, and rotation). Strains and sprains often reduce neck mobility, so make sure to target these movements to prevent lasting impairments. Finally, begin implementing cervical isometrics as an early strengthening tool. With muscle strains, add load gradually so that you don't reinjure the healing tissue. Isometrics are a great way to load the tissue in a gradual and controlled fashion. Push on your head with your hand in each of the directions demonstrated in the protocol, but use only as much force as your neck muscles can tolerate. Modify the resistance of your arm so that it provides some challenge without causing more than mild discomfort in the neck.

In phase 3, you focus on resistance training exercises that help make the neck and surrounding muscle tissue more resilient, which lowers your likelihood of suffering another strain. If an exercise causes more than mild discomfort, modify it by reducing the range of motion or remove it temporarily. You can test the exercise again in one to two weeks to see if your body has healed enough to add the movement back into your program.

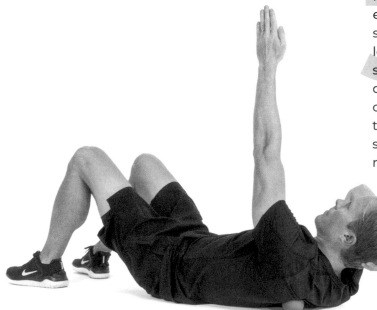

# CERVICAL SPONDYLOSIS (ARTHRITIS)

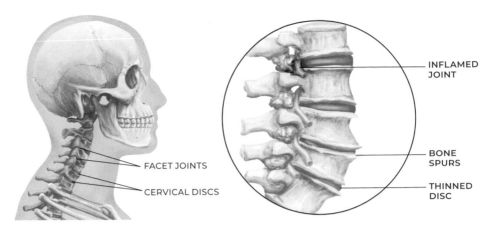

FACET JOINTS

CERVICAL DISCS

INFLAMED JOINT

BONE SPURS

THINNED DISC

**DESCRIPTION:** Spondylosis, or arthritis of the neck, is common as we age and often produces no pain.[8,9] The discs in our spine slowly lose water and shrink in height, applying more stress to the facet joints that connect our vertebrae (back bones). Increased stress on the joints and surrounding bones creates arthritic changes, including bone spurs. In some cases, these changes result in neck pain and stiffness.

With arthritis, you'll experience pain or stiffness when checking your blind spot, looking up at the ceiling, or performing any activity that requires the neck to move through its full ranges of motion. Arthritis is typically diagnosed via medical imaging after someone starts experiencing neck pain and losing range of motion.

**SIGNS AND SYMPTOMS:** Arthritis of the neck joints typically produces dull, achy pain and stiffness. In some cases, clicking and popping may occur when turning the head from side to side, or it will hurt at the ends of the range of motion, when trying to turn your head all the way to one side.

**AGGRAVATING FACTORS:** Looking all the way up (neck extension) or to the side (rotation); holding the head in one position for long periods (for example, driving or reading). General contributors include genetics, aging, previous injury, and pro-inflammatory lifestyle habits (many conditions are now being linked to underlying inflammation).

**PROGNOSIS:** While age-related changes to the tissue cannot be reversed, most pain associated with an arthritis flare-up improves significantly after four to six weeks of rehab.

**TREATMENT STRATEGY:** Pain due to arthritic changes is usually treated and managed with conservative care, such as soft tissue massage, stretching and mobility exercises, and resistance training.

Phase 1 focuses on soft tissue mobilization techniques that address the neck and scapular muscles and the thoracic region to reduce tension and pain and improve neck mobility. Because arthritis is a degenerative disorder, you should worry less about interfering with healing tissue (like in the neck strain section), but you should still pay attention to your symptoms and only apply a level of pressure that feels "therapeutic," which means having a positive effect. Too many people think that pushing harder is better. This isn't always true and can often exacerbate pain symptoms.

In phase 2, you stretch your neck and scapular muscles and add cervical mobility exercises. Arthritis in the neck not only causes pain but often results in reduced joint mobility. The stretches and mobility exercises take your neck through all available movements to address the directions of hypomobility (stiffness), help with pain, and improve functional capacity. Do not push past mild pain (three out of 10 on the pain scale) when performing the cervical mobility exercises, which could flare up arthritis-related pain. Phase 2 ends with cervical isometrics, which gradually rebuild neck muscle strength.

Phase 3 focuses on resistance training exercises that improve neck strength. For arthritis, resistance exercises complement the first two phases to reduce and manage pain and tension while protecting the neck from future injuries.

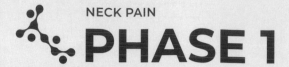

# PHASE 1

## GUIDELINES:

- Perform every day
- Tools: small massage ball, peanut tool, yoga block, foam roller
- Add phase 2 when you have no pain at rest and no more than mild pain (3/10) with the exercises

### GOOD FOR:

- Alleviating neck pain
- Relieving muscle tension
- Warm-up for phase 2 and 3 exercises

## SOFT TISSUE MOBILIZATIONS:

- Spend 1–2 minutes on each area
- Perform in any order on both sides
- Stop on tender points for 10–20 seconds

---

### levator scapulae mobilization

Position a small massage ball at the corner of your shoulder blade. Elevate your hips to increase the pressure. Add arm movements to further mobilize the muscle.

### upper trapezius mobilization

Position the ball between a doorframe or rack and your upper trapezius muscle. Work your way across the entire muscle from your shoulder to the base of your neck. Drive into the ball to increase the pressure. Move your arm (behind your back or in front of your body) and head (down and to the side) to further mobilize the muscle.

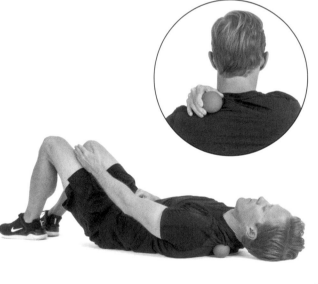

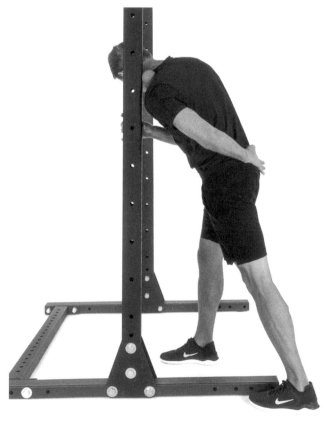

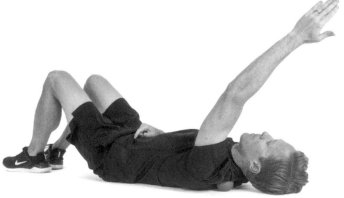

# cervical extensor mobilization

## with peanut tool

Place a peanut tool against the muscles on the back of your neck. Work slowly from the base of your skull down to the base of your neck, stopping on each spinal segment. Add movement by tucking your chin and extending your neck. Skip this exercise or replace it with the manual variation if it causes more than mild discomfort or you have a more severe neck sprain or strain.

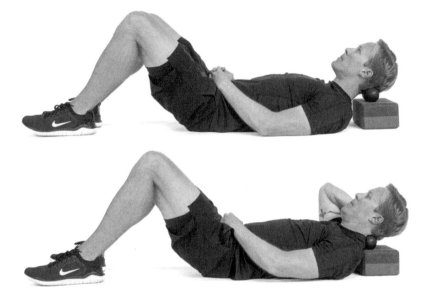

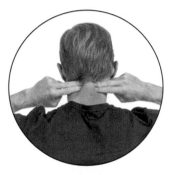

## manual variation

Press your index and middle fingers into your neck extensors and massage lightly when you find tender points.

# rhomboid mobilization

Place a small massage ball between your shoulder blade and spine. Work the entire area around the shoulder blade (rhomboids). Add arm movements and lift your head to further mobilize the muscles.

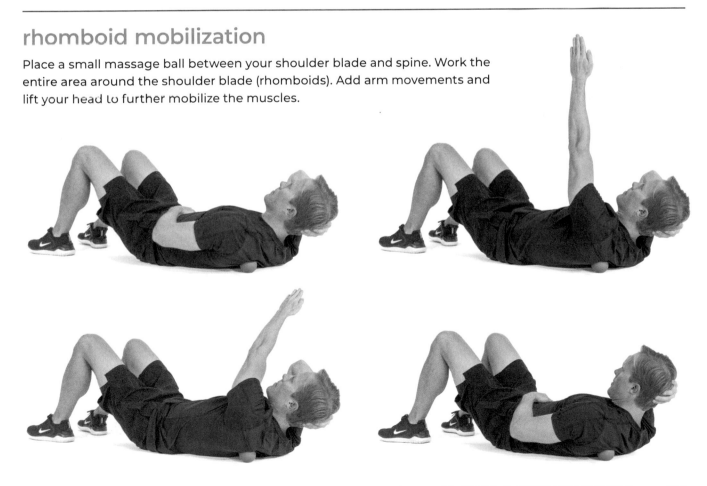

## thoracic mobilization
### roll up and down the spine

Position a foam roller perpendicular to your spine under your upper back. Cross your arms over your chest, lift your butt, and then drive off your heels to roll out your upper back region (not the low back or neck). If it hurts to stabilize your neck, cup the back of your head with your hands as shown in the next sequence.

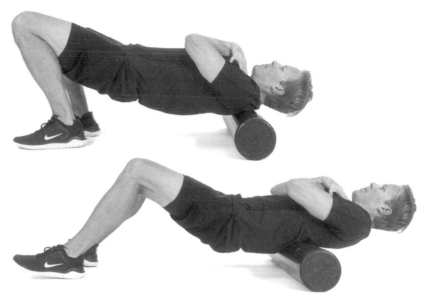

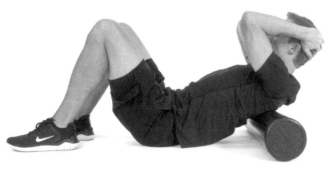

### flex and extend

Keeping your butt on the ground, extend over the roller by dropping your head toward the ground. You can hold this position or flex and extend (abdominal crunch) over the roller.

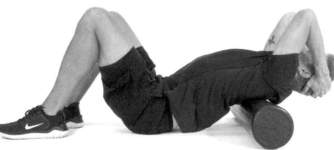

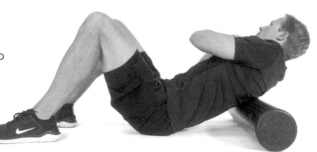

### rotate and roll side-to-side

Cross your arms over your chest or cup the back of your head with your hands and roll from side to side on stiff areas.

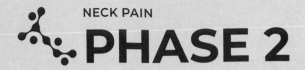

NECK PAIN

# PHASE 2

**GOOD FOR:**

- Improving neck range of motion
- Strengthening the neck
- Warm-up for phase 3 exercises

**GUIDELINES:**

- Perform every day
- Add phase 3 when you can do the exercises with no more than mild pain (3/10)

## STRETCHING EXERCISES:

- Do 3 reps with 30- to 60-second holds
- Perform in any order on both sides
- Don't stretch into pain

> Skip or move carefully with these stretches if you have a neck strain or sprain.

### pectoral stretch

Position your forearm against a doorframe or rack with your shoulder at about 90 degrees. Step forward until you feel a stretch in your chest region. Move your arm slightly higher to stretch the upper fibers of your pectoral muscles.

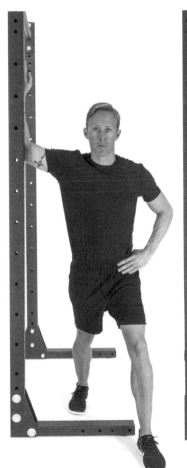
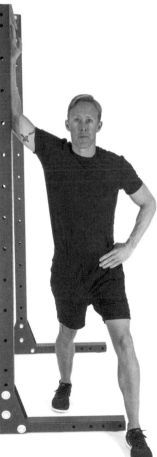

### upper trapezius stretch

Position one arm behind your back. Use the other arm to pull your head toward your opposite shoulder.

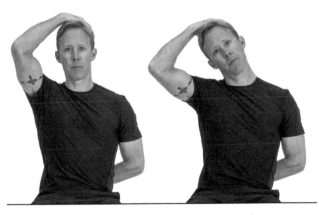

### levator scapulae stretch

With one arm behind your back, use your other hand to pull your head down at an angle so that you are looking at your opposite hip.

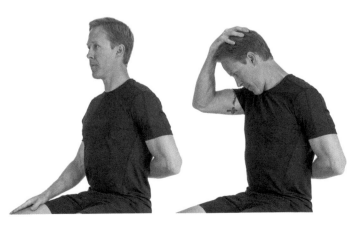

# MOBILITY EXERCISES:

- ▸ Do 3 sets of 10–15 reps
- ▸ Perform seated or standing
- ▸ Active range of motion (AROM)—move as far as you can without pain
- ▸ Pause at end range for 2–3 seconds

## cervical mobility

### flexion and extension

Start in a neutral position. Slowly lower your chin toward your chest, then tilt your head back.

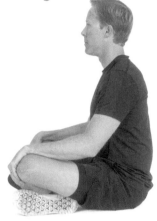 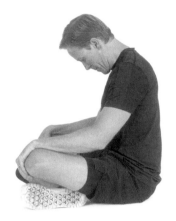 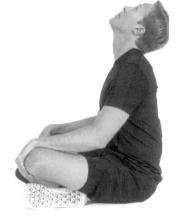

### rotation

Keeping your spine straight, slowly rotate your head toward one shoulder, then the other.

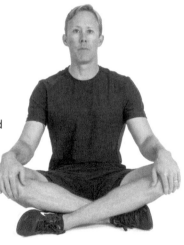 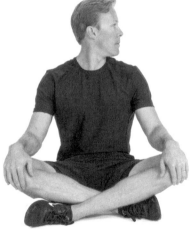 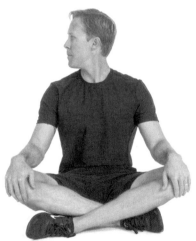

### side-bend

Slowly move your ear toward one shoulder, then the other.

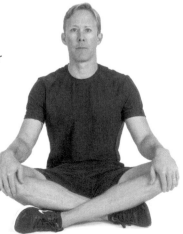 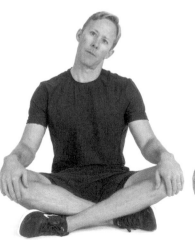 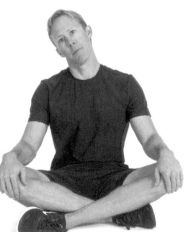

# ISOMETRIC EXERCISES:

► Do 4 or 5 reps with 30- to 45-second resisted holds
► Apply as much force as your neck can tolerate without pain
► Perform seated or standing

## cervical manual isometrics (four directions)

### flexion

Tilt your head forward. Push on your forehead with your hand and resist.

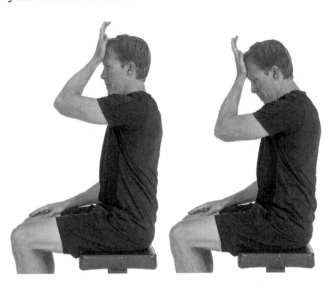

### extension

Tilt your head back slightly. Push on the back of your head with your hand and resist.

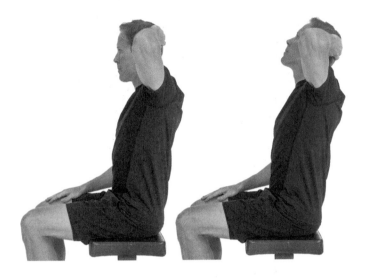

### lateral flexion (side-bend)

Tilt your head to the side. Push on that side of your head with your hand and resist. Perform on both sides.

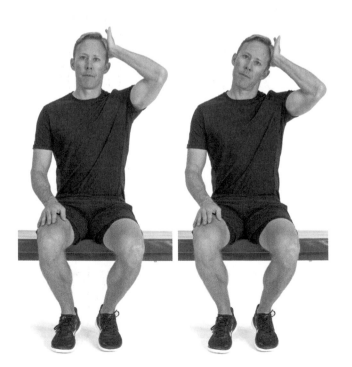

### rotation

Turn your head slightly. Push on the side of your head with your hand and resist. Perform on both sides.

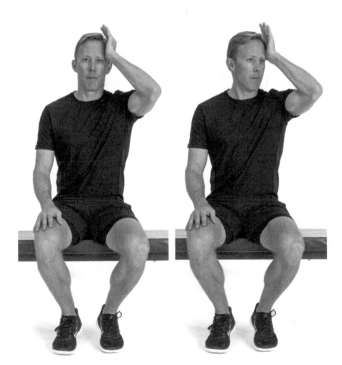

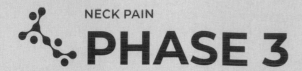
# PHASE 3

**GOOD FOR:**

- Strengthening the neck and surrounding muscles
- Preventing neck pain and injury

**GUIDELINES:**

- Perform 3 or 4 days a week
- Do 3 sets of 10–15 reps
- Push sets to fatigue
- Add load or reps to increase difficulty
- Tools: resistance band, dumbbells, bench

## cervical flexor curl

Lying on your back, slowly tuck your chin to your chest, moving as far as you can without pain. Lower just to the point where your head is barely touching the ground, then raise again.

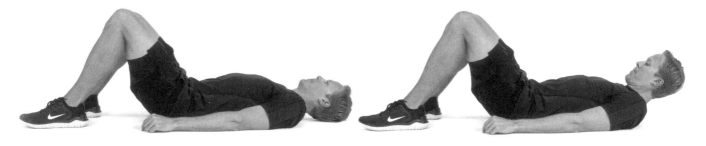

## cervical lateral flexor curl

Lying on your side, slowly move your ear toward your top shoulder, moving as far as you can without pain. Keep your head neutral; don't tuck your chin or tilt your head back. Perform on both sides.

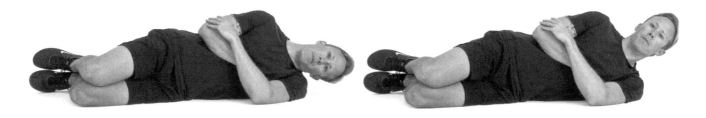

## cervical rotator curl

Slowly turn your head toward the ground, then rotate in the opposite direction by moving your chin toward your top shoulder. Keep your head neutral; don't tuck your chin or tilt your head back. Perform on both sides.

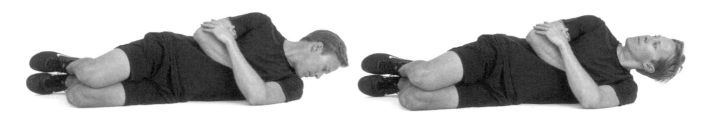

## banded cervical retraction

Wrap a band around the back of your head and hold the ends with both hands. Stretch the band to apply resistance. Starting with your head forward, move backward into retraction against the resistance.

## dumbbell row

Place one hand and knee on a bench with your spine neutral. Let your opposite arm hang down to the side of the bench, then bend your elbow and pull the dumbbell straight up toward your chest. You can do a banded, inverted, or machine row variation of this exercise.

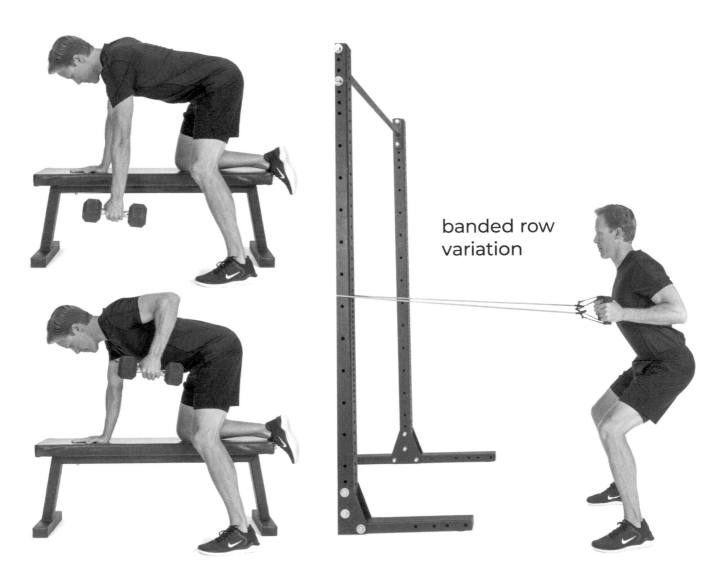

banded row variation

## dumbbell shrug

Holding dumbbells at your sides, slowly shrug your shoulders toward your ears while keeping your spine and head straight.

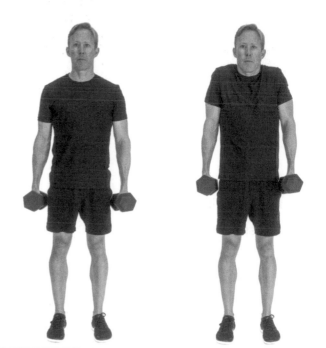

## lateral raise

Raise your arms with your palms facing down until they reach shoulder level.

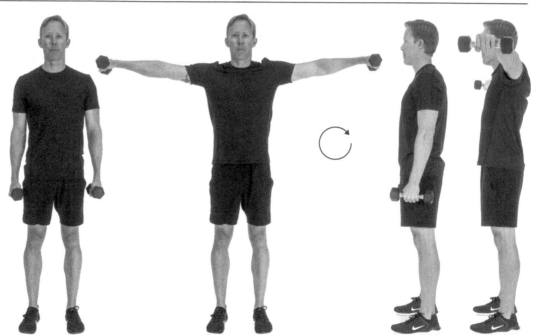

## bent-over lateral raise

Hinge from your hips and bend your knees—keeping your shins vertical and back flat—so that your torso is at a roughly 45-degree angle. With a slight bend in your elbows, raise your arms with your palms facing down until they reach shoulder level.

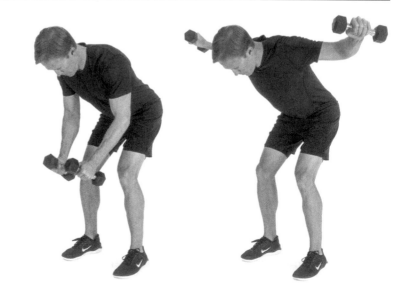

# NERVE PAIN (RADICULOPATHY)

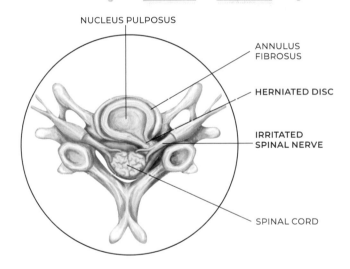

**Follow this program to treat:**

- Sharp neck pain
- Numbness and tingling radiating down the arm (radiculopathy)
- Disc herniation (disc bulge) and stenosis
- Thoracic outlet syndrome

## DISC HERNIATION (DISC BULGE) AND STENOSIS

**DESCRIPTION:** Nerve pain that radiates down the arm often originates in the neck, where the nerves that travel to the arm and hand begin. This type of pain can result from nerve inflammation, disc herniations, stenosis (a narrowing of the space through which the nerve travels), and prolonged postural positions that compromise nerve health (see Aggravating Factors). Essentially, the inner part of the disc (aka nucleus pulposus or disc nucleus) is pushed out toward the annulus, or disc wall. If the outward movement of the nucleus is forceful enough, the disc wall can tear and disc material will leak out, causing inflammation.

A lot of people have nerve pain not because a disc bulge is touching the nearby nerve but because inflammation has irritated and sensitized it. For instance, an MRI might show nothing wrong with a disc even though the patient has nerve pain, which could be caused by inflammation due to overuse, stress, diet, or other factors.

Other potential causes include traumatic injuries from whiplash-type car accidents, sport-related injuries, and any activity that uses the neck and shoulder muscles in a novel way, like a new weightlifting program.

**SIGNS AND SYMPTOMS:** Discomfort associated with nerve irritation can range from sharp pain, like a lightning bolt, to numbness and tingling sensations. Symptoms travel along the path of the nerve and may go all the way to the fingers.

NUCLEUS PULPOSUS

ANNULUS FIBROSUS

HERNIATED DISC

IRRITATED SPINAL NERVE

SPINAL CORD

**AGGRAVATING FACTORS:** Neck and arm movements or positions that stress the nerve. For example, rotating the head toward the painful side or looking up typically causes nerve discomfort that originates in the neck. You may also experience pain after holding a position that compromises the nerve for an extended period, such as falling asleep with your neck tilted to one side.

**PROGNOSIS:** Many disc injuries (bulges and herniations) and most radiculopathy cases resolve in eight to 12 weeks if you eliminate or modify aggravating activities and follow a rehab program.

**TREATMENT STRATEGY:** Radiculopathy associated with a disc herniation or bulge often improves with rehab. As stated in Chapter 7, nerve pain issues can cause mobility and flexibility impairments and muscle weakness if the nerve becomes more irritated. Over-the-counter pain medications and doctor-prescribed muscle relaxants may also be helpful during the early phases of rehab.

In phase 1, you perform soft tissue mobilizations that target the neck (cervical extensors and levator scapulae), pectoral muscles, and mid-back region. Each mobilization plays a key role in reducing tension and pain. The neck mobilizations can alleviate symptoms where pain is present. The pectoral mobilization may not seem intuitive when it comes to reducing neck pain, but it is important because tightness in this area can contribute to nerve pain that travels down the arm. Because the upper thoracic spine functions together with the neck, you need to address any areas of hypomobility (stiffness) in this region. Also, certain types of cervical radiculopathy can make pain radiate to the intrascapular region (between the shoulder blades), so mobilizing that area can reduce pain if you experience discomfort in your mid-back.

Phase 2 focuses on spine and peripheral nerve mobility. The thoracic rotation stretches and cervical mobility exercises help improve spinal mobility and reduce pain. The angel exercises dynamically stretch the pectoral muscles (the nerves run under the pecs) and generally mobilize the major peripheral nerves of the arm (median, ulnar, and radial). Next, you implement nerve slider exercises to mobilize the peripheral nerves individually. Slider or flossing techniques involve tensioning the nerve close to the neck and then alternating by tensioning the nerve down toward the hand. This causes the nerve to slide back and forth (like a strand of dental floss) and has been shown to reduce pain and improve nerve health.[10] Phase 2 finishes with a wall chin tuck exercise, which helps retrain a more neutral neck posture and teaches you how to correct the forward head position—a potential contributor to neck tension and pain.

Phase 3 introduces more intense nerve mobilizations called tensioners. These can be thought of as nerve stretches, but nerves can only stretch a little bit, so be careful about applying too much stretch force, which can flare up the nerve and make pain worse. Once your pain has resolved and your mobility improves, complete the exercises in phase 3 of the Neck Pain protocol to reduce future flare-ups. Those exercises will also strengthen muscles that may have been weakened by nerve irritation.

If pain persists or you observe muscle weakness, consult with a neurologist to rule out more severe issues (spinal tumor, fracture, or infection) that may compromise nerve health. You might consider a discectomy, which is the most common surgery for pain radiating from the neck—usually for a large disc herniation that's not getting better with conservative care (rehab). You could also use this protocol if you had a neck fusion, which is another common type of surgery for prolonged neck or nerve pain.

## WHEN SHOULD I CONSIDER SURGERY FOR A DISC HERNIATION?

Whether you need surgery usually depends on your symptoms and functional ability. If you've had pain for six months or longer, you are a candidate, especially if you tried physical therapy without improvement. If you have radiating nerve pain and are noticing a progressive loss of strength in your arm—you can't grip or lift things, bend your elbow, or lift your arm outward—or you suddenly have a muscle that isn't working, you should consult a doctor immediately and consider surgical intervention.

I've worked with people who have permanent or partial nerve paralysis because they didn't address the problem in time, so pay attention to your symptoms and whether they are getting better or worse.

# THORACIC OUTLET SYNDROME

**DESCRIPTION:** Thoracic outlet syndrome (TOS) describes a condition in which the nerves and/or blood vessels that run from the neck to the arm become irritated, injured, or compressed in the space between the first rib and collarbone, which is called the thoracic outlet. This condition often results from sports that involve repetitive shoulder movements (baseball, golf, swimming), postures that stress the nerves and blood vessels, and traumatic accidents (whiplash).

**SIGNS AND SYMPTOMS:** Pain in the neck, arm, or hand, often accompanied by numbness or tingling in the arm and hand. In severe cases, hand weakness (grip strength) can occur.

**AGGRAVATING FACTORS:** Repetitive shoulder or arm movements such as carrying heavy items. Stress, depression, and sleep disorders also can exacerbate symptoms.

**PROGNOSIS:** In many cases, symptoms improve within four to six weeks of implementing the appropriate rehab exercises.

**TREATMENT STRATEGY:** TOS is treated initially with physical therapy, which includes exercises that stretch the muscles of the neck and shoulders and teach postural modification (neutral head, neck, and spinal positions) to reduce nerve stress. Over-the-counter pain medications and doctor-prescribed muscle relaxants may also be helpful during the early phases of rehab.

Nerve pain associated with TOS creates mobility and flexibility impairments and muscle weakness that are very similar to nerve pain related to disc injuries and stenosis. TOS affects many of the same nerves as those conditions but farther downstream, so rehab is quite similar. This is why the Nerve Pain protocol includes symptoms related to disc injuries, stenosis, and TOS.

**1** In phase 1, you perform soft tissue mobilization techniques that target the neck, shoulder complex, and thoracic spine, which help reduce tension and pain and get your body ready for the more challenging mobility exercises in phase 2.

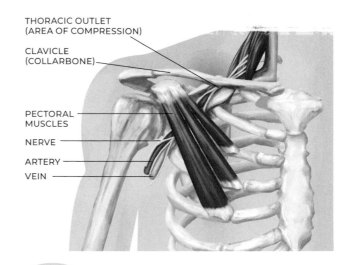

THORACIC OUTLET
(AREA OF COMPRESSION)

CLAVICLE
(COLLARBONE)

PECTORAL
MUSCLES

NERVE

ARTERY

VEIN

**2** Phase 2 focuses on spine and peripheral nerve mobility and introduces stretches and nerve mobilization techniques. These exercises will improve nerve health, reduce pain and improve neck and shoulder girdle mobility.[10]

**3** Phase 3 introduces tensioner nerve mobilizations, which challenge the nerves more than the slider exercises in phase 2. Be careful about applying too much stretch force because this can wind up the nerve and make pain worse.

Once your pain has resolved and your mobility improves, complete the exercises in phase 3 of the Neck Pain protocol to reduce the chances that your nerve pain returns. The exercises also strengthen muscles that may have been weakened by nerve irritation.

In the 10 to 20 percent of cases that do not improve with rehab, surgery may be suggested to reduce nerve stress. Such procedures may involve removing the first rib and/or sections of soft tissue (muscle or fascia) to stop them from interfering with nerve health.

**NOTE:** Individuals with vascular TOS (which occurs when veins or arteries become compromised) typically require surgery more often than individuals who suffer from TOS that affects the nerves. If you have nerve symptoms (pain, numbness, and tingling) and notice swelling or poor circulation in your hands—all signs of vascular compromise—talk with your doctor to ensure that a more serious issue like a blood clot does not occur.

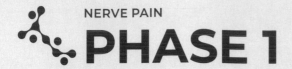

NERVE PAIN

# PHASE 1

**GOOD FOR:**

- Alleviating neck and arm nerve pain
- Relieving muscle tension
- Warm-up for phase 2 and 3 exercises

**GUIDELINES:**

- Perform every day
- Tools: small massage ball, peanut tool, yoga block, foam roller
- Add phase 2 when you have no pain at rest and no more than mild pain (3/10) with the exercises

## SOFT TISSUE MOBILIZATIONS:

- ▸ Spend 1–2 minutes on each area
- ▸ Perform in any order on both sides
- ▸ Stop on tender points for 10–20 seconds

## pectoral mobilization

Position a small massage ball between a doorframe or rack and your pectoral muscles near the front of your shoulder. Place that arm behind your back and add dynamic movement by reaching overhead to further mobilize the muscles.

## cervical extensor mobilization

Place a peanut tool against the muscles on the back of your neck. Work slowly from the base of your skull down to the base of your neck, stopping on each spinal segment. Add movement by tucking your chin or extending your neck. If this exercise is too painful, you can do the manual variation on page 153.

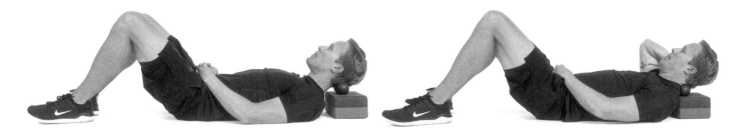

# thoracic mobilization

Position a foam roller perpendicular to your spine under your upper back. Keeping your butt on the ground, extend over the roller by slowly lowering your head toward the ground. You can hold this position or flex and extend (abdominal crunch) over the roller. You can also elevate your butt and roll up and down your upper back to massage the area (but not the low back or neck).

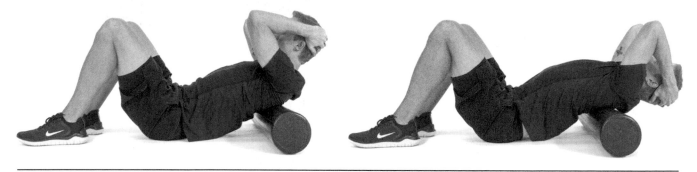

# levator scapulae mobilization

Position the ball at the corner of your shoulder blade. Elevate your hips to increase the pressure. Add arm movements to further mobilize the muscle.

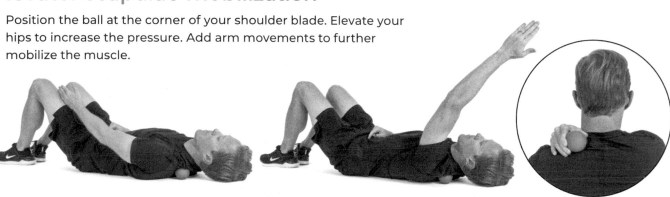

# rhomboid mobilization

Place the ball in the space between your shoulder blade and spine. Work up and down several inches around the shoulder blade (rhomboids). Add arm movements and lift your head to further mobilize the muscles.

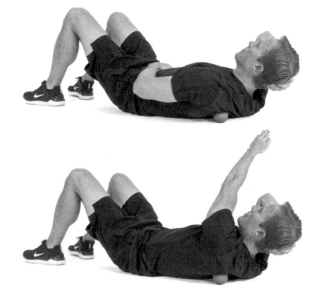
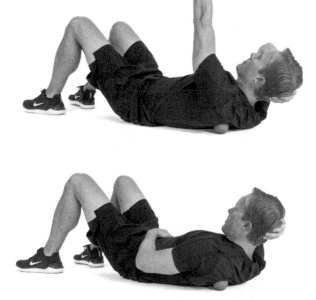

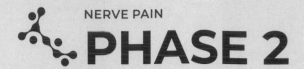

NERVE PAIN

# PHASE 2

## GOOD FOR:

- Improving spinal and nerve mobility
- Reducing nerve pain sensitivity
- Warm-up for phase 3 exercises

## GUIDELINES:

- Perform every day
- Tool: foam roller
- Add phase 3 when you can do the exercises with no more than mild pain (3/10)

## thoracic rotation stretch

Lie on your side and bend your hips to about 90 degrees. Grip the outside of your top knee with your bottom arm. Keeping your top arm straight, lower it toward the ground and rotate away from your knees as far as you can without pain. As you do, pull down on your knees and try to get both shoulders flush with the ground. Perform 3 reps with 15- to 20-second holds on both sides.

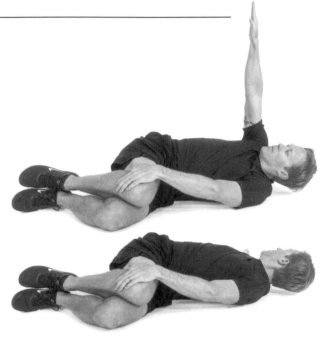

# MOBILITY EXERCISES:

- ▶ Do 3 sets of 10–15 reps
- ▶ Active range of motion (AROM)—move as far as you can without pain
- ▶ Pause at end range for 2–3 seconds

## angel

Position your spine over a foam roller so that your head and tailbone are supported. Start with your arms at your sides and palms up, then reach as far overhead as you can without pain.

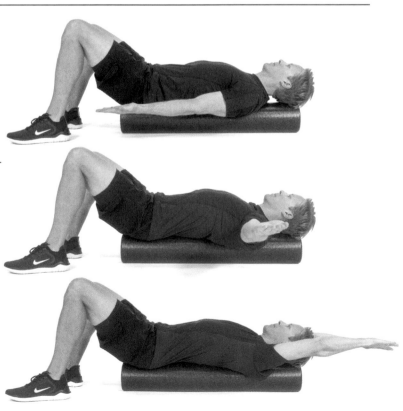

# cervical mobility

## flexion and extension

Start in a neutral position. Slowly move your chin toward your chest, then tilt your head back.

## rotation

Keeping your spine straight, slowly rotate your head toward one shoulder, then the other.

## side-bend

Slowly move your ear toward one shoulder, then the other.

## protraction and retraction

Slowly move your chin forward and then backward.

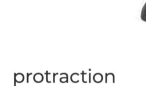
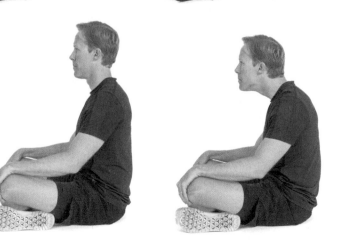
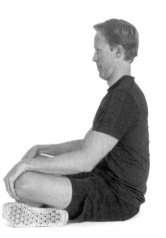

# NERVE MOBILIZATIONS:

▸ Start with 1 set of 10–15 reps
▸ Add 1–2 more sets if symptoms don't flare up

## median nerve slider mobility

Start with your arm out to your side with your shoulder at 90 degrees, your elbow and wrist bent, and your head titled away from your elevated arm. In one fluid motion, straighten your elbow, extend your wrist, and move your head toward your arm. Go back and forth between these positions to mobilize the median nerve.

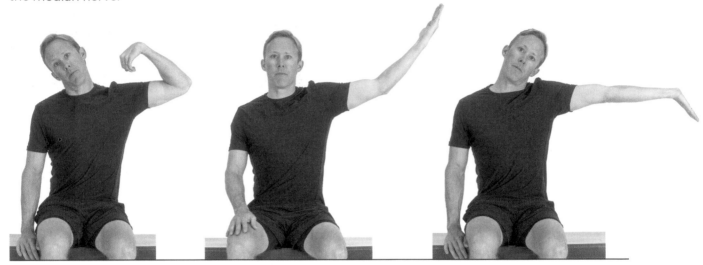

## radial nerve slider mobility

Start with your arm out to your side and your palm facing behind you. Flex your wrist and tilt your head toward your outstretched arm. In one fluid motion, bend your head away from your arm and extend your wrist. Go back and forth between these positions to mobilize the radial nerve.

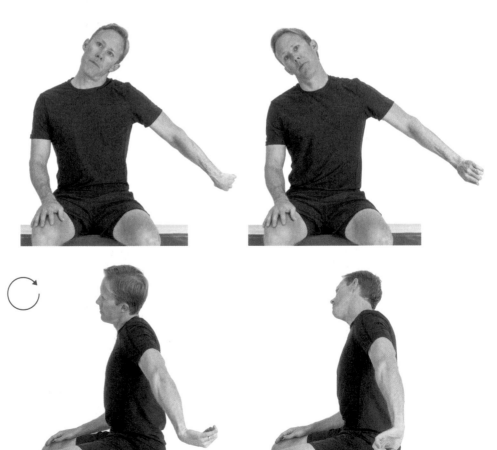

## ulnar nerve slider mobility

Start with your arm out to your side with your shoulder at 90 degrees, your elbow bent, your wrist extended with palm facing up, and your head tilted toward your arm. In one fluid motion, straighten your elbow, bend your wrist, and move your head away from your arm. Go back and forth between these positions to mobilize the ulnar nerve.

## wall chin tuck

Stand with your head and back against a wall or rack. Slide the back of your head up the wall while tucking your chin to your chest. Go back and forth between these positions.

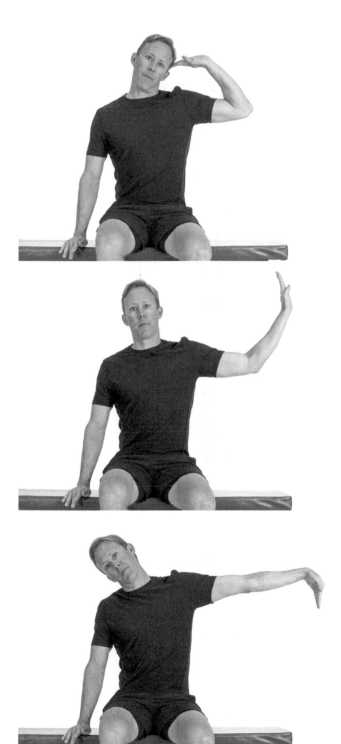

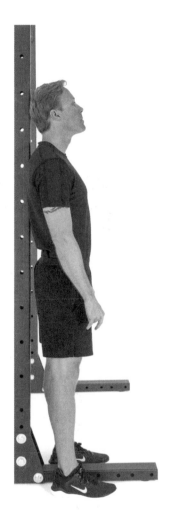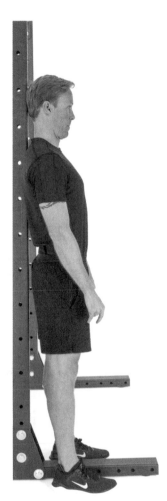

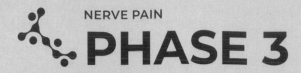

# PHASE 3

## GOOD FOR:

- Reducing nerve pain sensitivity
- Improving nerve mobility and stretch tolerance
- Preventing nerve-related neck pain and injury

## GUIDELINES:

- Perform 3 or 4 days a week
- Do 3 reps with 5- to 10-second holds
- Stop or back off the stretch if you feel tingling, numbness, or shooting pain
- Once nerve sensitivity calms down, add phase 3 exercises from the Neck Pain protocol (pages 158–160) to prevent future flare-ups

## median nerve tensioner

Lift your arm out to your side so that your shoulder is at 90 degrees and your palm is facing up. Extend your wrist (fingers toward the ground). Keeping your elbow straight and wrist bent, slowly tilt your head away from your extended arm by moving your ear toward your opposite shoulder without rotating or moving your head up or down. Hold this position at maximum tension without pain for 5–10 seconds, then go back to the start position and repeat 3 times.

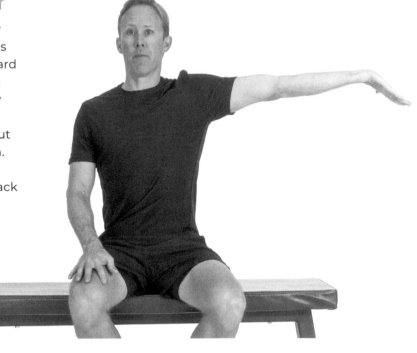

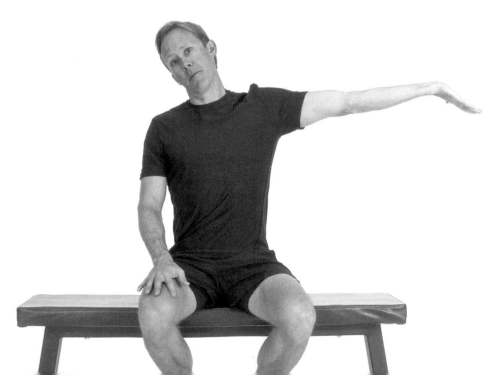

# radial nerve tensioner

Bend your elbow and position your thumb near the center of your upper chest. Start to extend your elbow out to the side of your body. As you extend, slowly bend your head by moving your ear toward your opposite shoulder and flex your wrist. Hold this position at maximum tension without pain for 5–10 seconds, then go back to the start position and repeat 3 times.

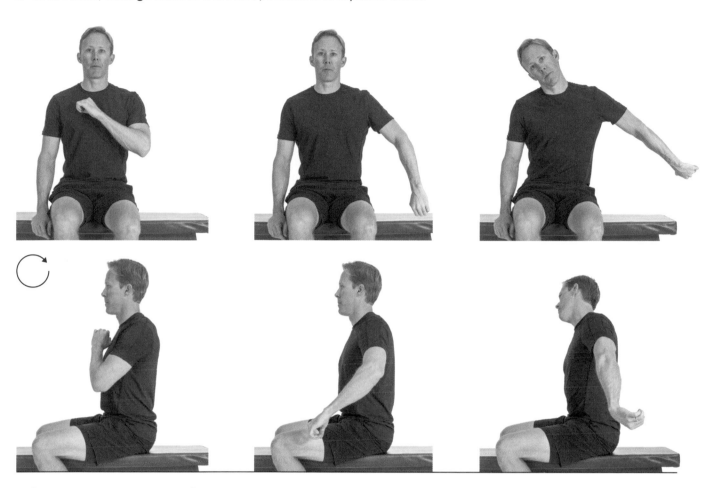

# ulnar nerve tensioner

Start with your arm extended out to your side with your palm facing down and your shoulder at 90 degrees. Simultaneously bend your elbow, get your palm to face the ceiling, and reach toward your head. At the same time, bend your head toward your opposite shoulder. Hold this position at maximum tension without pain for 5–10 seconds, then go back to the start position and repeat 3 times.

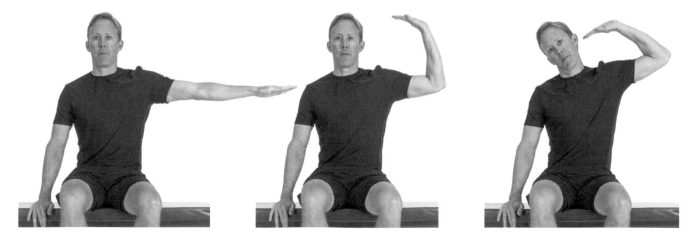

# HEADACHE PAIN

**Follow this program to treat:**

- Pain in the front of the head and/or face
- Tension headaches stemming from the neck
- Cervicogenic headache

## CERVICOGENIC HEADACHE

**DESCRIPTION:** Cervicogenic headaches originate from the upper cervical spine (neck) and can cause referred pain in regions of the head and/or face. Tissues that contribute to the development of this type of headache include the muscles, joints, and discs in the region between the skull and the upper cervical vertebrae (C1–3). In most cases, cervicogenic headaches are caused by activities that create tension in the neck: stress; holding certain static positions, such as looking at a computer screen; and sleep difficulties, which may include your neck position while sleeping or any factors interfering with getting adequate sleep.

**SIGNS AND SYMPTOMS:** The primary symptom is steady, non-throbbing pain on one side of the neck near the base of the skull that can refer down the neck into the shoulder blade or up into the forehead. For most people, the pain radiates from the upper neck, over the head, and into one eye socket or the forehead, following that specific path. Neck stiffness and pain when sneezing or coughing also can occur.

**AGGRAVATING FACTORS:** The position that causes pain typically involves lower cervical flexion (looking down) with upper cervical extension (looking down and forward, with the back of the neck tightened in the upper cervical area). Put simply, the head comes forward and then the upper part of the neck extends so that the eyes are looking straight ahead, which is sometimes referred to as the "forward head on neck" position.

**PROGNOSIS:** Typically, pain resolves within a few weeks once you correct the triggering positions.

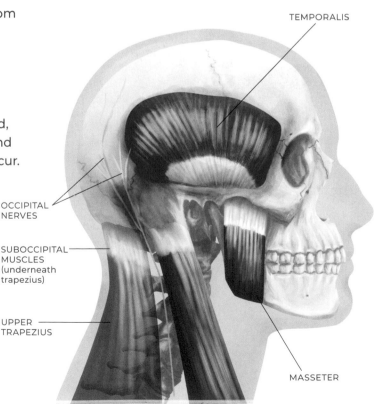

TEMPORALIS

OCCIPITAL NERVES

SUBOCCIPITAL MUSCLES (underneath trapezius)

UPPER TRAPEZIUS

MASSETER

**TREATMENT STRATEGY:** Cervicogenic headaches often resolve with conservative care (physical therapy and massage) and behavior modification (changing your work/desk position or getting a new pillow).

**1** Phase 1 focuses on mobilizing the suboccipital muscles at the base of the skull. The nerves that create neck-related headaches come from this area of the spine, so loosening them can reduce symptoms. However, be cautious when implementing this technique, as applying too much pressure can make headache symptoms worse. The key is to find a pressure that feels therapeutic (helps release muscle tension). You can also use your fingers to mobilize these muscles if the massage ball (the first variation) creates too much discomfort. In this phase, you mobilize the levator scapulae and upper trapezius muscles, which also attach to the skull and upper neck and can contribute to neck discomfort, tension, and headaches.

**2** In phase 2, you start by stretching the suboccipital muscles, the muscles in which headache symptoms originate. The other stretches and mobility exercises in phase 2 are designed to improve the mobility of the neck, thoracic spine, and shoulder blades, all of which have a mechanical influence on the upper neck. The wall chin tuck exercises create upper cervical (neck) flexion and lower cervical extension, teaching you how to correct the forward head position that may contribute to tightness in the region and irritate the upper neck nerves that run through the suboccipital region. Lastly, the neck flexor isometric hold builds neck strength in a neutral position (imagine a plank for the neck) and can be a helpful strategy for reducing the recurrence of headache symptoms.

**3** Phase 3 adds isometric contractions for the other neck movements to continue building strength in all planes of motion. Once your pain lessens significantly or goes away, implement the exercises in phase 3 of the Neck Pain protocol to strengthen your neck and the surrounding muscles so that you are less likely to have headaches in the future.

If conservative care isn't successful, you may need a nerve block (injection of a nerve-numbing medication). If you're a candidate for surgery but want to avoid it, go through the protocol. You won't risk making the problem worse. If you're not getting better after six to eight weeks, then consider the nerve block procedure more seriously.

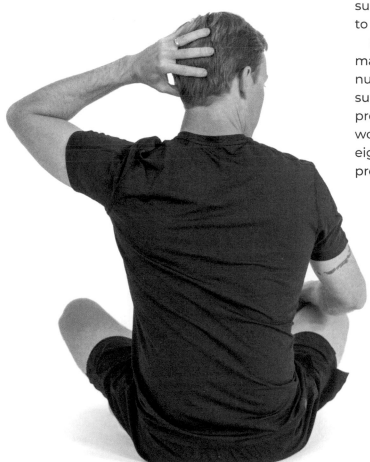

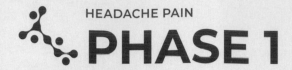

HEADACHE PAIN

# PHASE 1

## GOOD FOR:

- Alleviating upper neck and headache pain
- Relieving muscle tension
- Warm-up for phase 2 and 3 exercises

## GUIDELINES:

- Perform every day
- Tools: small massage ball, yoga block
- Add phase 2 when you have no pain at rest and no more than mild pain (3/10) with the exercises

## SOFT TISSUE MOBILIZATIONS:

- ▸ Spend 1–2 minutes on each area
- ▸ Perform in any order on both sides
- ▸ Stop on tender points for 10–20 seconds

---

## suboccipital mobilization

Place a small massage ball on a yoga block, positioning the ball at the base of your skull, just to the side of your cervical spine. Move slowly around this region to target the suboccipital muscles. You can rotate your head to the side or twist and adjust the ball with your opposite hand. If the pressure is too intense or you don't have the tools, do one of the manual variations.

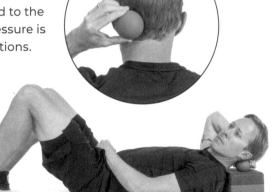

## manual variation 1

To do the manual variation using both hands, cup your hands around your skull just above your ears and press your thumbs into your suboccipital muscles around the base of your skull. Gently massage the area. Apply pressure and move your chin to your chest.

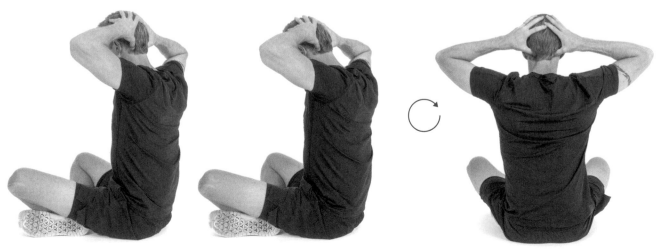

## manual variation 2

You can also do the manual variation using one hand. While pressing your thumb into your suboccipital muscles, rotate your head to the side by moving your chin toward your opposite shoulder.

## upper trapezius mobilization

Position a small massage ball between a doorframe or rack and your upper trapezius muscle. Work your way across the entire muscle from your shoulder to the base of your neck. Drive into the ball to increase the pressure. Move your arm behind your back or in front of your body and your head down and to the side to further mobilize the muscle.

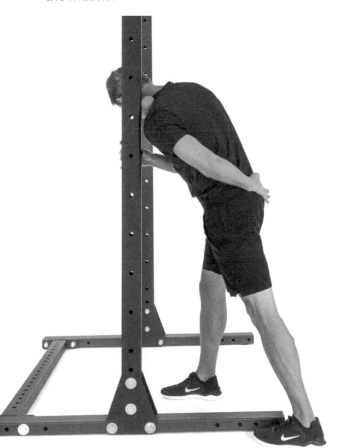

## levator scapulae mobilization

Position the ball at the corner of your shoulder blade. Elevate your hips to increase the pressure. Add arm movements to further mobilize the muscle.

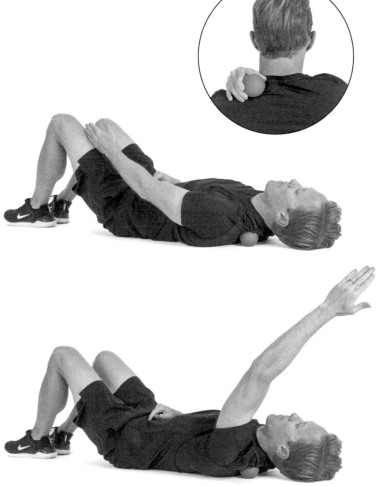

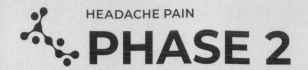

# PHASE 2

**GOOD FOR:**

- Improving neck range of motion
- Alleviating headache symptoms
- Building neck flexor strength
- Warm-up for phase 3 exercises

**GUIDELINES:**

- Perform every day
- Tool: foam roller
- Add phase 3 when you can do the exercises with no more than mild pain (3/10)

## STRETCHING EXERCISES:

- ▸ Do 3 reps with 30- to 60-second holds
- ▸ Don't stretch into pain

### suboccipital stretch

Make a fist with one hand and position it underneath your chin. With your other hand, grab the back of your head and pull up and forward until you feel a moderate stretch on the back of your neck.

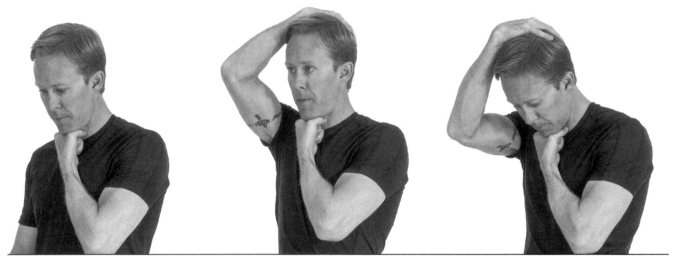

### thoracic extension stretch

Position a foam roller perpendicular to your spine under your upper back. Cup the back of your head with your hands to support your neck. Keeping your butt on the ground, extend slowly over the roller. Relax and hold for 15–20 seconds to improve thoracic extension.

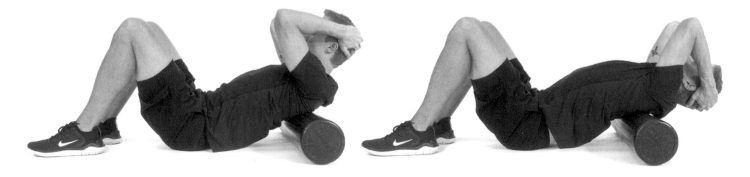

# MOBILITY EXERCISES:

- ▶ Do 3 sets of 10–15 reps unless otherwise noted
- ▶ Active range of motion (AROM)—move as far as you can without pain
- ▶ Pause at end range for 2–3 seconds

## angel

Position your spine over the roller so that your head and tailbone are supported. Start with your arms at your sides and palms up, then reach as far overhead as you can without pain.

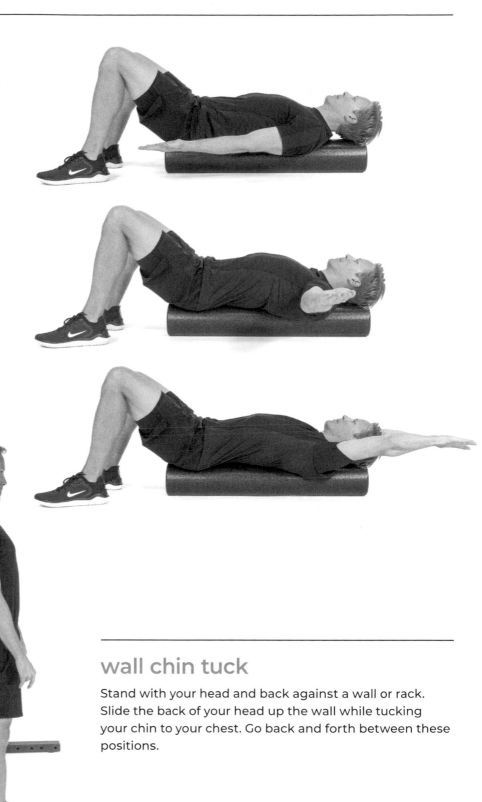

## wall chin tuck

Stand with your head and back against a wall or rack. Slide the back of your head up the wall while tucking your chin to your chest. Go back and forth between these positions.

## cervical protraction and retraction mobility

Start with your head and neck in a neutral position. Slide your head forward into protraction (stick your chin out) and backward into retraction (tuck your chin) without looking up or down.

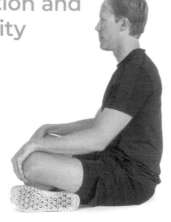
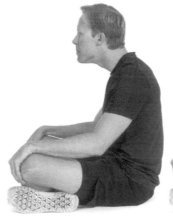
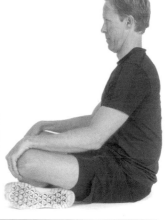

## scapular protraction and retraction mobility

Start with your shoulders in a neutral position. Round your shoulder blades forward into protraction and then backward into retraction without lifting your shoulders or moving your spine.

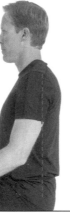
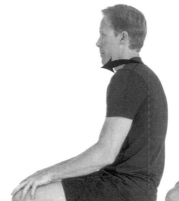
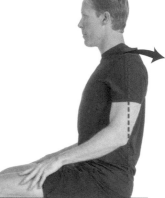

## cervical flexor isometric hold

Tuck your chin and elongate your neck. Keeping your head neutral, lift it just high enough to clear the ground and hold. Stop if you cannot maintain the chin tuck or you start lifting your head higher to reduce fatigue. Do 3 sets of 3–5 reps and work up to 20- to 30-second holds.

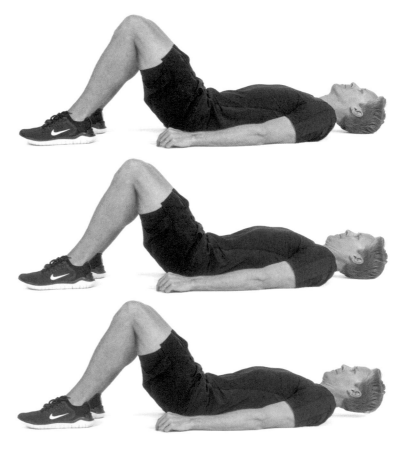

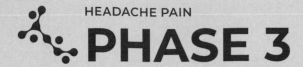

# PHASE 3

**GOOD FOR:**

- Strengthening the neck and surrounding muscles
- Preventing headache pain

**GUIDELINES:**

- Perform every day
- Once your symptoms improve and you can do the isometric exercises without causing flare-ups, add phase 3 exercises from the Neck Pain protocol (pages 158–160)

## cervical manual isometrics (four directions)

- Do 4 or 5 reps with 30- to 45-second resisted holds
- Apply as much force as your neck can tolerate without pain
- Perform seated or standing, on both sides (side-bend and rotation)

### flexion

Tilt your head forward. Push on your forehead with your hand and resist.

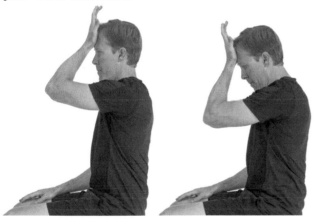

### extension

Tilt your head back slightly. Push on the back of your head with your hand and resist.

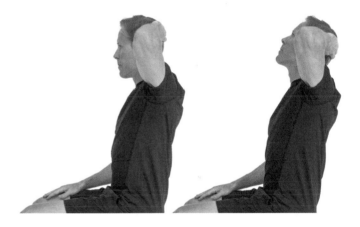

### lateral flexion (side-bend)

Tilt your head to the side. Push on the side of your head with your hand and resist.

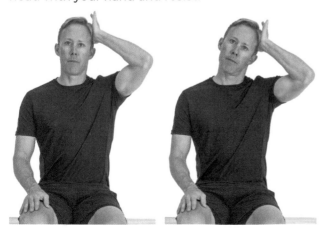

### rotation

Turn your head slightly. Push on the side of your head with your hand and resist.

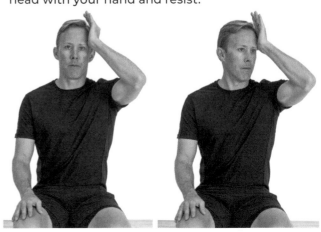

# JAW PAIN

**Follow this program to treat:**

- Temporomandibular joint (TMJ) pain
- Temporomandibular disorder (TMD)

## TEMPOROMANDIBULAR DISORDER (TMD)

**DESCRIPTION:** The temporomandibular joints (TMJs) connect the mandible (jawbone) and the temporal bones (skull) and allow for complex hinging and gliding movements. The TMJs are composed of synovial fluid, cartilage, and a joint capsule, like other joints in the body, but they also contain a unique fibrocartilaginous disc. This makeup allows for several movements that contribute to various tasks such as eating, breathing, and speaking. TMJ disorders can result from a direct injury (blunt force trauma), inflammation of the joints, and/or overuse of the region. Sleep issues related to the jaw (grinding, clenching, and so on) and neck sprains and strains also can contribute to TMD.

**SIGNS AND SYMPTOMS:** TMD typically creates an aching pain near the joint or in the ear and may cause difficulty chewing. You may also experience locking or catching while moving your jaw.

**AGGRAVATING FACTORS:** Grinding teeth, clenching jaw muscles, and chewing hard or chewy foods.

**PROGNOSIS:** This disorder can persist for months or even years if the true cause is not identified. Rehabilitation exercises are important, but it is crucial to see a dental provider to ensure dental problems aren't causing the issue.

**TREATMENT STRATEGY:** In most cases, TMD is treated conservatively with a combination of physical therapy and dental interventions (use of a bite plate or splint).

The rehab exercise program focuses on soft tissue mobilization and mobility exercises for the jaw and upper neck.

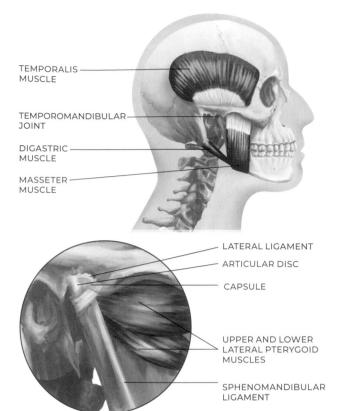

TEMPORALIS MUSCLE

TEMPOROMANDIBULAR JOINT

DIGASTRIC MUSCLE

MASSETER MUSCLE

LATERAL LIGAMENT

ARTICULAR DISC

CAPSULE

UPPER AND LOWER LATERAL PTERYGOID MUSCLES

SPHENOMANDIBULAR LIGAMENT

In phase 1, you mobilize the masseter and temporalis muscles, which are your primary jaw muscles and common sites of tightness and tension. This phase also features suboccipital mobilization because the upper neck muscles and joints are often linked to jaw pain.

Phase 2 incorporates active mobility exercises that capture the primary jaw movements. The goal of these exercises is to move slowly and improve jaw coordination. Movements like lateral deviation, protraction, and retraction require mental focus when you start, so take your time and be intentional about working on your neuromuscular control and range of motion.

Phase 3 implements jaw-specific strengthening exercises for the opening and closing movements introduced in phase 2. Once your pain has improved, I recommend completing the exercises in phase 3 of the Neck Pain protocol. Again, the neck is often linked to jaw pain, and improving neck mobility and strength can reduce the likelihood that your jaw pain comes back.[11,12]

In cases that are resistant to conservative care, surgery may be appropriate. But it's important to give rehab at least six to eight weeks while addressing any aggravating factors before exploring surgical interventions.

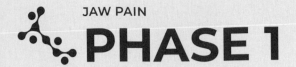

JAW PAIN

# PHASE 1

## GOOD FOR:

- Alleviating jaw pain
- Relieving muscle tension
- Warm-up for phase 2 and 3 exercises

## GUIDELINES:

- Perform every day
- Tools: small massage ball, yoga block
- Add phase 2 when you have no pain at rest and no more than mild pain (3/10) with the exercises

## SOFT TISSUE MOBILIZATIONS:

- ▸ Spend 1–2 minutes on each area
- ▸ Perform in any order on both sides
- ▸ Stop on tender points for 10–20 seconds

---

## masseter mobilization

Using your fingers or thumb, push into the muscle that connects your jawbones. Gently massage the area. Apply pressure on tender spots while opening and closing your jaw.

### manual variation 1

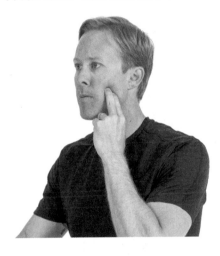
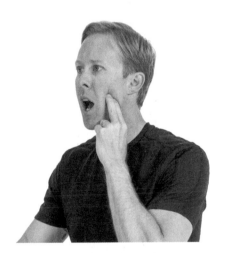
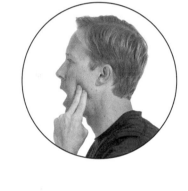

### manual variation 2

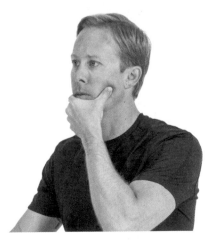
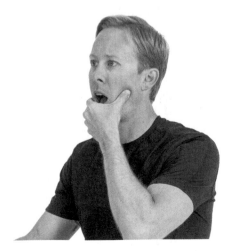
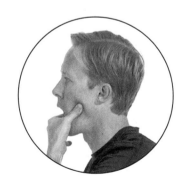

## temporalis mobilization

Using your fingers or a small massage ball, push on the temporalis muscles on the side of your forehead. Gently massage the area. Apply pressure on tender spots while opening and closing your jaw.

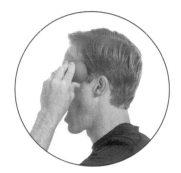

### manual variation

### ball variation

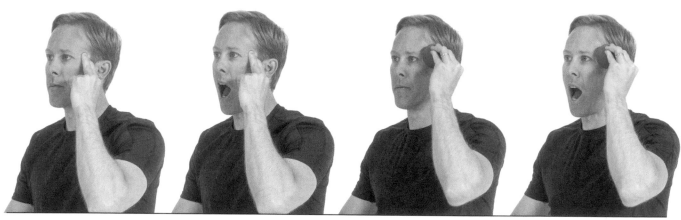

## suboccipital mobilization

Place a small massage ball on a yoga block, positioning the ball at the base of your skull, just to the side of your cervical spine. Slowly move around this region to target the suboccipital muscles. You can rotate your head to the side or twist and adjust the ball with your opposite hand. You can also do the manual variations on pages 174 and 175.

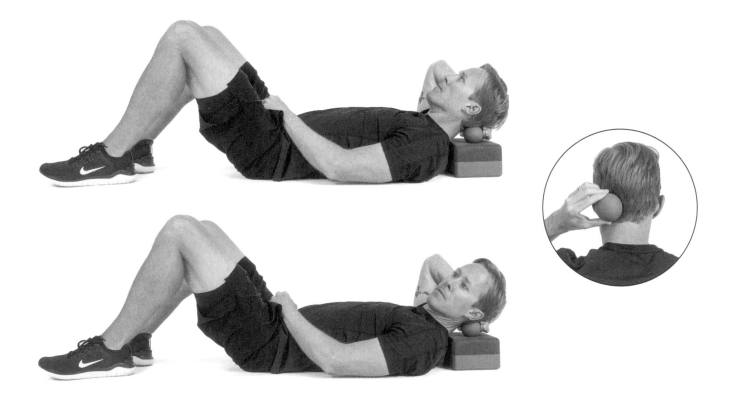

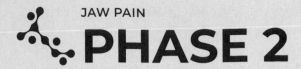

JAW PAIN

# PHASE 2

### GOOD FOR:

- Improving jaw and neck range of motion
- Warm-up for phase 3 exercises

### GUIDELINES:

- Perform every day
- Add phase 3 when you can do the exercises with no more than mild pain (3/10)

## MOBILITY EXERCISES:

- ▸ Do 3 sets of 10–15 reps
- ▸ Active range of motion (AROM)—move as far as you can without pain
- ▸ Pause at end range for 2–3 seconds
- ▸ Perform seated or standing

---

## tmj mobility

### opening and closing

Open your jaw as far as you can without pain. Use your fingers to gently stretch the joint.

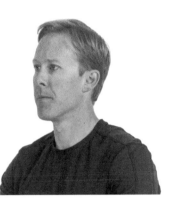 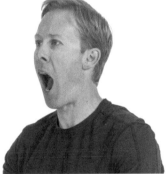 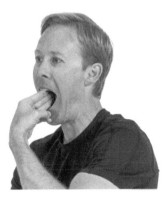

### lateral deviation

Open your mouth slightly, then slide your lower jawbone from right to left.

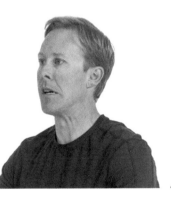 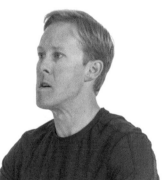

You can position a pen between your teeth to gauge the distance.

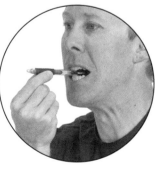

### protraction and retraction

Open your mouth slightly, then slide your lower jawbone forward and backward.

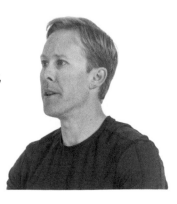 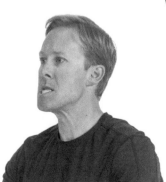

# cervical mobility

## flexion and extension

Start in a neutral position. Slowly move your chin toward your chest, then tilt your head back.

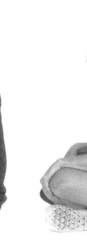
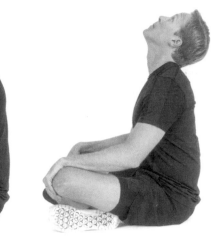

## rotation

Keeping your spine straight, slowly rotate your head toward one shoulder, then the other.

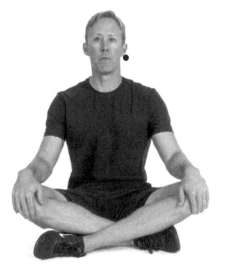
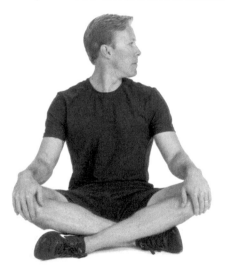
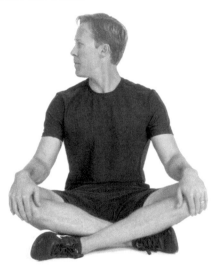

## side-bend

Slowly move your ear toward one shoulder, then the other.

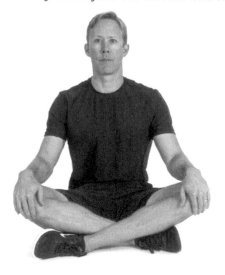
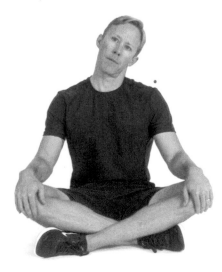
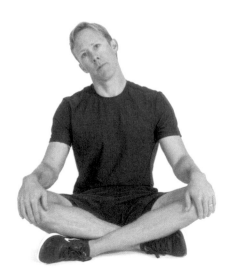

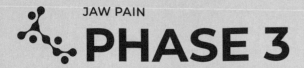

# PHASE 3

## GOOD FOR:

- Strengthening the jaw and neck
- Preventing jaw pain

## GUIDELINES:

- Perform 3 or 4 days a week
- Do 3 sets of 10–15 reps unless otherwise noted
- Add phase 3 exercises from the Neck Pain protocol (pages 158–160) to prevent future jaw pain flare-ups

## resisted opening

Push up on the bottom of your chin with your thumb. Applying steady resistance with your thumb, slowly open and close your jaw.

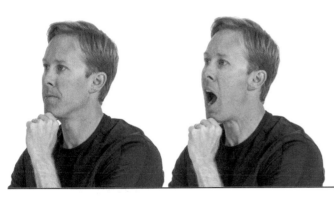

## resisted closing

Pull down on your chin with your fingers. Applying steady resistance with your fingers, slowly open and close your jaw.

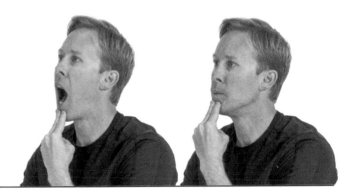

## cervical flexor isometric hold

Tuck your chin and elongate your neck. Keeping your head neutral, lift it just high enough to clear the ground and hold. Stop if you cannot maintain the chin tuck or you start lifting your head higher to reduce fatigue. Perform 4 or 5 reps and work up to 30- to 45-second holds.

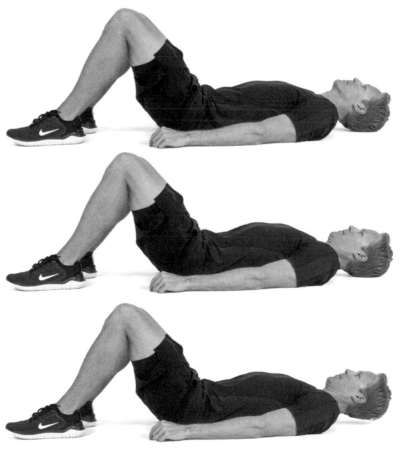

## CHAPTER 16

# SHOULDER
# PROTOCOLS

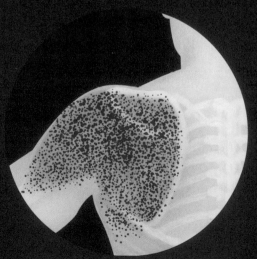

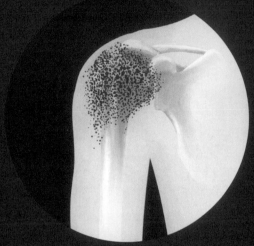

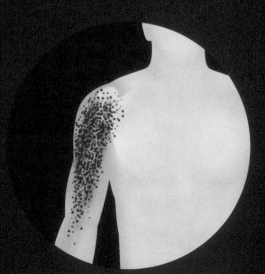

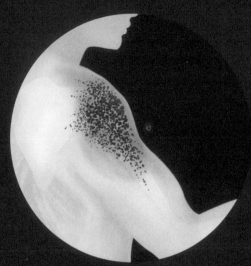

**SHOULDER PAIN**
**(p. 187)**

**SHOULDER INSTABILITY**
**(p. 204)**

**FROZEN SHOULDER**
**(p. 216)**

**BICEPS TENDINOPATHY**
**(p. 224)**

# SHOULDER PAIN

## Follow this program to treat:

- Pain at the top, side, and/or front of the shoulder
- Pain when reaching away from the body and overhead
- Rotator cuff injury (tear/tendinopathy)
- Shoulder impingement (subacromial pain syndrome)
- Shoulder bursitis

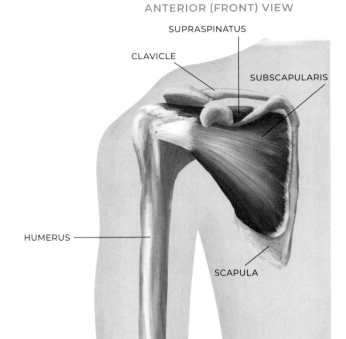

SUPRASPINATUS

CLAVICLE

SUBSCAPULARIS

HUMERUS

SCAPULA

## ROTATOR CUFF INJURY (TEAR/TENDINOPATHY)

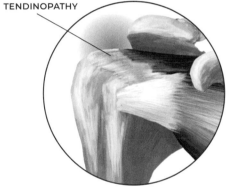

TENDINOPATHY

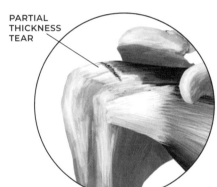

PARTIAL THICKNESS TEAR

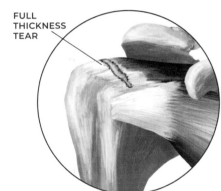

FULL THICKNESS TEAR

**DESCRIPTION:** The rotator cuff includes four muscles that stabilize and rotate the shoulder joint: the supraspinatus on the top of the shoulder, the subscapularis on the front side of the shoulder, and the infraspinatus and teres minor on the back side. These muscles and their tendons are susceptible to tears and irritation (aka tendinopathy or tendinitis). The supraspinatus is the most commonly injured of the four, but any of them can be injured if enough force is applied to the shoulder joint.

Rotator cuff injuries can happen to people of any age. In a younger person, it's usually the result of trauma from an impact, fall, or overuse—any movement that forces the arm away from the body (such as a fall) or repeated movements that stress the muscles beyond their workload capacity (such as high-volume throwing).

Degenerative tears are more common as we age and almost always affect the supraspinatus.[1,2] To reduce your susceptibility to a degenerative tear, start and maintain a resistance training program, such as the one outlined in phase 3 of the rehab protocol.

**SIGNS AND SYMPTOMS:** Because the supraspinatus is prone to injury, most people experience pain at the top or side of the shoulder, and it may refer down the side of the upper arm. This pain is typically close to the surface and can be triggered by sleeping on the painful side, reaching above the level of the shoulder (such as to grab something from a high shelf), or playing sports that involve repeated overhead motions, such as swimming and tennis. If you injure one of the other rotator cuff muscles, you may experience pain on the back of the shoulder (infraspinatus and teres minor) or the front of the shoulder and/or the armpit (subscapularis). Pain is typically dull and achy but becomes sharp when the muscles are active.

**AGGRAVATING FACTORS:** Reaching overhead and/or away from the body, sleeping on the painful side, and lifting objects with an extended arm. Postural positions, such as rounding your shoulders, also can exacerbate pain.

**PROGNOSIS:** This depends on the severity of the injury. Tendinopathy usually resolves within four to 12 weeks with appropriate rehab. Small tears can take up to six months to heal, and large tears often require surgery.

**TREATMENT STRATEGY:** Tendinopathy and small tears in the rotator cuff are treated conservatively with mobility and strengthening exercises. Large tears are usually treated surgically with a rotator cuff repair, which involves sewing the injured tendon back together.[3-5]

In phase **1**, you start by implementing soft tissue mobilization techniques that target the posterior rotator cuff (infraspinatus and teres minor), levator scapulae, rhomboids, upper trapezius, pectoral muscles, and thoracic spine. All of these can reduce pain and tension in not only the rotator cuff but also some of the major muscles that influence scapular (shoulder blade) movement and position.

Next, you add shoulder isometrics to reduce tendon pain and start building strength in the rotator cuff muscles and tendons in order to begin strengthening them in a very low-load manner. Lastly, you start working shoulder joint mobility with passive range of motion (PROM) drills using a dowel or similar object. These exercises allow the rotator cuff muscles to remain relatively relaxed while your uninjured arm guides the injured arm through different movements. Start with PROM drills because implementing active range of motion (AROM) exercises too early can flare pain up and worsen some rotator cuff tears. You should begin passive mobility exercises early in the rehab process to reduce the likelihood of developing a joint contracture, frozen shoulder, or similar range of motion impairments.

In phase **2**, you add thoracic flexion-extension and scapular protraction-retraction mobility exercises, which complement the soft tissue mobilizations from phase 1. By loosening those areas in phase 1, you laid the groundwork to move your shoulder actively—meaning the muscles of the injured arm do the work—which improves mobility and motor control. If this is too challenging or creates too much pain, use the dowel, but don't let the injured arm be fully passive; instead, allow it to do 50 percent of the work while the uninjured arm does the other half (referred to as active assisted range of motion, or AAROM).

You will also perform the angel, a shoulder mobility exercise that dynamically stretches the pectoral muscles, helping you assume a more upright and less rounded posture. Phase 2 ends with the first strengthening exercise, the prone T. This exercise strengthens your scapular retractors, which are located between the shoulder blades and, like the muscles used in the angel exercise, help you maintain a neutral shoulder position.

**Phase 3** focuses on building rotator cuff and scapular muscle strength with resistance training exercises. Because this injury affects a contractile element, improving tissue strength can reduce the likelihood of reinjury.

This phase starts with two row variations that strengthen the scapular retractors by pulling the shoulder blades back.

The next group of exercises focus on external rotation and are arguably the most important for rotator cuff health. I recommend choosing one of the options listed. For most people, the side-lying banded option is a good place to start. The 90/90 variation places the shoulder in abduction, a naturally challenging position that improves strength and control when the arm is away from the body, which is especially important for athletes who throw.

To strengthen your subscapularis—the only muscle that internally rotates the shoulder joint—you will also perform the banded internal rotation exercise.

Next, the shoulder raise options train the deltoid muscle and rotator cuff, especially the supraspinatus. These exercises build strength with movements that involve lifting the arm out and away from the body, which is important because the rotator cuff muscles play a vital role in stabilizing and moving the shoulder in that way. As stated in the protocol, choose one raise option when going through your workout. Then, at your next workout, try a different raise variation to make sure that you practice each one. The D2 variation is like pulling a sword from its sheath and combines shoulder elevation with external rotation. The scaption raise is one of the best exercises for activating the supraspinatus muscle. The lateral and frontal raises continue to build strength with movements that involve lifting the arm out away from the body, which is important because the rotator cuff muscles play a vital role in stabilizing and moving the shoulder joint in that way.

Various pressing exercises are next, working the pectoral and serratus anterior muscles, the latter of which is an important upward rotator of the shoulder blade.

The push-up plus exercise adds to the standard push-up and targets the serratus anterior. If you're interested in variations, you can also do a banded press or standard dumbbell bench press. Sometimes the full-range pressing exercises stress the shoulder and biceps tendon and cause pain (when the arm extends past your trunk in shoulder extension). In this scenario, I recommend reducing the range of motion by performing the floor press and then adding in a full-range pressing exercise once your injury has healed.

The supinated curl is the final exercise in this phase and is designed to strengthen the biceps brachii muscle. One of the tendons of the biceps muscle runs up into the shoulder joint—right next to the supraspinatus tendon. Because of this, many people with rotator cuff pain also have problems with their biceps tendon. The supinated biceps curl can strengthen the biceps muscle and its tendons to reduce shoulder pain. However, if your pain is primarily on the front of your shoulder, I recommend reading the Biceps Tendinopathy protocol, which may be better suited to treat your symptoms.

## WHEN SHOULD I CONSIDER SURGERY?

A full-thickness rotator cuff tear doesn't usually heal from rehab alone; there is always a risk of reoccurring pain and a gradual loss of function. In fact, evidence shows that having an unrepaired full-thickness tear can increase and accelerate your chances of developing shoulder osteoarthritis.[6] If osteoarthritis becomes severe, a total shoulder replacement may be recommended. For this reason, I generally encourage people to consider rotator cuff repair for full-thickness tears and partial-thickness tears that don't improve sufficiently after six months of healing and rehab. The surgery has a high success rate—meaning people regain function and have less pain—and it may lower your chances of needing a total shoulder replacement later in life.

# SHOULDER IMPINGEMENT (SUBACROMIAL PAIN SYNDROME)

**DESCRIPTION:** The term "shoulder impingement" has been replaced with "subacromial pain syndrome," which occurs when the structures underneath the acromion (the bone at the top of the shoulder) become sensitive.[7] These structures include the supraspinatus (a rotator cuff muscle and tendon), the biceps long head tendon, and the subacromial bursa. This pain typically occurs when reaching away from the body with an extended arm, especially when reaching above shoulder level or sleeping on the painful side.

Subacromial pain syndrome differs from a rotator cuff tear because, while a tear could involve any of the four rotator cuff muscles, shoulder impingement involves only the supraspinatus. Shoulder impingement isn't usually caused by a traumatic injury and doesn't always mean anything's torn. Inflammation and irritation also can cause pain when you use those structures. Another possibility is a bone spur, which can occur because of genetics or from overuse injuries.

**SIGNS AND SYMPTOMS:** Pain is usually dull and achy at rest and becomes sharp when stressing the structures in the subacromial space. Pain is experienced on the top, side, or front of the shoulder and may refer down the side of the upper arm. Usually, it is painful at certain points in the range of motion when reaching overhead, even in the absence of trauma.

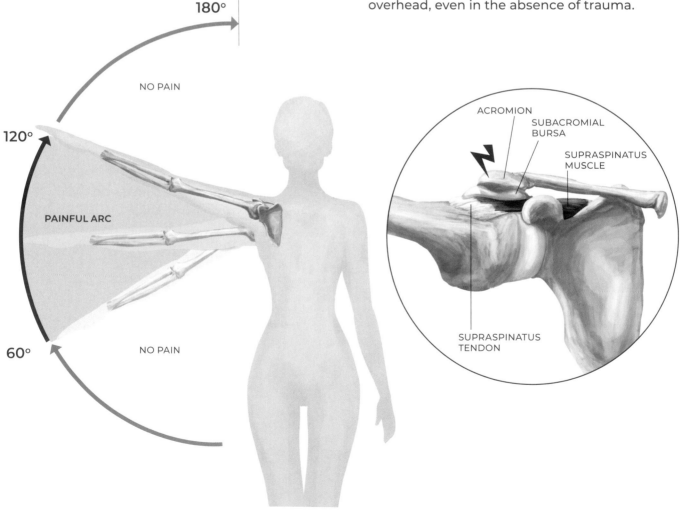

180°
NO PAIN
120°
PAINFUL ARC
60°
NO PAIN

ACROMION
SUBACROMIAL BURSA
SUPRASPINATUS MUSCLE
SUPRASPINATUS TENDON

**AGGRAVATING FACTORS:** Reaching overhead, sleeping on the painful side, and lifting objects with an extended arm. With a repetitive overuse injury, sometimes pain is caused by overhead use of the arm. It doesn't need to be a traumatic injury; you just irritated the area. In the worst-case scenario, you might have a small rotator cuff or biceps tear, but for most people it's just inflammation.

**PROGNOSIS:** Pain and function typically return to normal within four to 12 weeks of implementing an appropriate rehab program.

**TREATMENT STRATEGY:** Rehab should serve as the primary treatment option for subacromial pain syndrome.[8,9] Shoulder mobility work and rotator cuff strengthening are the most common treatments for this condition. A doctor may recommend surgery if they identify a bone spur or a large tear in the supraspinatus or biceps tendons, or if symptoms don't improve with rehab.

If you do undergo surgery—say, to remove a bone spur or repair a tear—you can still implement the rehab exercises if they don't cause pain. The phases are very similar to a post-surgical protocol, so you could implement the rehab exercises before surgery to make the tissues more resilient or after surgery to recover if you don't have access to personalized care.

When it comes to the rehab program—and the reasons for performing the prescribed exercises—the Shoulder Impingement protocol is similar to the rotator cuff treatment strategy (see page 188) in that it involves the structures in the subacromial space, which are the rotator cuff (supraspinatus) and biceps tendons.

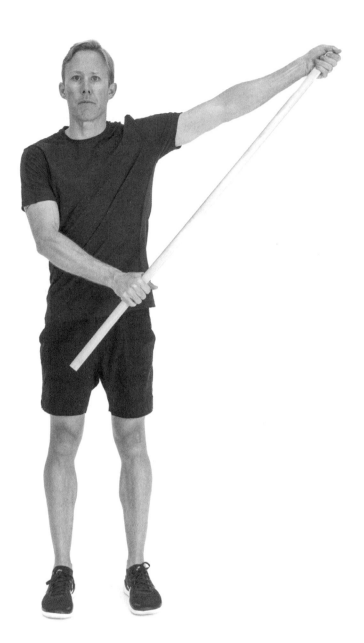

## WHEN SHOULD I SEEK MEDICAL ATTENTION OR CONSIDER SURGERY?

For shoulder impingement, consider speaking with your doctor if you've modified all aggravating activities and tried rehab for at least eight to 12 weeks and you're still not getting better. A doctor can order imaging, which can help determine if you have a bone spur or full-thickness tear, which will not usually heal with rehab alone. Surgical intervention is often required to get back to full function, alleviate pain, and avoid more severe issues later in life.

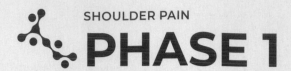

# PHASE 1

## GOOD FOR:

- Alleviating shoulder pain
- Relieving muscle tension
- Improving shoulder range of motion
- Warm-up for phase 2 and 3 exercises

## GUIDELINES:

- Perform every day
- Tools: small massage ball, foam roller, dowel
- Add phase 2 when you have no pain at rest and no more than mild pain (3/10) with the exercises

## SOFT TISSUE MOBILIZATIONS:

- ▸ Spend 1–2 minutes on each area
- ▸ Perform in any order on both sides
- ▸ Stop on tender points for 10–20 seconds
- ▸ Avoid exercises and arm movements that flare up your symptoms

---

## posterior rotator cuff mobilization

Lying on your side, position a small massage ball on the back of your shoulder just below your shoulder blade. Control the pressure with your upper body: roll into the ball to increase the pressure; rotate away from the ball to decrease the pressure. Move your shoulder into internal rotation with your other arm to dynamically mobilize the muscles. You can also do this exercise standing against a wall.

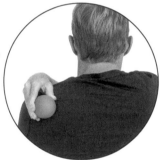

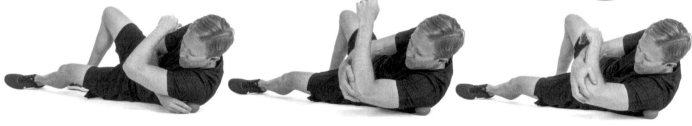

---

## levator scapulae mobilization

Position the ball at the corner of your shoulder blade. Elevate your hips to increase the pressure. Add arm movements to further mobilize the muscle.

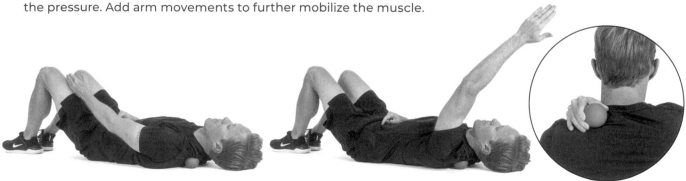

## rhomboid mobilization

Place the ball in the space between your shoulder blade and spine. Work up and down several inches around the shoulder blade (rhomboids). Add arm movements and lift your head to further mobilize the muscles.

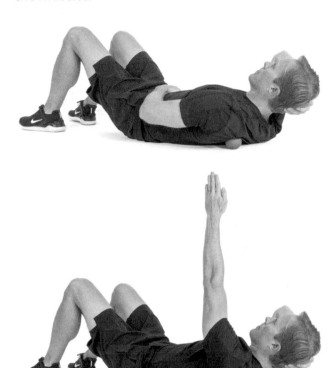

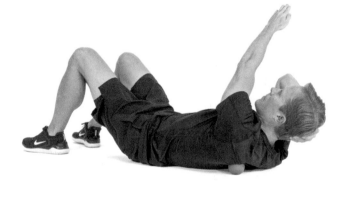

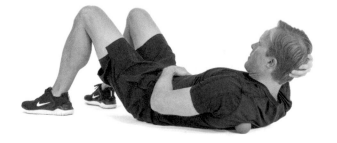

## upper trapezius mobilization

Position the ball between a doorframe or rack and your upper trapezius muscle. Work your way across the entire muscle from your shoulder to the base of your neck. Drive into the ball to increase the pressure. You can move your arm behind your back or in front of your body and your head down and to the side to further mobilize the muscle.

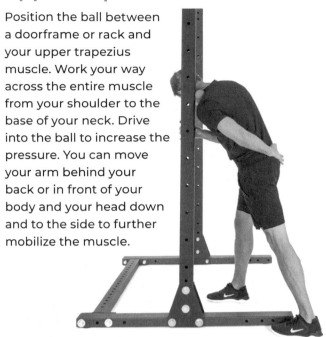

## pectoral mobilization

Position the ball between the doorframe or rack and your pectoral muscles near the front of your shoulder. Place that arm behind your back and add dynamic movement by reaching overhead to further mobilize the muscles.

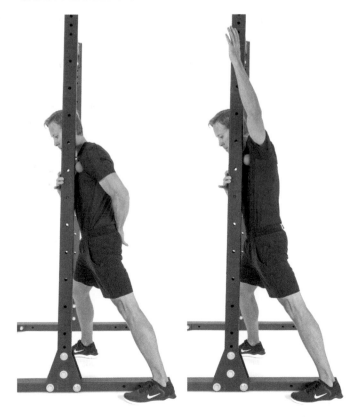

# thoracic mobilization

Position a foam roller perpendicular to your spine under your upper back. Cross your arms over your chest, lift your butt, and then drive off your heels and slowly roll over your mid-back region (not the low back or neck). You can also roll from side to side on stiff areas or flex and extend over the roller (see page 154 for those variations).

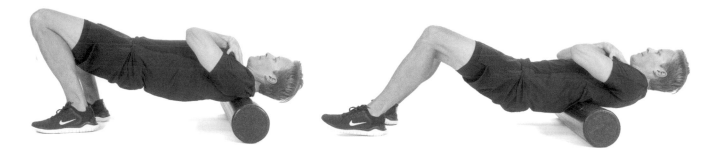

## ISOMETRIC EXERCISES:

▸ Do 4 or 5 reps with 30- to 45-second resisted holds

▸ Apply as much force as your shoulder can tolerate with no more than mild pain

▸ Bend your elbow to 90 degrees and push into a wall or rack

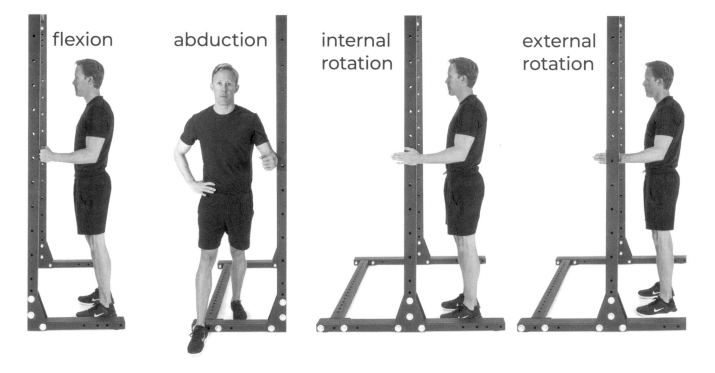

flexion    abduction    internal rotation    external rotation

## MOBILITY EXERCISES:

▸ Do 3 sets of 10–15 reps

▸ Passive range of motion (PROM)—move slowly and as far as you can with no more than mild pain

▸ Pause at end range for 2–3 seconds

▸ Add active assisted range of motion (AAROM) as pain decreases

## shoulder flexion (PROM/ AAROM) mobility

Grip one end of a dowel with your injured arm so that your thumb is facing up. Use your uninjured arm to guide your injured arm straight out in front of you into the overhead position.

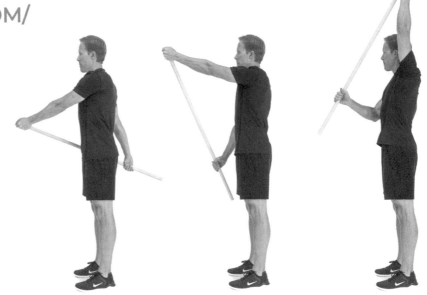

## shoulder abduction (PROM/AAROM) mobility

Start with your injured arm at your side with your palm facing forward. Form your grip by wrapping your thumb over the end of the dowel with your injured arm. Use your uninjured arm to guide your injured arm out to the side into the overhead position.

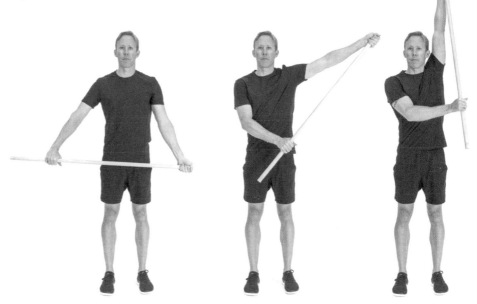

## internal and external rotation (PROM/AAROM) mobility

Grip the dowel with your hands shoulder width apart and palms facing up. Keeping your elbows close to your body, use your uninjured arm to guide your injured arm along a horizontal path to one side—one shoulder will move into external rotation while the other moves into internal rotation. Repeat in the opposite direction.

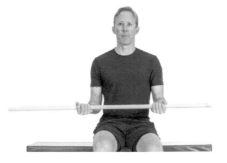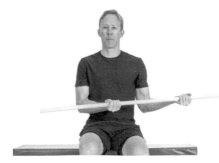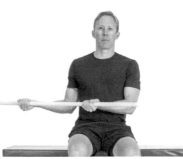

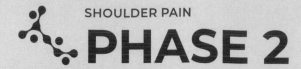

SHOULDER PAIN

# PHASE 2

**GOOD FOR:**

- Improving range of motion
- Building early scapular strength
- Warm-up for phase 3 exercises

**GUIDELINES:**

- Perform every day
- Tools: foam roller, bench
- Add phase 3 when you can do the exercises with no more than mild pain (3/10)

## MOBILITY EXERCISES:

- ▸ Do 3 sets of 10–15 reps
- ▸ Active range of motion (AROM)—move as far as you can with no more than mild pain
- ▸ Pause at end range for 2–3 seconds

## thoracic flexion and extension mobility

Get into the quadruped position—knees aligned under your hips and shoulders over your wrists. Flex (round) your mid-back and neck, then extend. Try to isolate your mid-back and limit movement through your lower back.

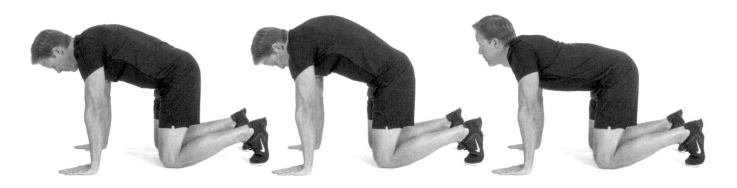

## shoulder protraction and retraction mobility

With your posture upright and your spine neutral, protract your shoulders by pushing them forward, then retract by pulling them back—squeezing your shoulder blades together and tucking your chin slightly at end range.

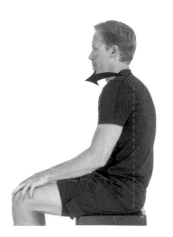
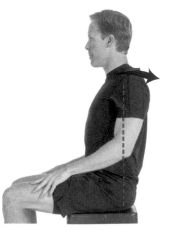

## shoulder flexion mobility

Stand or sit with your arm at your side and your palm facing inward (thumb up). Keeping your arm straight and leading with your thumb, reach your hand out in front of your body and over your head.

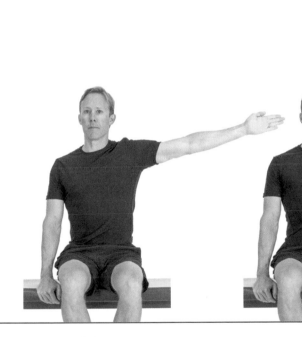

## abduction mobility

Stand or sit with your arm at your side and your palm facing forward. Keeping your arm straight and leading with your thumb, reach your hand out to the side and over your head.

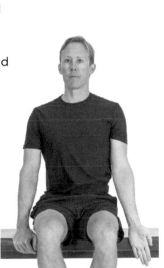

## internal and external rotation mobility

Start with your arm at your side, elbow bent at 90 degrees and thumb facing upward. Keeping your elbow close to your body and thumb up, rotate from your shoulder and move your hand outward and then inward.

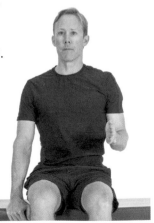
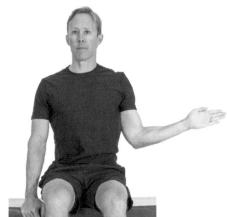
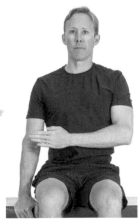

## angel

Position your spine over a foam roller so that your head and tailbone are supported. Start with your arms at your sides and palms up, then reach as far overhead as you can without pain.

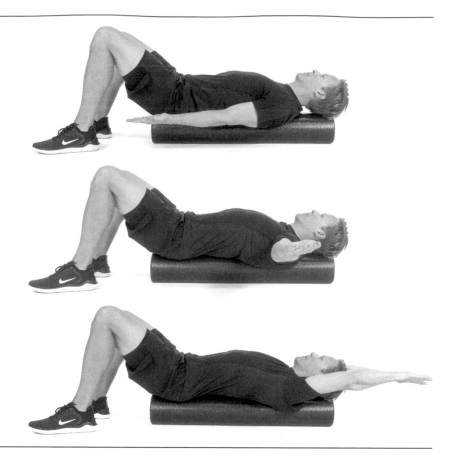

## prone t

Lie facedown on a bench with your arms hanging down, your wrists positioned just behind your shoulders, and your palms facing forward. Leading with your thumbs and keeping your elbows straight, lift your arms out to the side and make a "T" shape. Squeeze your shoulder blades together at the top of the motion.

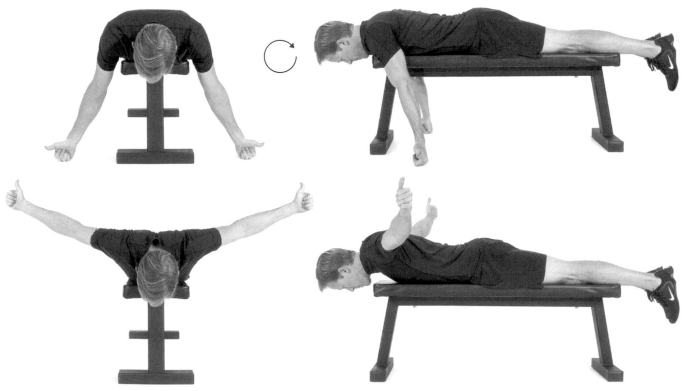

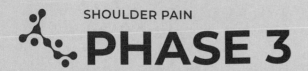

## SHOULDER PAIN
# PHASE 3

**GOOD FOR:**

- Strengthening the shoulder and surrounding muscles
- Preventing shoulder pain and injury

**GUIDELINES:**

- Perform 3 or 4 days a week
- Do 3 sets of 10–15 reps
- Push sets to fatigue
- When there are multiple exercise options, choose a variation based on your injury type, equipment availability, and personal preference
- Tools: bench, dumbbells, resistance bands, towel
- All banded exercises can be done using a cable machine

---

### row *(choose one)*

## dumbbell row

Place one hand and knee on a bench with your spine neutral. Let your opposite arm hang down to the side of the bench, then bend your elbow and pull the dumbbell straight up toward your chest.

## banded row

Kneel on the ground and position a band at shoulder height. Start with your arm extended in front of your body, then draw your elbow back and pull the handle toward your armpit, keeping your thumb facing upward.

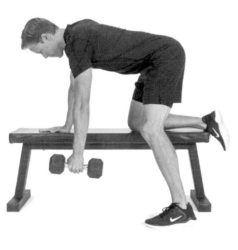

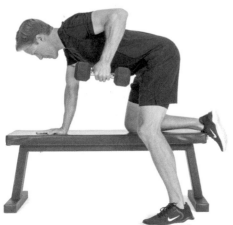

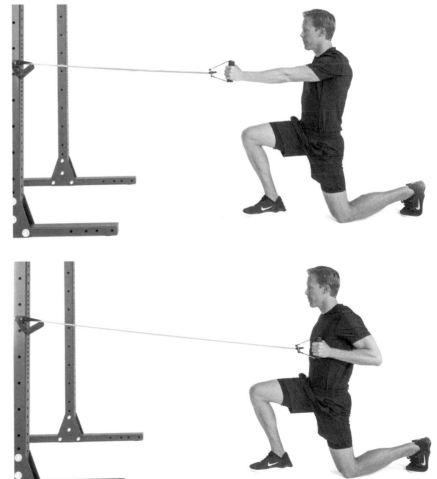

# external rotation *(choose one)*

## side-lying dumbbell

Lie on your side on the bench with your injured arm on top. Position a folded/rolled-up towel between your elbow and body. Keep your elbow at 90 degrees and start with your hand next to your stomach. Keeping your elbow pinned to your side, lead with your knuckles and lift the dumbbell by externally rotating from your shoulder.

## prone 90/90

Lie facedown on the bench. Start with your shoulder and elbow at 90 degrees. Keeping your elbow bent, lift the dumbbell by externally rotating your shoulder until your arm is parallel with the ground.

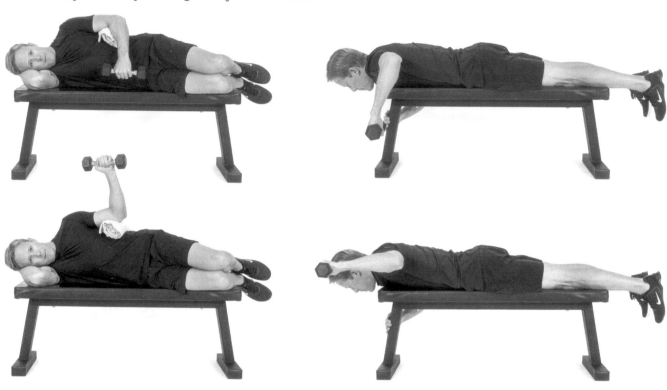

## banded variation

Anchor a band at about belly button level. With a folded/rolled-up towel positioned between your elbow and body, bend your arm to 90 degrees and grip the handle near your stomach. Keeping your elbow pinned to your side, lead with your knuckles and pull the band outward by externally rotating from your shoulder.

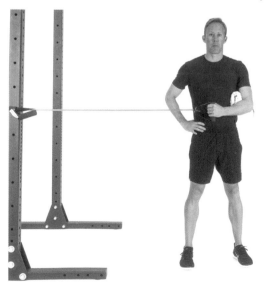 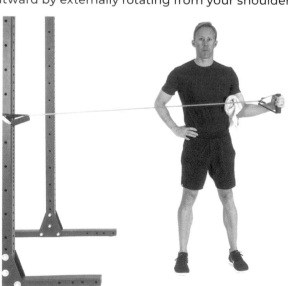

# banded internal rotation

Anchor a band just above hip height. With a folded/rolled-up towel positioned between your elbow and body, bend your arm to about 90 degrees. Keeping your elbow pinned to your side, internally rotate your shoulder and slowly pull the handle to your stomach.

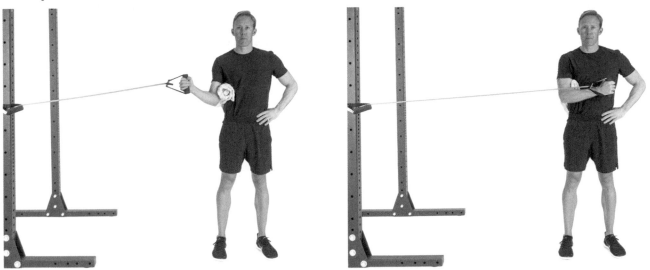

## raise *(choose one)*

### d2 raise

Secure an overhand grip on a resistance band so that it's in front of your body with your arms at your sides. Start by moving your injured arm across your body, positioning your hand near your centerline with your thumb down. Keeping your uninjured arm at your side, move your injured arm out and away from your body while externally rotating your shoulder. Finish with your arm overhead and your thumb up.

### scaption raise

Hold dumbbells at your sides with your palms facing forward. Keeping your elbows straight and leading with your thumbs, lift your arms out to the side and slightly in front of your body, creating a "V" shape. Stop the movement at shoulder level. Do not lift your shoulder blades (shrug your shoulders toward your ears).

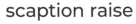
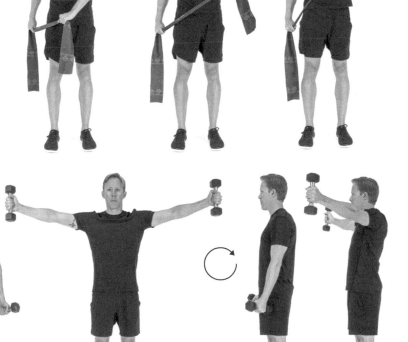

## lateral raise

With your thumbs facing forward, lift your arms out to the side to shoulder level. You can also do this variation with one arm using a resistance band or cable machine.

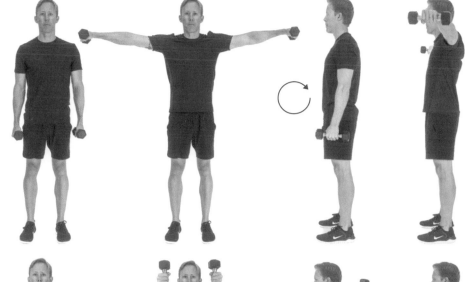

## frontal raise

With your thumbs facing forward, raise your arms to shoulder level.

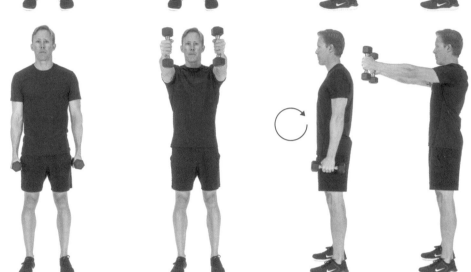

## press *(choose one)*

## push-up plus

Get into the plank position: hands shoulder width apart, shoulders aligned over your wrists, and back flat. Perform a standard push-up by lowering your chest to the ground. Try to keep your elbows in (about 45 degrees from your body), forearms vertical, and back flat as you lower into the bottom position. As you reverse the movement and return to the start position with your elbows extended, protract your shoulder blades by pushing your shoulders toward the ground. This should raise your body a few inches.

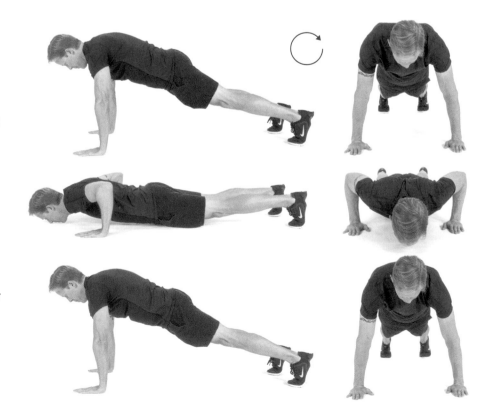

## floor press

Lie on the floor, position the dumbbells over your lower chest with your palms facing your legs, and get your triceps flush with the ground. Position your elbows slightly away from your body (at a 45-degree angle) and keep your forearms vertical. As you press the dumbbells straight up, rotate your shoulders so that your palms are facing each other at the top of the movement.

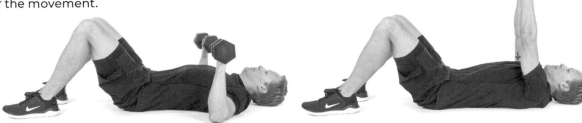

## bench press

Lie on a bench and position the dumbbells over your lower chest with your palms facing your legs. Position your elbows slightly away from your body (at a 45-degree angle) and keep your forearms vertical. As you press the dumbbells straight up, rotate your shoulders so that your palms are facing each other at the top of the movement.

## banded press with protraction

Anchor the band at about chest height. Press your arms straight out. As you extend your elbows, rotate your palms toward the ground and protract your shoulders (push your shoulder blades forward).

## single-arm supinated curl

Hold a dumbbell with your arm at your side and your palm facing inward. Keeping your elbow close to your side, lift the dumbbell toward your shoulder. As you curl your arm, rotate your palm upward and toward your body (supination).

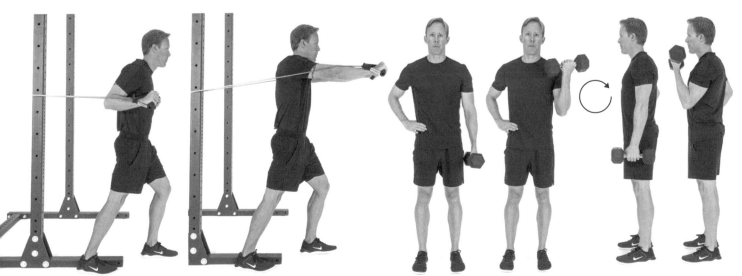

# SHOULDER INSTABILITY

**Follow this program to treat:**

- Pain deep in the shoulder joint
- Dislocations/subluxations
- Labral tears
- Hypermobility

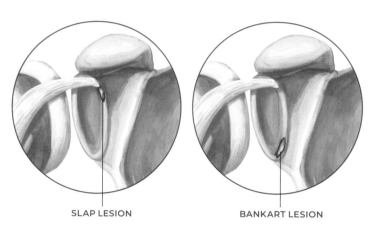

SLAP LESION

BANKART LESION

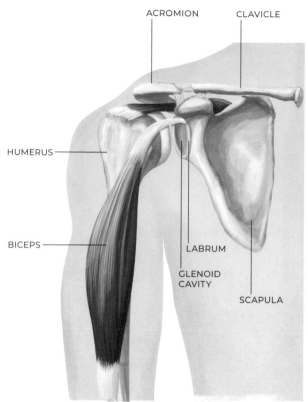

ACROMION

CLAVICLE

HUMERUS

BICEPS

LABRUM

GLENOID CAVITY

SCAPULA

## LABRAL TEARS AND DISLOCATIONS/SUBLUXATIONS

**DESCRIPTION:** Labral tears (SLAP and Bankart lesions are two types) involve injuries to the fibrocartilaginous rim that covers the periphery of the shoulder joint. These injuries can result in shoulder instability, a condition of increased joint mobility that often leads to dislocations and/or subluxations.

One common injury type is anterior dislocation, where the ball pops forward out of the socket, toward the front of the body. Usually, it involves reaching away from the body—often with the arm out and externally rotated—and losing control, such as while incline bench pressing or falling on an outstretched arm. Maybe you're putting on a sweatshirt, and when you put your arm up through the hole, you experience sharp pain or a sensation that your shoulder is going to dislocate. You can reproduce the pain by reaching away from your body and may experience apprehension with unstable shoulder positions.

A previous injury makes people more susceptible to labral tears and dislocations. For example, if you dislocate your shoulder and have a labral tear, you are at a higher risk of reinjury because you may have damaged the passive restraints (ligaments, labrum, and joint capsule) that protect the joint. So, if it's a more substantial injury—such as a tear, a severe stretch of the ligaments around the shoulder, or an injured labrum—you'll have less stability in the joint. What's more, some people are born with hypermobile joints, making them more susceptible to labral tears and dislocations. Following this protocol will increase neuromuscular control and strength, reducing not only the pain but also the likelihood of reinjury.

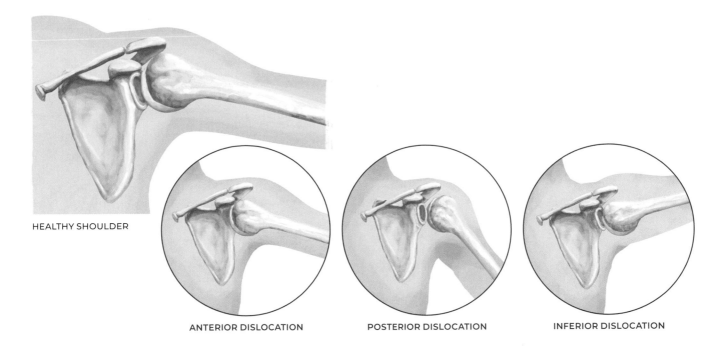

HEALTHY SHOULDER

ANTERIOR DISLOCATION      POSTERIOR DISLOCATION      INFERIOR DISLOCATION

**SIGNS AND SYMPTOMS:** A labral tear often causes sharp, catching pain with certain movements—such as rotating the shoulder externally, reaching overhead, and moving the arm out or across the body—followed by a deep aching sensation for several hours after the provocative movement. This dull pain feels as though it's coming from deep inside the joint—as in, you can't touch it. The shoulder might also pop, click, or grind, and you may feel weakness, looseness, or instability in the shoulder, as if the joint could slip out of place when you reach away from your body or rotate your arm.

**AGGRAVATING FACTORS:** Overhead motions like lifting and throwing or any shoulder motion that involves reaching up, out, or across the body combined with rotation.

**PROGNOSIS:** With some cases of shoulder instability, especially those that don't involve trauma, you see significant improvements in pain and function within eight to 12 weeks. Some traumatic instability cases improve with rehab, but recurrent dislocations often require surgical repair of the labrum.

**TREATMENT STRATEGY:** Labral tears and shoulder instability are usually treated with eight to 12 weeks of physical therapy focused on improving shoulder stability and strength.

People who are born with hypermobility or have shoulder instability without a preexisting traumatic injury have a 50 to 85 percent success rate with rehab.[10-12] Following the rehab exercises to strengthen the shoulder and surrounding muscles improves stability and decreases occurrences of shoulder dislocation.

However, people who had a traumatic injury have only a 15 percent success rate with rehab.[12] For example, say you never had shoulder issues before, but your shoulder dislocated in a car accident, and now it dislocates frequently. Your chances of getting back to full function with rehab are not promising, and you should consider surgical repair.

In phase 1, start with soft tissue mobilization techniques that target the rotator cuff and many of the other major muscles that move and influence the shoulders and shoulder blades. People with shoulder instability often also have pain and tension in the surrounding muscles, which are working overtime to help stabilize the joint and compensate for the ineffective passive restraints (especially the labrum). After mobilizing these muscles, perform the active range of motion (AROM) drills for the shoulder complex.

Because shoulder instability affects the passive subsystem rather than contractile structures (muscles and tendons), lifting the arm usually causes less pain than with a rotator cuff injury. This means you can start AROM exercises earlier, skipping the passive range of motion (PROM) techniques. Also, AROM exercises require the neuromuscular system to be active, which is an essential ingredient in reducing shoulder instability. Phase 1 ends with shoulder isometrics, which begin increasing joint stability by activating and strengthening the shoulder muscles in multiple planes of motion.

Phase 2 jumps into lower load resistance training exercises. Don't do any stretching because, when the joint is already hypermobile, stretching can increase instability. Instead, focus on building motor control and strength in the muscles that surround the shoulder joint and shoulder blade.

In this phase, you perform pulling (banded row) and pushing (banded press) exercises, which work antagonistic (opposing) shoulder blade muscles. The lateral raise works the shoulder in the frontal plane and targets the middle deltoid and supraspinatus (a rotator cuff muscle). The bench liftoff strengthens the rotator cuff muscles and many other scapular muscles.

The remainder of phase 2 focuses on targeted rotator cuff strengthening (banded internal and external rotation) because stabilizing the shoulder joint is one of the rotator cuff's primary functions. Additionally, internal rotation strengthening can help reduce future anterior dislocations by targeting the subscapularis rotator cuff muscle, which runs across the front of the shoulder.

Phase 3 provides more advanced resistance training exercises with the goal of teaching the neuromuscular system to compensate for the instability caused by either laxity in the passive subsystem or instability from a traumatic injury. You start with a supinated biceps curl to strengthen the biceps brachii muscle, which runs across the front of the shoulder joint, and to protect against future dislocations (especially anterior ones). To continue building shoulder stability and strength, you will perform D2 flexion and prone 90/90 external rotation raises. Most dislocations and subluxations happen when someone reaches out away from the body, so it is important to build strength in that position.

Continuing with the program, you move on to a series of closed-chain drills (hands fixed to the ground), which include the shoulder tap, clock, and dolphin press. Each exercise requires you to use your muscles to stabilize the ball of the humerus bone in the shoulder socket. Shoulder taps come first because they are the most straightforward. Stabilize the joint and then lift the other arm and tap the unstable shoulder, working the joint when your body weight is on that arm. The clock takes things up a level by requiring dynamic movements and resistance from the band. You do this exercise on both sides to make your injured shoulder both stabilize itself and move against the resistance of the band. The dolphin press strengthens the serratus anterior muscle, an important mover and stabilizer of the shoulder blade.

Last is the shoulder press, an open-chain exercise. This one comes at the end because it puts the joint in a position where injury is more likely if you don't possess the necessary strength and motor control. Start with a light dumbbell and make sure your neuromuscular control is dialed in before adding weight.

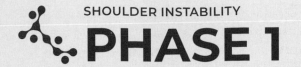

# PHASE 1

## GOOD FOR:

- Alleviating shoulder pain
- Improving neuromuscular control
- Warm-up for phase 2 and 3 exercises

## GUIDELINES:

- Perform every day
- Tool: small massage ball
- Add phase 2 when you have no pain at rest and no more than mild pain (3/10) with the exercises

## SOFT TISSUE MOBILIZATIONS:

▸ Spend 1–2 minutes on each area

▸ Perform in any order on both sides

▸ Stop on tender points for 10–20 seconds

## posterior rotator cuff mobilization

Lying on your side, position a small massage ball on the back of your shoulder just below your shoulder blade. Control the pressure with your upper body: roll into the ball to increase the pressure; rotate away from the ball to decrease the pressure. Move your shoulder into internal rotation with your other arm to dynamically mobilize the muscles. You can also do this exercise standing against a wall.

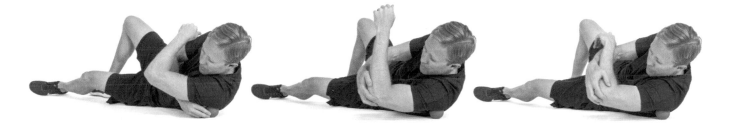

## rhomboid mobilization

Place the ball in the space between your shoulder blade and spine. Work up and down several inches around the shoulder blade (rhomboids). Add arm movements and lift your head to further mobilize the muscles.

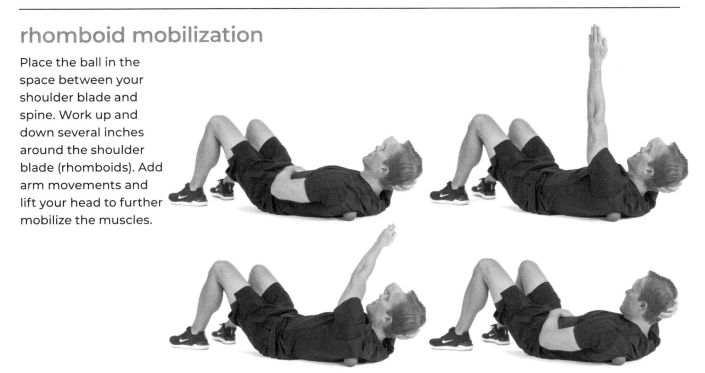

## pectoral mobilization

Position the ball between a doorframe or rack and your pectoral muscles near the front of your shoulder. Place that arm behind your back and add dynamic movement by reaching overhead to further mobilize the muscles. Skip the arm movements if they flare up your symptoms.

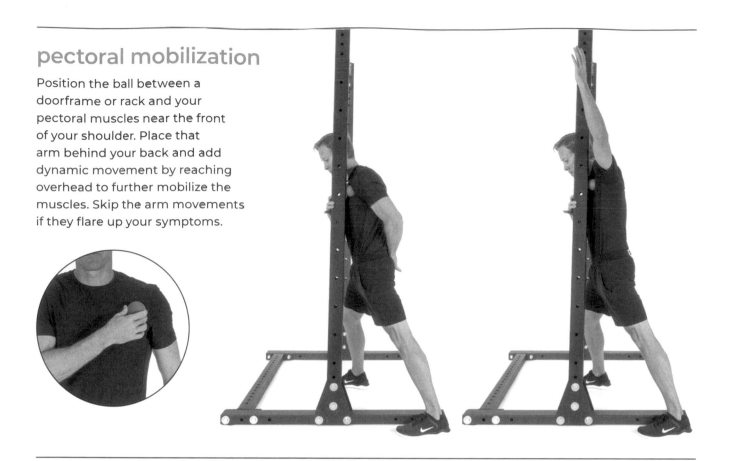

## MOBILITY EXERCISES:

- ▸ Do 3 sets of 10–15 reps
- ▸ Active range of motion (AROM)—move as far as you can without pain
- ▸ Pause at end range for 2–3 seconds

## shoulder flexion mobility

Stand or sit with your arm at your side and your palm facing inward. Keeping your arm straight and leading with your thumb, reach your hand out in front of your body and over your head.

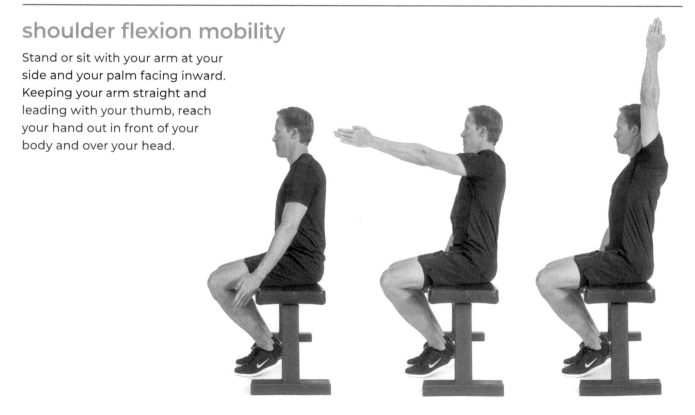

## abduction mobility

Stand or sit with your arm at your side and your palm facing forward. Keeping your arm straight and leading with your thumb, reach your hand out to your side and over your head.

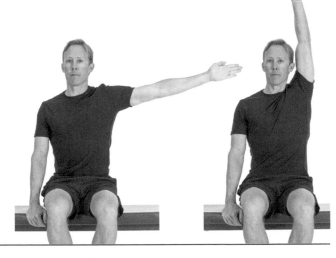

## internal and external rotation mobility

Bend your elbow at 90 degrees with your thumb facing upward. Keeping your elbow close to your body and thumb up, rotate from your shoulder and move your hand outward and then inward.

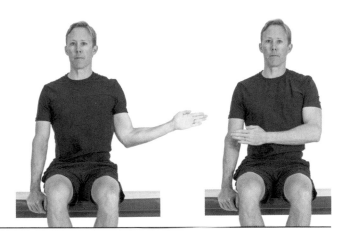

## ISOMETRIC EXERCISES:

▸ Do 4 or 5 reps with 30- to 45-second resisted holds

▸ Apply as much force as you can tolerate with no more than mild pain

▸ Bend your elbow to 90 degrees and push into a wall or rack

flexion     abduction     internal rotation     external rotation

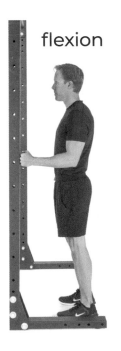
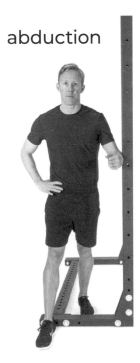
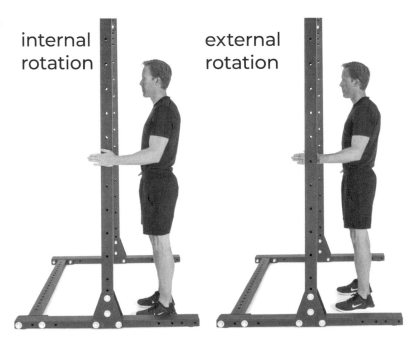

# PHASE 2

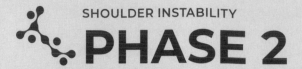

## GOOD FOR:

- Improving shoulder stability and neuromuscular control
- Warm-up for phase 3 exercises

## GUIDELINES:

- Perform 3 or 4 days a week
- Do 3 sets of 10–15 reps
- Tools: resistance tube band, dumbbells, bench, towel
- All banded exercises can be done using a cable machine
- Add phase 3 when you can do the exercises with control and no more than mild pain (3/10)

## kneeling banded single-arm row

Kneel on the ground and anchor a band at shoulder height. Start with your arm extended in front of your body, then draw your elbow back and pull the handle toward your armpit, keeping your thumb facing upward. Keep your shoulders square and don't lean back as you pull.

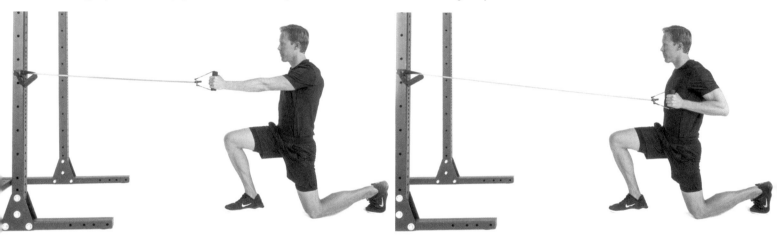

## kneeling banded single-arm press

Facing away from the rack, press your arm straight out in front of your body. As you extend your elbow, rotate your palm toward the ground.

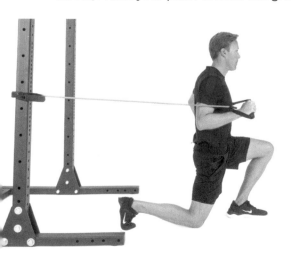
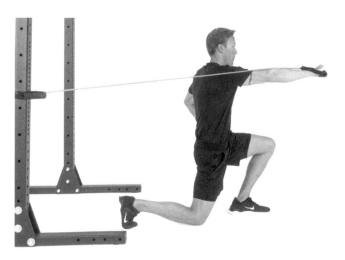

## lateral raise

Holding dumbbells at your sides, raise your arms to shoulder level with your palms facing downward and elbows straight.

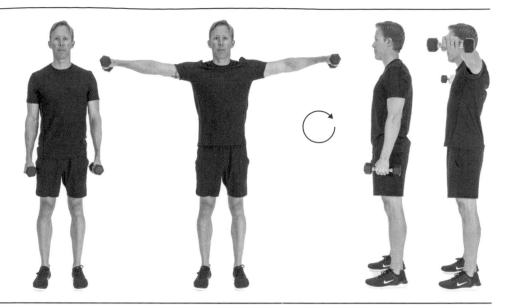

## bench lift-off

Sit on a bench and grip the edge with both hands. Tilt your torso forward, drive through your palms, and push your shoulders toward the ground. Hold this position for 2–3 seconds. You can keep your knees bent and lift your entire body off the ground or keep your feet on the floor to help support your weight.

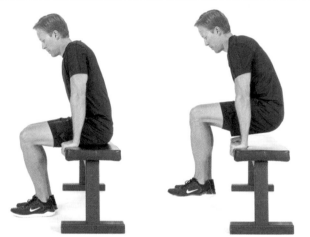

## banded internal rotation

Anchor the band just above hip height. With a folded/rolled-up towel positioned between your elbow and body, bend your arm to about 90 degrees. Keeping your elbow pinned to your side, internally rotate your shoulder and slowly pull the handle to your stomach.

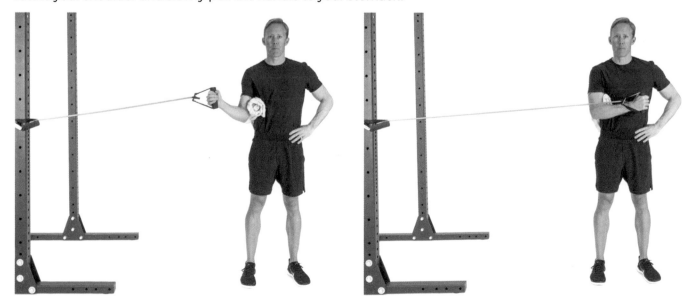

# banded external rotation

With a folded/rolled-up towel positioned between your elbow and body, bend your arm to 90 degrees and grip the handle near your stomach. Keeping your elbow pinned to your side, lead with your knuckles and pull the band outward by externally rotating from your shoulder.

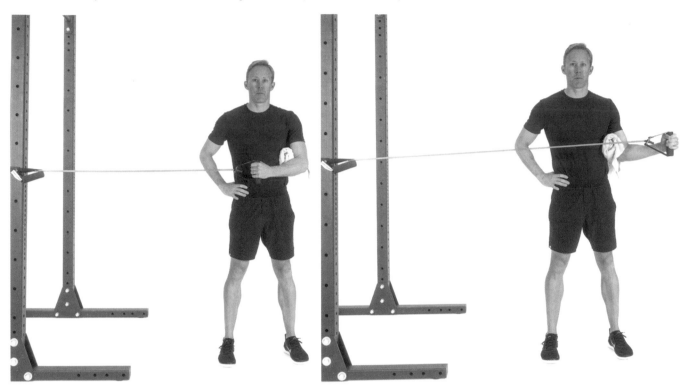

## side-lying dumbbell variation

Lie on your side with your injured arm on top. Position a folded/rolled-up towel between your elbow and body. Keep your elbow at 90 degrees and start with your hand next to your stomach. Keeping your elbow pinned to your side, lead with your knuckles and lift the dumbbell by externally rotating from your shoulder.

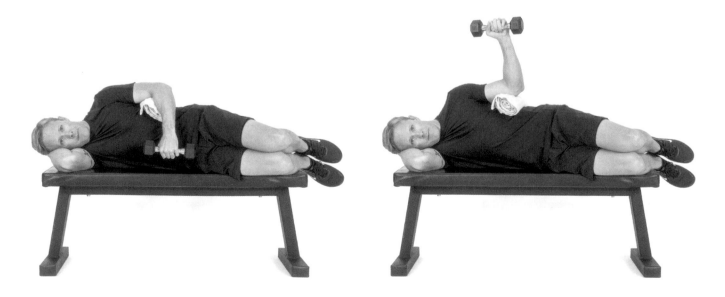

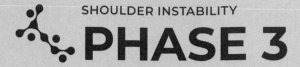

# PHASE 3

## GOOD FOR:

- Strengthening the shoulder with higher stabilization demands
- Improving shoulder stability and neuromuscular control

## GUIDELINES:

- Perform 3 or 4 days a week
- Do 3 sets of 10–15 reps
- Push sets to fatigue
- Tools: dumbbell, resistance band, bench, resistance loop

## single-arm supinated curl

Hold a dumbbell with your arm at your side and your palm facing inward. Keeping your elbow close to your side, lift the dumbbell toward your shoulder. As you curl your arm, rotate your palm upward and toward your body (supination).

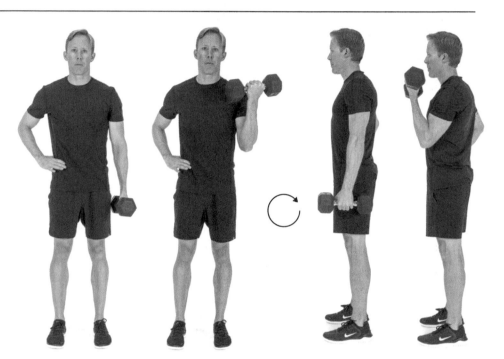

## d2 flexion

Secure an overhand grip on a resistance band so that it's in front of your body with your arms at your sides. Start by moving your injured arm across your body, positioning your hand near your centerline with your thumb down. Keeping your uninjured arm at your side, move your injured arm out and away from your body while externally rotating your shoulder. Finish with your arm overhead and your thumb up.

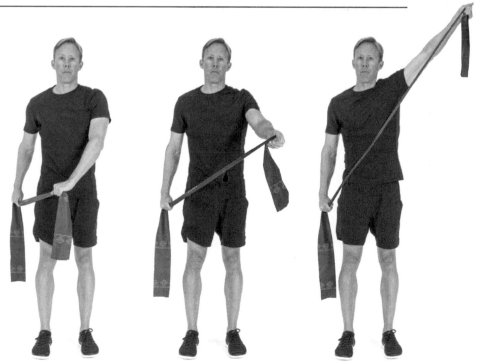

## prone 90/90 external rotation

Lie facedown on a bench with your shoulder and elbow at 90 degrees and your hand pointed toward the ground. Maintaining your shoulder and elbow position and leading with your knuckles, lift the dumbbell by externally rotating your shoulder so that your arm is parallel with the ground.

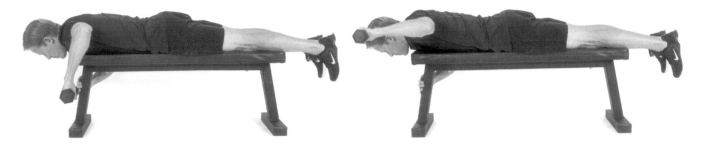

## shoulder taps

Get into the plank position (top of a push-up): hands shoulder width apart, shoulders aligned over your wrists, and back flat. Shifting your weight on to one side, reach your opposite hand across your body, touch the shoulder of your supporting arm (quick tap), and then go back to the start position. Immediately repeat on the other side, and that's one rep.

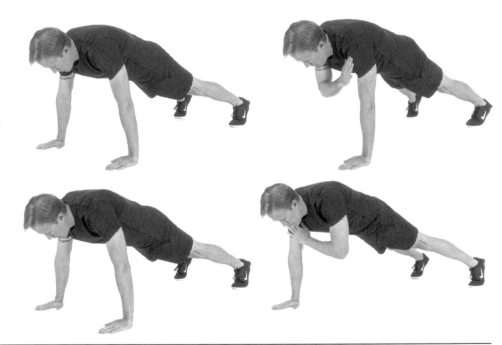

## shoulder clock

With a resistance loop around your wrists, get into plank position. The idea is to move your hand forward, outward, and toward your hips, returning to the start position after every step. Add diagonal steps to hit every clock position to make the exercise more challenging. If you're moving your left hand, you would go 12 o'clock, 11 o'clock, and so on until you get to 7 o'clock.

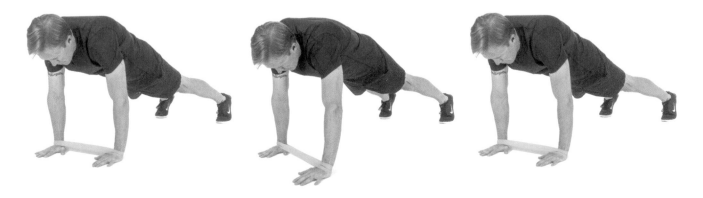

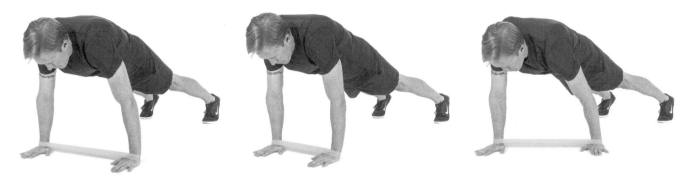

Repeat on the opposite side. Each hand movement—out and back—counts as a rep. Aim for 12–18 reps with each arm.

## dolphin press

Get into the plank position with your elbows positioned underneath your shoulders and your forearms flush with the ground. Walk your feet forward and elevate your hips, keeping your back as flat as possible. Lower your head to the ground and allow your shoulders to retract. Maintaining your back and hip angle, protract your shoulders (push your shoulders toward the ground) and lift your body.

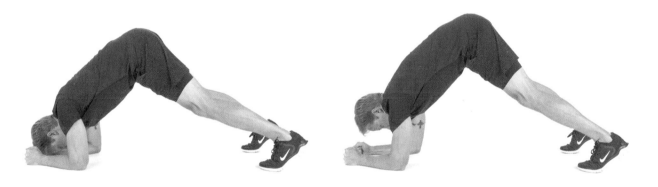

## shoulder press

Start in a kneeling position with your lead shin vertical and torso upright. Position a dumbbell over one shoulder, keeping your elbow tight to your body and palm facing inward. Push the weight straight up and fully lock out your elbow. Return to the start position slowly and with control.

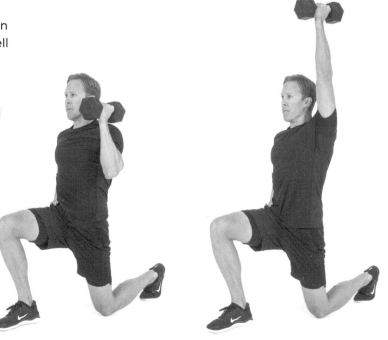

# FROZEN SHOULDER (ADHESIVE CAPSULITIS)

**Follow this program to treat:**

- Shoulder joint stiffness and pain
- Shoulder range of motion restriction
- Adhesive capsulitis

**DESCRIPTION:** Adhesive capsulitis, or frozen shoulder, describes a progressive condition in which the shoulder joint capsule tightens, leading to progressive stiffness, pain, functional limitations, and mobility restrictions. It is most common in people between the ages of 40 and 65, especially women and anyone who has already experienced frozen shoulder. Diseases that lead to systemic inflammation (such as diabetes and thyroid disease) also increase the risk of developing this issue and injuries such as rotator cuff or labral tears.[13]

If you have shoulder pain and start to lose range of motion—as in, you can't turn your arm outward or lift it all the way overhead—you should start rehab. There are three phases for this condition:

- **FREEZING:** It hurts and is getting tight (two to nine months).
- **FROZEN:** Your range of motion is stuck. The pain usually isn't as bad in this phase, but the arm won't move (four to 12 months).
- **THAWING:** It slowly starts loosening up, which tends to happen spontaneously and can take 12 to 24 months to occur.[13]

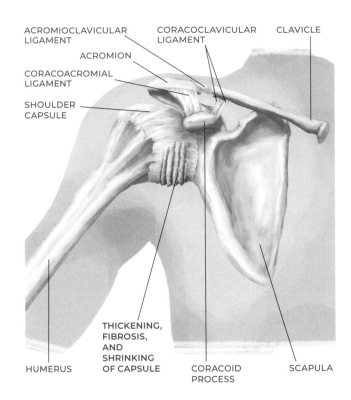

ACROMIOCLAVICULAR LIGAMENT
CORACOCLAVICULAR LIGAMENT
CLAVICLE
ACROMION
CORACOACROMIAL LIGAMENT
SHOULDER CAPSULE
THICKENING, FIBROSIS, AND SHRINKING OF CAPSULE
HUMERUS
CORACOID PROCESS
SCAPULA

**SIGNS AND SYMPTOMS:** Mobility restrictions and pain are the most common symptoms associated with frozen shoulder. The mobility restrictions worsen over time and typically follow a capsular pattern, where range of motion is lost in a particular order (external rotation, then abduction, then flexion). Pain may be the first thing you notice, but then your arm stops turning outward. One side will be normal, but the other side will be stuck, as if there's a wall, and you can't turn your arm away from your body or lift it out to the side. The hallmark symptom is that it just won't move. The pain associated with this condition is typically deep and vague and affects the whole joint, unlike point-specific pain. Frozen shoulder has a very specific set of symptoms, and it's one of the only conditions where you lose range of motion completely.

**AGGRAVATING FACTORS:** Pain and mobility restrictions are often noted when attempting to move the shoulder through its normal range of motion, especially into external rotation, abduction, and flexion.

**PROGNOSIS:** When treated early with physical therapy and cortisone injections, frozen shoulder can resolve within six months.[14,15] If it is not addressed early, it can persist for one to three years.

**TREATMENT STRATEGY:** Frozen shoulder treatment usually combines physical therapy (joint mobilizations and stretching), anti-inflammatory medication, and steroid injections. The rehab protocol mainly focuses on progressively improving range of motion; it does not include any soft tissue mobilizations because you should focus on regaining shoulder mobility and function. If you are looking for strategies to reduce pain and muscle tension, use the phase 1 soft tissue mobilizations from the Shoulder Pain protocol on pages 192 to 194.

Phase 1 focuses on passive range of motion (PROM) exercises where you use a dowel or similar tool and the healthy arm to stretch the affected arm. PROM exercises let you stretch the shoulder farther than moving the arm on its own (active range of motion) and can help reduce pain. The key is to push the affected shoulder to the point where you feel a moderate stretch but not severe pain. The table slide is another shoulder flexion mobility variation where the painful arm stays mostly relaxed as you lean your trunk forward and stretch the joint.

Phase 1 ends with shoulder isometrics, which activate the shoulder muscles and build early strength. Because frozen shoulder causes severe impairments in joint range of motion, the shoulder muscles can atrophy; the isometric exercises help offset some of these negative changes.

Phase 2 adds stretches that employ many of the same movements from phase 1, but now you're holding the positions longer to challenge your mobility. With each stretch, move to the point of moderate stretch and hold it for as long as you can tolerate (up to five minutes), as joints often respond better to longer hold times.[16] These are referred to as low-load, long-duration (LLLD) stretches because you are not applying tons of force (low load) but are performing longer hold times (long duration). Think of a kid who gets braces on their teeth. The orthodontist tightens the braces to the point of mild to moderate discomfort, and then that position is held for a long period (months to years) to slowly shift the teeth. This is how we think about improving joint mobility, as joints are supported and restrained by dense connective tissues that are very similar to the ligaments surrounding our teeth.

Each phase 2 stretch is static, which means you are relaxed and holding a stretch without movement, except for the last exercise in phase 2, the shoulder flexion eccentrics. This exercise is designed to improve shoulder flexion but uses a slow eccentric contraction to improve joint mobility and the length of the working muscle. This exercise also starts building neuromuscular control and strength in overhead positions.

Phase 3 focuses on rebuilding shoulder strength once mobility has started improving. Because frozen shoulder takes so long to heal, I recommend adding the phase 3 exercises as soon as you have the mobility to complete them. Don't wait until your mobility has returned to normal, as your shoulder muscles will have become deconditioned and atrophied. Even if you can perform only part of the range of motion demonstrated in the phase 3 exercises, add them to your program as soon as you can do them with no more than mild pain (three out of 10 on the pain scale).

If you have pain and you're losing shoulder range of motion, see a doctor early because a cortisone injection in the freezing stage can really help. If the joint is severely limited and not improving with the exercises in this protocol, your doctor may recommend surgery and/or manipulation under anesthesia to break up scar tissue and loosen the joint capsule.

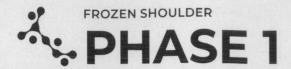

## FROZEN SHOULDER
# PHASE 1

**GOOD FOR:**

- Improving shoulder range of motion
- Building early tendon strength
- Warm-up for phase 2 and 3 exercises

**GUIDELINES:**

- Perform every day
- Tool: dowel
- Add phase 2 when you have no pain at rest and no more than mild pain (3/10) with the exercises

## MOBILITY EXERCISES:

- ▸ Do 3 sets of 10–15 reps
- ▸ Passive range of motion (PROM)—move slowly and as far as you can with no more than mild pain
- ▸ Pause at end range for 2–3 seconds
- ▸ Add active assisted range of motion (AAROM) as pain decreases

---

## internal and external rotation (PROM/AAROM) mobility

Hold a dowel with your hands shoulder width apart and palms facing up. Keeping your elbows near your sides, move the dowel along a horizontal path from one side to the other—one shoulder will move into external rotation while the other moves into internal rotation.

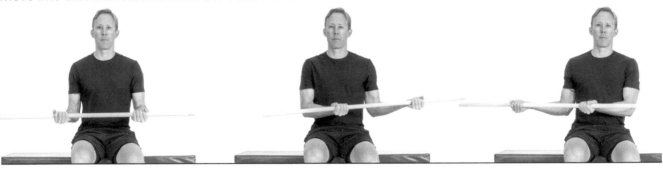

## shoulder flexion (PROM/AAROM) mobility

Grip the end of the dowel with your injured arm so that your thumb is facing up. Use your uninjured arm to guide the injured arm straight out in front of you into the overhead position.

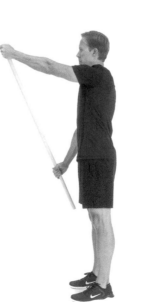
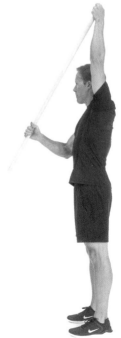

## shoulder abduction (PROM/AAROM) mobility

Start with your injured arm at your side with your palm facing forward. Form your grip by wrapping the thumb of your injured arm over the end of the dowel. Use your uninjured arm to guide the injured arm out to the side and into the overhead position.

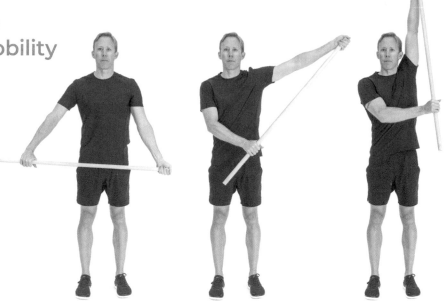

## table slide flexion mobility

Place your injured arm on a table with your thumb facing up. Keeping your arm relaxed, lean forward so that your arm slides overhead into flexion.

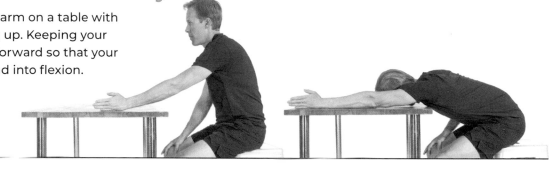

## ISOMETRIC EXERCISES:

▸ Do 4 or 5 reps with 30- to 45-second resisted holds

▸ Apply as much force as you can tolerate with no more than mild pain

▸ Bend your elbow to 90 degrees and push into a wall or rack

flexion    abduction    internal rotation    external rotation

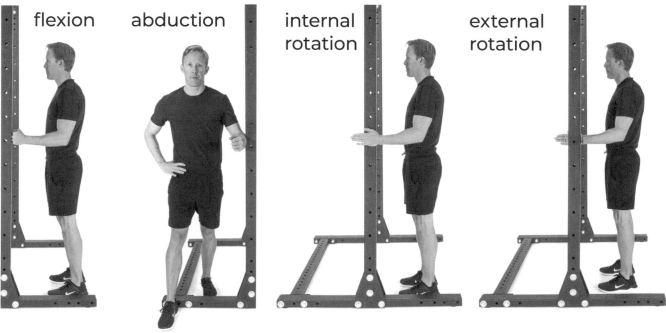

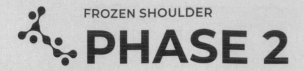

# FROZEN SHOULDER
# PHASE 2

**GOOD FOR:**

- Improving shoulder range of motion with increased mobility demands

**GUIDELINES:**

- Perform every day, 2 or 3 times per day
- Tools: towel, dowel, dumbbell
- Add phase 3 when you can do the exercises with no more than mild pain (3/10)

## shoulder external rotation stretch

Start with your elbow at 90 degrees. Place the palm of your hand against a doorframe or rack. Rotate your body away from your arm so that your shoulder moves into external rotation. Perform 3 reps with 30- to 60-second holds and work up to 2–5 minutes.

## shoulder flexion stretch

Stand facing a doorframe, wall, or rack. Place the outside edge (blade) of your hand against the wall, then slide your arm straight up over your head. Step forward through the doorway as your mobility improves. Perform 3 reps with 30- to 60-second holds and work up to 2–5 minutes.

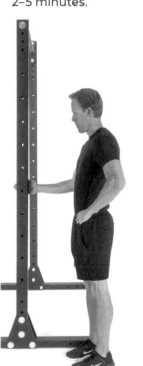
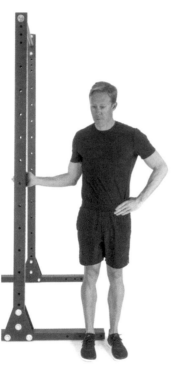
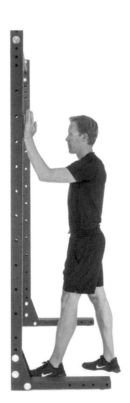
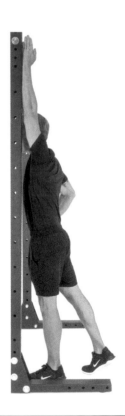

## horizontal adduction stretch

Elevate your arm to about 90 degrees and reach across your body. Keeping your shoulders square, place your opposite hand over your elbow and pull it toward your shoulder. Perform 3 reps with 30- to 60-second holds and work up to 2–5 minutes.

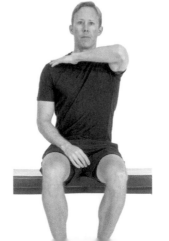
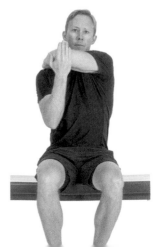

## shoulder abduction stretch

Standing with the side of your body facing a wall or rack, place the blade of your hand against the wall, then slide your arm straight up over your head. Step toward the wall as your mobility improves. Perform 3 reps with 30- to 60-second holds and work up to 2–5 minutes.

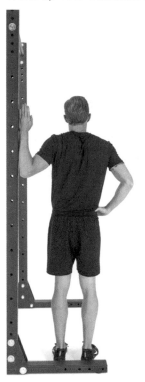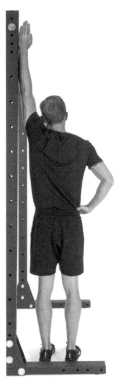

## shoulder internal rotation stretch

Holding a towel with one hand, throw it over your shoulder and grip it behind your back with the opposite hand with your palm facing away from your body. Use your top hand to slowly pull the towel, pulling your opposite arm up the center of your back. You can also do this stretch using a dowel. Perform 3 reps with 30- to 60-second holds and work up to 2–5 minutes.

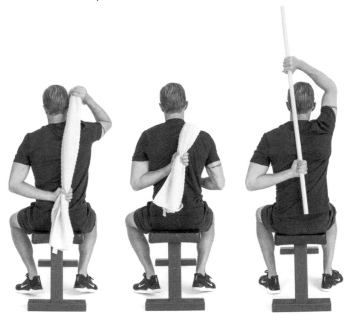

## shoulder flexion eccentrics

Lie on a bench while holding a dumbbell in the press position. Keeping your elbow straight, slowly lower your arm into the overhead position. Hold for 2–3 seconds, then bend your elbow and return to the start position. Do 2–3 sets of 10–15 reps.

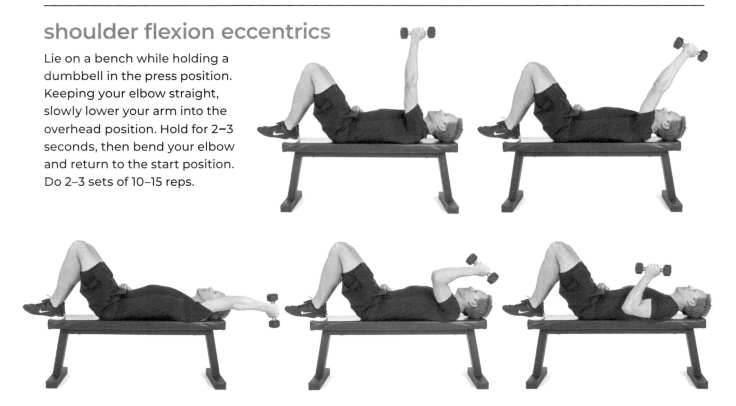

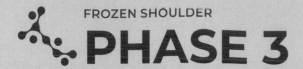

# PHASE 3

## GOOD FOR:

- Strengthening the shoulder and surrounding muscles
- Maintaining shoulder range of motion and mobility
- Preventing shoulder pain and injury

## GUIDELINES:

- Perform 3 or 4 days a week
- Do 3 sets of 10–15 reps
- Push sets to fatigue
- Tools: resistance tube band, towel, dumbbell
- All banded exercises can be done using a cable machine
- You can also follow phase 3 of the Shoulder Pain protocol for a more comprehensive shoulder strengthening program

## kneeling banded single-arm row

Kneel on the ground and anchor a band at shoulder height. Start with your arm extended in front of your body, then draw your elbow back and pull the handle toward your armpit, keeping your thumb facing upward. Keep your shoulders square and don't lean back as you pull.

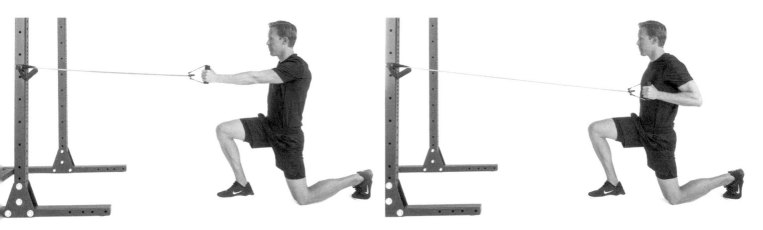

## kneeling banded single-arm press

Facing away from the rack, press your arm straight out in front of your body. As you extend your elbow, rotate your palm toward the ground.

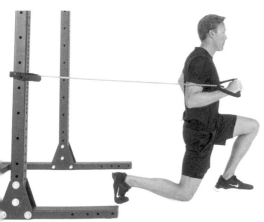
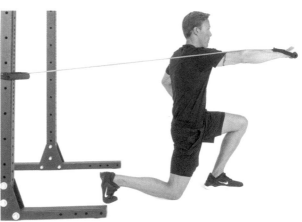

## side-lying external rotation

Choose either the dumbbell or banded variation. To perform the dumbbell variation, lie on your side with your injured arm on top. Position a folded/rolled-up towel between your elbow and body. Keep your elbow at 90 degrees and start with your hand next to your stomach. Keeping your elbow pinned to your side, lead with your knuckles and lift the dumbbell by externally rotating from your shoulder.

## banded external rotation variation

To do the banded variation, anchor the band at about belly button level. With a folded/rolled-up towel positioned between your elbow and body, bend your arm to 90 degrees and grip the handle near your stomach. Keeping your elbow pinned to your side, lead with your knuckles and pull the band outward by externally rotating from your shoulder.

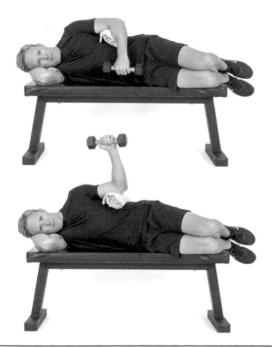

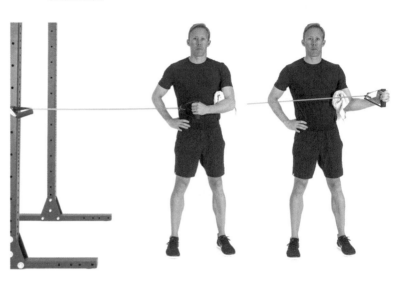

## banded internal rotation

Anchor the band to belly button level. With a folded/rolled-up towel positioned between your elbow and body, bend your arm to about 90 degrees. Keeping your elbow pinned to your side, internally rotate your shoulder and slowly pull the handle to your stomach.

## shoulder press

Start in a kneeling position with your lead shin vertical and torso upright. Position a dumbbell over one shoulder, keeping your elbow tight to your body and palm facing inward. Push the weight straight up and fully lock out your elbow. Return to the start position slowly and with control.

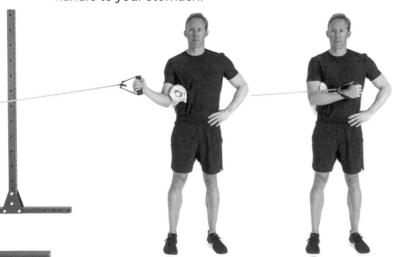

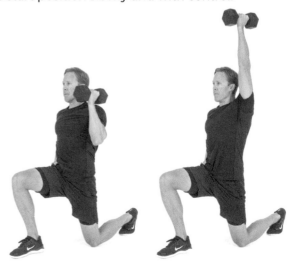

# BICEPS TENDINOPATHY

**Follow this program to treat:**

- Pain at the front of the shoulder
- Pain when moving your arm overhead and/or out in front of your body
- Biceps tendon tear

**DESCRIPTION:** The tendon of the "long head" of the biceps brachii muscle (aka the long head biceps or LHB tendon) runs vertically along the upper arm and attaches to the shoulder blade at the top of the shoulder joint. The LHB tendon often develops tendinopathy and pain at the front of the shoulder, and the region is typically irritated by activities that involve repetitive shoulder stress, such as racquet sports, golf, swimming, and throwing. Injury can also occur when your arm reaches behind your body, like at the bottom of a bench press or dip. Pain comes on either gradually or suddenly from these activities, often as an overuse injury. A tendon tear is usually caused by long-standing wear and tear or a high-acceleration movement.

**SIGNS AND SYMPTOMS:** The dull, achy, generalized pain associated with biceps tendinopathy typically affects the front of the shoulder and can become sharp with aggravating movements or activities, such as lifting your arm out to the front. Other factors can cause this type of pain—sometimes the labrum hurts there, for example—but this pain is different in that your shoulder doesn't feel unstable.

**AGGRAVATING FACTORS:** Reaching, lifting, or pulling overhead; sleeping on the painful side; and moving your arm behind your body.

**PROGNOSIS:** In most cases, biceps tendinopathy resolves within six to 12 weeks if you modify provocative activities and implement an appropriate recovery and rehab program.

**TREATMENT STRATEGY:** Treatment involves allowing the tendon to calm down and then implementing a progressive strengthening program that targets the shoulder and scapula (shoulder blade) muscles.[17,18] If a tendon tear is limiting necessary functions (such as lifting objects and sleeping) or, for an elite-level athlete, your ability to perform in your sport, surgical repair may be appropriate. If you're not an athlete, however, most surgeons won't recommend reconstructive surgery. Most people can tear their biceps, not have surgery, and be fine (unless the pain doesn't get better after 12 to 16 weeks and is interfering with your life).

If you're unsure which protocol to complete (shoulder impingement or biceps tendinopathy), pick the one that matches your symptoms more closely and get started. The exercises for these conditions are very similar, so either protocol will help.

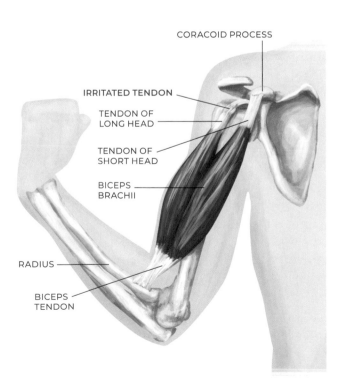

CORACOID PROCESS

IRRITATED TENDON

TENDON OF LONG HEAD

TENDON OF SHORT HEAD

BICEPS BRACHII

RADIUS

BICEPS TENDON

In phase 1, you start by performing soft tissue mobilizations of the elbow flexors, pectorals, and levator scapulae muscles. Because the biceps muscle is also an elbow flexor, mobilizing these muscles can often reduce pain and tension in the arm. The pectoral and levator scapulae techniques help improve shoulder and shoulder blade mobility, which takes stress off the healing biceps tendon.

After the soft tissue mobilization techniques, you use a physio ball to improve shoulder flexion mobility in a passive manner. When the biceps tendon is irritated or injured, lifting the shoulder into flexion can be quite painful. With the ball exercise, the muscle and tendon are kept in a relaxed state, so you can stretch the joint to preserve range of motion during the healing process.

Phase 1 concludes with shoulder flexion and external rotation isometrics. The shoulder flexion isometric directly loads the LHB tendon and can reduce pain and begin building strength. The external rotation isometric loads the rotator cuff and has been added to the protocol because biceps tendon and rotator cuff injuries often occur together. Many individuals with LHB tendon–related pain report reduced symptoms when also implementing rotator cuff exercises.

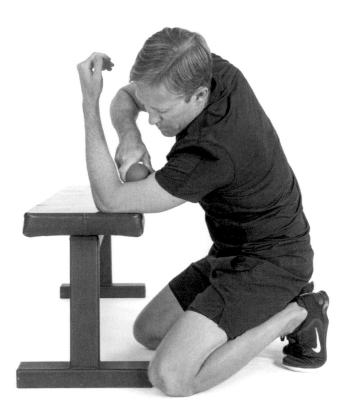

In phase 2, you implement active range of motion (AROM) exercises for shoulder flexion and abduction, both of which activate the biceps tendon and enable you to gradually begin strengthening the tendon while also making sure you can actively achieve full overhead mobility.

Next, phase 2 jumps into early biceps and rotator cuff resistance exercises. Loaded movements are added earlier in this program because resistance training has the best scientific evidence for resolving tendon issues.[19] The biceps curl focuses on the elbow action of the biceps brachii, but this movement strengthens the entire muscle, including the tendons near the shoulder region. The banded internal and external rotation exercises target the rotator cuff and can help with biceps-related pain.

The final exercise in phase 2 is the floor press, which loads the biceps tendon while limiting shoulder extension in the bottom of the movement and avoiding putting stress on the healing biceps tendon. The partial range of motion strategy also protects the tendon from being compressed against adjacent bony structures.

In phase 3, resistance exercises directly challenge the shoulder and biceps tendons. Start by building shoulder strength in the frontal plane with the lateral raise. Next, target the biceps brachii muscle with the supinated frontal raise, which includes two biceps actions (supination and flexion) in one movement. This exercise is one of the best options for targeting the LHB tendon.

The push-up plus, banded press, and bench press are progressions from the floor press and take the shoulder into deeper ranges of motion. If you have pain with these movements, shorten your range of motion until the tendon has sufficiently healed and you can move farther. The final exercise is the dolphin press, which strengthens the shoulder and shoulder blade muscles, including the serratus anterior, in a position of increased flexion. This position is more stressful for the biceps tendon, which is why you save it for the final stage of rehab.

# BICEPS TENDINOPATHY
# PHASE 1

## GOOD FOR:

- Alleviating anterior shoulder pain
- Relieving muscle tension
- Warm-up for phase 2 and 3 exercises

## GUIDELINES:

- Perform every day
- Tools: small massage ball, physio (exercise) ball
- Add phase 2 when you have no pain at rest and no more than mild pain (3/10) with the exercises

## elbow flexor mobilization

Lay your arm out straight on a bench or table with your palm facing up. Press a small massage ball into your elbow flexor muscles (lower biceps) and message around the area. Add dynamic movement by bending your arm to further mobilize the muscle. Spend 1–2 minutes massaging the area, stopping on tender points for 10–20 seconds.

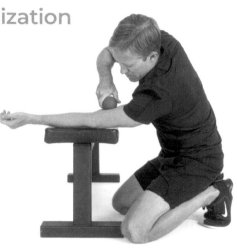

## pectoral mobilization

Position the ball between a doorframe or rack and your pectoral muscles near the front of your shoulder. Place that arm behind your back and add dynamic movement by reaching overhead to further mobilize the muscles. Spend 1–2 minutes massaging the area, stopping on tender points for 10–20 seconds. Skip the arm movements if they flare up your symptoms.

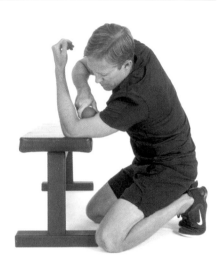

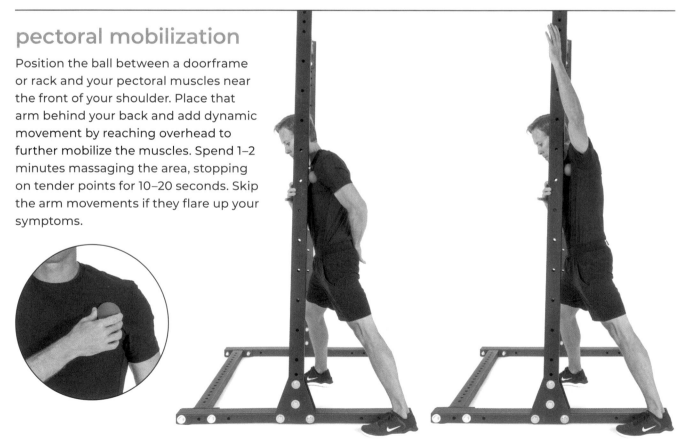

## levator scapulae mobilization

Position the ball at the corner of your shoulder blade. Elevate your hips to increase the pressure. Add arm movements to further mobilize the muscle (skip if this flares up symptoms). Spend 1–2 minutes massaging the area, stopping on tender points for 10–20 seconds.

## shoulder flexion mobility with exercise ball

Place your arms on a physio ball with your elbows straight and your thumbs pointing up. Lean forward so that the ball rolls forward and your shoulders move overhead into flexion. Perform 2–3 reps with 20- to 30-second holds.

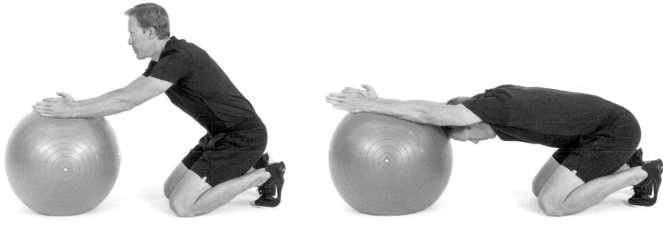

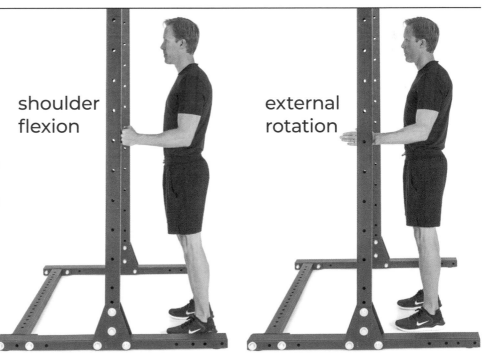

## ISOMETRIC EXERCISES:

▸ Do 4 or 5 reps with 30- to 45-second resisted holds

▸ Apply as much force as you can tolerate with no more than mild pain

shoulder flexion

external rotation

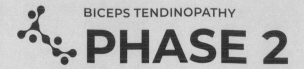

## BICEPS TENDINOPATHY
# PHASE 2

**GOOD FOR:**

- Improving shoulder range of motion
- Strengthening the shoulder and biceps tendon
- Warm-up for phase 3 exercises

**GUIDELINES:**

- Perform the mobility exercises every day and the resistance exercises 3 or 4 times a week
- Tools: dumbbell, resistance tube band, towel
- Add phase 3 when you can do the exercises with no more than mild pain (3/10)

## MOBILITY EXERCISES:

▸ Do 3 sets of 10–15 reps

▸ Active range of motion (AROM)—move as far as you can without pain

▸ Pause at end range for 2–3 seconds

## shoulder flexion mobility

Stand or sit with your arm at your side and your palm facing inward. Keeping your arm straight and leading with your thumb, reach your hand out in front of your body and over your head.

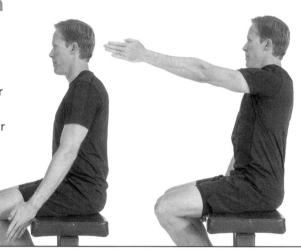
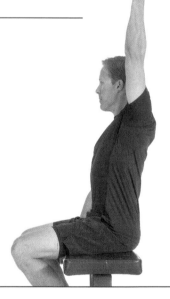

## abduction mobility

Stand or sit with your arm at your side and your palm facing forward. Keeping your arm straight and leading with your thumb, reach your hand out to your side and over your head.

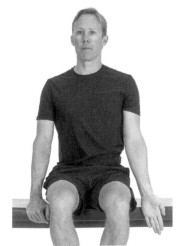
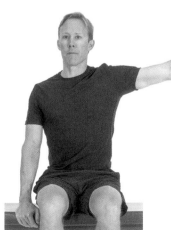
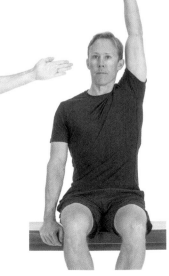

# RESISTANCE EXERCISES:

- ▸ Do 3 sets of 10–15 reps
- ▸ Push sets to fatigue
- ▸ All banded exercises can be done using a cable machine

## single-arm supinated curl

Hold a dumbbell with your arm at your side and your palm facing inward. Keeping your elbow close to your side, lift the dumbbell toward your shoulder. As you curl your arm, rotate your palm upward and toward your body (supination).

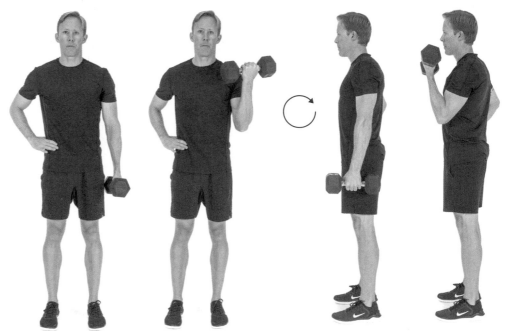

## banded internal rotation

Anchor a band just above hip height. With a folded/rolled-up towel positioned between your elbow and body, bend your arm to about 90 degrees. Keeping your elbow pinned to your side, internally rotate your shoulder and slowly pull the handle to your stomach.

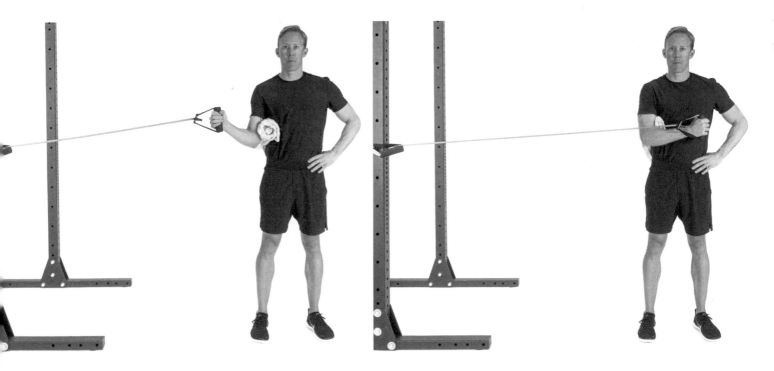

## banded external rotation

Anchor a band at about belly button level. With a folded/rolled-up towel positioned between your elbow and body, bend your arm to 90 degrees and grip the handle near your stomach. Keeping your elbow pinned to your side, lead with your knuckles and pull the band outward by externally rotating from your shoulder.

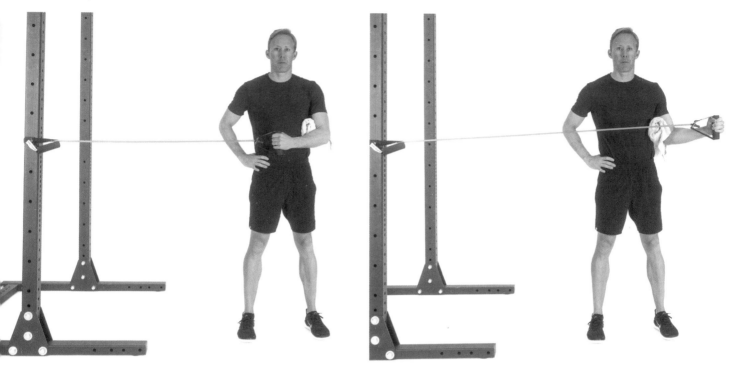

## floor press

Lie on the floor, position the dumbbells over your lower chest with your palms facing your legs, and get your triceps flush with the ground. Position your elbows slightly away from your body (at a 45-degree angle) and keep your forearms vertical. As you press the dumbbells straight up, rotate your shoulders so that your palms are facing each other at the top of the movement.

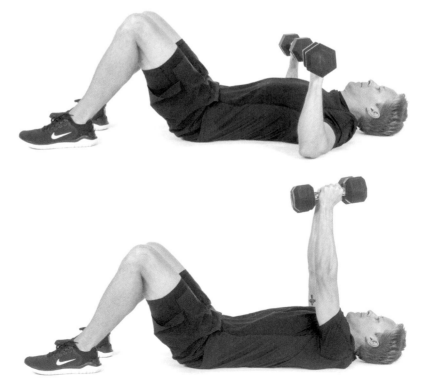

# PHASE 3

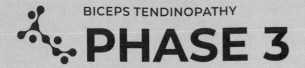

**GOOD FOR:**

- Strengthening the shoulder and biceps tendon
- Preventing pain and injury

**GUIDELINES:**

- Perform 3 or 4 days a week
- Do 3 sets of 10–15 reps
- Push sets to fatigue
- Tools: dumbbells, resistance tube band, bench

## lateral raise

Holding dumbbells at your sides, raise your arms to shoulder level with your palms facing down. You can also do this exercise with one arm using a resistance band or cable machine.

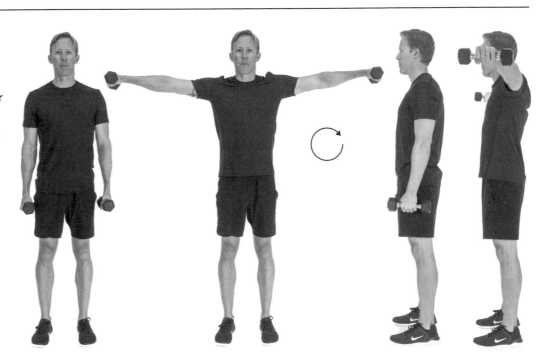

## supinated frontal raise

With your palms facing forward, raise your arms to shoulder level. You can also do this exercise using a resistance band or cable machine.

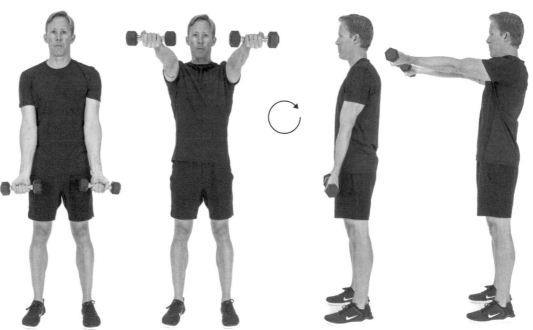

## push-up plus

Get into the plank position: hands shoulder width apart, shoulders aligned over your wrists, and back flat. Perform a standard push-up by lowering your chest to the ground. Try to keep your elbows in (about 45 degrees from your body), forearms vertical, and back flat as you lower into the bottom position. As you reverse the movement and reach the start position with your elbows extended, protract your shoulder blades by pushing your shoulders toward the ground. This should raise your body a few inches higher.

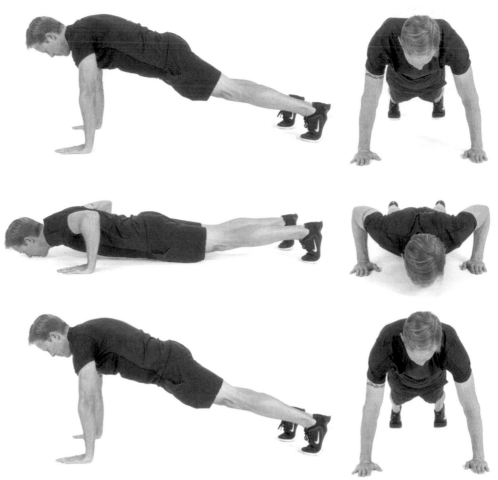

## banded press with protraction

Anchor a band at about chest height. Press your arms straight out. As you extend your elbows, rotate your palms toward the ground and protract your shoulders (push your shoulder blades forward).

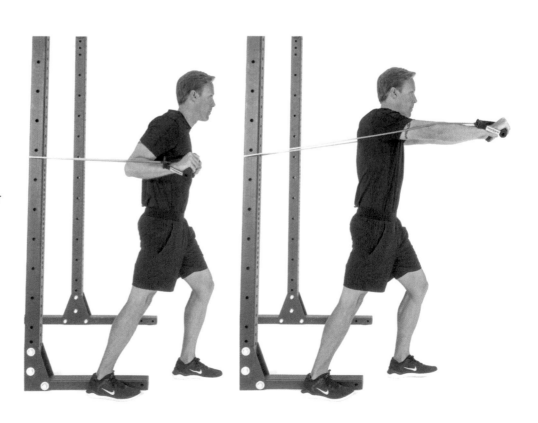

# bench press

Lie on a bench and position the dumbbells over your lower chest with your palms facing your legs. Position your elbows slightly away from your body (at a 45-degree angle) and keep your forearms vertical. As you press the dumbbells straight up, rotate your shoulders so that your palms are facing each other at the top of the movement.

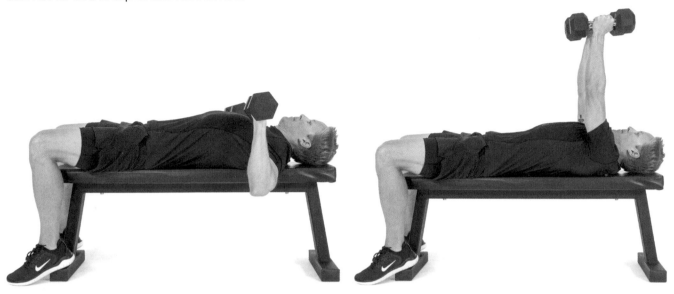

# dolphin press

Get into the plank position with your elbows positioned underneath your shoulders and your forearms flush with the ground. Walk your feet forward and elevate your hips, keeping your back as flat as possible. Lower your head to the ground and allow your shoulders to retract. Maintaining your back and hip angle, protract your shoulders (push your shoulders toward the ground) and lift your body.

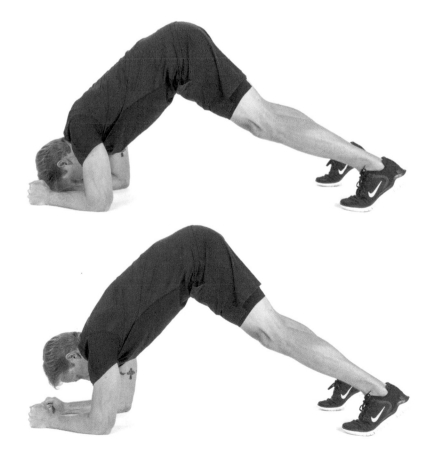

## CHAPTER 17

# ELBOW
# PROTOCOLS

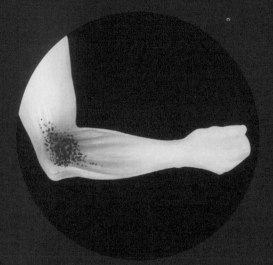

**TENNIS ELBOW**
(p. 235)

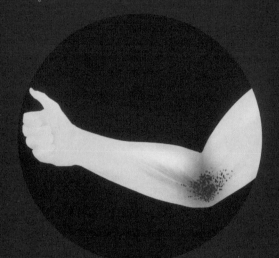

**GOLFER'S ELBOW**
(p. 243)

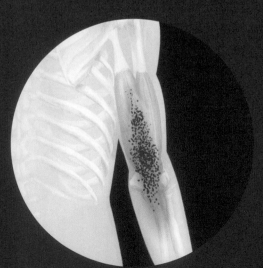

**TRICEPS TENDINOPATHY**
(p. 251)

# TENNIS ELBOW (LATERAL EPICONDYLALGIA)

**Follow this program to treat:**

- Pain on the outside or lateral aspect of the elbow (where the forearm connects to the elbow)

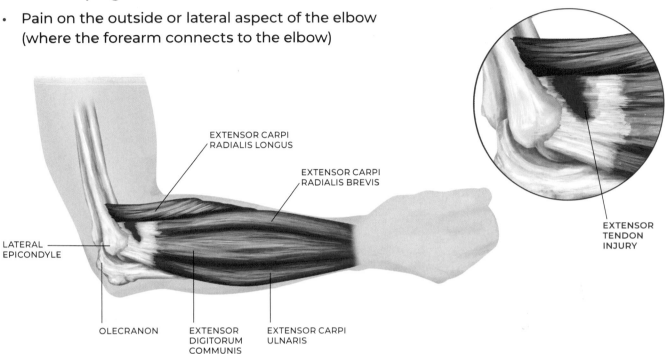

EXTENSOR CARPI RADIALIS LONGUS

EXTENSOR CARPI RADIALIS BREVIS

LATERAL EPICONDYLE

OLECRANON

EXTENSOR DIGITORUM COMMUNIS

EXTENSOR CARPI ULNARIS

EXTENSOR TENDON INJURY

**DESCRIPTION:** Lateral epicondylalgia, or tennis elbow, typically involves an irritation of the tendon of the extensor carpi radialis brevis (ECRB) muscle, which attaches to the outside of the elbow.[1] This tendon becomes irritated when you overuse the finger and wrist extensor muscles with grip-intensive activities like gardening, typing, cooking, and tennis.

Tennis elbow is like many tendon issues in that it often happens following repeated eccentric contractions. In tennis, that's usually when you are following through with the racquet—the wrist is bending into flexion, and the wrist extensors act as a brake to slow it down. The wrist extensor muscles are slowing the wrist as it bends, placing tension on the upper forearm tendons. It's like running downhill, during which you can get quadriceps tendinopathy because your quads must contract eccentrically to slow you down.

Tennis elbow usually occurs when the tendon is used with high force or at high volume, but it can also result from repetitive overuse if the finger extensors are constantly opening the hand.

**SIGNS AND SYMPTOMS:** Tennis elbow produces pain on the outside of the elbow that worsens when extending the fingers and/or wrist or performing activities that activate these muscles (such as bending your wrist toward your arm). Pain is typically dull and achy at rest and becomes sharp during aggravating tasks. Weakness in the hand and forearm is also common.

With this condition, you can palpate or press on the meaty area where the forearm attaches to the elbow, that should reproduce your pain.

**AGGRAVATING FACTORS:** Any activity that causes the finger and wrist extensor muscles to contract repetitively or for long periods—for example, lifting your wrist and fingers into extension to type on a keyboard or opening, closing, or squeezing your hands while pruning plants.

**PROGNOSIS:** Most cases of tennis elbow resolve within two to 12 weeks of starting the appropriate recovery and rehab program.

**TREATMENT STRATEGY:** Tennis elbow usually responds well to rehab, which should focus on building wrist extensor muscle and tendon strength.[2] Cortisone injections can significantly reduce inflammation but must be used with caution, as steroids are known to weaken connective tissue, including tendons. Tennis elbow braces also can reduce pain but should only be used as a temporary strategy, as they can lead to muscle and tendon deconditioning with prolonged use. If symptoms persist after six to 12 months, surgical debridement (removal of diseased tissue) and repair of the tendon may be an option. However, this treatment route should be a last resort.

In phase 1, you focus on soft tissue mobilizations that target the wrist and finger extensor muscles on the back side or posterior surface of the forearm, which can help reduce pain on the outside of the elbow. Phase 1 also includes several exercises (pectoral mobilization, radial nerve slider and angel) that target the nerves that travel to the outside of the elbow, which also help reduce pain and improve mobility.

In phase 2, you start by stretching the pectoral and wrist and finger extensor muscles to further reduce pain and improve mobility. After that, you begin loading the affected tendons with an isometric wrist extensor contraction. This and the next finger extensor exercise begin strengthening the tendons and can reduce pain. Phase 2 finishes with a wrist flexion and extension active mobility exercise, which trains the muscles and tendons in a low-load fashion through a full range of motion before you add weight in phase 3.

Phase 3 focuses on strengthening the forearm muscles because resistance training has the best evidence for healing tendinopathy.[3,4] The first exercise is a continuation of the last exercise in phase 2—a loaded wrist extensor curl with a dumbbell. Next, the pronator and supinator curls strengthen the muscles that rotate the forearm. The supinator muscle attaches to the lateral epicondyle with the wrist extensors and can contribute to tennis elbow pain, so make sure to address it. The radial deviator curl strengthens the muscles that lift the wrist on the thumb side, which run up the lateral forearm and, in some cases, attach to the lateral epicondyle.

The last two exercises in phase 3 involve grip training, especially the farmer's carry, which can help rehabilitate forearm injuries. Even though grip training works the wrist and finger flexors, it can help with lateral elbow pain as well. The bent-over reverse fly involves some grip force, but the wrist extensor muscles work isometrically to keep the wrist joint in a neutral position during the movement.

## WHAT IF I HAVE BOTH TENNIS AND GOLFER'S ELBOW?

It is possible to have tennis elbow and golfer's elbow simultaneously. If you do, you can combine the phases of the two protocols because they target opposite sides of the forearm and different muscle groups, meaning they won't interfere with each other. If there are redundant movements, do them just once.

Also, the phased approach doesn't need to be linear. For example, if you're in phase 3 and you start playing tennis or golf again but immediately experience the same acute pain, go back to phase 1 and be mindful of the aggravating factors so that you can calm the tissue down. Repeat the process until you have strengthened the tissue enough that it doesn't become a recurring problem.

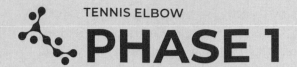

# PHASE 1

## GOOD FOR:

- Alleviating lateral elbow pain
- Relieving muscle tension
- Warm-up for phase 2 and 3 exercises

## GUIDELINES:

- Perform every day
- Tools: small massage ball, foam roller
- Add phase 2 when you have no pain at rest and no more than mild pain (3/10) with the exercises

## SOFT TISSUE MOBILIZATIONS:

- ▸ Spend 1–2 minutes on **each area**
- ▸ Perform in any order **on both sides**
- ▸ Stop on tender points for **10–20 seconds**

## wrist extensor mobilization

Lay your arm out straight on a bench or table with your palm facing down. Press a small massage ball into your forearm extensor muscles (where the top of your forearm connects to your elbow) and massage above and below the area. Add dynamic movement on tender points by flexing your wrist while applying steady pressure with the ball.

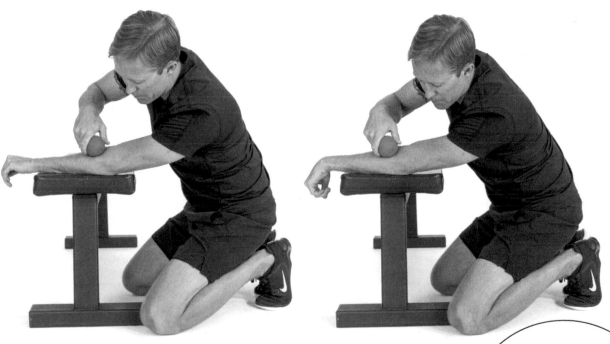

## manual variation

The manual variation shares the same technique, but instead of applying pressure with a ball, you use your fingers.

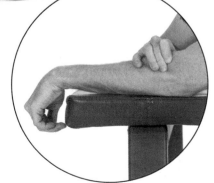

## pectoral mobilization

Position the ball between a doorframe or rack and your pectoral muscles near the front of your shoulder. Place that arm behind your back and add dynamic movement by reaching overhead to further mobilize the muscles.

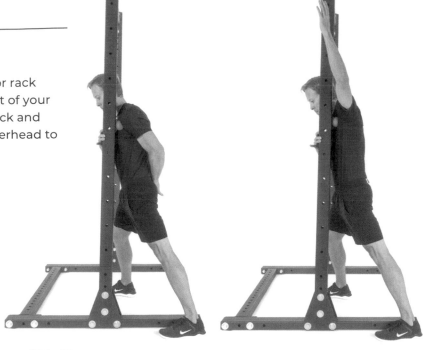

# MOBILITY EXERCISES:

- ▸ Do 3 sets of 10–15 reps
- ▸ Move as far as you can with no more than mild pain
- ▸ Pause at end range for 2–3 seconds

## radial nerve slider mobility

Starting with your arm out to your side and your palm facing behind you, flex your wrist and tilt your head toward your outstretched arm. In one fluid motion, bend your head away from your arm and extend your wrist. Go back and forth between these positions to mobilize the radial nerve.

## angel

Position your spine over a foam roller so that your head and tailbone are supported. Start with your arms at your sides and palms facing up, then reach overhead as far as you can without pain.

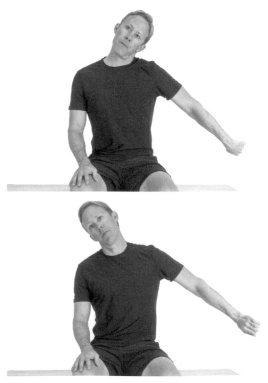

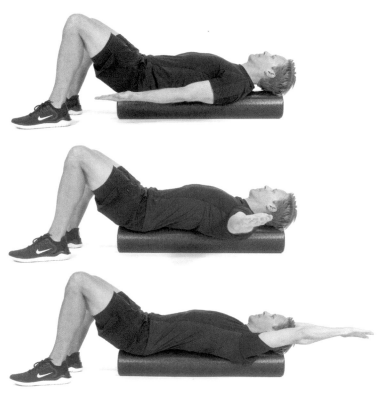

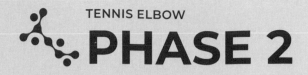

TENNIS ELBOW

# PHASE 2

**GOOD FOR:**

- Alleviating lateral elbow pain
- Improving wrist mobility
- Early tendon strengthening
- Warm-up for phase 3 exercises

**GUIDELINES:**

- Perform every day
- Tools: dumbbell, finger exerciser
- Add phase 3 when you can do the exercises with no more than mild pain (3/10)

## pectoral stretch

Position your forearm against a doorframe or rack with your shoulder at about 90 degrees. Step forward until you feel a stretch in your chest region. Move your arm slightly higher to stretch the upper fibers of your pectoral muscles. Perform 3 reps with 30- to 60-second holds.

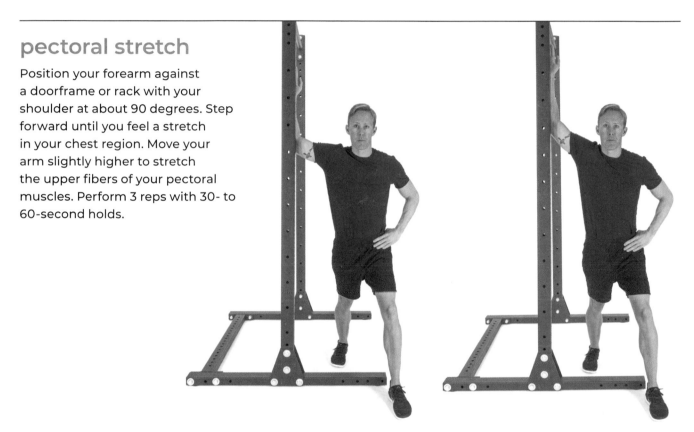

## wrist extensor stretch

Straighten your elbow out in front of your body with your palm facing down. Form a grip around your knuckles with your opposite hand, then pull down until you feel a stretch on the top of your forearm. Perform 3 reps with 30- to 60-second holds.

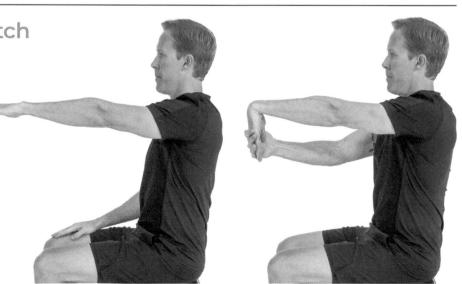

## wrist extensor isometrics

Rest your arm on a table so that only your hand is hanging over the edge and your palm is facing down. Hold a dumbbell out straight so that your wrist is in a neutral position. Perform 4 or 5 reps with 30- to 45-second holds.

## resisted finger extensor

Place your fingers in the holes of a finger extensor resistance exerciser, then splay and extend your fingers and thumb. Do 3 sets of 10–15 reps.

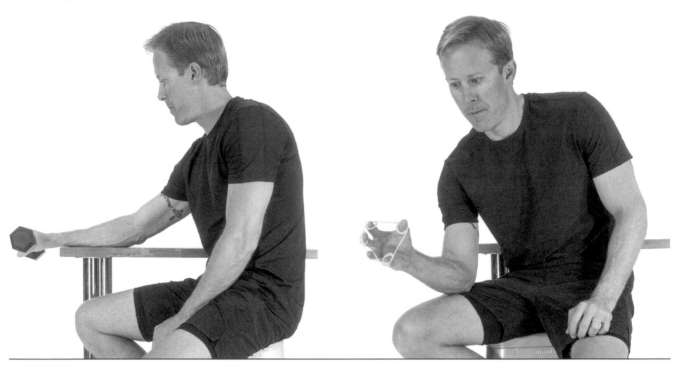

## wrist flexion and extension mobility

With your arm supported, flex and extend your wrist as far as you can, pausing for 2–3 seconds in both flexion and extension. Do 3 sets of 10–15 reps.

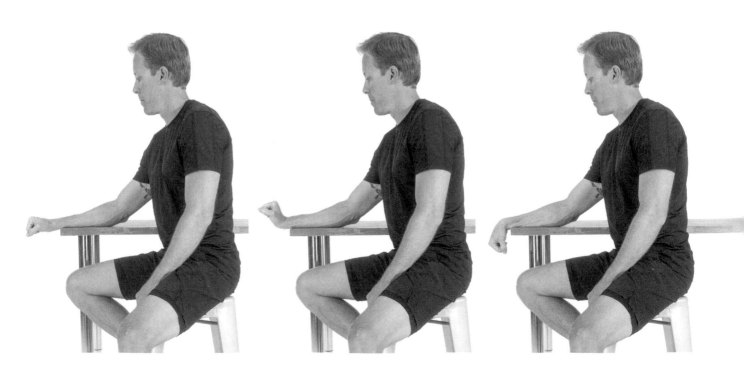

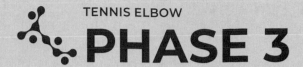

# PHASE 3

**GOOD FOR:**

- Strengthening the extensor tendons and forearm muscles
- Preventing tennis elbow–related pain

**GUIDELINES:**

- Perform 3 or 4 days a week
- Do 3 sets of 10–15 reps unless otherwise noted
- Push sets to fatigue
- Tools: dumbbells

## wrist extensor curl

Support your arm on a table so that only your hand is hanging over the edge and your palm is facing down. Holding a dumbbell, slowly bend your wrist, then extend (lift up). Momentarily pause in the top position before transitioning to the next rep.

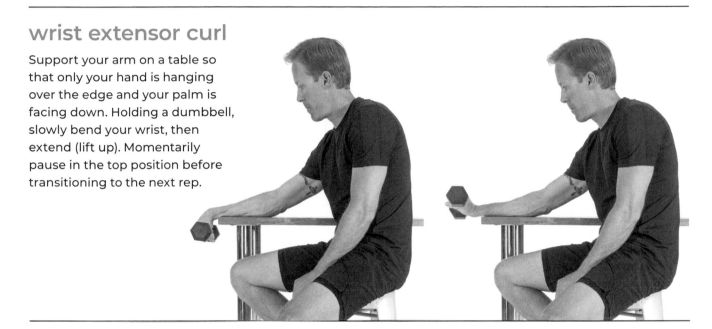

## supinator and pronator curl

With your arm supported, hold one end of the dumbbell and rotate through pronation and supination. Keep your elbow on the table, isolate the movement through your wrist and forearm, and focus on slowly rotating from a palm-up to a palm-down position.

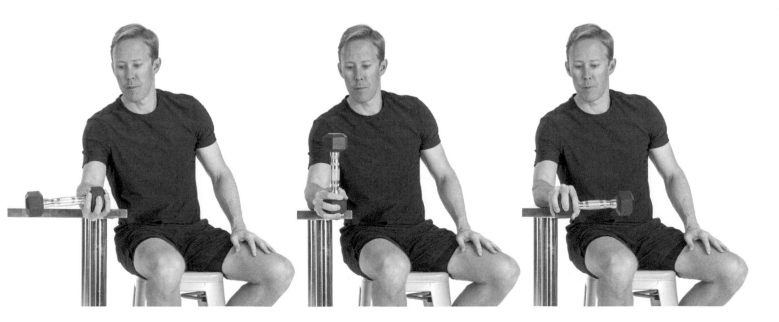

## radial deviator curl

Keeping the outside of your forearm and back of your elbow in contact with the table and the inside of your wrist facing up, lower the top of the dumbbell toward the ground, then lift it toward your body (bending only at the wrist).

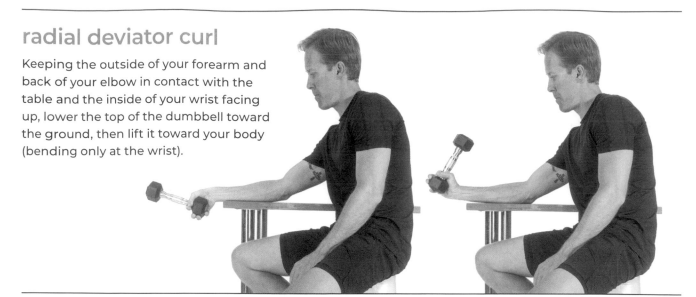

## farmer's carry

Hold a heavy dumbbell at your side and walk 15–20 meters (or take 20–30 steps), then turn around and return to the starting point. Do this 3 times on each arm.

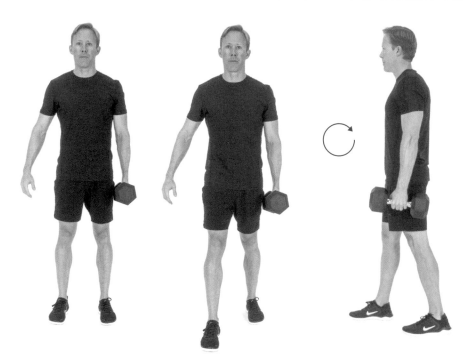

## bent-over lateral raise

Holding dumbbells at your sides, hinge from your hips and bend your knees—keeping your shins vertical and back flat—so that your torso is at a roughly 45-degree angle. With a slight bend in your elbows, raise your arms to about shoulder level with your palms down.

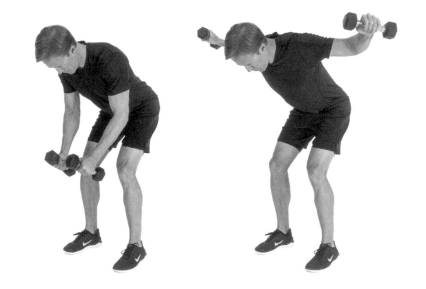

# GOLFER'S ELBOW

**Follow this program to treat:**

- Pain on the inside or medial side of the elbow

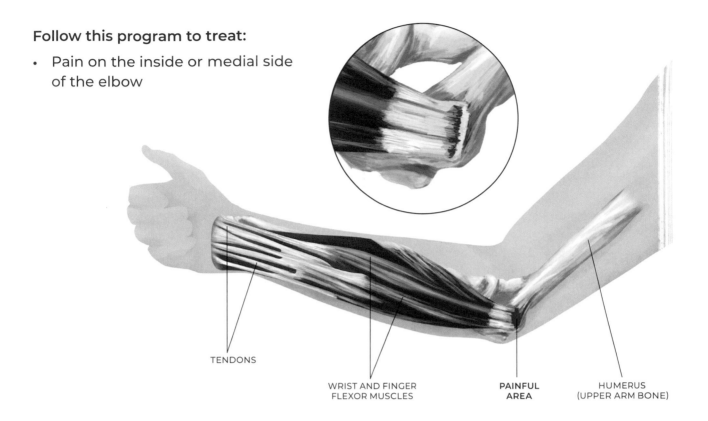

TENDONS

WRIST AND FINGER
FLEXOR MUSCLES

**PAINFUL
AREA**

HUMERUS
(UPPER ARM BONE)

**DESCRIPTION:** Medial epicondylalgia or golfer's elbow is a condition where the wrist and finger flexor muscles become irritated at their attachment site on the inside or medial side of the elbow. Pain is usually associated with activities that require repetitive, forceful use of the flexor muscles, including climbing, playing golf or racquet sports, and gripping tools for gardening or carpentry.[5]

This condition is like tennis elbow but on the opposite side of the forearm, affecting the wrist and finger flexors rather than the extensors. As such, it affects the squeezing part of the movement instead of the opening of the hand. Golfer's elbow is less common than tennis elbow because the forearm and finger flexors are twice as strong as the extensors, so they're less prone to overuse issues.

You can get golfer's elbow even if you don't play golf. The flexion movement has more than one eccentric part, so you can even get golfer's elbow from playing tennis, but it's usually on the serve, when the arm moves overhead and the wrist goes into extension—the wrist flexors slow the movement before coming forward and hitting the ball. In golf, this occurs on the backswing, as your arms come back and prepare to go forward; you need to slow the club to change direction, and that's what stresses the tendon of your wrist flexors and the inside of your elbow. Overhead throwers may also experience this condition because they accelerate and decelerate their arm while simultaneously holding an object that places increased stress on their tissues.

**SIGNS AND SYMPTOMS:** A dull, achy pain on the inside of the elbow that becomes sharp with certain tasks. You may also notice reduced grip strength. With this condition, you can palpate and reproduce the pain. Touching next to the bone (medial epicondyle) on the inside of the elbow will trigger pain. Wrist flexion with resistance may also hurt.

**AGGRAVATING FACTORS:** Activities that work the wrist and finger flexor muscles, such as flexing and extending the wrist and performing grip-related tasks.

**PROGNOSIS:** Golfer's elbow usually resolves within two to 12 weeks when you modify or temporarily eliminate aggravating activities and implement a phased approach to rehab exercise.

**TREATMENT STRATEGY:** Most cases of golfer's elbow improve with physical therapy focused on gradually improving wrist and finger flexor strength. Like with tennis elbow, elbow braces that tighten around the upper forearm can reduce pain but should be used temporarily, as prolonged use can lead to muscle and tendon deconditioning and other problems. In rare cases where symptoms have not improved after six to 12 months, surgical repair of the tissue may be an option. These types of operations are performed infrequently and should be a last resort.

In phase 1, you focus on mobilizing the wrist and finger flexor muscles, which are located on the front or anterior side of the forearm. Mobilizing these muscles can help reduce tension and pain on the inside of the elbow. After that, you mobilize the elbow flexors, which share fascial connections with and often assist in the movements of the wrist flexors. In this phase, you also mobilize the pectoral muscles and median and ulnar nerves, as these techniques improve nerve health and mobility and can help reduce pain.

In phase 2, you initially stretch the pectoral muscles and wrist and finger flexor muscles, which will continue to improve mobility and reduce pain. Then you begin loading the affected tendons with isometric contractions (wrist flexor isometric and grip strengthener) and active mobility exercises (wrist flexion and extension). Both of these exercises train the tendons in a relatively low-load fashion, so that strength can be increased without causing a flare-up in pain.

In phase 3, you focus on strengthening the forearm muscles, especially those that attach on the medial epicondyle (wrist and finger flexors and pronator teres), because resistance training has the best evidence for rehabilitating tendon injuries.[6,7] The last three exercises in phase 3 all involve grip training, especially the farmer's carry, which can help rehabilitate forearm and elbow injuries. The bent-over row and biceps curl also work the elbow flexors and other pulling muscles that often serve as synergists for the wrist and finger flexors, so strengthening these parts of the kinetic chain is important to the rehabilitation process.

**NOTE:** If you suspect that you have both golfer's elbow and tennis elbow, refer to page 236 for guidance.

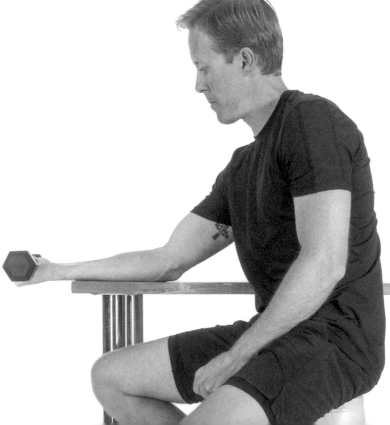

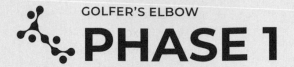

# PHASE 1

## GOOD FOR:

- Alleviating medial elbow pain
- Relieving muscle tension
- Warm-up for phase 2 and 3 exercises

## GUIDELINES:

- Perform every day
- Tools: small massage ball, foam roller
- Add phase 2 when you have no pain at rest and no more than mild pain (3/10) with the exercises

## SOFT TISSUE MOBILIZATIONS:

▸ Spend 1–2 minutes on each area
▸ Perform in any order on both sides
▸ Stop on tender points for 10–20 seconds

---

## wrist flexor mobilization

Lay your arm out straight on a bench or table with your palm facing up. Press a small massage ball into your forearm flexor muscles (where the bottom of your forearm connects to your elbow) and massage around the area. Add dynamic movement by extending your wrist while applying steady pressure with the ball.

## manual variation

The manual variation shares the same technique, but instead of applying pressure with a ball, you use your thumb and palm.

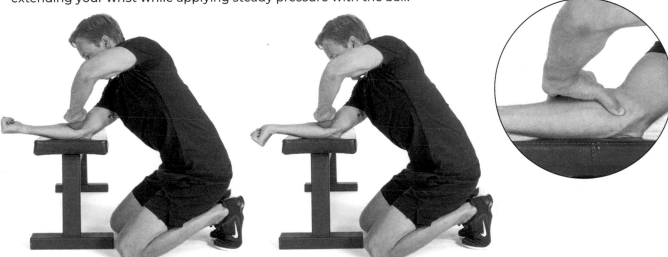

---

## elbow flexor mobilization

Lay your arm out straight on a bench or table with your palm facing up. Press the ball into your elbow flexor muscles (lower biceps) and message around the area. Add dynamic movement by bending your arm to further mobilize the muscle.

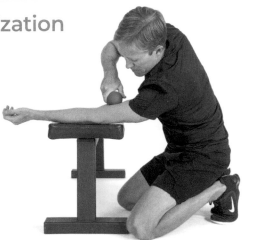
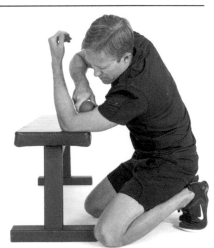

## pectoral mobilization

Position the ball between a doorframe or rack and your pectoral muscles near the front of your shoulder. Place that arm behind your back and add dynamic movement by reaching overhead to further mobilize the muscles.

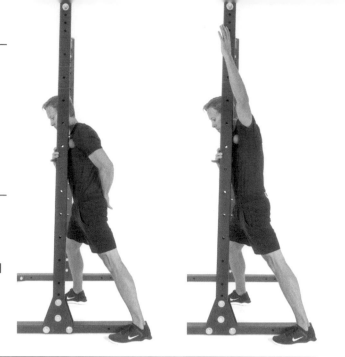

## MOBILITY EXERCISES:

▸ Do 3 sets of 10–15 reps

▸ Move as far as you can with no more than mild pain

▸ Pause at end range for 2–3 seconds

## median nerve slider mobility

Start with your arm out to your side with your shoulder at 90 degrees, your elbow and wrist bent, and your head titled away from your elevated arm. In one fluid motion, straighten your elbow, extend your wrist, and move your head toward your arm. Go back and forth between these positions to mobilize the median nerve.

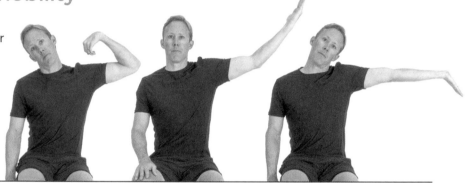

## ulnar nerve slider mobility

Start with your arm out to your side with your shoulder and elbow at roughly 90-degree angles, your wrist extended with your palm facing up, and your head titled toward your elevated arm. In one fluid motion, bend your wrist so that your palm is facing the ground and tilt your head away from your arm. Go back and forth between these positions to mobilize the ulnar nerve.

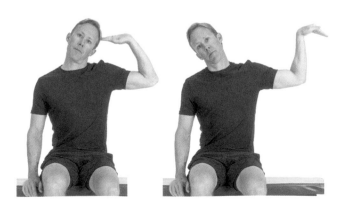

## angel

Position your spine over a foam roller so that your head and tailbone are supported. Start with your arms at your sides and palms up, then reach as far overhead as you can without pain.

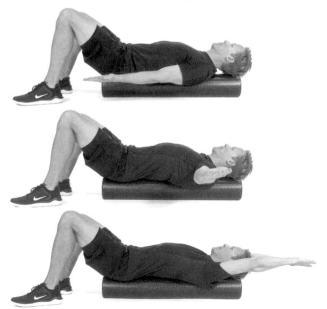

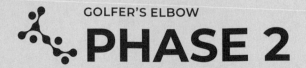
# PHASE 2

**GOOD FOR:**

- Alleviating medial elbow pain
- Early tendon strengthening
- Warm-up for phase 3 exercises

**GUIDELINES:**

- Perform every day
- Tools: dumbbell, grip strengthener
- Add phase 3 when you can do the exercises with no more than mild pain (3/10)

## pectoral stretch

Position your forearm against a doorframe or rack with your shoulder at about 90 degrees. Step forward until you feel a stretch in your chest region. Move your arm slightly higher to stretch the upper fibers of your pectoral muscles. Perform 3 reps with 30- to 60-second holds.

## wrist flexor stretch

Straighten your arm out in front of your body with your palm facing up. Form a grip around your palm with your opposite hand, then pull down until you feel a stretch on the bottom of your forearm. Perform 3 reps with 30- to 60-second holds.

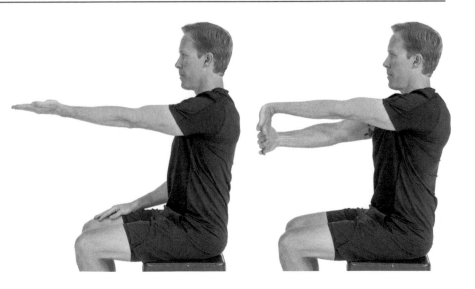

## wrist flexor isometrics

Support your arm on a table so that only your hand is hanging over the edge and your palm is facing up. Hold a dumbbell out straight so that your wrist is in a neutral position. Perform 4 or 5 reps with 30- to 45-second holds.

## grip strengthener

Use a grip strengthening device (resistance hand gripper, finger exerciser, or grip ring) to improve your forearm and hand strength. You can use any tool that provides resistance while closing your hand. Do 3 sets of 10–15 reps.

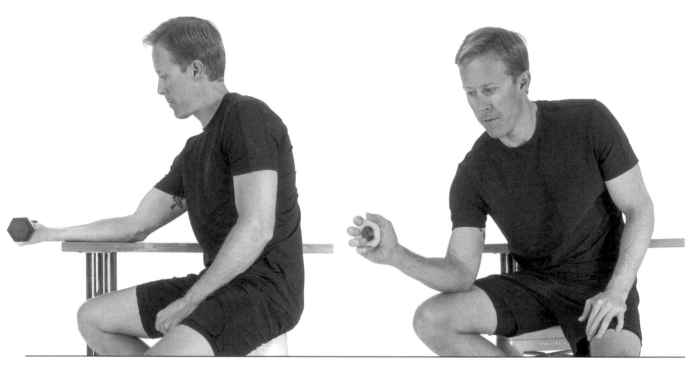

## wrist flexion and extension mobility

With your arm supported, flex and extend your wrist as far as you can, pausing for 2–3 seconds in both flexion and extension.

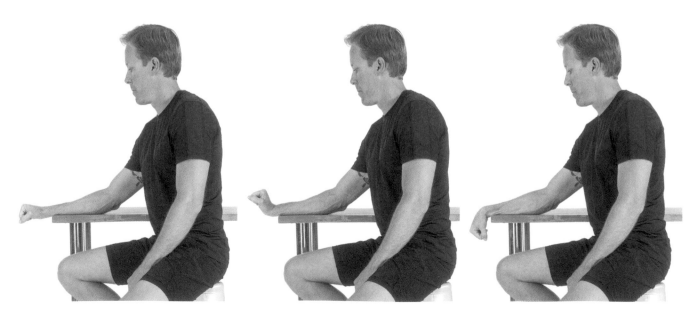

# PHASE 3

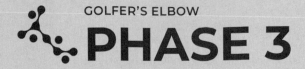

## GOOD FOR:

- Strengthening the flexor tendons and forearm muscles
- Preventing golfer's elbow–related pain

## GUIDELINES:

- Perform 3 or 4 days a week
- Do 3 sets of 10–15 reps unless otherwise noted
- Push sets to fatigue
- Tools: dumbbell, bench

## wrist flexor curl

Support your arm on a table so that only your hand is hanging over the edge and your palm is facing up. Holding a dumbbell, slowly extend your wrist, then flex (curl toward your body). Momentarily pause in the top position before transitioning to the next rep.

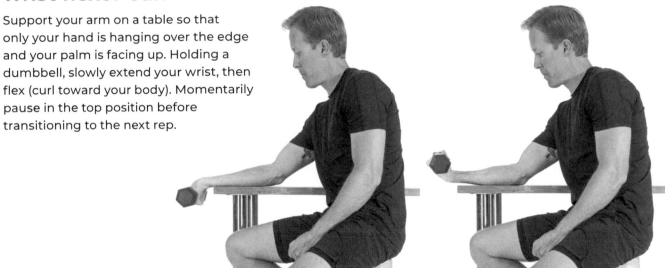

## supinator and pronator curl

With your arm supported, hold one end of the dumbbell and rotate through pronation and supination. Keep your elbow on the table, isolate the movement through your wrist and forearm, and focus on slowly rotating from a palm-up to a palm-down position.

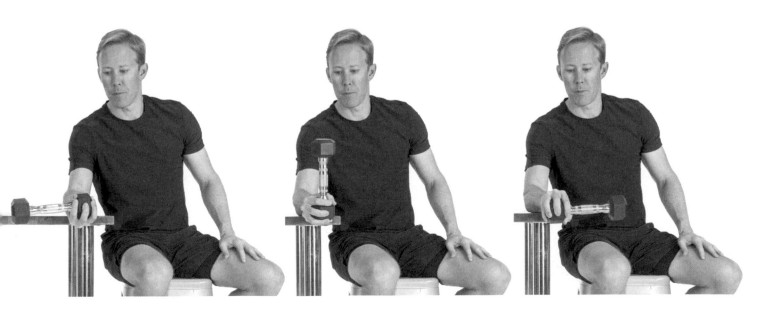

## dumbbell row

Place one hand and knee on a bench with your spine neutral. Let your opposite arm hang down to the side of the bench, then bend your elbow and pull the dumbbell straight up toward your chest.

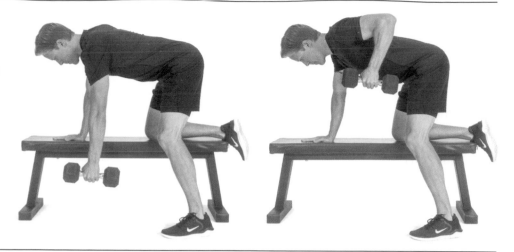

## single-arm supinated curl

Hold a dumbbell with your arm at your side and your palm facing inward. Keeping your elbow close to your side, lift the dumbbell toward your shoulder. As you curl your arm, rotate your palm upward and toward your body (supination).

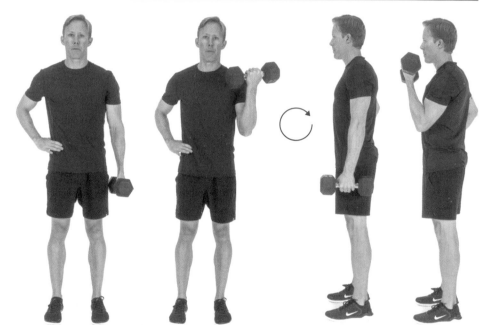

## farmer's carry

Hold a heavy dumbbell at your side and walk 15–20 meters (or take 20–30 steps), then turn around and return to the starting point. Do this 3 times on each arm.

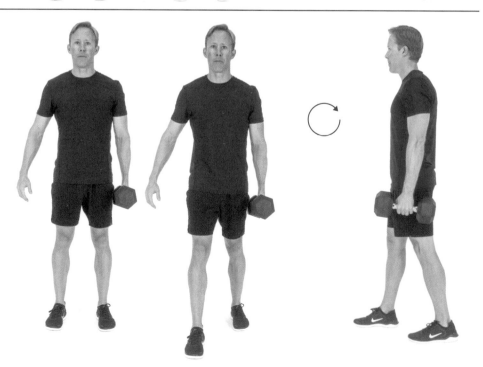

# TRICEPS TENDINOPATHY

**Follow this program to treat:**

- Pain on the back of the elbow

**DESCRIPTION:** The triceps brachii is a large muscle on the posterior (back side) of the upper arm that extends the elbow. Irritation of the triceps tendon near its insertion point at the elbow can occur when training demand surpasses the tendon's capacity (think overuse or repetitive stress injuries).[8]

For instance, say you do a workout that includes a lot of burpees. Perhaps you haven't done them in a while, you're new to the exercise, you've been doing burpees every day and you're already sore, or you simply do more than you've ever attempted before. Whether the problem is a novel stressor or aggregate volume, the stress on the triceps irritates the tendon, resulting in pain on the back of the elbow. Burpees can be particularly problematic because, during the eccentric loading phase, the triceps act as a brake to slow the body as you drop to the ground and lower into the push-up.

All pressing motions that involve extending the elbow under force or load can create a triceps tendon flare-up. These overuse injuries can result from doing too many push-ups, heavy bench presses, dips, or overhead movements like military presses and handstands.

**SIGNS AND SYMPTOMS:** Dull, achy pain at rest and sharp pain on the back side of the elbow occur when working the triceps with pushing activities like push-ups, bench presses, or other triceps-specific exercises.

**AGGRAVATING FACTORS:** Activities that require extending the elbow or contracting the triceps muscles forcefully or rapidly (such as pressing motions).

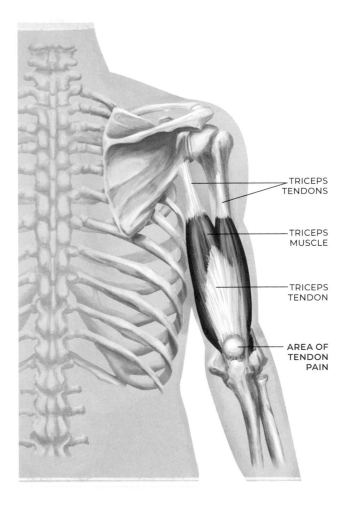

TRICEPS TENDONS

TRICEPS MUSCLE

TRICEPS TENDON

AREA OF TENDON PAIN

**PROGNOSIS:** Triceps tendinopathy typically resolves within two to 12 weeks when you modify or temporarily eliminate aggravating activities and implement an appropriate rehab program.

**TREATMENT STRATEGY:** In most cases, this condition improves when you reduce or temporarily eliminate the aggravating factors and implement physical therapy focused on gradually strengthening the triceps tendon. This involves slowly loading the tendon, first with isometric exercises and then with eccentric exercises and heavy, slow, full range of motion movements.

In phase 1, you start by mobilizing the triceps muscles directly to reduce tension and pain in the area. You can add elbow flexion and extension to this mobilization to dynamically mobilize the muscle. The latissimus dorsi muscle (aka lat) mobilization is implemented in this protocol because of how closely it attaches to the upper triceps and because the lats often act as synergists with the triceps. After this mobilization, you perform a lat stretch with a dowel to improve not only lat flexibility but also thoracic spine mobility. You can bend your elbows more than is demonstrated in the photos to add a bit of triceps stretch to the exercise.

Phase 1 finishes with a triceps isometric exercise designed to reduce tendon pain and begin loading/strengthening the tendon in a gradual and controlled fashion. Isometric contractions can reduce tendon pain, which is why this exercise appears in phase 1.

Phase 2 begins focusing on resistance training, which has the best evidence for supporting tendinopathy rehab.[6] The first exercise is a push-down eccentric, which involves using the uninjured arm during the concentric portion of the exercise (the push-down) and then completing the eccentric portion with the injured arm only. The bent-over reverse raise targets the upper portion of the triceps, which contributes to shoulder extension and requires the elbow portion of the triceps to maintain an isometric contraction, making it another good early strengthening exercise.

Phase 2 wraps up with the shoulder tap exercise, which is the first closed-chain (hands fixed on the floor) exercise and again requires the triceps to hold an isometric contraction, but this time you must support a portion of your body weight.

In phase 3, you implement the targeted and challenging triceps exercises that focus on making the tendon stronger and more resilient. Every exercise in this phase requires the triceps on the injured side to complete concentric and eccentric contractions without the assistance of the uninjured arm. Exercises like the triceps kickback and push-down are triceps focused, while other exercises that incorporate the triceps include the shoulder press, push-up, bench press, and banded press. The final exercise is the bench dip, which is usually the most challenging due to the high degree of load placed on the triceps muscles.

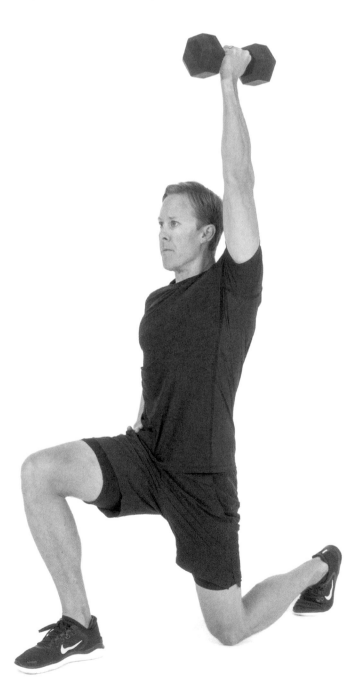

## TRICEPS TENDINOPATHY
# PHASE 1

### GOOD FOR:

- Alleviating posterior elbow and triceps pain
- Relieving muscle tension
- Warm-up for phase 2 and 3 exercises

### GUIDELINES:

- Perform every day
- Tools: small massage ball, foam roller, dowel
- Add phase 2 when you have no pain at rest and no more than mild pain (3/10) with the exercises

## elbow extensor mobilization

With your arm straight on a bench or table, place a small massage ball (or peanut tool) under your triceps muscles. Massage the entire length of the muscles from the back of your elbow up to the base of your shoulder (armpit region). Add dynamic movement by bending, straightening, and rotating your arm on stiff areas. Spend 1–2 minutes massaging the area, stopping on tender points for 10–20 seconds.

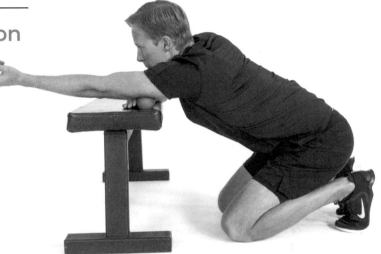

## foam roller variation

You can also use a foam roller. Lie on your side, raise your arm overhead, and mobilize the triceps using the same technique as you would with a ball.

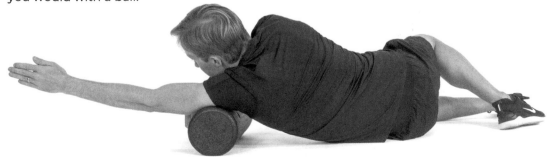

## lat mobilization

With your weight over a roller, start at your armpit and work your way down the lat muscle toward your low back. Put your hand behind your head to stretch and expose more of the muscle and roll from side to side on tight spots. Spend 1–2 minutes massaging the area.

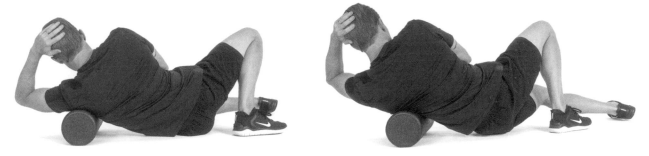

## lat stretch with dowel

In a kneeling position, hold a dowel with your palms facing up and place your elbows on the bench or table. Sit your hips back toward your heels and lower your head through your arms to create a stretch through your lats and triceps. This stretch also works thoracic extension mobility. Perform 3 reps with 30- to 60-second holds.

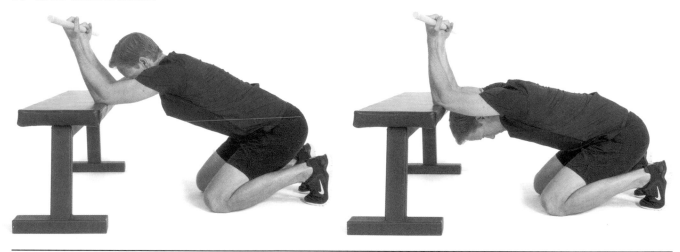

## elbow extensor isometrics

In a sitting or standing position, place your elbows on a table with your arms bent, then grip the back of one wrist with the other hand. Straighten your elbow with moderate force while holding your arm in place with the opposite hand, which is providing resistance. Do this exercise at a variety of elbow angles to strengthen the triceps tendon. Perform 1 or 2 reps with 30- to 45-second holds at 2 or 3 different angles.

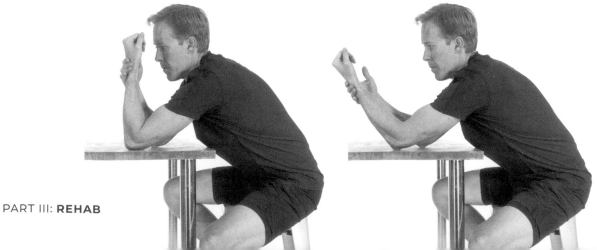

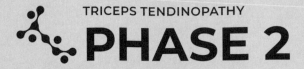

## TRICEPS TENDINOPATHY
# PHASE 2

**GOOD FOR:**

- Alleviating posterior elbow pain
- Strengthening the elbow extensor tendon
- Warm-up for phase 3 exercises

**GUIDELINES:**

- Perform every day
- Do 3 sets of 10–15 reps
- Tools: resistance tube band, dumbbell
- Add phase 3 when you can do the exercises with no more than mild pain (3/10)

## push-down eccentrics

Stand or kneel in front of a rack and grip the handle of the resistance band or cable with your injured elbow bent and palm facing down. Use your uninjured arm to pull down on the band, straightening your injured arm at your side.

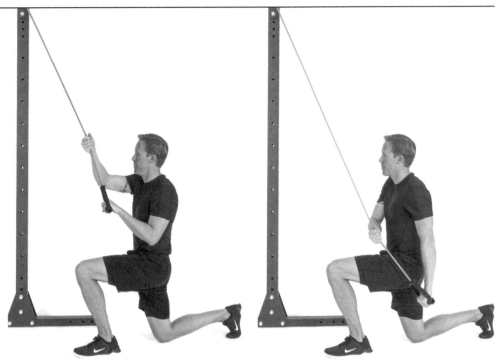

Release your grip on the band with your uninjured arm and perform a slow eccentric contraction with your injured arm back to the start position.

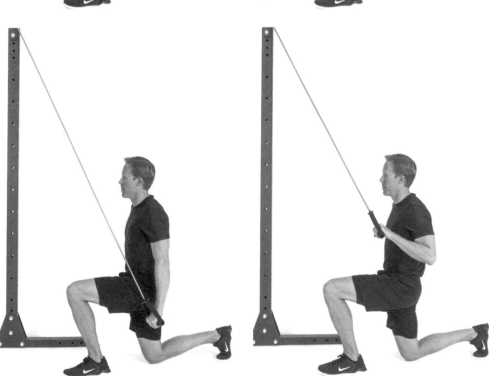

## bent-over reverse raise

Holding dumbbells at your sides, hinge from your hips and tilt your torso forward while maintaining a neutral spine. Keeping your arms close to your sides and elbows slightly bent (almost straight), extend your arms behind your body.

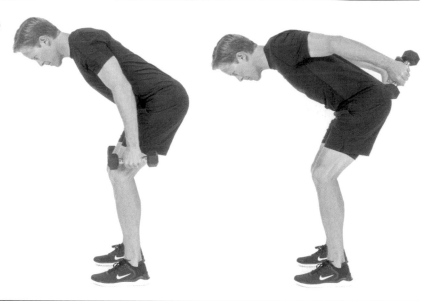

## skull crusher

Grip a dumbbell with the insides of your hands (your thumbs and index fingers) wrapped around the handle and your palms cupped around one end of the dumbbell. Straighten your arms and position the dumbbell over your forehead. Slowly bend your elbows and lower the dumbbell over your head.

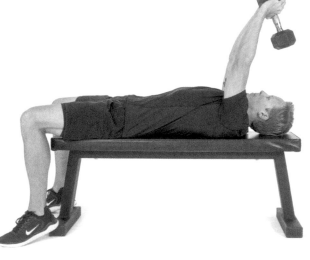

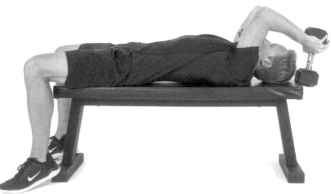

## shoulder taps

Get into the plank position: hands shoulder width apart, shoulders aligned over your wrists, and back flat. Shifting your weight to one side, reach your opposite hand across your body, touch the shoulder of your supporting arm (quick tap), and then go back to the start position. Immediately repeat on the other side, and that's one rep.

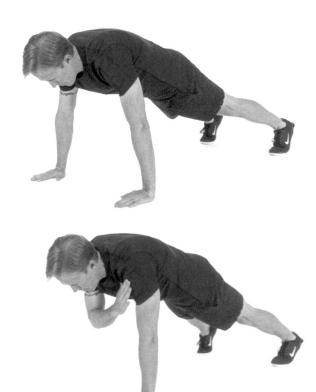

# PHASE 3

## GOOD FOR:

- Strengthening the triceps, shoulders, and pecs
- Preventing triceps pain and injury

## GUIDELINES:

- Perform 3 or 4 days a week
- Do 3 sets of 10–15 reps
- Push sets to fatigue
- Add load or reps to increase difficulty
- Tools: dumbbells, bench, resistance tube band

## triceps kickback

Start with one hand and knee on a bench and your back straight. With your other arm holding a dumbbell at your side, bend your elbow to about 90 degrees. Keeping your arm close to your body, straighten your elbow into full extension.

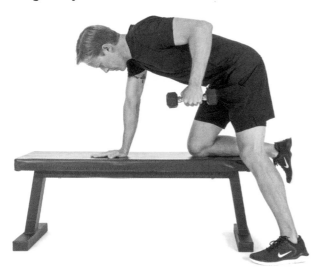 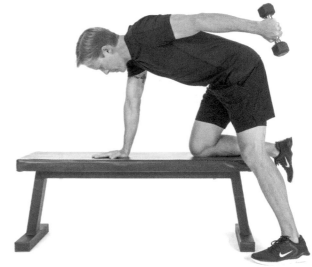

## triceps push-down

You can do this exercise in a standing or kneeling position with either a resistance band or a cable machine. With your palm facing down and your elbow bent, drive your hand toward the ground and extend your elbow while keeping your arm close to your side.

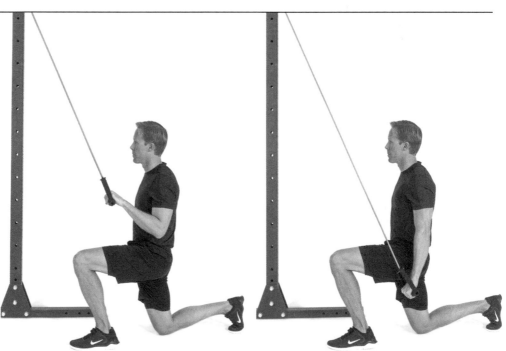

## shoulder press

Start in a kneeling position with your lead shin vertical and torso upright. Position a dumbbell over one shoulder, keeping your elbow tight to your body and palm facing inward. Push the weight straight up and fully lock out your elbow. Return to the start position slowly and with control.

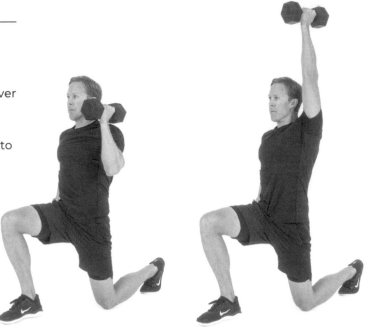

---

## press *(choose one)*

### bench press

Lie on a bench and position dumbbells over your lower chest with your palms facing your legs. Position your elbows slightly away from your body (at a 45-degree angle) and keep your forearms vertical. As you press the dumbbells straight up, rotate your shoulders so that your palms are facing each other at the top of the movement.

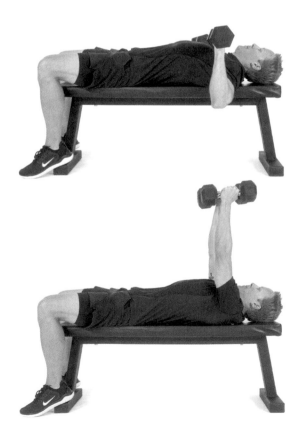

### push-up

Get into the plank position: hands shoulder width apart, shoulders aligned over your wrists, and back flat. Keeping your elbows in (about 45 degrees from your body), forearms vertical, and back flat, slowly lower your chest to the ground. Reverse the movement and reach the start position with your elbows extended.

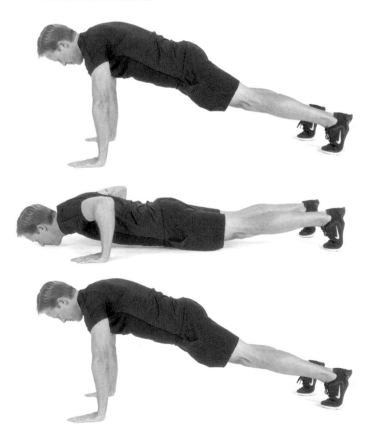

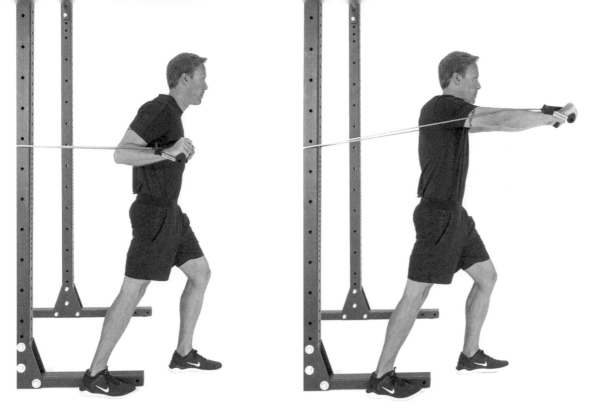

## banded press

Anchor a band at about chest height. Press your arms straight out.
As you extend your elbows, rotate your palms toward the ground.

## bench dip

Grip the edge of a bench with your elbows straight. Walk your feet out, position your legs together, and get your back flat. Slowly lower yourself as far as you can without pain, then return to the start position. If you can't complete the full movement due to pain, stick with partial range of motion repetitions.

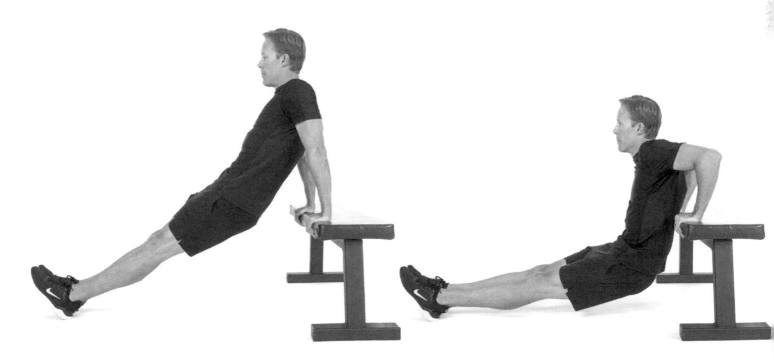

## CHAPTER 18

# WRIST & HAND
# PROTOCOLS

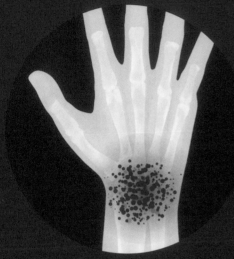

**WRIST PAIN**
(p. 261)

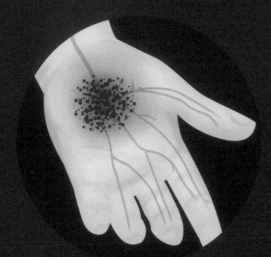

**CARPAL TUNNEL SYNDROME**
(p. 271)

# WRIST PAIN

**Follow this program to treat:**

- General wrist pain (posterior, anterior, medial, and lateral)
- Wrist sprain
- Wrist fracture
- De Quervain's tenosynovitis (thumb tendon pain)

## WRIST SPRAIN

**DESCRIPTION:** Wrist sprains typically result from a blunt force trauma such as a fall where you reach out to catch yourself and incur a FOOSH (fall onto an outstretched hand) injury. Like other sprains, wrist sprains are ligament injuries, which harm the connective tissue structures that attach bone to bone and provide joint stability.

Wrist sprains often occur alongside wrist fractures, which are cracks in the bone. The wrist bone usually breaks at the end of the radius or in one of the carpal bones. Sprains and fractures can both hurt a lot, so if you fall on your wrist and have pain or deformation, go to the doctor and get an X-ray. If the wrist is fractured, they may put you in a cast or splint or even insert pins to put the bone back together. If you wait without treatment, you might permanently lose some range of motion in your wrist.

The rehab exercise protocol is the same for either injury except for the timing of when to start the protocol. For a sprain, you can begin as soon as you are out of the acute pain phase. For a fracture, prioritize the rehab exercises provided by your physical therapist because those will be designed for the type of fracture you have. For example, your protocol might differ based on whether you had a surgery involving pins or you were simply placed in a cast. After you complete the prescribed regimen—or if you were unable to get physical therapy—the rehab exercises in this protocol should serve you well.

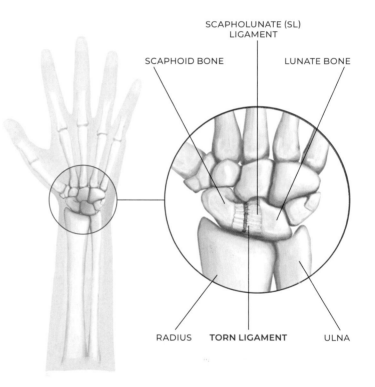

SCAPHOLUNATE (SL) LIGAMENT

SCAPHOID BONE

LUNATE BONE

RADIUS  **TORN LIGAMENT**  ULNA

**SIGNS AND SYMPTOMS:** Typical symptoms include sharp pain (especially with movements that stress the involved ligament), swelling, and weakness (the inability to grasp and pick up objects).

**AGGRAVATING FACTORS:** Moving the wrist (flexing, extending, and twisting); picking up or squeezing objects.

**PROGNOSIS:** First, rule out a fracture, as that will affect healing time. Hairline fractures typically heal in six to eight weeks. Most wrist sprains heal within two to 12 weeks, depending on severity.

**TREATMENT STRATEGY:** Most sources of wrist pain (including sprains) respond well to physical therapy involving a combination of temporary bracing (in severe cases), gradual mobility, and strengthening exercises.

Phase 1 focuses on reducing tension and pain in the wrist flexor and extensor muscles and regaining joint mobility in all planes of motion. The soft tissue mobilization techniques can reduce pain and tension because the muscles in the forearm attach to the wrist and fingers and are responsible for moving these joints. The active mobility exercises in phase 1 will not only help reduce pain but also ensure that you don't lose range of motion while the area is healing. You can also use the uninjured arm to help stretch the injured wrist. Respect your injury and only move as far as you can without pain. If you practice consistently as your body heals, you should gradually regain range of motion.

In phase 2, you perform stretches for the wrist flexor and extensor muscles, which you mobilized in phase 1. These stretches not only help with mobility but also reduce pain and tension in the forearm and wrist. Next, you begin implementing gradual strengthening work with wrist flexor and extensor isometrics and finger flexor (grip strength) and extensor exercises. These exercises use a low load so that you don't aggravate the healing tissues, but they help you prepare for the more challenging strengthening exercises in phase 3.

Phase 3 focuses on regaining wrist muscle and tendon strength and making the entire wrist and hand region more resilient. You will revisit all the motions from phase 1 while adding resistance, which will strengthen key wrist muscles and reduce the likelihood of reinjury.

## WHAT IS THE DIFFERENCE BETWEEN SPRAINS AND FRACTURES WHEN IT COMES TO TREATMENT STRATEGY?

With sprains and fractures, there are still three grades of severity, but the approach to the protocol phases is very similar. For a sprained wrist or post-surgery hairline fracture, you might require a splint until you're able to start phase 1. Whatever the condition, this protocol can work.

The primary difference between sprains and fractures is the risk of losing range of motion in the joint. Fractures stiffen as they heal, so you may need to work on passive range of motion stretches (see phases 1 and 2). Be aware of your normal range of motion, which you can usually determine by checking how far your other wrist can bend. If you have significantly less range of motion in the injured wrist, you may need to stretch the joint capsule, connective tissue, and scar tissue.

With a sprain, you probably won't need to do that. Instead of forceful stretching, focus on maintaining range of motion with active movements and strengthening exercises for the muscles that control the joint. Even for a more severe sprain, such as a grade II or III injury, or a fracture that doesn't require surgery, you shouldn't stay immobilized for too long. If the sprain is severe, you might be in a splint for a week or two to calm it down before starting phase 1.

Unlike with a fracture, you should let sprained connective tissue heal in a stiffer way so that it restabilizes the joint. A lot of people want to wear a splint for most of the day and then take it off to perform the phase 1 range of motion exercises, but be careful. You don't want the wrist to stiffen completely because you can also develop a contracture, which means the wrist can't move.

If you have a hairline fracture, see a doctor for guidance, but if you have a bad sprain, consider wearing a splint for a week or two and taking it off throughout the day to do the phase 1 exercises, especially if you think your daily activities are going to irritate the injury and slow the healing process. This also applies if you just had surgery, but in that case, work with your doctor and physical therapist to ensure the exercises are right for you.

# DE QUERVAIN'S TENOSYNOVITIS (THUMB TENDON PAIN)

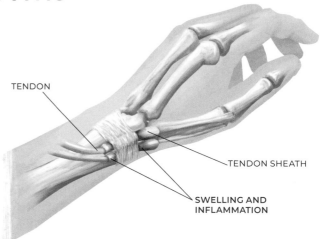

TENDON

TENDON SHEATH

SWELLING AND INFLAMMATION

**DESCRIPTION:** De Quervain's tenosynovitis is a condition in which the sheath that surrounds some of the tendons that attach to the thumb—specifically the abductor pollicus longus and extensor pollicus brevis—become irritated, causing pain on the side of the wrist near the base of the thumb. Not all tendons have a sheath, but those that do can get inflamed with repetitive use. In the case of de Quervain's tenosynovitis, texting and typing without regular breaks can cause flare-ups.

**SIGNS AND SYMPTOMS:** This issue typically produces dull, achy pain on the side of the wrist near the base of the thumb. It can become sharp with provocative movements and positions of the wrist and hand (such as bending the wrist to one side).

**AGGRAVATING FACTORS:** Excessive use of the thumb abductor and extensor muscles, such as with activities like picking up your child, video gaming, texting, gardening, and racquet sports.

**PROGNOSIS:** In most cases, this issue resolves within four to six weeks of implementing a rehab program and modifying or temporarily eliminating aggravating behaviors.

**TREATMENT STRATEGY:** Full recovery is usually possible with conservative strategies, including avoiding aggravating activities (you may need to rest and use a splint) and performing rehab exercises that help the tendon and sheath move more efficiently. In severe cases, an injection with steroid medication or an anesthetic (numbing medication) can reduce pain. Surgery for this condition is rare (it involves cutting the tendon sheath so that it can move more freely) and is recommended only when pain becomes unmanageable and the tendon does not respond to rehab or other treatment options.

**1** Phase 1 starts with wrist flexor and extensor soft tissue mobilizations. These techniques, especially the wrist extensor mobilization, can help the thumb abductor and extensor muscles, which run through this area of the forearm. The wrist mobility exercises in phase 1 also help the thumb tendons move and stretch, which can reduce pain and promote healing. The ulnar deviation movement targets the thumb tendons involved with de Quervain's tenosynovitis, so take that one slowly and move only as far as you can without pain.

**2** In phase 2, you stretch the wrist/finger extensor and flexor muscles, which partially involves the thumb tendons, especially when stretching the extensors. Phase 2 also includes several wrist and finger strengthening exercises. The resisted finger extension exercise is by far the most important one to focus on, as it involves the thumb extensor and abductor muscles.

**3** In phase 3, you perform strengthening exercises for all the available wrist movements. Although these exercises are more specific to wrist muscles, they do require the thumb tendons to move and glide, and a strong hand/wrist will help protect your thumb from future injuries. In addition to wrist exercises, I recommend that you continue the finger extension strengthening exercises from phase 2 and any mobility exercises from phase 1 that were helpful.

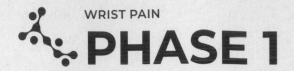

# PHASE 1

## GOOD FOR:

- Alleviating wrist pain
- Relieving muscle tension
- Improving wrist and forearm mobility
- Warm-up for phase 2 and 3 exercises

## GUIDELINES:

- Perform every day
- Tool: small massage ball
- Add phase 2 when you have no pain at rest and no more than mild pain (3/10) with the exercises

## SOFT TISSUE MOBILIZATIONS:

- ▸ Spend 1–2 minutes on each area
- ▸ Perform in any order on both sides
- ▸ Stop on tender points for 10–20 seconds

## wrist flexor mobilization

Lay your arm out straight on a bench or table with your palm facing up. Press a small massage ball into your forearm flexor muscles (where the bottom of your forearm connects to your elbow) and massage around the area. Add dynamic movement by extending your wrist while applying steady pressure with the ball.

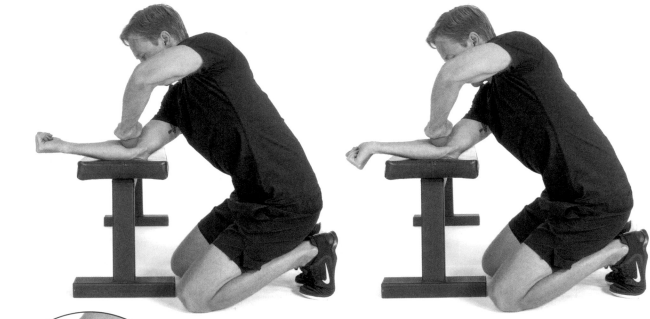

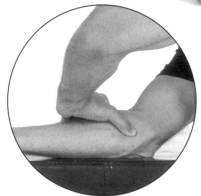

## manual variation

The manual variation shares the same technique, but instead of applying pressure with a ball, you use your thumb and palm.

## wrist extensor mobilization

With your palm facing down, press the ball into your forearm extensor muscles (where the top of your forearm connects to your elbow) and massage around the area. Add dynamic movement by flexing your wrist while applying steady pressure with the ball.

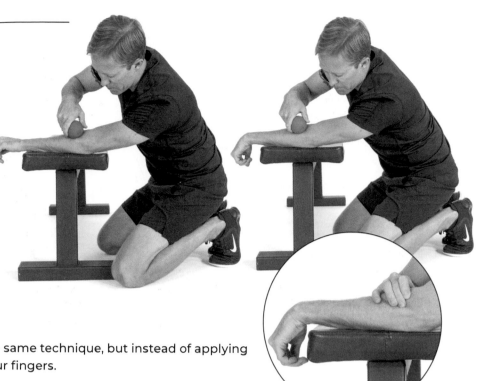

### manual variation

The manual variation shares the same technique, but instead of applying pressure with a ball, you use your fingers.

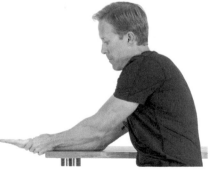

## MOBILITY EXERCISES:

- ▶ Do 3 sets of 10–15 reps
- ▶ Move as far as you can with no more than mild pain
- ▶ Pause at end range for 2–3 seconds
- ▶ Be careful with the stretches (holding end range) if you have a strain or sprain, as they can flare up symptoms

## forearm pronation and supination

With your arm supported on a table and your hand open, rotate your forearm as far as you can in each direction. Turn your palm up and then down, isolating your wrist and forearm. Once you reach end range, you can use your free hand to increase the stretch, pausing for 2–3 seconds before rotating in the opposite direction.

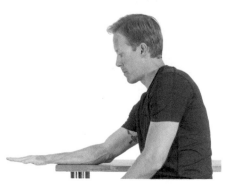

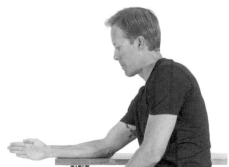

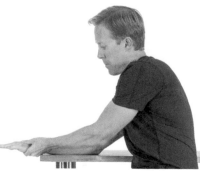

# wrist flexion and extension mobility

With your hand in a fist, extend your wrist as far as you can. Once you reach end range, you can use your opposite hand to increase the range of motion, pausing for 2–3 seconds in extension.

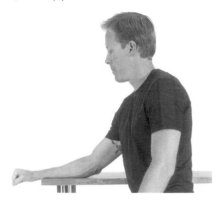 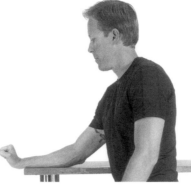 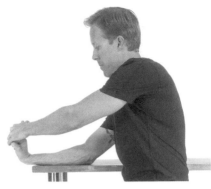

After passing through extension, flex your wrist as far as you can. Again, once you reach end range, you can use your opposite hand to increase the range of motion, pausing for 2–3 seconds in flexion.

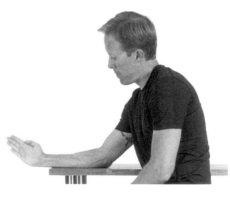 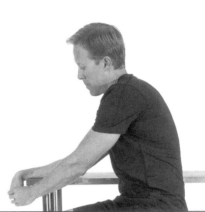

# wrist ulnar and radial deviation mobility

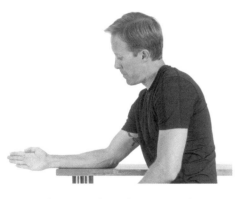 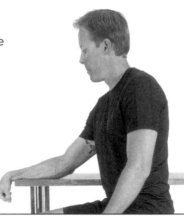 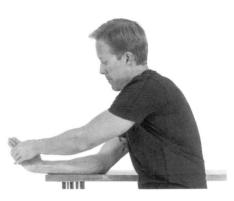

With your hand open and your thumb pointing up, move your wrist up and down as far as you can in each direction. Once you reach end range, you can use the opposite hand to hold and increase the stretch, pausing for 2–3 seconds in both positions.

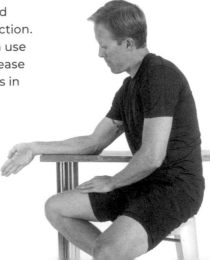 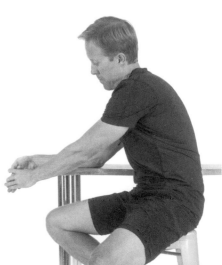

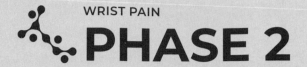

WRIST PAIN

# PHASE 2

## GOOD FOR:

- Alleviating wrist pain
- Improving forearm muscle flexibility
- Early wrist and finger strengthening
- Warm-up for phase 3 exercises

## GUIDELINES:

- Perform every day
- Tools: dumbbell, grip strengthener, finger exerciser
- Add phase 3 when you can do the exercises with no more than mild pain (3/10)

---

## wrist flexor stretch

Straighten your arm out in front of your body with your palm facing up. Form a grip around your palm with your opposite hand, then pull down until you feel a stretch on the bottom of your forearm. Perform 3 reps with 30- to 60-second holds.

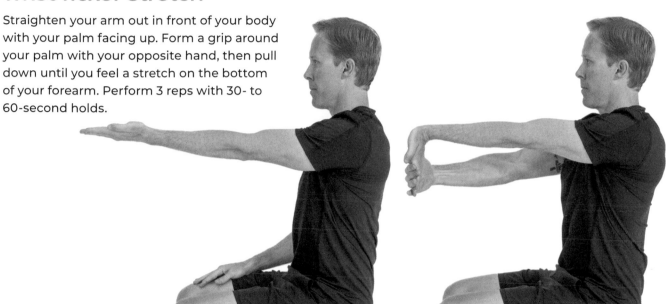

---

## wrist extensor stretch

With your palm facing down, form a grip around your knuckles with your opposite hand, then pull down until you feel a stretch on the top of your forearm. Perform 3 reps with 30- to 60-second holds.

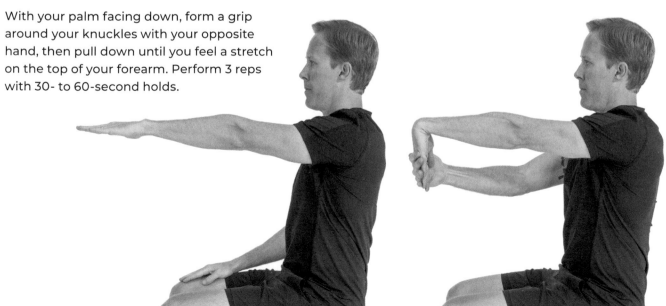

## wrist flexor isometrics

Support your forearm on a table so that only your hand is hanging over the edge and your palm is facing up. Hold a dumbbell out straight with your wrist in a neutral position. Perform 4 or 5 reps with 30- to 45-second holds.

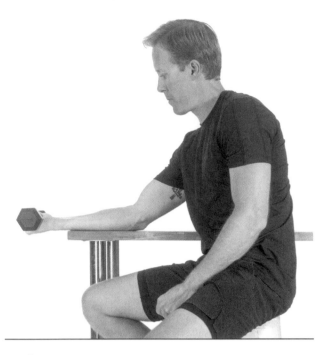

## wrist extensor isometrics

With your palm facing down, hold the dumbbell out straight with your wrist in a neutral position. Perform 4 or 5 reps with 30- to 45-second holds.

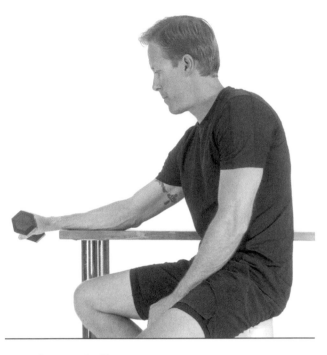

## grip strengthener

Use a grip strengthening device (resistance hand gripper, finger exerciser, or grip ring) to improve your forearm and hand strength. You can use any tool that provides resistance while closing your hand. Do 3 sets of 10–15 reps.

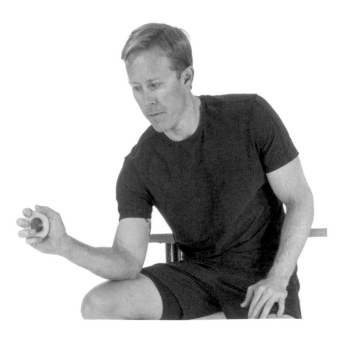

## resisted finger extensor

Place your fingers in the holes of a finger extensor resistance exerciser, then splay and extend your fingers and thumb. Do 3 sets of 10–15 reps.

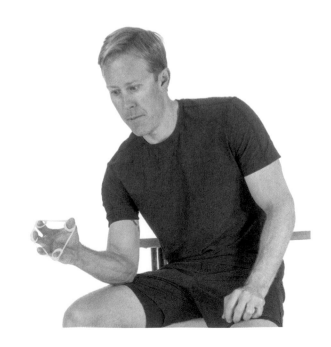

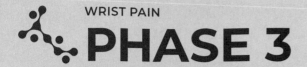

# PHASE 3

## GOOD FOR:

- Strengthening the wrist and forearm muscles
- Preventing wrist pain and injury

## GUIDELINES:

- Perform 3 or 4 days a week
- Do 3 sets of 10–15 reps
- Push sets to fatigue
- Add load or reps to increase difficulty
- Tools: dumbbell, resistance band

## wrist flexor curl

Support your arm on a table so that only your hand is hanging over the edge and your palm is facing up. Holding a dumbbell, slowly extend your wrist, then flex (curl toward your body). Momentarily pause in the top position before transitioning to the next rep.

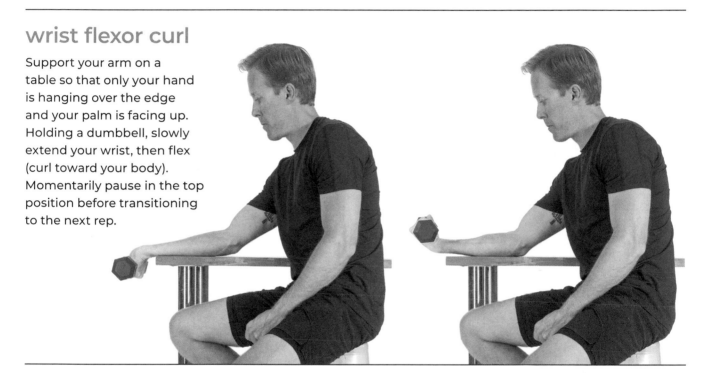

## wrist extensor curl

With your arm supported and your palm facing down, slowly flex your wrist, then extend (lift up). Momentarily pause in the top position before transitioning to the next rep.

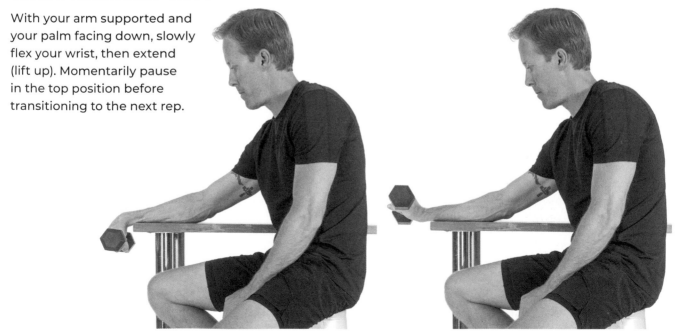

# supinator and pronator curl

With your arm supported, hold one end of the dumbbell and rotate through pronation and supination. Keep your elbow on the table, isolate the movement through your wrist and forearm, and focus on slowly rotating from a palm-up to a palm-down position.

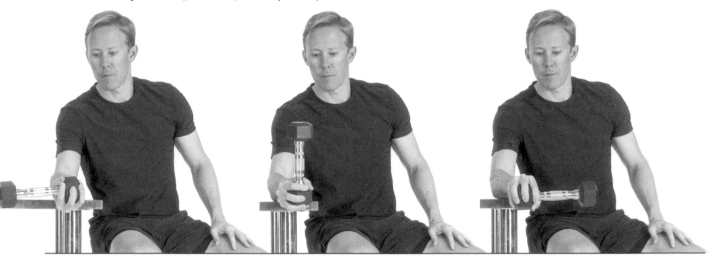

# radial deviator curl

Keeping the outside of your forearm and back of your elbow in contact with the table and the inside of your wrist facing up, lower the top of the dumbbell toward the ground, then lift it toward your body (bending only at the wrist).

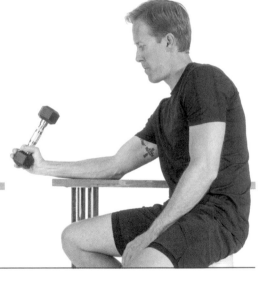

# ulnar deviator curl

Wrap a band around the pinky side of your hand with your palm facing down. Apply tension to the band with your other arm. Slowly move your hand from side to side against the resistance to strengthen the ulnar deviator muscles.

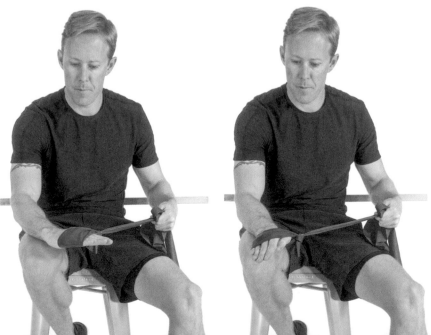

# CARPAL TUNNEL SYNDROME

**Follow this program to treat:**

- Nerve pain, numbness, and tingling in the thumb, index, middle, and half of the ring finger

**DESCRIPTION:** Carpal tunnel syndrome is the most common compression neuropathy in the peripheral nervous system and is found in 3 to 6 percent of the general population.[1,2] This issue involves stress on the median nerve on the front or anterior side of the wrist. Although the condition isn't fully understood, recent research consistently observes edema or swelling inside the nerve, which can have irreversible consequences to nerve health if not treated.[3]

This is because the median nerve—one of the largest peripheral nerves—runs through a narrow space called the carpal tunnel, which can become inflamed. This tiny tunnel also houses eight tendons that attach to your finger flexor muscles. If you are flexing your fingers a lot—moving them quickly with repetitive actions such as typing or writing, for example—those tendons slide and create friction in the tunnel, which can cause inflammation and put pressure on the median nerve.

If that pressure exists for too long or is too intense, it's as if the nerve is slowly choking. Nerves have their own microcirculation, so when you choke a nerve, you stop blood flow to it. A lack of blood flow leads to hypoxia, which is a lack of oxygen, and that can cause cell death, which stops the nerve from healing. Thankfully, carpal tunnel syndrome is preventable and treatable if you remain cognizant of the aggravating factors and follow the rehab exercises provided in this protocol.

ANTERIOR WRIST (PALM SIDE OF HAND)

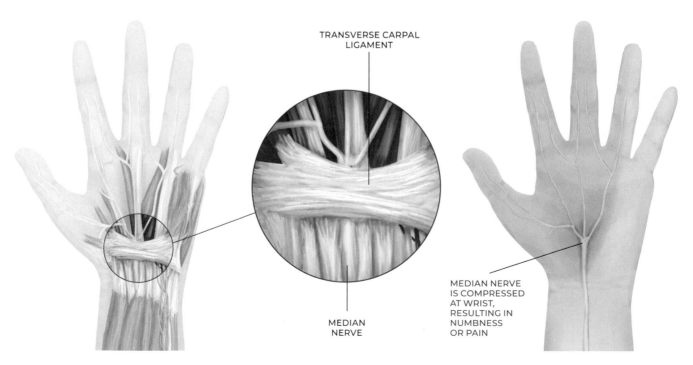

TRANSVERSE CARPAL LIGAMENT

MEDIAN NERVE

MEDIAN NERVE IS COMPRESSED AT WRIST, RESULTING IN NUMBNESS OR PAIN

**SIGNS AND SYMPTOMS:** Carpal tunnel syndrome typically produces pain, numbness, and tingling in the thumb, index finger, middle finger, and thumb-side half of the ring finger. Hand weakness and difficulty with fine motor tasks may also occur as the condition worsens.

**AGGRAVATING FACTORS:** Forceful gripping,[4] holding an object for prolonged periods, or keeping the wrists bent forward or backward, such as when typing, driving, or reading a book.

**PROGNOSIS:** If treated within six months of development, carpal tunnel syndrome typically resolves within eight to 12 weeks. However, if symptoms have persisted for more than six months or muscle atrophy and weakness are present, surgical intervention might be necessary (see Treatment Strategy). This is why you should pay attention to signals from your body (such as pain and weakness in the hand) and employ a prehab or exercise regimen to keep the surrounding tissue strong and resilient to avoid reoccurring flare-ups.

**TREATMENT STRATEGY:** In the early phases, carpal tunnel syndrome is treated primarily with conservative techniques, including wrist splints (which keep the wrists in a neutral position and reduce nerve irritation), nerve gliding exercises, steroid injections, and changing sleep and work habits.

Carpal tunnel is a tricky condition because people can't always take time off from the aggravating activity to recover. The solution is to boost nerve health, which requires getting more blood to the nerve. This does not mean doing a clump of exercise once a day; rather, you should perform activities that boost the nerve's health frequently throughout the day. Take breaks to work on increasing blood flow. You could be on phase 3 and out of pain but still benefit from implementing phase 1 or 2 exercises as a maintenance protocol. So, for every 90 minutes you're on the computer, go quickly through the phase 1 exercises, repeating that process to alleviate pain symptoms or prevent them from reoccurring.

In phase 1, you start by mobilizing the pectoral and wrist/finger flexor muscles, as the median nerve runs through these regions, and muscle tension can compress the nerve and reduce blood flow. After that, you perform two median nerve mobilization techniques to help improve nerve mobility and blood flow. The first technique is a standard nerve mobilization exercise used by rehab practitioners; the second is a new technique based on emerging research that has proved effective at targeting the carpal tunnel.[5] I recommend trying both and seeing which one is the most helpful. Phase 1 finishes with the angel exercise, which is an amazing option for dynamically improving mobility in the anterior chest wall (pectoral muscles), shoulder joint, and arm nerves.

## WHEN SHOULD I CONSIDER SURGERY, AND WHAT DOES IT ENTAIL?

Surgery for carpal tunnel syndrome is rare but necessary when symptoms become severe and do not improve sufficiently with rehab. This typically occurs in people who struggle to modify or eliminate aggravating factors because they have a job or some other activity they can't stop doing that progressively worsens the problem.

During surgery, the doctor cuts the ligament that goes over the top of the carpal tunnel, releasing the roof and relieving pressure on the nerve. This intervention is only appropriate if you are experiencing signs of irreversible nerve damage, such as weakness or atrophy in your hand. If you have only numbness, tingling, and pain, surgery might not be necessary. Those are early signs that you need to address your work conditions or other factors so that you can prioritize rehab.

In phase 2, you transition to stretching your pecs and wrist flexors, which you mobilized in phase 1. Again, the goal is to loosen these muscles so that the median nerve can move more freely. Next, you perform a wrist flexion and extension mobility exercise to mobilize the median nerve at the carpal tunnel space on the front side of your wrist.

Phase 2 finishes with two neck or cervical exercises because the median nerve is formed by nerves that originate in the neck (C5–T1). The wall chin tuck teaches a neutral cervical posture, which can reduce stress on the cervical nerve roots. The cervical flexor isometric hold works many of the same muscles involved in the wall chin tuck, but this time you are lifting against gravity, which means you are strengthening the muscles on the front of your neck. Improving the strength of these muscles will improve neck health and control, and this often reduces pain associated with the nerves that exit the neck and run through the arms.

In phase 3, you strengthen the affected wrist and finger muscles. The median nerve can weaken some of the wrist and finger flexor muscles and the pronator teres muscle. Adding these exercises will ensure that you aren't left with strength impairments. It's important to work on grip strength if your carpal tunnel issues are severe, as this is usually where people become the weakest.

The farmer's carry is a great exercise for strengthening your grip in a functional way. The last exercise in phase 3 is the banded cervical retraction, which is similar to the cervical exercises in phase 2. It strengthens the muscles that allow you to maintain an upright and neutral neck posture, which can reduce stress on the cervical nerve roots.

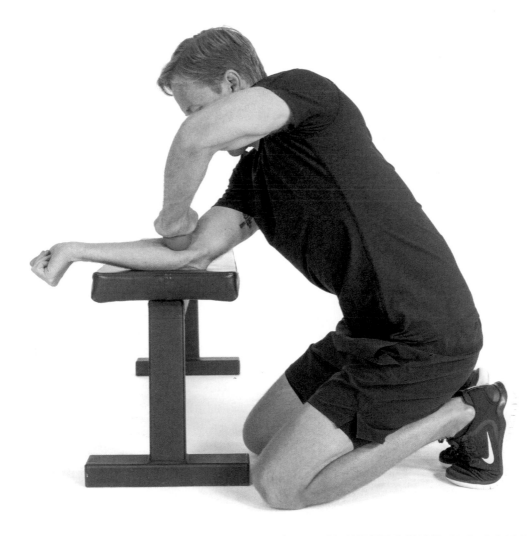

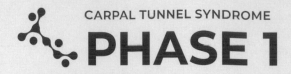

# PHASE 1

**GOOD FOR:**

- Alleviating nerve pain in the wrist and hand
- Relieving muscle tension
- Warm-up for phase 2 and 3 exercises

**GUIDELINES:**

- Perform every day
- Tools: small massage ball, foam roller
- Add phase 2 when you have no pain at rest and no more than mild pain (3/10) with the exercises

## SOFT TISSUE MOBILIZATIONS:

- ‣ Spend 1–2 minutes on each area
- ‣ Perform in any order on both sides
- ‣ Stop on tender points for 10–20 seconds

### pectoral mobilization

Position a small massage ball between a doorframe or rack and your pectoral muscles near the front of your shoulder. Place that arm behind your back and add dynamic movement by reaching overhead to further mobilize the muscles.

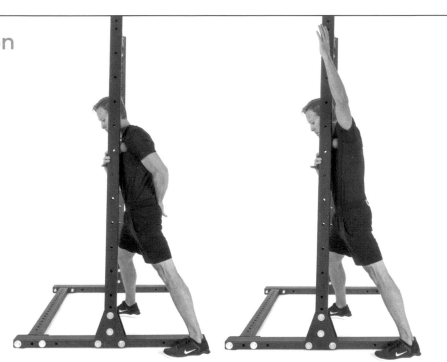

### wrist flexor mobilization

Lay your arm out straight on a bench or table with your palm facing up. Press the ball into your forearm flexor muscles (where the bottom of your forearm connects to your elbow) and massage around the area. Add dynamic movement by extending your wrist while applying steady pressure with the ball.

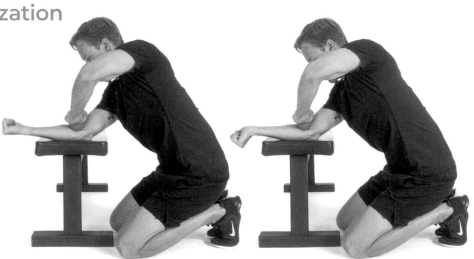

# MOBILITY EXERCISES:

▸ Do 3 sets of 10–15 reps

▸ Active range of motion (AROM)—move as far as you can without pain

▸ Pause at end range for 2–3 seconds

## median nerve slider mobility 1

Start with your arm out to your side with your shoulder at 90 degrees, your elbow and wrist bent, and your head titled away from your elevated arm. In one fluid motion, straighten your elbow, extend your wrist, and move your head toward your arm. Go back and forth between these positions to mobilize the median nerve.

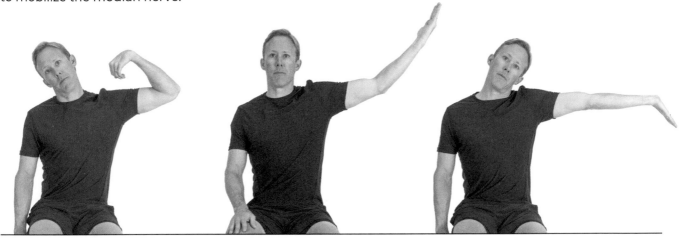

## median nerve slider mobility 2

Position your shoulder and elbow at 90-degree angles with your palm facing forward. Splay your fingers and thumb, then bring them together to mobilize the median nerve.

## angel

Position your spine over a foam roller so that your head and tailbone are supported. Start with your arms at your sides and palms up, then reach as far overhead as you can without pain.

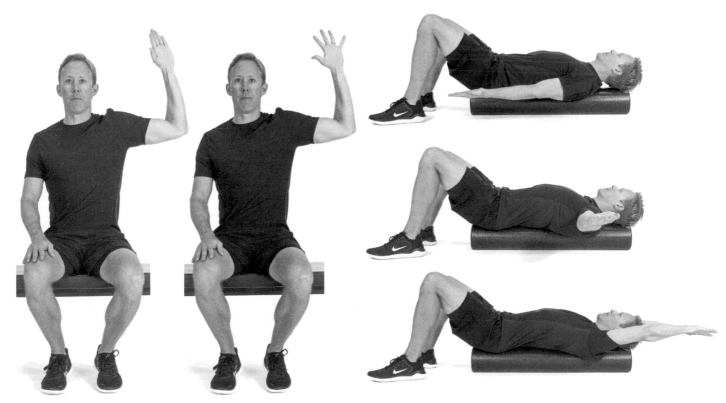

# PHASE 2

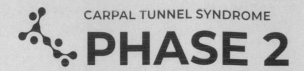

## GOOD FOR:

- Alleviating nerve pain in the wrist and hand
- Improving wrist range of motion
- Warm-up for phase 3 exercises

## GUIDELINES:

- Perform every day
- Add phase 3 when you can do the exercises with no more than mild pain (3/10)

## pectoral stretch

Position your forearm against a doorframe or rack with your shoulder at about 90 degrees. Step forward until you feel a stretch in your chest region. Move your arm slightly higher to stretch the upper fibers of your pectoral muscles. Perform 3 reps with 30- to 60-second holds.

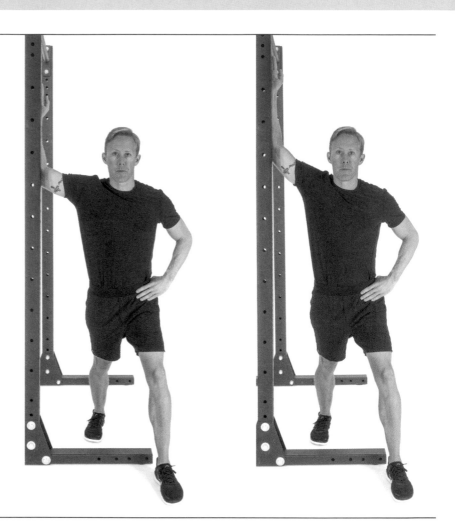

## wrist flexor stretch

Straighten your arm out in front of your body with your palm facing up. Form a grip around your palm with your opposite hand, then pull down until you feel a stretch on the bottom of your forearm. Perform 3 reps with 30- to 60-second holds.

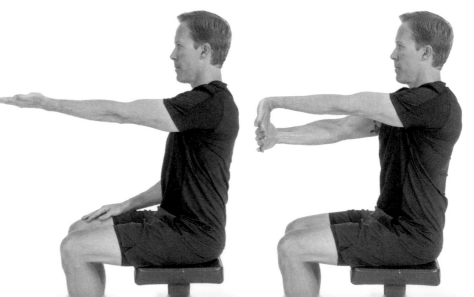

# wrist flexion and extension mobility

With your arm supported on a table and your palm facing down, flex and extend your wrist as far as you can, pausing for 2–3 seconds in both flexion and extension. Do 3 sets of 10–15 reps.

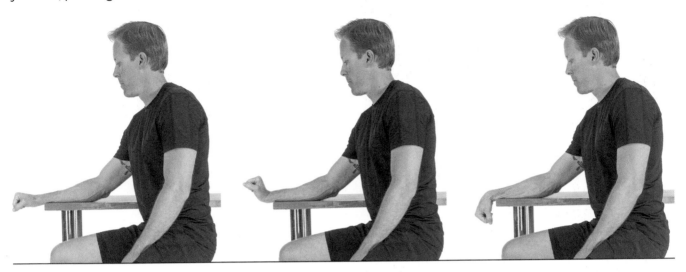

## wall chin tuck

Stand with your head and back against a wall or rack. Slide the back of your head up the wall while tucking your chin to your chest. Go back and forth between these positions. Do 3 sets of 10–15 reps.

## cervical flexor isometric hold

Tuck your chin and elongate your neck. Keeping your head neutral, lift it just high enough to clear the ground and hold. Stop if you cannot maintain the chin tuck or you start lifting your head higher to reduce fatigue. Do 3 sets of 3–5 reps and work up to 20- to 30-second holds.

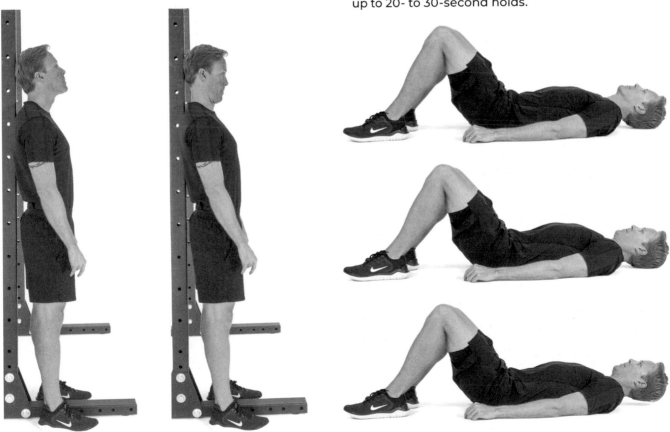

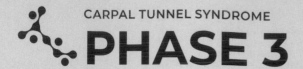

# PHASE 3

**GOOD FOR:**

- Strengthening the wrist, hand, forearm, and neck muscles
- Preventing hand and wrist nerve pain

**GUIDELINES:**

- Perform 3 or 4 days a week
- Do 3 sets of 10–15 reps
- Push sets to fatigue
- Tools: dumbbell, grip strengthener, finger exerciser, resistance band

## wrist flexor curl

Support your arm on a table so that your palm is facing up and only your hand is hanging over the edge. Holding a dumbbell, slowly extend your wrist, then flex (curl toward your body). Momentarily pause in the top position before transitioning to the next rep.

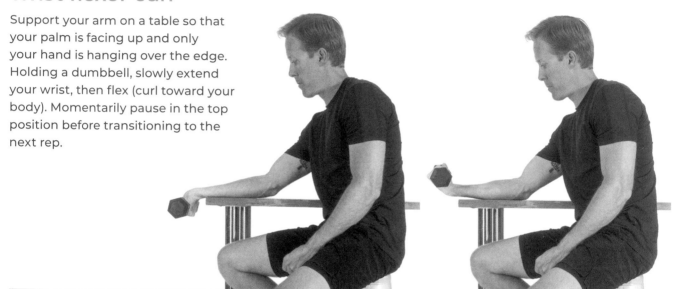

## supinator and pronator curl

With your arm supported, hold one end of the dumbbell and rotate through pronation and supination. Keep your elbow on the table, isolate the movement through your wrist and forearm, and focus on slowly rotating from a palm-up to a palm-down position.

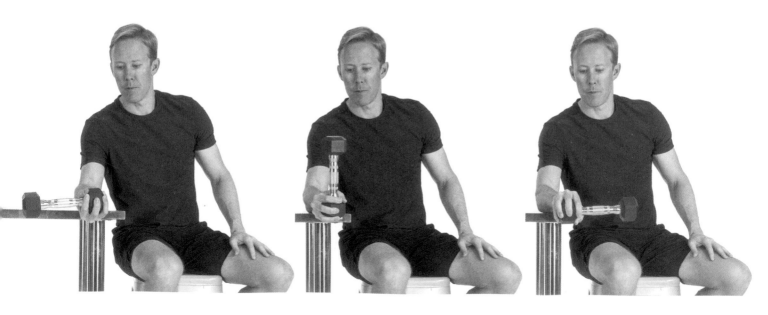

## grip strengthener

Use a grip strengthening device (resistance hand gripper, finger exerciser, or grip ring) to improve forearm and hand strength. You can use any tool that provides resistance while closing your hand.

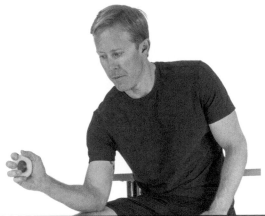

## resisted finger extensor

Place your fingers in the holes of a finger extensor resistance exerciser, then splay and extend your fingers and thumb.

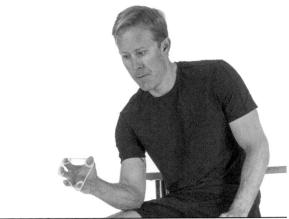

## farmer's carry

Hold a heavy dumbbell at your side and walk 15–20 meters (or take 20–30 steps), then turn around and return to the starting point. Do this 3 times with each arm.

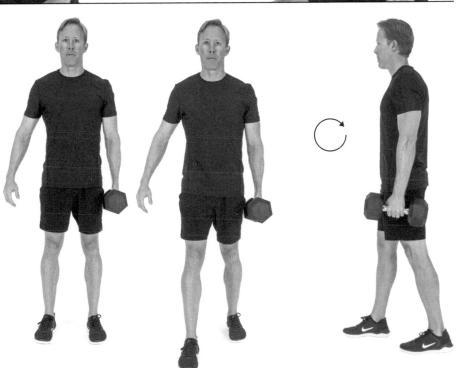

## banded cervical retraction

Wrap a band around your head and hold it with both hands. Stretch the band to apply resistance on the back of your head. Start with your head forward and move it backward into retraction against the resistance.

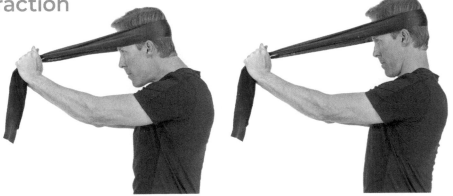

## CHAPTER 19

# BACK & SPINE
## PROTOCOLS

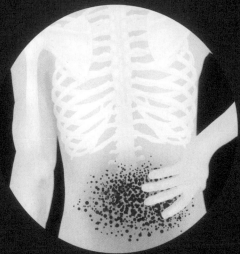

**LOW BACK PAIN**
(p. 281)

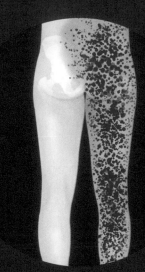

**NERVE PAIN**
(p. 304)

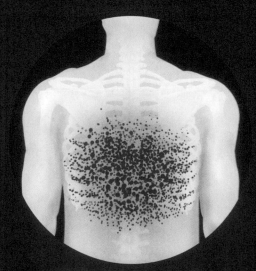

**MID-BACK AND
RIB CAGE PAIN**
(p. 317)

# LOW BACK PAIN

**Follow this program to treat:**

- Non-specific low back pain (acute and chronic)
- Sharp, achy pain in the low back
- Lumbar flexion and hyperextension sensitivity
- Pain on one side of the back
- Muscle strain
- Facet joint sprain
- Spondylolysis and spondylolisthesis
- Sacroiliac (SI) joint pain

## NON-SPECIFIC LOW BACK PAIN (ACUTE AND CHRONIC)

**DESCRIPTION:** Non-specific back pain, which accounts for 90 to 95 percent of back pain cases, describes a type of pain where a specific nociceptive source for a person's symptoms (disc, muscle, joint, etc.) cannot be determined. Medical and rehab providers chose the term *non-specific* to describe general pain that exists when an obvious source cannot be linked to the person's pain.[1,2]

Such a diagnosis often leaves people feeling frustrated because being able to link pain to something on an image makes it seem like a definitive explanation has been reached, and we can move forward with confidence. When an MRI is inconclusive and a diagnosis like non-specific low back pain is made, many people end up feeling like they won't get better because the practitioner doesn't know what is going on with their body. However, you must remember that while pain and injury often occur together, they are different and can occur independently. Low back pain is the premier example of this since most cases do not involve injury. Trust that most cases resolve in four to six weeks, especially when you implement graded doses of movement and exercise and address any other contributing factors (stress, sleep, nutrition, etc.).

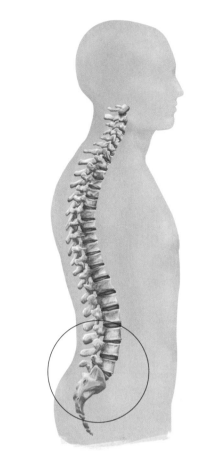

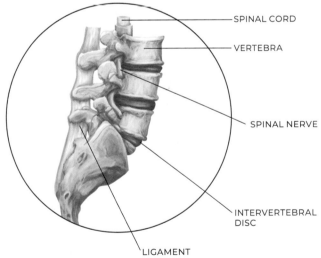

SPINAL CORD

VERTEBRA

SPINAL NERVE

INTERVERTEBRAL DISC

LIGAMENT

**SIGNS AND SYMPTOMS:** Non-specific back pain typically causes dull, achy pain along one or both sides of the low back. In some cases, pain radiates into the buttock. Symptoms can become sharp with certain movements and can limit range of motion and the ability to carry out functional tasks. However, the location and type of symptoms can vary quite a bit from one person to the next.

**AGGRAVATING FACTORS:** Non-specific pain is usually less mechanical than a straightforward back injury (strain, sprain, etc.) and is often influenced by factors such as stress, sleep, and general physical activity. So, it is important to pay attention not only to physical factors that make your back pain worse but also to factors that may not be on your radar. To learn more about other factors that can be associated with musculoskeletal pain, read Chapter 4.

**PROGNOSIS:** Most non-specific back pain resolves within four to six weeks when you implement the appropriate recovery and treatment regimen. If you leave it untreated and do not modify aggravating factors, it can last much longer and even become chronic.

**TREATMENT STRATEGY:** Rehab for non-specific back pain combines manual therapy (massage, joint mobilization) and mobility, sensorimotor control, and resistance training exercises.[3-5] If symptoms become chronic, psychological and emotional interventions (counseling, sleep studies, etc.) may be added to the treatment plan. With chronic pain, you don't want to let fear or anxiety deter you from moving and exercising. You want to respect your symptoms while confronting the pain with gradual doses of movement so that you don't lose mobility, strength, or functional capacity. As you do the protocol, pay attention to your body and tweak the sets, reps, and exercise variations to match your symptoms. Consistent training should desensitize your system and improve your mobility, strength, and function.

Phase 1 starts with spine and hip soft tissue mobilizations that can reduce low back pain and muscle tension. Then hip-biased stretches target muscles that attach to either the pelvis or the spine (hip flexors), which can effectively combat low back pain. The last exercise in phase 1, quadruped flexion and extension, introduces low-load active mobility. If your low back pain flares up when performing flexion and/or extension movements, skip the exercise and add it to the next phase.

Phase 2 features more advanced mobility and stretching drills that take the spine deeper into available ranges of motion. Go slowly and stop if you experience more than mild discomfort. Then comes a series of gluteal activation and strengthening exercises (bridge, side-lying hip abduction, and lateral squat walk). The last phase 2 exercise, the Pallof press, is the first resistance exercise that targets the spinal musculature. This exercise makes your trunk muscles keep your spine in a neutral position and resist the rotation being imposed by the band, which reduces the likelihood of low back aggravation and starts to rebuild muscle strength.

Phase 3 focuses on building hip (especially gluteal) and trunk/core strength and control. The fire hydrant and single-leg hip extension variations are included as progressions from the phase 2 exercises because increasing gluteal strength often reduces pain and protects the low back from injury. The following exercises challenge the spinal muscles through all planes of motion, which makes the spine more resilient. The last two exercises, the squat and deadlift, are commonly encountered compound movement patterns that involve the hip and spinal muscles. Strengthening these patterns will prepare you to resume the activities of daily living. If you have pain with the bilateral squat or deadlift, you can substitute split-stance and single-leg loading options like split squats, lunges, and single-leg deadlifts to keep your spine in a neutral position while training your trunk/core muscles, which can be helpful for sensitive or healing spinal structures.

# MUSCLE STRAIN

**DESCRIPTION:** Muscle strains in the low back are common and typically happen when lifting or catching something heavy unexpectedly. The muscles surrounding the low back must generate force rapidly and are more likely to be strained if they do not have the strength to handle the external load. However, strains can also happen with slower movements if you are heavily loaded or with lower loads if your back is rounded or twisted. They can even happen when doing something mundane, like bending over to pick something up or standing up from a chair. It's not something any of us like to confess, but it's common to complete a movement when your tissues are not warm and end up with a muscle strain.

Low back pain can vary in severity from a legitimate muscle strain to tender or achy general pain that might result from sleeping in an odd position, prolonged sitting, wearing heels, or holding a child in an awkward position for extended periods. Whether it's a strain or a minor ache, this protocol contains exercises that alleviate pain and prevent future flare-ups.

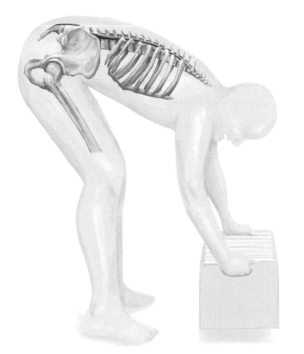

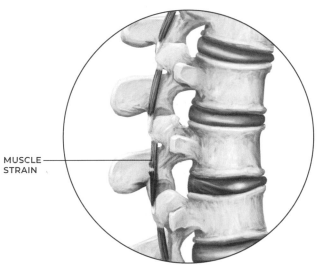

MUSCLE STRAIN

## DOES ROUNDING YOUR BACK INCREASE THE CHANCES OF A MUSCLE STRAIN?

We often teach people with low back strains how to bend from their hips, which activates the glutes and hamstrings and reduces stress on the low back muscles. However, flexion or rounding of the back is a part of normal biomechanics and not something to be feared. Once your back has healed and you have built strength with the exercises in this protocol, you can return to normal movement. Of course, the heavier the load, the more you need to think about spinal mechanics, especially if you haven't developed the capacity to handle the load you're lifting. For example, if you're performing a heavy deadlift, the hip hinge strategy is good to use, and it might be safer to lift with your back in a neutral (somewhat flat) position.

**SIGNS AND SYMPTOMS:** When a muscle is strained, it typically produces pain when it is working (contracting), being stretched, or being palpated or touched. With a low back strain, you often experience pain when you return to standing after bending over. Imagine bending to tie your shoe. As you stand, the extensor muscles of your low back must contract to lift your trunk, and this is when many people feel pain.

Pain is often sharp when the tissue is stressed. You can have a strain on both sides, but people usually feel it more on one side or the other. The pain typically remains in the back and does not radiate down the leg. The muscle may ache and feel tight or like it is spasming at rest.

**AGGRAVATING FACTORS:** Pain typically ignites when contracting or stretching the low back muscles—bending at the waist, lifting an object from the floor, or even carrying or bracing from an upright position.

**PROGNOSIS:** Again, the severity of the strain (grade I–III) dictates how long the healing process will ultimately take, but because back muscle tissue has a good blood supply, three to six weeks is a fair range.

**TREATMENT STRATEGY:** Muscle strains are usually treated with rehab exercises rather than medical management such as injections or surgery, except when a prescription muscle relaxant may help with severe pain. Rehab exercises can improve muscle strength, which helps the injury heal and reduces the likelihood of reinjury. In cases of longtime one-sided back pain, the nervous system can inhibit muscles, causing them to atrophy.[6,7] You can change this pattern with training. Strengthening the extensors and surrounding tissues will trigger hypertrophy and reduce the likelihood of another strain.

**1** Strengthening is important for muscle strain rehab, but loading the tissues can be difficult when pain is acute. So, phase 1 focuses on alleviating pain using soft tissue mobilization and stretching exercises, but be careful with techniques that target the healing tissues. Applying too much pressure with the lumbar extensor and QL mobilizations could aggravate the area and delay healing. If those techniques create more than mild discomfort, remove them.

**2** It's important to gradually work on spinal mobility as your pain decreases to avoid this area becoming stiff. The quadruped flexion and extension mobility exercise at the end of phase 1 and most of the movements and stretches in phase 2 are designed to help you regain full spinal range of motion. Again, move only as far as your body can tolerate. As your muscle strain heals, you will regain mobility in your spine.

**3** By phase 3, your pain should be minimal or absent with most daily tasks, so you can start adding more resistance. The exercises target the gluteal and spinal muscles to improve their strength, which increases their capacity to handle force without damage, maximizing tissue integrity and reducing the likelihood of a future strain.

# FACET JOINT SPRAIN

**DESCRIPTION:** Facet joints are small joints that connect one vertebra (back bone) to the next. They allow you to bend, twist, and extend your spine and create the "crack" sound when you twist your back. Like other joints in the body, each facet joint is surrounded by a fibrous joint capsule that provides stability and holds in joint fluid. When the spine is injured by being jarred (such as in a car accident or sports-related trauma) or forced to move beyond its normal mobility, facet joints can be sprained.

## HOW IS A FACET JOINT SPRAIN DIFFERENT FROM A MUSCLE STRAIN?

A strain typically occurs when force is applied to the muscle, such as when performing a heavy deadlift. Sprains, on the other hand, happen when the joints are in an end-range position and then twisted or jarred. Although the pain might be similar, the mechanism of injury is different, and the treatment strategy varies slightly.

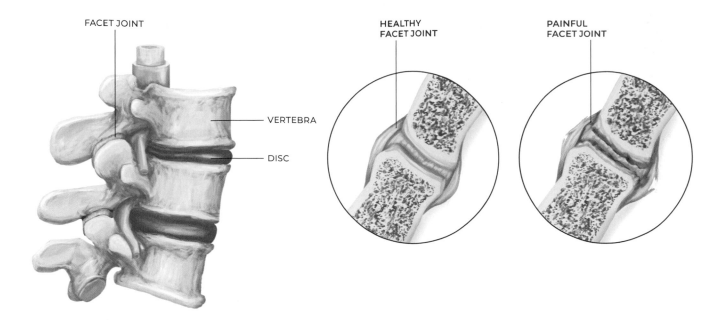

FACET JOINT

VERTEBRA

DISC

HEALTHY
FACET JOINT

PAINFUL
FACET JOINT

**SIGNS AND SYMPTOMS:** Facet joint sprains typically happen in the low back and produce pain on only one side (unilateral pain) that is reproduced with twisting, extending, or arching the back in a way that stresses the inflamed facet joint. Pain is often sharp in these provocative positions and then achy at rest, especially in the acute phase.

**AGGRAVATING FACTORS:** Pain typically comes on when arching the low back or bending or twisting to one side. Individuals also report pain when transitioning from one position to another, such as going from seated to standing.

**PROGNOSIS:** Facet joint sprains typically heal within four to six weeks, assuming the inflamed joint capsule is not irritated by aggravating activities that stress the area.

**TREATMENT STRATEGY:** Facet joint sprains respond well to rehab exercises designed to reduce pain and restore spinal range of motion and strength. A prescription muscle relaxant may be helpful for severe pain.

With a sprain, you approach the protocol as if you have a strain but with the goal of regaining full spinal mobility. The strengthening exercises are important because your muscles support and protect your joints, but you aren't using them to directly rehabilitate injured tissue as with a muscle strain.

**1** The phase 1 exercises, which include soft tissue mobilizations and stretches, can reduce muscle pain, tension, or spasming caused by the surrounding low back and hip muscles tightening to protect the injured joints, which compresses the spine. The hip stretches target muscles that commonly affect the low back because they attach either to the pelvis (hamstrings and glutes) or the spine (hip flexors).

**2** Once your pain decreases, working on spinal joint mobility becomes important. The quadruped flexion and extension mobility exercise at the end of phase 1 and most of the movements and stretches in phase 2 can help you regain full spinal range of motion. Move only as far as your body can tolerate. As the facet joints heal, you will regain spinal mobility.

**3** Phase 3 focuses on building hip and low back muscle strength once your mobility is back to normal and your pain is gone. While a sprain doesn't involve an injury to a muscle, improving neuromuscular strength and control allows you to better protect your joints. Muscles act like shock absorbers, so optimal function means less force is transferred to your joints, whereas weakness or impaired control increases the risk of injury.

# SPONDYLOLYSIS AND SPONDYLOLISTHESIS

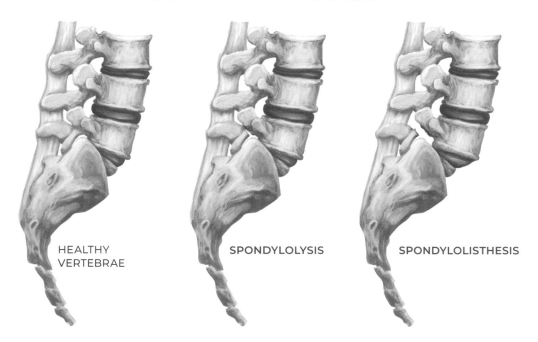

HEALTHY VERTEBRAE     SPONDYLOLYSIS     SPONDYLOLISTHESIS

**DESCRIPTION:** Spondylolysis and spondylolisthesis are common causes of low back pain, especially in children and adolescents who participate in sports that apply repetitive force to the spinal column, such as gymnastics, football, and weightlifting.[8-11]

Spondylolysis describes a situation in which a stress fracture occurs in the vertebrae (small bones that make up the spine). With spondylolisthesis, the bone becomes weakened—usually due to an accumulation of stress and a lack of recovery—to the point that it begins to shift out of position either backward (retrolisthesis) or forward (anterolisthesis). A spondylolisthesis is graded from I to IV based on how far the bone has moved from its original position.

Although there are differences between spondylolysis and spondylolisthesis, the signs and symptoms, aggravating factors, prognosis, and treatment strategies are the same.

**SIGNS AND SYMPTOMS:** In most cases, people experience only general low back pain, and the cause is usually not identified unless an X-ray is ordered. Symptoms may include pain that radiates into the buttock, back stiffness, back muscle spasms, and hamstring tightness. With a higher-grade spondylolisthesis that affects a nerve in the low back, numbness, tingling, and weakness in the legs may occur.

**AGGRAVATING FACTORS:** Arching or extending the spine beyond neutral and under force (such as backbends and back handsprings in gymnastics or weight over shoulders in weightlifting).

**PROGNOSIS:** Most individuals return to full function after six to 12 weeks of rest from aggravating activities, which gives the weakened bone time to heal.

**TREATMENT STRATEGY:** Behavior modification (avoiding or limiting aggravating activities) and physical therapy stretches and exercises are the preferred treatments, but a low back brace may be recommended to take stress off the healing bones.[12,13] If symptoms are not improving or the vertebral slippage is worsening, doctors may recommend surgery to stabilize the injury.

The stretches in the protocol, particularly the hip flexor and hamstring stretches in phase 1, often reduce back pain associated with a spondylolisthesis. At the beginning of phase 2, be cautious with the lumbar extension mobility drills; many spondylolisthesis injuries are related to repeated lumbar extension. So, perform only partial range of motion with these drills or skip them entirely. When you get to the dead bug and abdominal rollout in phase 3, avoid letting your low back extend. If any other exercises cause back pain or radiating nerve pain in your legs, omit them.

# SACROILIAC (SI) JOINT PAIN

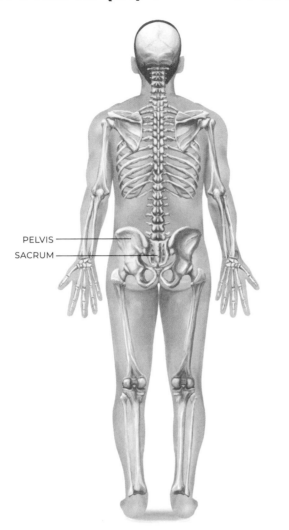

PELVIS

SACRUM

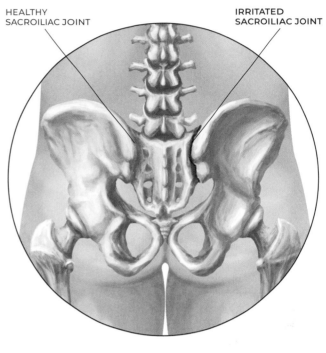

HEALTHY
SACROILIAC JOINT

IRRITATED
SACROILIAC JOINT

**DESCRIPTION:** The sacroiliac (SI) joints are two small synovial joints located on the right and left sides of the low back between the sacrum and the ilium bones of the pelvis. They are surrounded by ligaments, which makes them very strong and capable of supporting body weight. Injury to an SI joint typically stems from an abnormal one-sided trauma, such as falling on your tailbone or stepping off a curb without realizing it and jarring your leg and one side of your pelvis. It is also common in pregnancy. The reproductive hormone relaxin loosens and relaxes the ligaments around the pelvis, which can create SI joint pain.

Because of their shape and the surrounding ligaments, the SI joints move little and are thought to account for just 15 to 30 percent of back pain cases.[14,15] This means many people think they have SI pain when it's actually their low back, such as the lower lumbar vertebrae

L5–S1 and L4–L5, which are only a few centimeters apart, making it easy to mistake them for the SI joint. Luckily, there are specific tests (administered by a professional) that can help determine whether this region is the source of your pain. The good news is that the SI Joint protocol and the Low Back Pain protocol contain similar exercises, and you are likely to improve regardless of which one you do.

**SIGNS AND SYMPTOMS:** Pain is usually located on one side of the low back and may radiate into the buttock or back of the thigh. Low back stiffness is often reported, and some people feel a sense of instability, as if their back is going to give out or buckle. SI joint pain usually does not cause pain that radiates into the lower leg and foot, so if you are experiencing this or if the pain goes down the back of your leg, refer to the Nerve Pain protocol beginning on page 304.

## I'M NOT SURE IF I HAVE SI JOINT PAIN OR SOMETHING ELSE. HOW DO I CHOOSE THE RIGHT PROTOCOL?

Don't focus too much on the tissue and what's causing your symptoms. Focus instead on getting out of pain. Even if you aren't sure your pain is caused by SI irritation, the rehab program will help. There are minor differences between SI joint pain, sciatica, and back strains, but the key is to find movements that reduce your symptoms. If you're in the right region and picking things that don't make you feel worse, chances are high that you're going to get better over time.

**AGGRAVATING FACTORS:** Placing pressure on the joint, such as when climbing stairs, running or jogging, standing on one leg, or lying on one side, often brings on SI joint pain.

**PROGNOSIS:** In most cases, SI joint pain resolves within four to six weeks once you modify aggravating activities.

**TREATMENT STRATEGY:** You manage SI joint pain by modifying aggravating activities and performing rehab exercises that target the hip and low back muscles.[16] If pain persists, a healthcare practitioner can administer an injection to reduce inflammation and pain. Injections can serve as a diagnostic tool; if you get one and your pain goes away, the pain was coming from the SI joint. For pregnant or hypermobile people, SI joint stability belts, which wrap around and tighten the pelvis, might provide some benefit and pain relief when performing the lumbar-pelvic stability exercises in the protocol, especially in phases 2 and 3.

Most people with SI joint–related pain find relief with gluteal mobilizations and stretches (knee to opposite shoulder and figure-four) and exercises that activate and strengthen these muscles (bridge with adduction, banded bridge, lateral squat walk, etc.). Many of the other spine-focused exercises help, too, so I recommend working through the entire protocol and seeing which movements are most effective for you. If something causes pain, take it out and try adding it again later. For instance, stick with double-leg bridges until your joint desensitizes and then try the single-leg variation again.

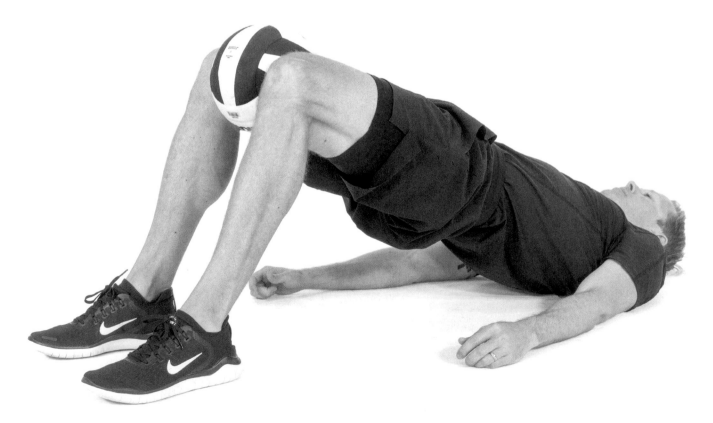

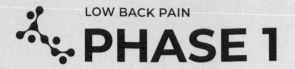

# PHASE 1

## GOOD FOR:

- Alleviating low back pain
- Relieving muscle tension
- Warm-up for phase 2 and 3 exercises

## GUIDELINES:

- Perform every day
- Tools: foam roller, peanut tool, massage ball, stretch strap, balance pad
- Skip any exercises that cause more than mild pain (3/10) and add them to phase 2
- Add phase 2 when you have no pain at rest and no more than mild pain with the exercises

## SOFT TISSUE MOBILIZATIONS:

▸ Spend 1–2 minutes on each area
▸ Perform in any order on both sides
▸ Stop on tender points for 10–20 seconds

### glute/piriformis mobilization

Sit on a foam roller and lean to one side, putting your weight over your glute muscles. Roll throughout the gluteal region: up, down, and side to side. To increase the pressure, stretch the muscles by crossing your leg over your opposite knee. For more precise pressure, use a large or small massage ball.

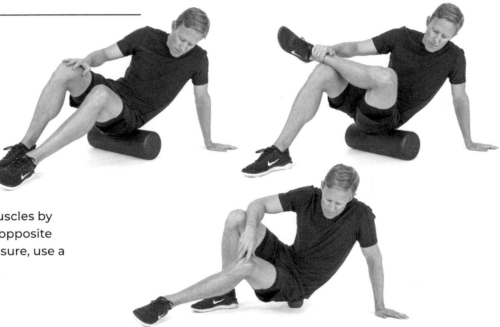

### lumbar extensor mobilization

Lie on your back with your feet on a bench or chair. Position a peanut tool under your low back. Press your heels into the bench to control the pressure. Keep your low back neutral and your butt off the ground (don't hyperextend or tilt your pelvis). You can roll up and down or rock from side to side. You can also use a small massage ball and work each side of the extensors, focusing on the area just above your hip.

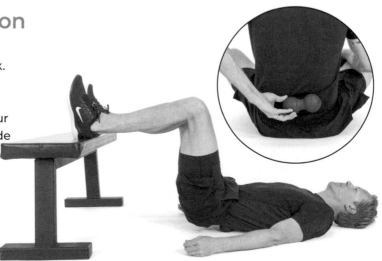

> Be careful with or skip this exercise if you have a lumbar muscle strain.

# ql mobilization

Be careful with or skip this exercise if you have a lumbar muscle strain.

Lie on your side with the roller or a large massage ball positioned under the muscles along the side of your lower back. Roll from the top of your pelvis to your lower rib. You can also roll from side to side by rotating your chest toward the ground. Try to keep your spine neutral. If you're using a ball, you can do this mobilization standing against a wall.

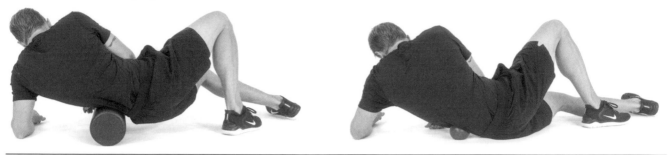

# hamstring mobilization

Sit on a bench or chair and place a large or small massage ball under your hamstring muscles. Roll up and down the entire length of your hamstring. Flex and extend your knee to dynamically mobilize the muscles.

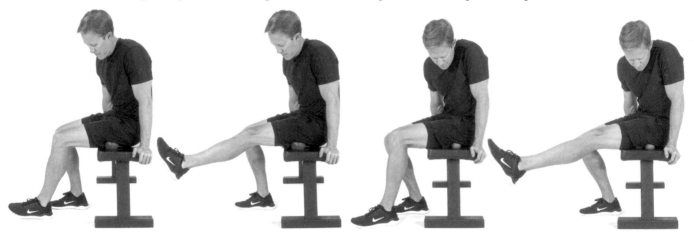

# STRETCHING EXERCISES:

- ▸ Do 3 reps with 30- to 60-second holds
- ▸ Perform on both sides
- ▸ Don't stretch into pain

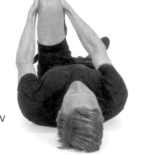
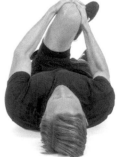

## knee to opposite shoulder

Lie on your back and bring one knee toward your chest. Interlock your fingers over your lower knee and upper shin. Keeping your low back flush with the ground, use your arms to pull your knee across your body toward your opposite shoulder.

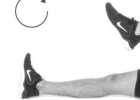
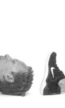
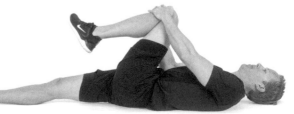

## hamstring stretch with strap

Hook a strap around the arch of your foot. Keeping your leg completely relaxed, use your arms to pull your foot toward your head and hold it in place once you feel a moderate stretch.

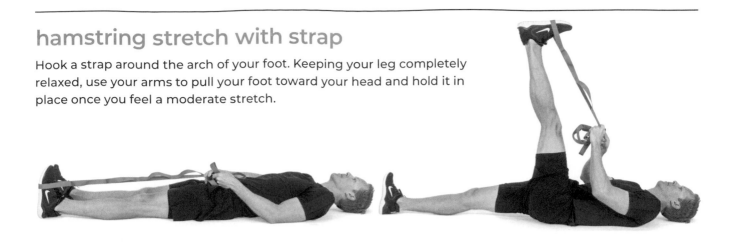

## hip flexor stretch

In a kneeling position, squeeze your abdominals and glutes to rotate your pelvis backward (posteriorly). If you are kneeling on a hard surface, use a balance pad to protect your knee.

Keeping your back neutral, shift your body forward slightly until you feel a stretch on the front of your hip and leg.

Bend your knee and grab your ankle to increase the intensity of the stretch. You can also prop your foot on a bench or chair or position your shin flush against a wall.

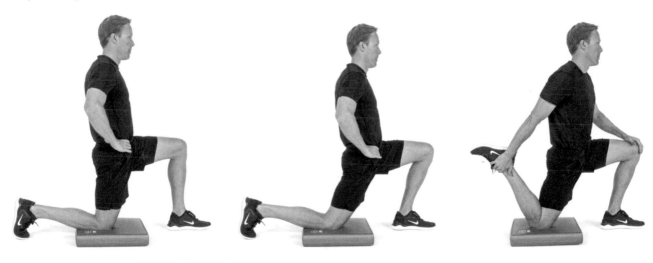

## quadruped lumbar flexion and extension mobility

In the quadruped position, round (flex) and arch (extend) through your low back. Move slowly and as far as you can without pain. Do 3 sets of 10–15 reps. Pause at end range for 2–3 seconds. Skip this exercise or save it for phase 2 if it flares up your symptoms.

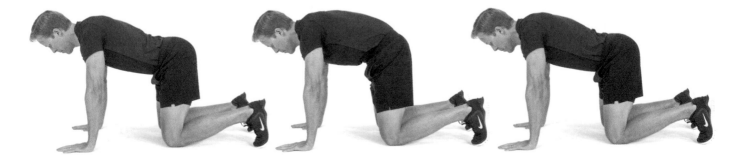

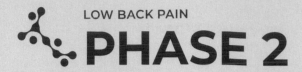

LOW BACK PAIN

# PHASE 2

## GOOD FOR:

- Alleviating low back pain
- Improving hip and back mobility
- Early glute and core strengthening
- Warm-up for phase 3 exercises

## GUIDELINES:

- Perform every day
- When there are multiple exercise options, start with the easiest (first) option and replace with the more advanced variations as your pain decreases
- Tools: bench, resistance loop, sports ball, resistance tube band
- Skip any exercises that create more than mild pain (3/10) and add them to phase 3
- Add phase 3 when you can do the exercises with no more than mild pain

## MOBILITY EXERCISES:

▸ Do 3 sets of 10–15 reps

▸ Active range of motion (AROM)—move as far as you can without pain

▸ Pause at end range for 2–3 seconds

▸ Skip exercises that flare up pain symptoms

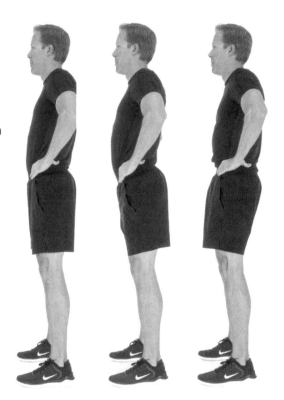

### standing pelvic tilt

Stand with your feet straight and spaced shoulder width apart. Place your hands on your hips so that your thumbs are touching the backs of your hip bones. Use your back muscles to slowly tilt your pelvis forward (anteriorly), then squeeze your glutes to rotate your pelvis backward (posteriorly). Control the range of motion and don't push into pain.

### lumbar flexion *(choose one)*

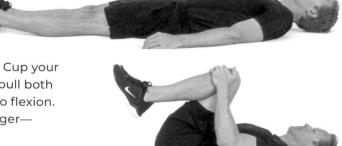

### knees to chest

Lie on your back, then bring your knees to your chest. Cup your hands around your upper shins and use your arms to pull both knees toward your chest, stretching your low back into flexion. Pause at end range—holding for a few seconds or longer—release the stretch, and then repeat.

## chest to knees (child's pose)

Get into the quadruped position. Keeping your palms on the ground, drop your butt toward your heels and lower your head through your arms.

You can hold the stretch or return to the start position and repeat the movement as a mobility exercise.

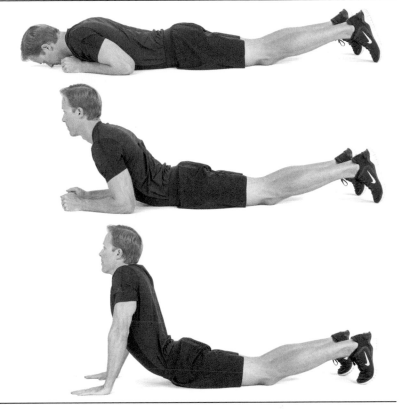

## lumbar extension

Lie on your stomach with your forearms positioned underneath your shoulders. Keeping your back relaxed and hips on the ground, push through your forearms (or climb up to your hands) and arch your back as far as you can without pain. Pause at end range—holding for a few seconds or longer—go back to the start position, and then repeat.

**Be careful with or skip this exercise if you have spondylolysis or spondylolisthesis.**

## lumbar rotation

Lie on your back with your knees bent and your feet on the ground. Rock your knees slowly from side to side, moving as far as you can without pain.

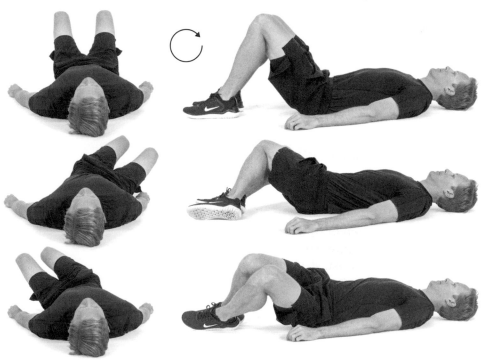

# STRETCHING EXERCISES:

- Do 3 reps with 30- to 60-second holds
- Perform in any order on both sides
- Don't stretch into pain

## glute/hip rotator stretch *(choose one)*

### seated figure-four stretch

Sit on a bench or chair, cross one leg over the opposite knee, and then hinge forward from the hips until you feel a stretch in your glute region.

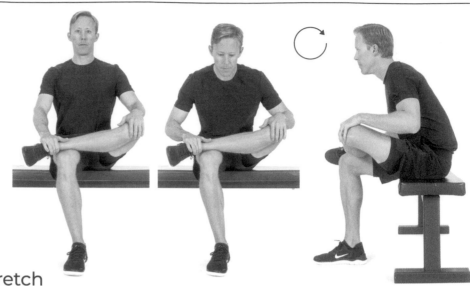

### supine figure-four stretch

Lie on your back with your legs bent and feet on the floor. Cross one leg over the opposite knee. Reach one arm between your legs, the other arm around the outside of your leg, and then interlock your fingers around the front of your knee. Now use your arms to pull your knee toward your chest.

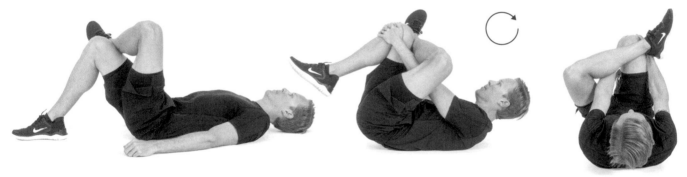

### pigeon stretch

Position your knee flush on the bench with your lower leg perpendicular to your body, then slide your rear foot back. Hinge forward from your waist until you feel a stretch in your glutes. If you feel pain in your knee or are unable to get into the start position comfortably, place a pillow under your knee or elevate one side of the bench (on the same side as your bent knee). To increase the stretch, do this exercise on the floor.

## lumbar rotation stretch

Lie on your back and bend your knee and hip to about 90 degrees. Reach across your body and cup your hand around the outside of your elevated knee. Keeping both shoulders on the floor, use your hand to pull your knee across your body and toward the floor. Rotate as far as your spine will comfortably allow.

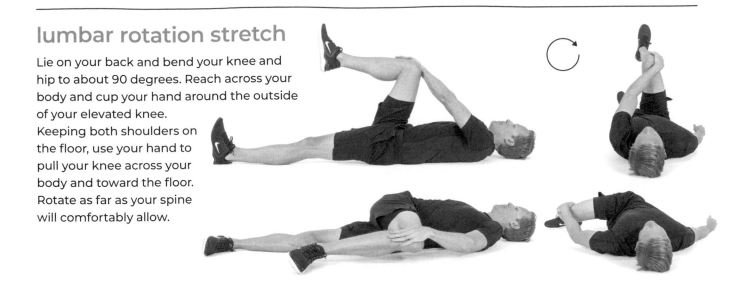

## RESISTANCE EXERCISES:

- ▸ Do 3 sets of 10–15 reps
- ▸ Push sets to fatigue
- ▸ Add load or reps to make the exercises more challenging

## bridge *(choose one)*

### bodyweight

Lie on your back with your knees bent and your feet flat on the floor. Push into the floor and lift your butt, fully extending your hips—a straight line runs from your shoulders to your knees. Squeeze your glutes as you reach full hip extension and pause in the top position for 1–2 seconds.

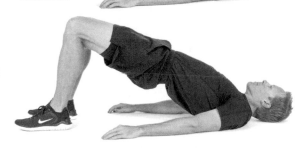

### banded

To increase glute activation and make the exercise more challenging, position a resistance loop just above your knees. Perform a bridge—drive your heels into the floor and extend your hips—while driving your knees out into the band. Maintain abduction resistance (knees out) throughout the entire range of the movement.

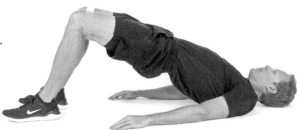

### with adduction (for si joint pain)

Position a volleyball, soccer ball, or basketball between your knees. Perform a bridge while squeezing your knees into the ball and contracting your glutes. Maintain pressure on the ball during the entire movement.

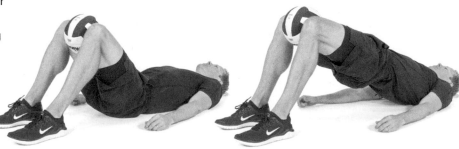

## side-lying hip abduction

Lie on your side, rotate your hips toward the floor slightly, and internally rotate your top leg so that your big toe is angled toward the arch of your bottom foot. Lift your top leg up and at a backward angle. Keep your spine neutral and pause in the top position for 1–2 seconds. Reduce the range of motion if you start to arch your back excessively. Add a resistance loop above your knees to increase glute activation and make the exercise more challenging.

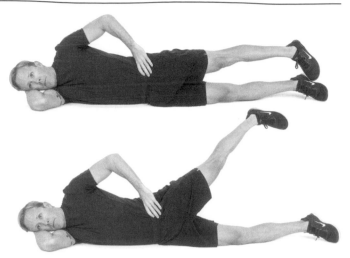

## lateral squat walk

Wrap a resistance loop above your knees. Position your feet shoulder width apart and bend your hips and knees slightly. Take a wide lateral step so there is a full stretch in the band. You can either walk along a line and then switch after a given number of steps or stay in one area by switching back and forth between legs. Choose a distance or rep range that is challenging—you feel your upper glutes burn—usually 15–20 steps in each direction. Don't pause between steps, and keep tension in the band during the entire movement.

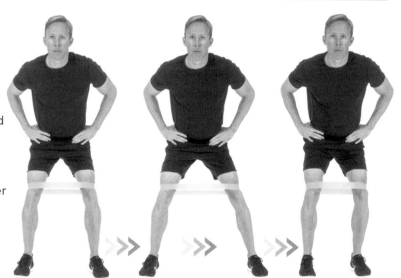

## pallof press

Anchor a resistance band to about hip level and step away to create tension in the band. Get into a kneeling position and grip the handle with both hands positioned at the center of your chest. Keeping your core tight, press the band straight out. The goal is to prevent the band from rotating your spine by contracting your abdominal and back muscles.

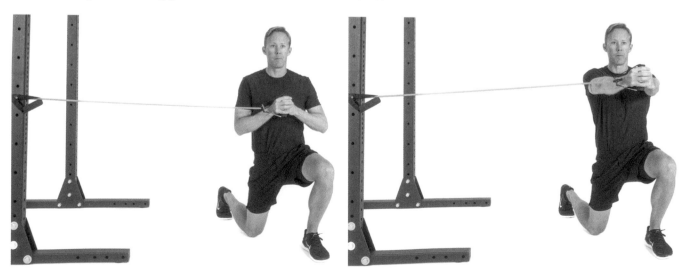

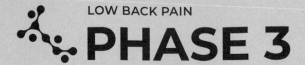

# PHASE 3

**GOOD FOR:**

- Strengthening the core (back and abdominal muscles) and lower body
- Preventing low back pain and injury

**GUIDELINES:**

- Perform 3 or 4 days a week
- Do 3 sets of 10–15 reps unless otherwise noted
- Push sets to fatigue
- When there are multiple exercise options, choose a variation based on experience, fitness level, equipment availability, and personal preference
- Tools: resistance loop, bench, physio (exercise) ball, dumbbells

## fire hydrant *(choose one)*

## bodyweight

Get into the quadruped position with your shoulders aligned over your wrists and hips over your knees. Keeping your knee bent, raise one leg back and out to the side—like a dog peeing on a fire hydrant. Do not rotate your spine and move only as far as your hip will allow.

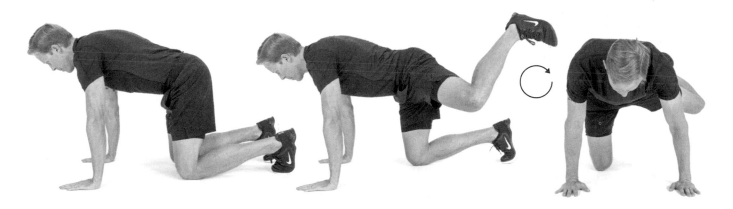

## banded

If the bodyweight variation is not challenging enough or you don't feel your glutes working, add a resistance loop above your knees to increase the resistance.

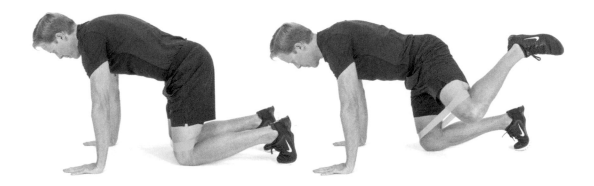

# single-leg hip extension *(choose one)*

## single-leg bridge

Get into the bridge start position and elevate one leg—you can either straighten it or keep it bent at about 90 degrees. Push into the floor and extend your hips. Focus on squeezing your glutes as you reach full hip extension, holding the contraction for 1–2 seconds.

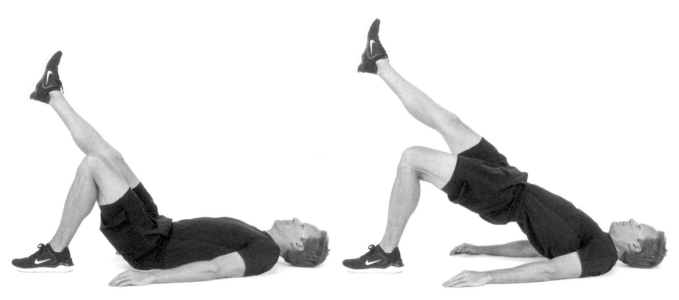

## single-leg hip thrust

Position your mid-back on the edge of a bench and lift one leg—you can either straighten it or keep it bent at about 90 degrees. Push into the floor and extend your hips. Focus on squeezing your glutes as you reach full hip extension, holding the contraction for 1–2 seconds.

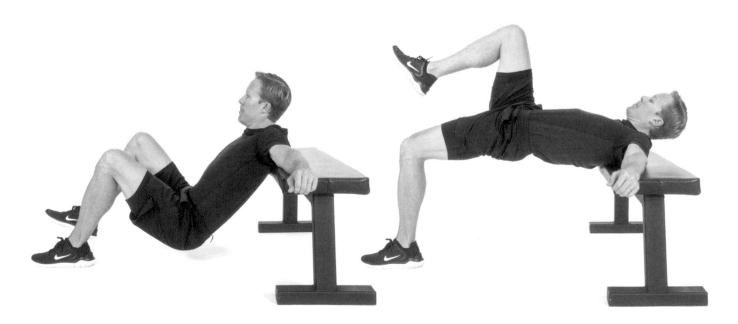

# lumbar flexion *(choose one)*

## dead bug

Lie on your back, bend your knees and hips to about 90 degrees, and straighten your arms above your body. Extend one leg and reach overhead with the opposite arm while keeping your abs tight and your low back flat on the floor. Stop if your low back arches. Repeat on the opposite side. If this version is too hard, move only your legs.

## abdominal rollout

Start on your knees with your hands on a physio ball. Keeping your abs tight, roll forward until you reach full hip extension—form a straight line from your shoulders to your knees. If you arch, struggle to maintain a neutral spine, or feel pain, perform partial range of motion repetitions. Return to the start position by reversing the movement while maintaining the same form (flat back).

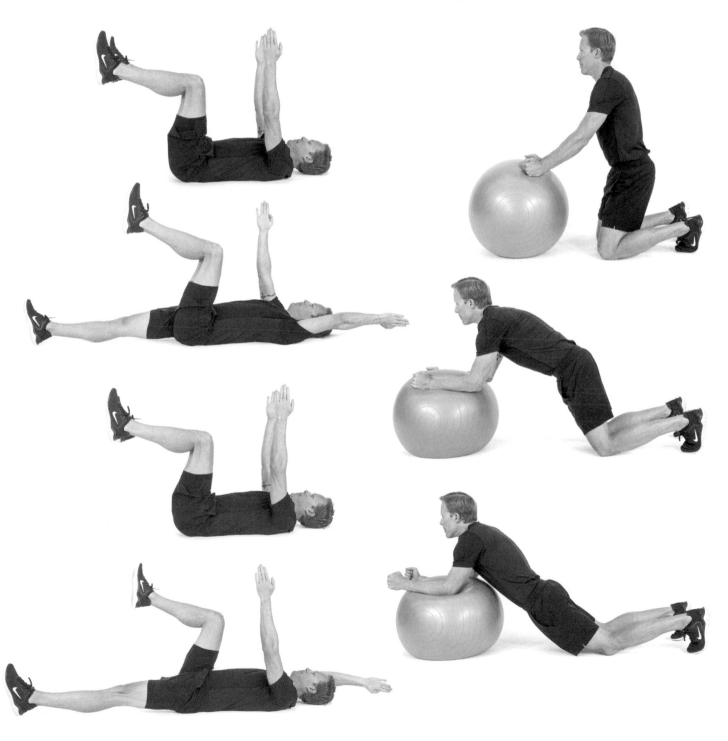

## lateral flexion *(choose one)*

### side plank offset

Lie on your side, position your elbow underneath your shoulder to elevate your upper body, and cross your top leg over your bottom leg. Use your trunk and core muscles to lift your hips. Perform 3 reps with 20- to 30-second holds.

### farmer's carry

Hold a heavy dumbbell at your side. Walk 15–20 meters (or take 20–30 steps), keeping your spine straight (try not to lean to the side). Then turn around and return to the starting place. Do this 3 times on each arm.

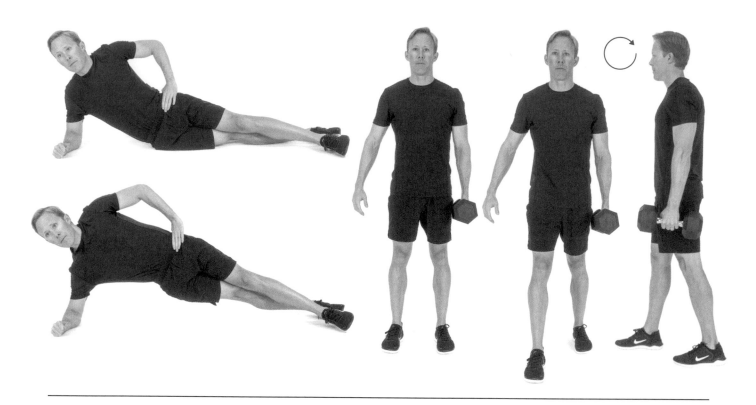

## lumbar extension *(choose one)*

### bird dog

Get into the quadruped position with your shoulders aligned over your wrists and hips over your knees. Extend one arm while extending the opposite leg. Keep your spine neutral and avoid arching your back during the movement. Repeat on the opposite arm and leg.

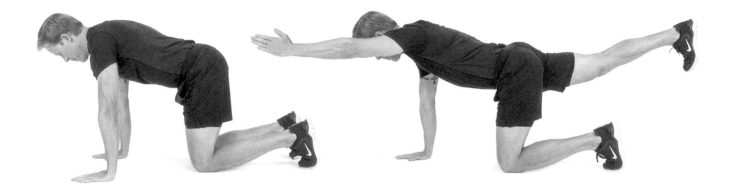

## skydiver

Lie on your stomach with your arms at your sides. Use your low back extensors to lift your lower and upper body segments off the floor. As you arch, squeeze your glutes and pull your shoulders back while maintaining a neutral neck position.

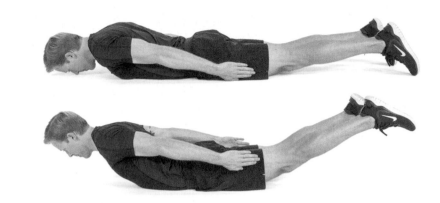

## superman

Lie on your stomach with your arms reaching overhead. Use your low back extensors to lift your lower and upper body segments off the floor. Keep your neck neutral (don't look up), keep your arms straight, and squeeze your glutes as you elevate your legs.

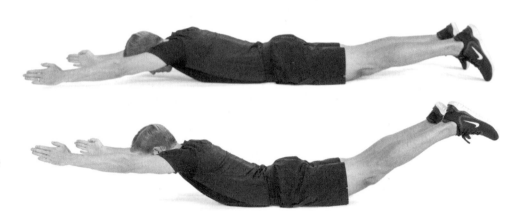

## spinal extensor curl

Position the physio ball under your stomach and push your feet into a wall while keeping your knees on the floor. Use your low back extensors to lift your chest, squeezing your glutes as you arch. Cross your arms over your chest to make the exercise easier, or place your hands on the back of your head to make it harder.

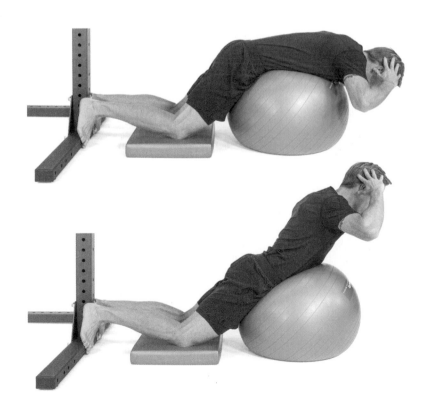

## goblet squat

Stand with your feet roughly shoulder width apart. When it comes to foot flare, you can orient your feet straight or turn them out slightly—whichever feels better and allows you to reach the lowest depth without discomfort. Cup the end of a dumbbell with both hands at the center of your chest. To perform the movement, reach your hips back slightly and sit straight down. As you lower into the bottom position, keep your spine in the neutral zone (not excessively arching or rounding), your knees aligned over your toes, and the weight close to your body. The goal is to keep your torso as upright as possible and lower as far as you can while maintaining good form.

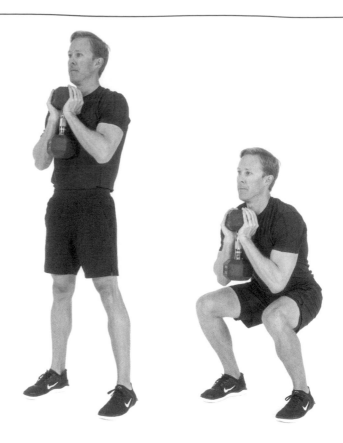

## air squat

If the goblet squat is too difficult—even with a light dumbbell—stick with the air squat variation. To perform the air squat, extend your arms in front of you as you reach your hips back and lower into the squat.

## box/chair squat

If you're new to squatting or have trouble controlling the movement, use a chair or box to gauge depth. Reverse the movement the moment your butt touches the chair; do not pause in the bottom position.

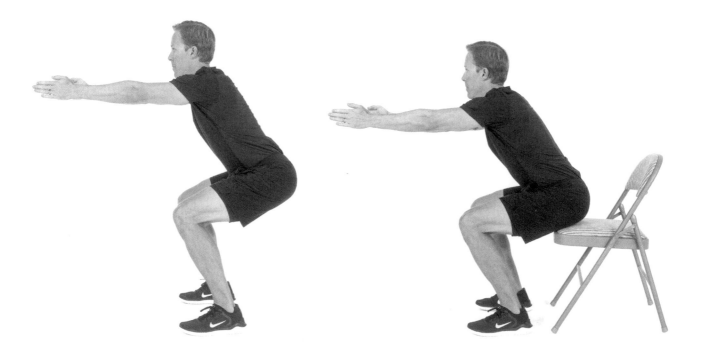

# deadlift/rdl *(choose one)*

## dumbbell deadlift

Hold dumbbells in front of your thighs with your palms facing your body, or with the dumbbells at a 45-degree angle relative to your body. Position your feet underneath your hips or just inside shoulder width. Keeping your back flat and arms relaxed, sit your hips back, bend your knees, and allow your torso to tilt forward—you should feel tension in your hips, hamstrings, and back. Keep the dumbbells close to your body (aligned over the centers of your feet), keep your shins as vertical as possible, and go as low as you can without rounding your back. To perform the upward movement, drive through your heels while extending your hips and knees.

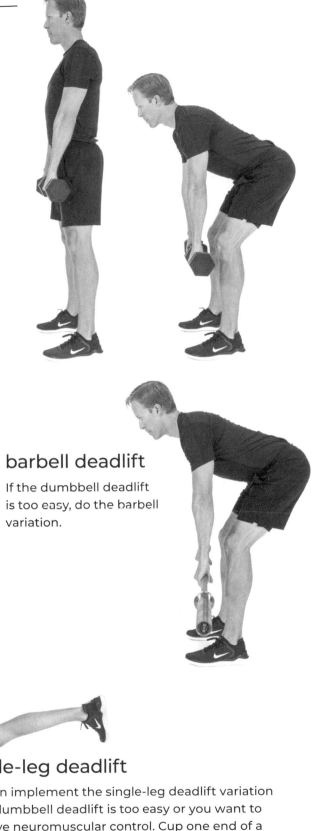

## bodyweight (dowel) deadlift

If the dumbbell deadlift is too challenging, perform the same hip hinge movement but hold a dowel instead of dumbbells.

## barbell deadlift

If the dumbbell deadlift is too easy, do the barbell variation.

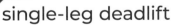

## single-leg deadlift

You can implement the single-leg deadlift variation if the dumbbell deadlift is too easy or you want to improve neuromuscular control. Cup one end of a dumbbell with both hands and shift the majority of your weight onto one leg. In one motion, hinge from your hips and bend your loaded knee slightly. As you lower your torso and the weight toward the floor, keep your back flat, grounded shin vertical, arms relaxed, and shoulders and hips square (try not to twist or rotate).

# NERVE PAIN

**Follow this program to treat:**

- Numbness and/or tingling that radiate into the buttock, back of the thigh, and down the leg
- Sciatica (from the low back)
- Disc herniation
- Lumbar stenosis

## SCIATICA (FROM THE LOW BACK)

**DESCRIPTION:** Sciatica describes an irritation of the sciatic nerve or its branches that originates in the low back (lumbar spine). Many factors can cause this type of irritation, including prolonged pressure on the nerve (sitting on a hard surface or for too long), a low back injury that causes inflammation around the nerves, and low back stenosis (narrowing of the passageway through which the nerves travel).

There are many types and causes of sciatica, and it can be debilitating. Lumbar-based cases come primarily from the low back and the nerve roots of the spine. The problem could be a disc herniation that is either touching the nerve roots or resulting in inflammation that's irritating the nerve roots. Sometimes sciatica comes from the glute region—we call it deep gluteal pain syndrome now, but it used to be known as piriformis syndrome. If you have pain radiating from your hip (not your lower back), you can also follow the Nerve Pain protocol for the hip beginning on page 344.

**SIGNS AND SYMPTOMS:** Sciatica typically produces sharp pain and burning, numbness, and/or tingling sensations that radiate into the buttock and back of the thigh. Increased nerve irritation can make pain travel into the calf, shin, and foot and cause muscle weakness in the legs.

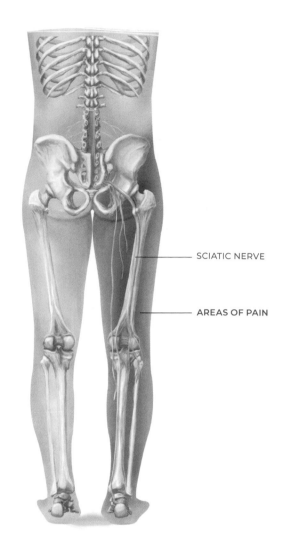

SCIATIC NERVE

AREAS OF PAIN

**AGGRAVATING FACTORS:** Pain is typically brought on by bending the back into flexion (such as bending over to tie your shoes) or extension (arching your spine), stretching the sciatic nerve (sitting and straightening your leg or bending over with your knees straight), prolonged sitting or driving, or lifting objects. Most people feel radiating nerve pain, especially in the low back, when the spine is in flexion.

You probably shouldn't stop working out, but keep in mind a concept called centralization. Try to identify the activities or tasks that make the pain from sciatica radiate farther down your leg. This pain is called peripheralization, and it means that activity is aggravating the nerve, so you should temporarily modify or eliminate it. Even within the rehab protocol, if an exercise makes your pain travel farther down your leg, you should take it out. Instead, you want to find activities and exercises that create centralization, where the pain moves toward your spine. If lying on your stomach or standing and arching your back makes the pain leave your leg—even if it makes your back hurt a bit more—that's a good sign. Such movements can serve as a test and a treatment exercise.

PROGNOSIS: Most cases resolve within four to six weeks if you modify or eliminate activities or positions that aggravate the nerve.

TREATMENT STRATEGY: Sciatica is managed with physical therapy exercises that improve nerve health and blood flow. If your symptoms do not improve after six weeks of rehab or you begin to notice leg weakness, see an orthopedic doctor for spinal imaging (MRI), as an injection or low back surgery may be necessary.[17]

## WHY DO I KEEP GETTING SCIATICA—AND WHAT CAN I DO ABOUT IT?

There are people who do everything right and still get sciatica. The good news about musculoskeletal pain is that it is usually cyclical, and with time and movement, it will resolve. You can do rehab and still have flare-ups (which is the case with all injuries and common pain symptoms), but I encourage you to remain optimistic and stick with the protocol. By avoiding or modifying the aggravating factors, listening to your body, and doing the rehab exercises, you can slow the cycle and reduce your likelihood of getting sciatica again.

It's also important to review the factors that influence pain and injury (Chapters 4 and 9) because you might think that your pain is solely exercise induced when it can be exacerbated by poor diet, lack of sleep, high stress, sitting or being static for long periods, inflammation, and so on.[18] Due to the complex nature of pain, and given the fact that sciatica can rear its ugly head spontaneously, you need to look at all the potential causes and take a multifactorial approach to alleviating and preventing the issue.

Besides the exercises outlined in this program, many people find relief with strategies such as low back traction (machine based or an inversion table), standing in chest-deep water in a swimming pool (spinal unloading), applying ice or heat to the low back, and taking anti-inflammatory medication.[19]

The phase 1 mobilizations often reduce back and nerve pain, as they target the nerve running through the buttock, down the hamstring region, and into the calf. Be cautious with the glute/piriformis and hamstring mobilizations; too much pressure can aggravate the sciatic nerve. The quad mobilizations target the path of the femoral nerve, so you should focus on these areas for nerve pain on the front or side of your thigh.

When doing the hamstring stretch with strap in phase 2, do not pull your leg too high, which can aggravate the sciatic nerve. Pull to the point where you feel a mild stretch and start there. When you get into lumbar flexion and extension mobility in phase 2, avoid movements that cause your nerve pain to peripheralize (travel farther down your leg), focusing instead on spinal mobility exercises that make the pain centralize (leave the leg). People often feel worse with lumbar flexion exercises and notice centralization with lumbar extension exercises, so test the movements and see how your body responds. Like the hamstring stretch, be gentle when performing the sciatic nerve mobilization at the end of phase 2. While it often reduces pain and improves nerve health, pulling the leg too high can make pain worse. The key is to find the position where your nerve begins to tighten without flaring up symptoms.

Phase 3 includes a more aggressive sciatic nerve mobilization (slump) and a femoral nerve mobilization. If your symptoms are primarily in the back of your leg, focus on the slump; if it causes more pain, stick with the sciatic nerve mobilization with strap from phase 2. The femoral nerve mobilization, like the quad mobilizations in phase 1, addresses nerve symptoms on the front of the thigh. The resistance exercises at the end of phase 3 target the gluteal muscles and often help with low back pain and sciatica.

# DISC HERNIATION

**DESCRIPTION:** Disc herniations in the low back occur when the inner material of a spinal disc (nucleus pulposus) pushes out through a tear in the wall of the disc (annulus fibrosus) and irritates nearby nerve roots. These injuries are most commonly observed in the last two segments of the low back (L4–5 and L5–S1) and can produce pain, numbness, and tingling that radiate into the leg (radiculopathy). However, disc herniations occur in a large chunk of the asymptomatic population, and having one does not necessarily mean you will have pain.[20,21] In fact, disc herniations are thought to account for only 1 to 3 percent of back pain cases.

Disc herniations most often occur when the low back is loaded in a flexed and rotated position, such as when bending over to pick up something heavy from the ground.

**SIGNS AND SYMPTOMS:** Disc herniations that produce pain typically do so in the low back and down the back of one leg, like sciatica. Leg symptoms usually travel into the buttock and hamstring region but can move into the calf, front of the shin, and foot. Pain can range from an ache in the back to sharp lightning-bolt pains, along with numbness, tingling, and weakness in the affected leg.

## DO DISC HERNIATIONS HEAL?

A common misconception is that herniations don't heal or reabsorb. In reality, research shows that around 66 percent do reabsorb and heal.[22] Even if the herniation isn't reabsorbed, pain typically goes away and function returns to normal. Again, having a disc herniation doesn't necessarily mean you will have pain or functional limitation. Many cases are asymptomatic.[20,21] That's why we think of disc herniations as a type of aging, such as when a disc gets flatter or has little bulges—it's almost like developing wrinkles as you grow older. It's simply part of how the disc changes over time and isn't something to worry about. This is why you shouldn't make diagnoses purely based on an MRI. You also need to assess your function and pain levels.

## DO HERNIATIONS GET WORSE WITH AGE?

Another misconception is that we become more susceptible to this kind of injury with age, but general back pain and disc herniation are reported more often in people aged 35 to 55 than in older people.[23] Back pain usually peaks around midlife and then drops. This may be due to activity levels; younger people tend to put more stress on their backs. But it nonetheless contradicts the idea that degeneration leads to pain. Older people have more degeneration but report less back pain. So, with age, degeneration goes up but pain goes down—an interesting but largely unknown fact.

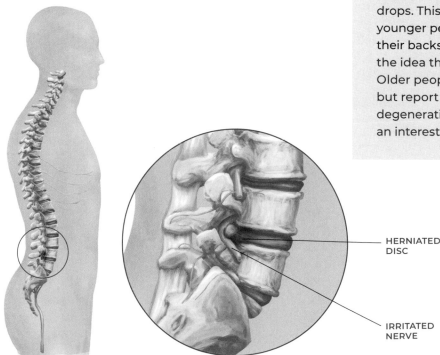

HERNIATED DISC

IRRITATED NERVE

## WHEN SHOULD I CONSIDER SURGERY?

If you've had pain for six months or longer, you are a candidate for surgery, especially if you've tried physical therapy and nothing has improved. If you have radiating nerve pain and are noticing a progressive loss of strength in your leg—as in, you can't do a calf raise, elevate your leg, or lift your leg outward—or you suddenly have a muscle that just isn't working, immediately consult with a doctor and consider surgical intervention.

I've worked with people who have permanent or partial nerve paralysis because they didn't address the problem in time. You really need to pay attention to your symptoms and whether they are getting better or worse.

**AGGRAVATING FACTORS:** In most cases, pain is triggered when the spine is flexed or rounded, such as when bending over to pick something up or sitting/driving, but it can also occur with prolonged standing.

**PROGNOSIS:** In most cases, pain resolves within several weeks to as long as three to four months if aggravating activities are modified.

**TREATMENT STRATEGY:** Anti-inflammatory medication, ice or heat on the low back, and traction units or inversion tables can ease pain.[19] But physical therapy is the best defense and the path to regain full function.[24] If your pain has not improved after three to four months or you have weakness in your leg muscles, see an orthopedic physician for possible injections or surgery, which can reduce inflammation and remove portions of the disc that are interfering with nerve function. Don't rush into surgery, but be mindful of nerve and muscle function and consult with a doctor or physical therapist if symptoms worsen over time.

The goal with the rehab exercises is to get out of pain and return to full function; the injury itself could be permanent and always show up on imaging. Focus on how you feel and move, and modify your behavior to accelerate healing.

Most symptomatic disc herniations cause sciatica, so you approach this injury in a similar fashion. Symptoms match the nerve that exits at the affected level of the spine. For instance, a herniation in the upper level of the lumbar spine (L1–3) tends to create pain on the front of the thigh, which means the phase 1 quadriceps mobilization and the phase 3 femoral nerve mobilization are likely to be most helpful. If the herniation is lower in the lumbar spine (L4, L5, S1), techniques that target the back of the thigh and glutes will be more effective. These include the glute, hamstring, and calf soft tissue mobilizations in phase 1 and the sciatic nerve mobilizations in phases 2 and 3.

With the flexion and extension mobility exercises in phase 2, one direction will typically be helpful, and the other won't help much or will make symptoms worse. Experiment with lumbar flexion and extension and eliminate a movement if it intensifies your nerve pain or causes it to travel farther down your leg.

# LUMBAR STENOSIS

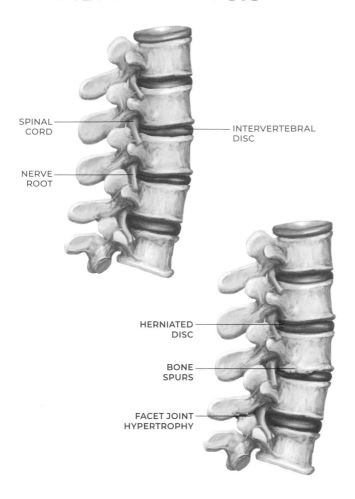

SPINAL CORD

INTERVERTEBRAL DISC

NERVE ROOT

HERNIATED DISC

BONE SPURS

FACET JOINT HYPERTROPHY

**DESCRIPTION:** Lumbar stenosis is a condition in which the pathway for the nerves in the low back narrows, leading to pain in the low back and legs.[25] Stenosis can occur anywhere in the spine but is most common in the low back. Anything that decreases space for the nerves, such as a herniated disc, arthritis in a facet joint, or a bone spur, can cause it. While it sounds scary, stenosis is common and generally not something to worry about unless you have neurological symptoms like numbness, tingling, or weakness. Most middle-aged people who get imaging have stenosis but not pain. Even if pain is present, people respond well to rehab and generally feel better after addressing aggravating factors and following an exercise program.

**SIGNS AND SYMPTOMS:** Pain and/or pressure in the low back and tingling and numbness that radiate into one or both legs. Weakness may also be present in the legs, and people may have difficulty walking longer distances.

Discomfort in the legs when walking is relieved by bending forward, which takes pressure off the low back nerves. With more severe nerve compromise, foot drop (weakness in the ankle muscles that causes the foot to slap down) can occur.

**AGGRAVATING FACTORS:** Extending or arching the low back (standing up straight, pushing the hips forward, being upright for too long, or walking) further narrows the nerve canal and increases pain and neurological symptoms.

**PROGNOSIS:** Most individuals can significantly reduce their symptoms within four to six weeks by modifying aggravating activities (reducing time standing and walking, maintaining a neutral spinal position) and implementing rehab exercises that target the hips and low back.

**TREATMENT STRATEGY:** Physical therapy that focuses on improving low back and hip mobility, strength, and endurance is the primary method of treatment. If symptoms are significant (radiating pain, leg weakness, foot drop, and so on), doctors may recommend surgery to remove any structures that are worsening the stenosis (such as bone spurs or disc bulges) and widen the neural canal.[26]

When progressing through the protocol, be careful with the lumbar extension mobility exercises, which tend to worsen stenosis-related nerve symptoms. Extending your low back closes the holes (intervertebral foramen) through which the nerve roots exit the spine, giving the nerves less room. This occurs naturally in a healthy spine, but structural changes related to stenosis allow even less space for the nerves, so extension can cause pain and other symptoms. To reduce pain, position your low back in flexion by bending forward slightly when performing exercises that involve an upright trunk position, such as the hip flexor stretch and lateral squat walk.

In addition to the low back extension exercise, be careful when mobilizing the nerves. While these techniques can reduce pain, you only want to stretch to the point where your symptoms begin. If you push too far, the nerve can flare up and increase pain for several days.

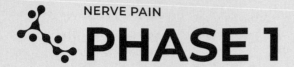

## NERVE PAIN
# PHASE 1

**GOOD FOR:**

- Alleviating nerve pain radiating down the low back, hip, and leg
- Relieving muscle tension
- Warm-up for phase 2 and 3 exercises

**GUIDELINES:**

- Perform every day
- Tools: foam roller, massage ball
- Add phase 2 when you have no pain at rest and no more than mild pain (3/10) with the exercises

## SOFT TISSUE MOBILIZATIONS:

- ▸ Spend 1–2 minutes on each area
- ▸ Perform in any order on both sides
- ▸ Stop on tender points for 10–20 seconds

### glute/piriformis mobilization

Sit on a foam roller and lean to one side, putting your weight over your glute muscles. Roll throughout the gluteal region: up, down, and side to side. To increase the pressure, stretch the muscles by crossing your leg over your opposite knee. For more precise pressure, use a large or small massage ball. Be cautious with this exercise and do not apply too much pressure if you have nerve pain that travels into the buttock and back of the leg.

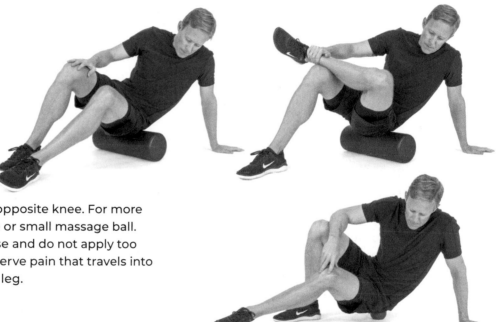

### quad mobilization

Lie on your stomach with your weight supported on your forearms or hands and one leg positioned over the roller with your toes pointed toward the floor. Supporting your weight with your grounded foot and arms, roll up and down to mobilize the quadriceps muscles on the front of your thigh—from hip to knee. Bend and straighten your knee to dynamically mobilize the muscles and femoral nerve.

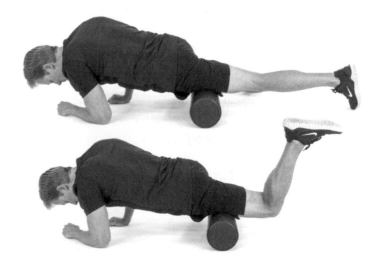

## lateral quad mobilization

The setup and execution are the same as in the quad mobilization: use your arms and grounded leg to control the pressure, roll up and down the entire thigh (from hip to knee), and stop on tender or stiff spots and bend and straighten your leg. But instead of mobilizing the front of your thigh, you target the lateral quadriceps along the outside of your leg.

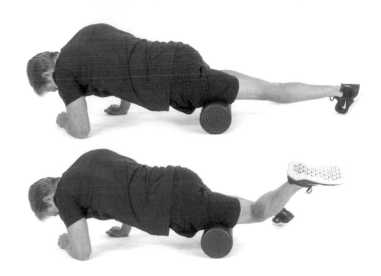

## calf mobilization

Sit on the floor with your calf positioned over the roller. Push off the floor with your hands and grounded foot—lifting your hips off the floor—to roll up and down your lower leg from ankle to knee.

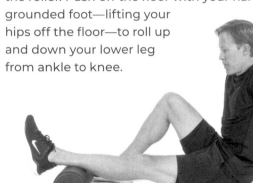

Stop on any tender or stiff spots and move your foot (flex, extend, and rotate from side to side).

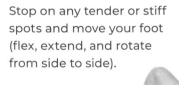

To increase the pressure, stack your other leg on top.

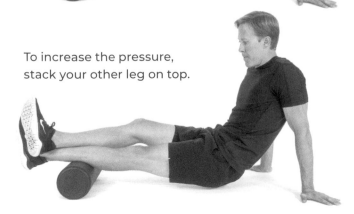

## hamstring mobilization

Sit on a bench or chair and place a large or small massage ball under your hamstring muscles. Roll up and down the entire length of your hamstring.

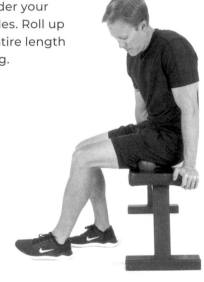

Flex and extend your knee to dynamically mobilize the muscles. Be cautious with this exercise and do not apply too much pressure if you have nerve pain that travels into the buttock and back of the leg.

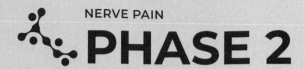

## NERVE PAIN
# PHASE 2

### GOOD FOR:

- Reducing nerve sensitivity
- Improving hip and lumbar flexion and extension range of motion
- Warm-up for phase 3 exercises

### GUIDELINES:

- Perform every day
- Tools: stretch strap, balance pad
- Add phase 3 when you can do the exercises with no more than mild pain (3/10)

## STRETCHING EXERCISES:

▸ Do 3 reps with 30- to 60-second holds

▸ Perform in any order on both sides

▸ Stop or back off the stretch if you feel tingling, numbness, or shooting pain

## knee to opposite shoulder

Lie on your back and bring one knee toward your chest. Interlock your fingers over your lower knee and upper shin. Keeping your low back flush with the floor, use your arms to pull your knee across your body toward your opposite shoulder.

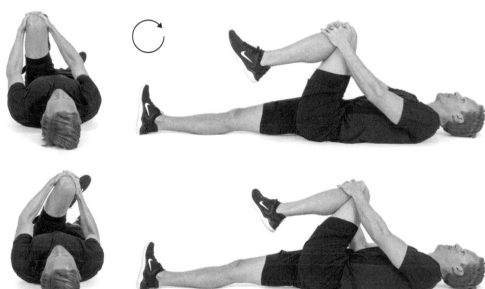

## hamstring stretch with strap

Hook a strap around your foot. Keeping your leg completely relaxed, use your arms to pull your foot toward your head and hold it in place once you feel a moderate stretch.

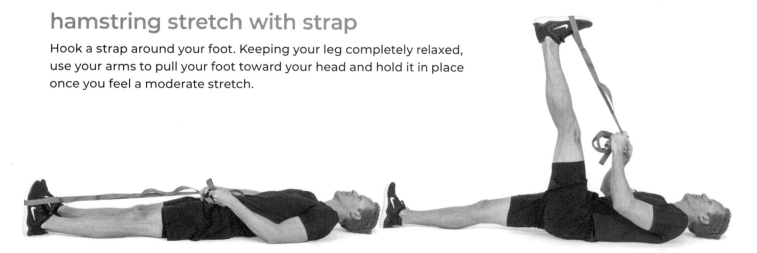

# hip flexor stretch

In a kneeling position, squeeze your abdominals and glutes to rotate your pelvis backward (posteriorly). Keeping your back neutral, shift your body forward slightly until you feel a stretch on the front of your hip and leg. To increase the intensity of the stretch, bend your knee and grab your ankle. You can also prop your foot on a bench or chair or position your shin flush against a wall. If you are kneeling on a hard surface, use a balance pad or cushion to protect your knee.

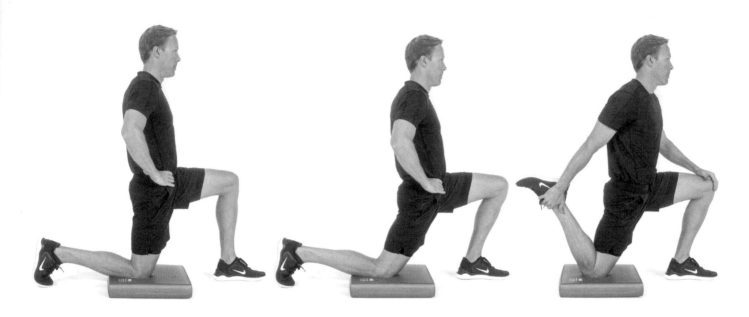

## MOBILITY EXERCISES:

- ▸ Do 3 sets of 10–15 reps
- ▸ Active range of motion (AROM)—move as far as you can without pain
- ▸ Pause at end range for 2–3 seconds

## lumbar flexion *(choose one)*

### knees to chest

Lie on your back and bring your knees to your chest. Cup your hands around your upper shins and use your arms to pull both knees closer to your chest, stretching your low back into flexion. Pause at end range—holding for a few seconds or longer—release the stretch, and then repeat.

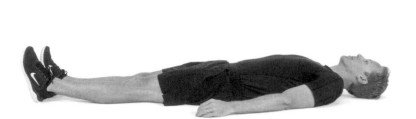
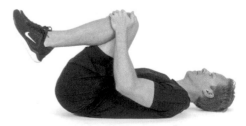

Be careful with or skip the lumbar flexion exercises if they make your back or nerve pain worse.

## chest to knees (child's pose)

Get into the quadruped position. Keeping your palms on the floor, drop your butt toward your heels and lower your head through your arms.

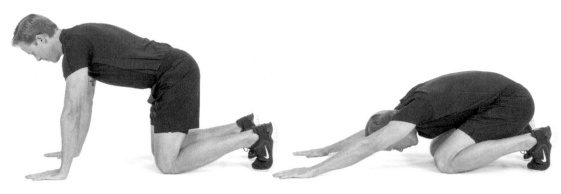

## lumbar extension

Lie on your stomach with your forearms positioned underneath your shoulders. Keeping your back relaxed and your hips on the floor, push through your forearms (or climb up to your hands) and arch your back as far as you can without pain. Pause at end range—holding for a few seconds or longer—then go back to the start position and repeat.

## sciatic nerve mobilization with strap

Lie on your back and hook a strap around your foot. Use your arms to lift your leg to the point where you feel tension or a stretch in the back of your leg. Alternate between pointing your foot and lifting your head (image 1) and flexing your foot toward your body (dorsiflexion) and laying your head back down (image 2).

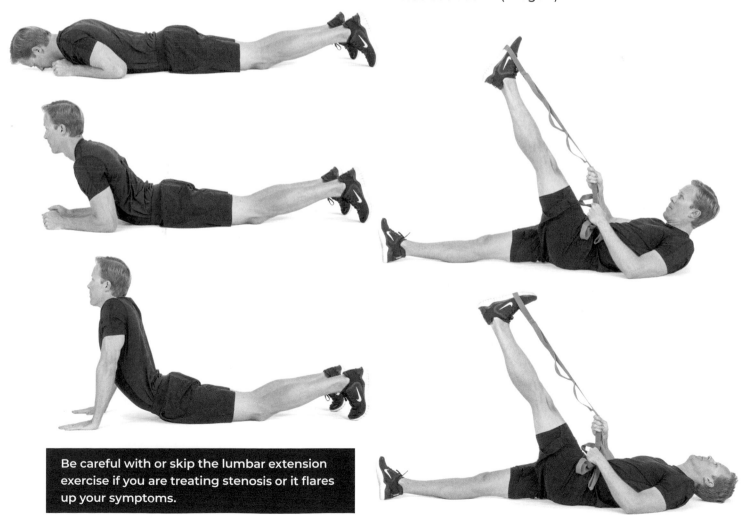

Be careful with or skip the lumbar extension exercise if you are treating stenosis or it flares up your symptoms.

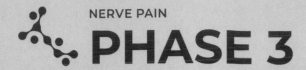

# PHASE 3

**GOOD FOR:**

- Reducing nerve sensitivity and preventing future flare-ups
- Improving glute and hip strength

**GUIDELINES:**

- Perform 3 or 4 days a week
- Tool: resistance loop
- Once nerve sensitivity calms down, add phase 3 exercises from the Low Back Pain protocol (pages 297–303)

## MOBILITY EXERCISES:

- ▸ Do 3 sets of 10–15 reps
- ▸ Active range of motion (AROM)—move as far as you can without pain
- ▸ Pause at end range for 2–3 seconds

## slump sciatic nerve mobilization

Sit on a stool or table so that your feet are off the floor. Slouch your shoulders and round your back. Slowly straighten one knee until you feel tension or a stretch in the back of your leg. Alternate between pointing your foot and looking down and lifting your foot and extending your neck (looking forward).

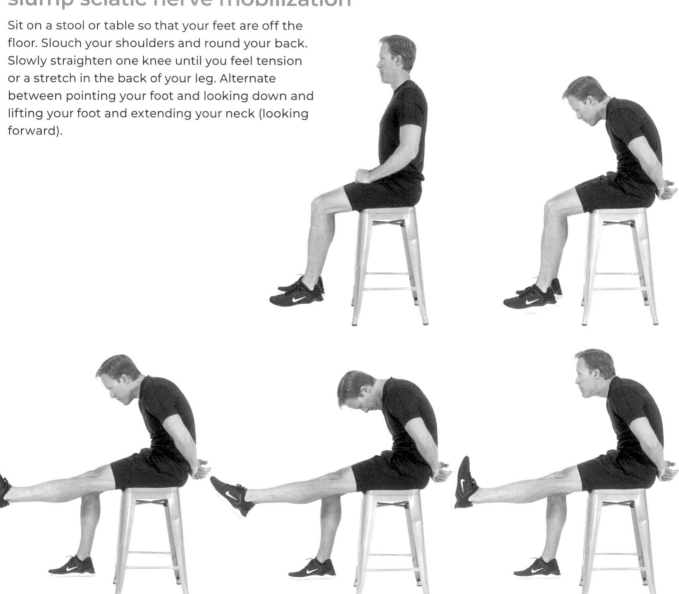

## femoral nerve mobilization

While standing, bend your knee and grip the outside of your ankle. Alternate between bringing your knee forward and your head down and pulling your leg back and lifting your head up.

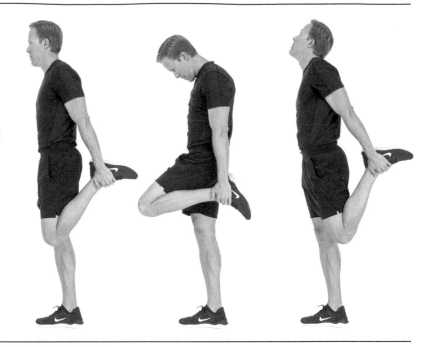

## RESISTANCE EXERCISES:

- ▸ Do 3 sets of 10–15 reps
- ▸ Push sets to fatigue
- ▸ Add load or reps to make the exercises more challenging

## bridge

Lie on your back with your knees bent and feet flat on the floor. Push into the floor and lift your butt, fully extending your hips—a straight line runs from your shoulders to your knees. Squeeze your glutes as you reach full hip extension and pause in the top position for 1–2 seconds.

## side-lying hip abduction

Lie on your side, rotate your hips toward the floor slightly, and internally rotate your top leg so that your big toe is angled toward the arch of your bottom foot. Lift your top leg up and at a backward angle. Reduce the range of motion if you start to arch your back excessively. Add a resistance loop above your knees to make the exercise more challenging.

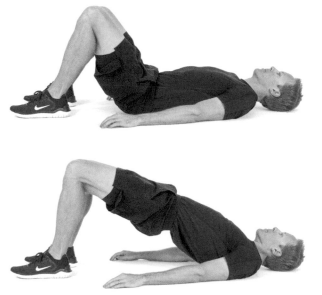

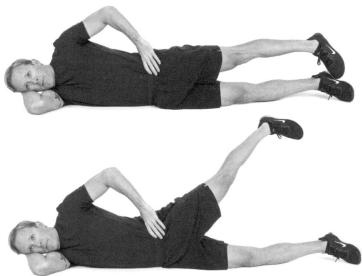

# lateral squat walk

Wrap a resistance loop above your knees. Position your feet shoulder width apart and bend your hips and knees slightly. Take a wide lateral step so there is a full stretch in the band. You can either walk along a line and then switch after a given number of steps or stay in one area by switching back and forth between legs. Choose a distance or rep range that is challenging—you feel your upper glutes burn—usually 15–20 steps in each direction. Don't pause between steps, and keep tension in the band during the entire movement.

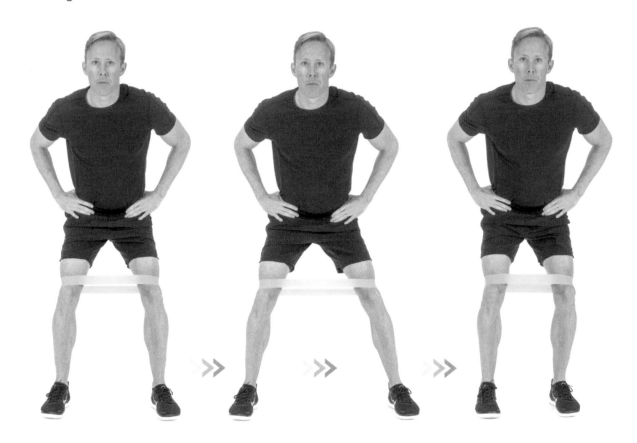

# clamshell

With the resistance loop above your knees, lie on your side with your hips bent to about 45 degrees, knees bent to about 90 degrees, and feet and legs stacked. Lift your top knee as far as you can without rotating your spine.

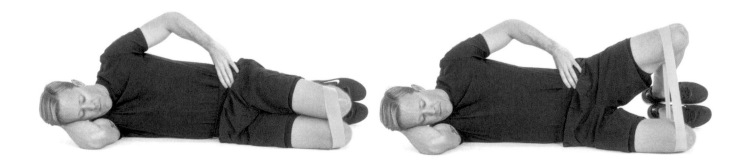

# MID-BACK AND RIB CAGE PAIN

**Follow this program to treat:**

- Pain and stiffness in the upper or mid-back
- Thoracic disc bulge
- Rib pain and injuries—sprain, fracture, or subluxation (dislocation)

## THORACIC DISC BULGE

**DESCRIPTION:** The thoracic spine is made up of 12 vertebrae (T1–T12) and naturally assumes a slightly rounded or kyphotic curve. Because the thoracic spine also has connections to the ribs, it is naturally more stable and less mobile than the lumbar and cervical spinal regions. This natural increase in stability means that issues like disc bulges and herniations are less common in this spinal region. Furthermore, many degenerative changes associated with the thoracic discs do not produce pain and occur unnoticed.[27] For example, a lot of people have degenerative thoracic disc bulges that show up on MRIs but cause no pain. So, the condition itself is not terribly uncommon; what's uncommon is a disc bulge that is symptomatic.

An injury to a spinal disc in this region that produces pain is usually the result of a trauma like a car crash or sudden force on the thoracic spine. Maybe you're bending over and rounded between your shoulder blades and ribs and then lift something heavy. Or maybe you cough or sneeze in a way that puts pressure on your thoracic cage. Injury could also occur when there is a heavy asymmetric load on the shoulders—a firefighter carrying a heavy ladder, for example.

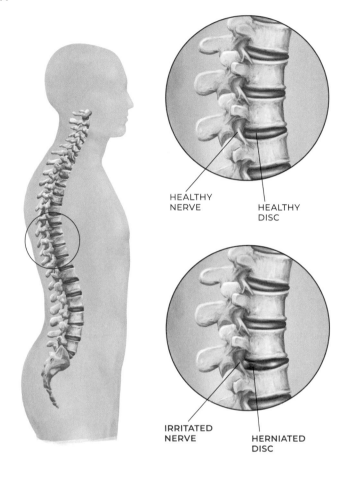

HEALTHY NERVE

HEALTHY DISC

IRRITATED NERVE

HERNIATED DISC

**SIGNS AND SYMPTOMS:** The most common symptom is sharp pain in the upper or mid-back, depending on which level of the spine is involved. If a nearby nerve root is also affected, pain may radiate around the side of the trunk in line with a rib. The thoracic spine is unique because the nerves don't go into the arms or legs; they only wrap around the ribs. As a result, pain is mainly isolated to the mid-back.

**AGGRAVATING FACTORS:** Activities that move the thoracic spine suddenly, such as sneezing or coughing, can exacerbate pain. Bending to lift something or rotating to look over one shoulder might also hurt.

**PROGNOSIS:** In most cases, this issue resolves with rest, general movement, and conservative care (physical therapy) directed at improving thoracic spine mobility. In rare instances where pain does not dissipate after six to eight weeks of rehab or the disc injury interferes with the spinal cord, decompression surgery may relieve pain and restore nerve health.

**TREATMENT STRATEGY:** If you have pain associated with a thoracic disc irritation, start with the mobilization, stretching, and mobility exercises in phases 1 and 2, which often reduce this type of pain. These exercises target either the thoracic spinal joints or the surrounding soft tissue structures that connect the thoracic spine and ribs to the shoulder complex. The rhomboid and pectoral mobilizations loosen up the major muscles that attach to the thoracic region, and then the thoracic extension mobilization and mobility exercises at the end of phase 1 improve joint and soft tissue mobility.

The thoracic rotation and extension stretches in phase 2 improve thoracic mobility and reduce mid-back–related pain. Stretching the pectoral muscles helps with pulling the shoulder blades back so that the shoulders are less rounded, which takes stress off the mid-back muscles. Once your pain has decreased, the resistance exercises at the end of phase 2 and in phase 3 can boost strength and control in the muscles on the anterior and posterior aspects of the thoracic cage. These exercises include pulling and pushing variations and are designed to not only reduce sensitivity and pain but also make your rib cage more resistant to injury.

# RIB INJURIES

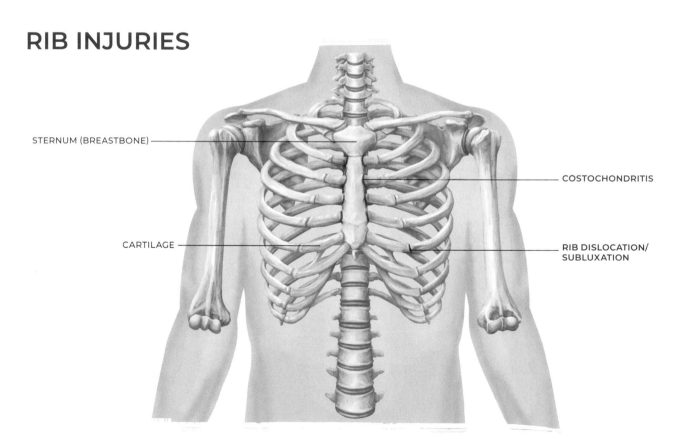

STERNUM (BREASTBONE)

CARTILAGE

COSTOCHONDRITIS

RIB DISLOCATION/ SUBLUXATION

**DESCRIPTION:** There are 12 sets of ribs in the human body, one for each of the 12 levels of the thoracic spine, and they are categorized based on how they attach. The first seven pairs, or "true" ribs, attach directly to the sternum (breastbone). The next three pairs are called "false" ribs because they do not attach directly to the sternum, but rather to the seventh rib via cartilage. Ribs 11 and 12 float and do not attach to the sternum. All ribs also attach to the spine via the costotransverse and costovertebral joints.

The types of rib injuries range from generalized pain and mild sprains to severe sprains (subluxation and dislocations), slipped rib syndrome, costochondritis, and fractures.

General rib pain does not involve trauma; a person reports pain after twisting to reach something or pick something up. This pain is usually associated with spasming of the surrounding muscles and not damage to the rib joints.

If the chest wall sustains a severe blunt-force trauma (such as the chest hitting the steering wheel in a car accident) or a severe sport-related insult, the rib joints can be severely stretched (sprains), torn (subluxation and dislocations), or fractured.[28]

Slipped rib syndrome, which is characterized when a rib "pops out," is common in sports like jiu-jitsu that involve rotating against a resisting opponent.[29] It feels like the rib tears away from the cartilage.

Another source of rib pain is costochondritis, which is a common diagnosis for pain along the sternum.[30] Most people who get this have sustained trauma to the rib cage—almost like a rib sprain—which causes inflammation that spreads and covers the entire sternum region.

While these conditions can vary when it comes to the mechanism of injury and pain symptoms, the treatment strategy and rehab exercises are similar to what's outlined below.

**SIGNS AND SYMPTOMS:** On the back side of the body, the costovertebral and costotransverse rib joints are often thought to be associated with sharp, nagging pain in the interscapular region, which is the zone between the spine and shoulder blade. On the front side, rib pain can be sharp with breathing, coughing, and sneezing and is typically experienced along the edge of the breastbone where the ribs attach. Again, rib pain and irritation along the sternum are often called costochondritis.

**AGGRAVATING FACTORS:** Most rib pain is exacerbated with movement of the rib cage, such as turning to look over one shoulder. Pain is also typically experienced when you apply pressure to the injured rib, chest, or back or use the muscles that attach to the rib.

**PROGNOSIS:** Most rib injuries, especially traumatic ones, require a fair bit of time to heal. Fractures typically take six to 12 weeks. The healing time for sprains depends on the severity but typically takes three to six weeks.

**TREATMENT STRATEGY:** Most rib injuries are treated by eliminating or modifying activities that would delay healing and implementing techniques that reduce muscle spasms and improve the mobility of the rib cage and thoracic spine.

**1** The soft tissue mobilizations in phase 1 reduce pain and tension in the pectoral, rhomboid, and portions of the trapezius muscles. Loosening these muscles can help you regain mobility when you move on to exercises like the thoracic extension mobilization. Because the thoracic spine naturally assumes a flexed (kyphotic) position, this mobilization can stretch you out of flexion and often reduces rib- and thoracic-related discomfort. The mobility exercises involve moving the thoracic spine and ribs through flexion and extension and the shoulders and shoulder blades through their movements (angel and scapular protraction and retraction mobility). These exercises are good for early rehab because they create relatively low stress while moving your rib and thoracic joints.

**2** **3** In phase 2, you implement more challenging stretches for the thoracic spine and rib cage (thoracic rotation and thoracic extension stretch). Don't push too hard if you've suffered a severe rib injury. Depending on the severity of the injury, you may need to spend more time in phase 1 or skip the more challenging stretches in phase 2 and add them to phase 3 once you can perform the other exercises with no more than mild discomfort. The resistance exercises at the end of phase 2 and in phase 3 are designed to make your thoracic spine and rib cage more resistant to injury. These exercises target muscles on the front and back of the rib cage and provide strength and stability to the entire region.

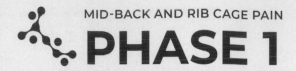

# PHASE 1

## GOOD FOR:

- Alleviating upper back pain
- Reducing muscle stiffness
- Improving range of motion
- Warm-up for phase 2 and 3 exercises

## GUIDELINES:

- Perform every day
- Tools: small massage ball, foam roller, peanut tool
- Add phase 2 when you have no pain at rest and no more than mild pain (3/10) with the exercises

## SOFT TISSUE MOBILIZATIONS:

- ▸ Spend 1–2 minutes on each area
- ▸ Perform in any order on both sides
- ▸ Stop on tender points for 10–20 seconds

---

## rhomboid mobilization

Place a small massage ball between your shoulder blade and spine. Work the entire area around the shoulder blade (rhomboids). Add arm movements and lift your head to further mobilize the muscles.

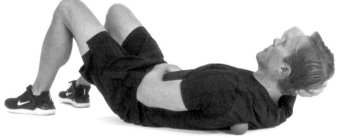

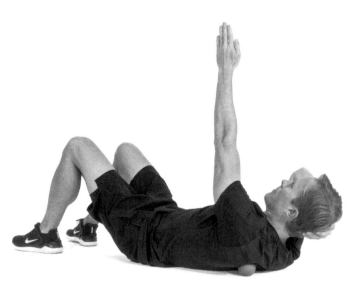

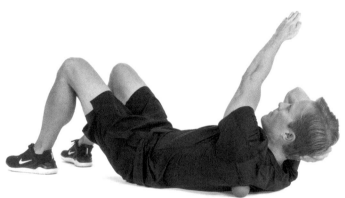

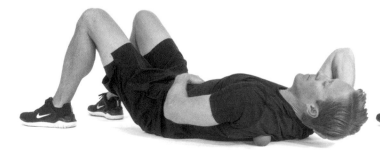

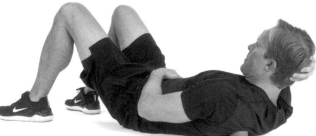

## pectoral mobilization

Position the ball between a doorframe or rack and your pectoral muscles near the front of your shoulder. Place your arm behind your back and add dynamic movement by reaching overhead to further mobilize the muscles.

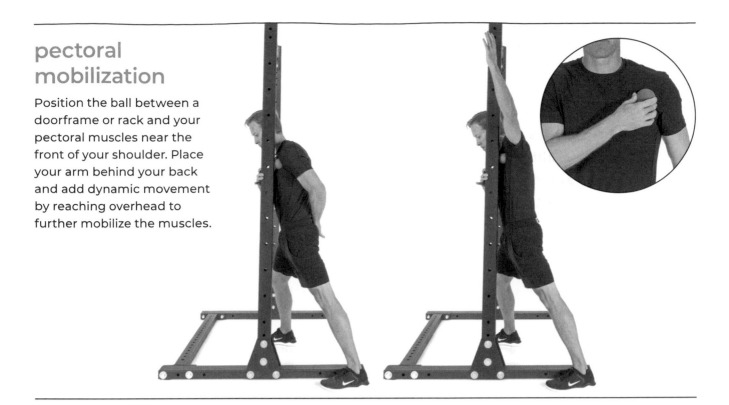

## thoracic extension *(choose one)*

### with foam roller

Position a foam roller perpendicular to your spine under your upper back. Keeping your butt on the floor, extend over the roller by slowly lowering your head toward the floor. You can hold this position or flex and extend (abdominal crunch) over the roller. You can also elevate your butt and roll up and down your upper back to massage the area (not the low back or neck).

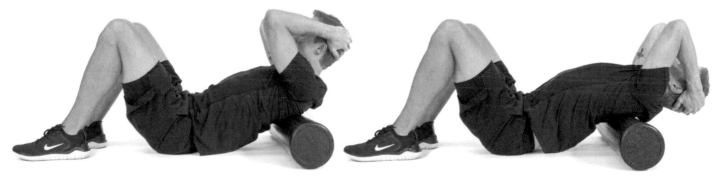

### with peanut tool

Position your upper back over a peanut tool. You can roll slowly from the base of your rib cage to your neck or flex and extend over the tool, stopping on each spinal segment.

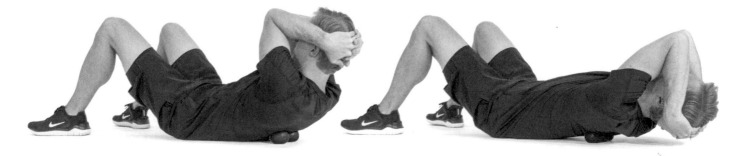

# MOBILITY EXERCISES:

▸ Do 3 sets of 10–15 reps

▸ Active range of motion (AROM)—move as far as you can without pain

▸ Pause at end range for 2–3 seconds

## thoracic flexion and extension

Get into the quadruped position—knees aligned under hips and shoulders over wrists. Flex (round) your mid-back and neck, then extend. Try to isolate your mid-back and limit movement through your low back.

## angel

Position your spine over the roller so that your head and tailbone are supported. Start with your arms at your sides and palms up. Reach overhead as far as you can without pain.

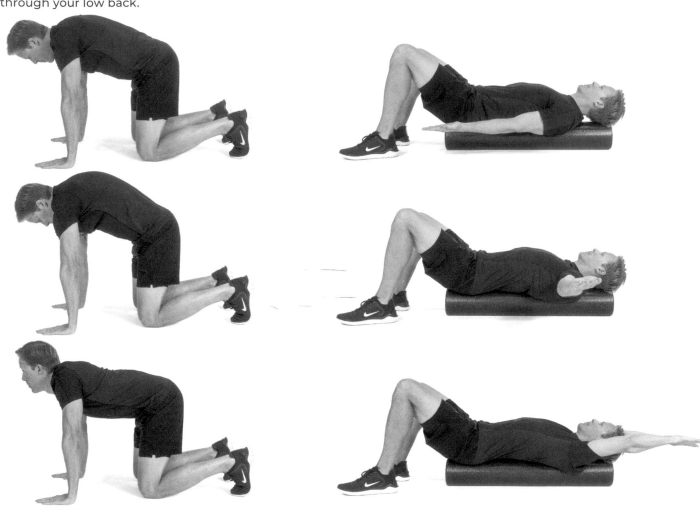

## shoulder protraction and retraction

With your posture upright and spine neutral, protract your shoulders by pushing them forward, then retract by pulling them back—squeezing your shoulder blades together and tucking your chin slightly at end range.

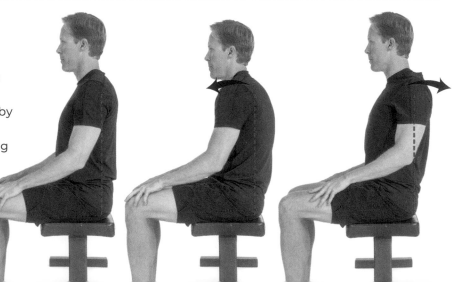

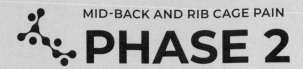

MID-BACK AND RIB CAGE PAIN

# PHASE 2

## GOOD FOR:

- Improving thoracic and rib mobility
- Early back and pec strengthening
- Warm-up for phase 3 exercises

## GUIDELINES:

- Perform every day
- Tools: dowel, resistance tube band
- Add phase 3 when you can do the exercises with no more than mild pain (3/10)

## STRETCHING EXERCISES:

- ▸ Do 3 reps with 30- to 60-second holds
- ▸ Perform in any order on both sides
- ▸ Don't stretch into pain

## thoracic rotation stretch

Lie on your side and bend your hips to about 90 degrees. Grip the outside of your top knee with your bottom arm. Keeping your top arm straight, lower it toward the ground and rotate away from your knees as far as you can without pain. As you do, pull down on your knees and try to get both shoulders flush with the ground.

## pectoral stretch

Position your forearm against a doorframe or rack with your shoulder at about 90 degrees. Step forward until you feel a stretch in your chest region. Move your arm slightly higher to stretch the upper fibers of your pectoral muscles.

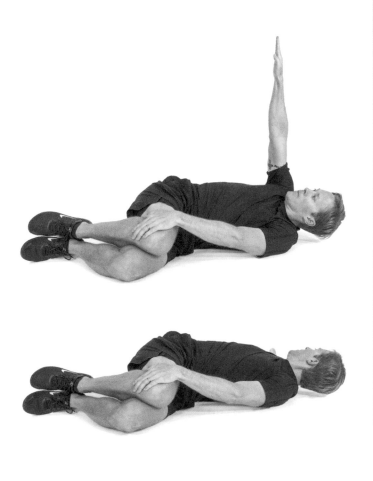

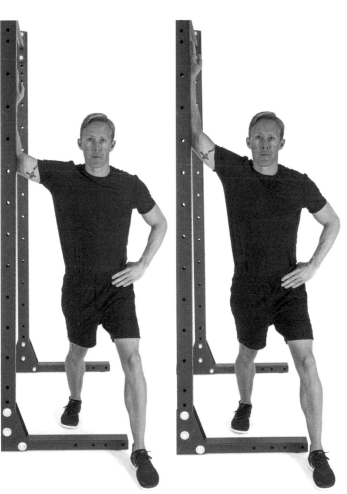

# lat/thoracic extension stretch with dowel

In a kneeling position, hold a dowel with your palms facing up and place your elbows on a bench. Sit your hips back toward your heels and lower your head through your arms to create a stretch through your lats and triceps. Hold for 20 to 30 seconds. This stretch also works thoracic extension mobility..

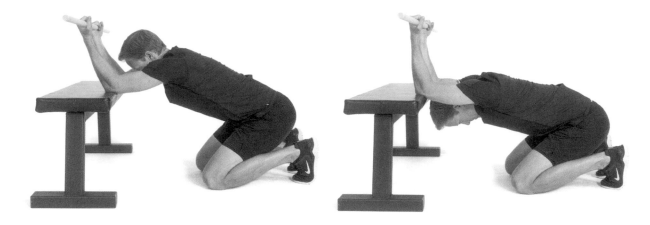

# RESISTANCE EXERCISES:

- ▸ Do 3 sets of 10–15 reps
- ▸ Push sets to fatigue
- ▸ Add load or reps to make the exercises more challenging

# banded row

Anchor a resistance band at chest height. Put tension in the band, lower into a quarter squat, and extend your arms in front of you. Keeping your thumbs facing upward, pull the handles toward your armpits. Keep your shoulders square and don't lean back as you pull. You can perform the dumbbell, inverted, or machine row variation in place of this exercise.

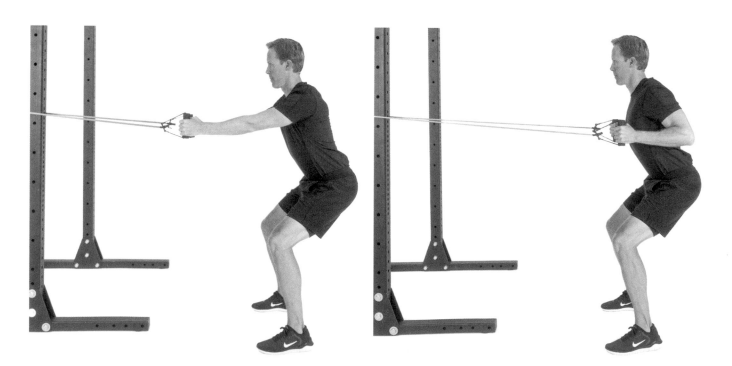

## press with protraction *(choose one)*

### push-up plus

Get into the plank position: hands shoulder width apart, shoulders aligned over your wrists, and back flat. Perform a standard push-up by lowering your chest to the floor. Keep your elbows in (about 45 degrees from your body), forearms vertical, and back flat as you lower into the bottom position. As you reverse the movement and reach the start position with your elbows extended, protract your shoulder blades by pushing your shoulders toward the floor. This should raise your body a few inches higher.

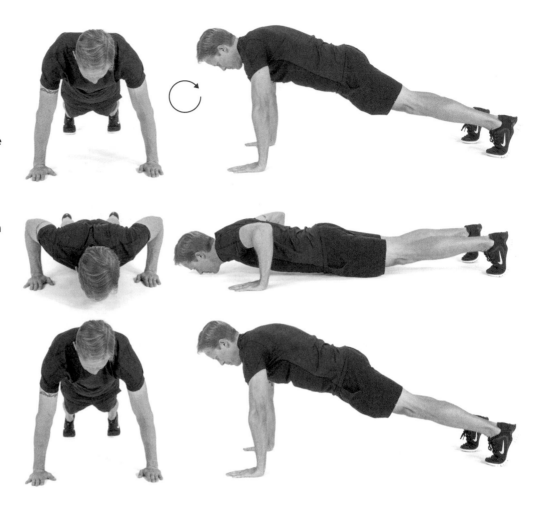

### banded press with protraction

Anchor the band to about chest height. Press your arms straight out. As you extend your elbows, rotate your palms toward the floor and protract your shoulders (push your shoulder blades forward).

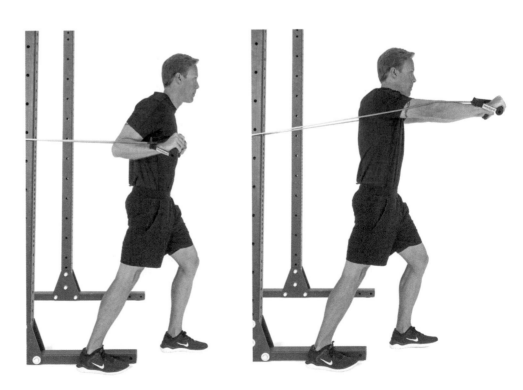

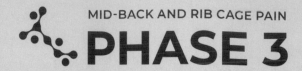

# PHASE 3

## GOOD FOR:

- Strengthening the upper back and abdominal muscles
- Preventing upper back and rib injuries

## GUIDELINES:

- Perform 3 or 4 days a week
- Do 3 sets of 10–15 reps
- Push sets to fatigue
- Add load or reps to increase difficulty
- Tools: bench, resistance tube band

## prone T

Lie facedown on a bench with your arms hanging down, wrists positioned just behind your shoulders, and palms facing forward. Lift your arms out to the sides and make a "T" shape. Lead with your thumbs and keep your elbows straight. Squeeze your shoulder blades together at the top of the motion.

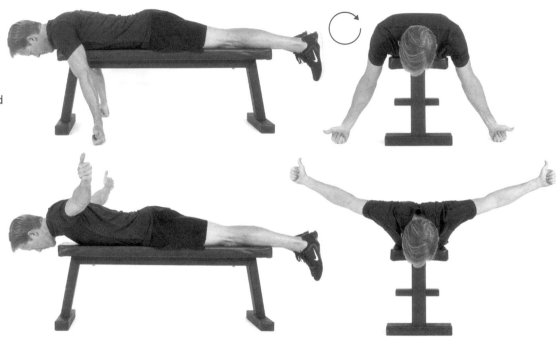

## pallof press

Anchor a band to about hip level and step away to create tension in the band. Get into a kneeling position and grip the handle with both hands positioned at the center of your chest. Keeping your core tight, press the band straight out. The goal is to prevent the band from rotating your spine by contracting your abdominal and back muscles.

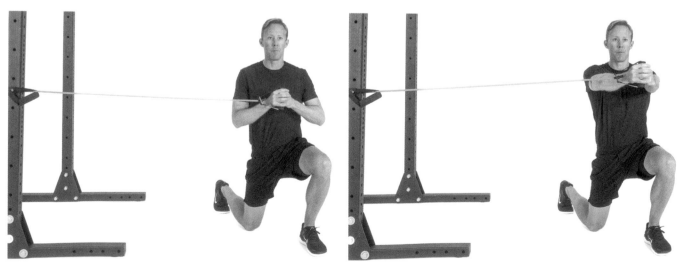

## prone reach

Lie on your stomach with your hands by your head (palms down) and elbows tight to your body. Lift your arms and squeeze your shoulder blades together, keeping your forearms parallel to the floor. Maintaining thoracic extension, straighten your elbows and reach your arms overhead. Keep your neck neutral (don't look up) throughout the entire range of motion. Reverse the sequence: pull your elbows back, squeeze your shoulder blades together while maintaining thoracic extension, and then lower your arms to the floor. That counts as one rep.

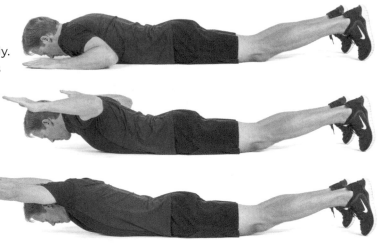

## skydiver

With your arms at your sides, use your low back extensors to lift your lower and upper body segments off the floor. As you arch, squeeze your glutes and pull your shoulders back while maintaining a neutral neck position.

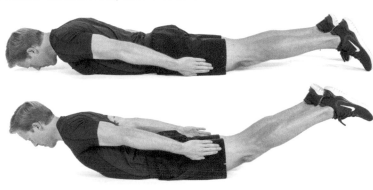

## plank crawl

Lie on your side, position your elbow underneath your shoulder, stack your feet, and use your trunk muscles to lift your hips. Keeping your core tight and your back as flat as possible, roll toward your stomach, placing your elbow on the floor below your opposite hand. Shift your weight onto your other arm and get into a side plank—start position on the opposite side.

## CHAPTER 20

# HIP
# PROTOCOLS

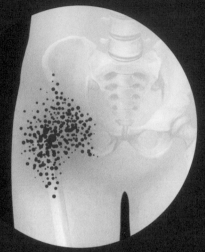

**HIP PAIN**
(p. 329)

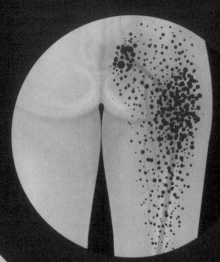

**NERVE PAIN**
(p. 344)

**HIP FLEXOR PAIN**
(p. 354)

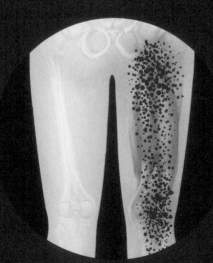

**HAMSTRING PAIN**
(p. 362)

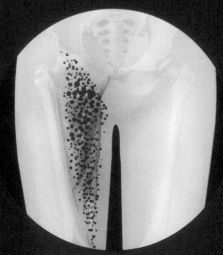

**GROIN STRAIN**
(p. 373)

# HIP PAIN

**Follow this program to treat:**

- General hip joint pain
- Hip impingement (pain on the inside of the hip and groin when squatting or sitting)
- Labral tear (sharp pain in the groin or front of the hip)
- Osteoarthritis (hip arthritis)
- Gluteal tendinopathy (pain in the gluteal region or lateral hip)

## HIP IMPINGEMENT

**DESCRIPTION:** Femoroacetabular impingement, or FAI, describes a condition in which premature contact between the ball of the femur and the roof of the acetabulum (hip socket) occurs.[1] Hip impingement is divided into two categories based on how the bones are affected:

- Cam deformities refers to changes in the shape of the femoral head neck junction.
- Pincer deformities are bony overgrowths on the acetabular rim that cover aspects of the femoral head.

In either case, hip impingement tends to create pain on the front or inside of the groin or hip when the hip is in an end-range flexion position. For example, you feel pain at the bottom of a squat. Some patients also report clicking, locking, catching, stiffness, or feeling like their hip might give way.

With a true hip impingement, the bone is shaped differently. You have a little bump on your femur, in the socket, or both, and those bumps are hitting each other. These bony growths form over time due to stress on the tissue. Stressed tissue—even bone—will adapt and hypertrophy. You may have anteversion or retroversion, where your sockets are shaped differently and moving makes the bones touch, causing them to hypertrophy. Another theory is that these conditions can be present at birth but not discovered until later in life when they start producing pain. It's difficult to determine because people typically aren't studied until they have symptoms. But most professionals believe that bones contacting each other causes hypertrophy, which can create friction within the joint or even rub the labrum and cause a labral tear.

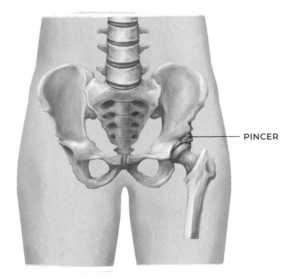

PINCER

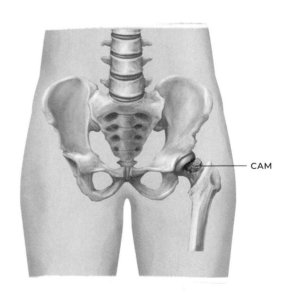

CAM

**SIGNS AND SYMPTOMS:** FAI tends to create pain in the groin region but can create pain on the outside of the hip, too. Patients also report hip stiffness and limping. Pain is typically sharp when the hip is forced into deep flexion (squatting) and/or end-range adduction or internal rotation. The hallmark symptom is that you feel a pinch in the front of your hip and groin when you are in deep hip flexion.

**AGGRAVATING FACTORS:** Activities that move the joint into end-range flexion and internal rotation positions, such as squatting, lunging, and twisting or turning the leg inward, trigger FAI. It is often provoked by sitting in low chairs or in deep hip flexion for long periods.

**PROGNOSIS:** Many cases of FAI can be managed with behavior modification, such as changing your squat and deadlift stance and depth and avoiding prolonged sitting and low chairs, along with rehab exercises designed to strengthen the hip muscles in all planes of motion.

**TREATMENT STRATEGY:** FAI is treated with physical therapy and anti-inflammatory medication first.[2,3] If conservative treatment is unsuccessful, arthroscopic surgery can correct bony deformities or a torn labrum.[4] Because FAI is rooted in anatomy, physical therapy is helpful for modifying behavior, especially for weightlifting form (e.g., foot position, stance width, and range of motion). People with long-standing pain often experience multiplanar hip weakness, probably because they've been avoiding certain positions or movements, so physical therapy also focuses on strengthening the hip in a multiplanar fashion.

Whether you have a true hip impingement, a bony overgrowth, a labral tear, or some other condition, pushing into the pain will flare it up, so it's better to modify movements to accommodate anatomical variations. For example, when doing squats or deadlifts, rotate one foot a little or adopt a wider stance. The key is to experiment and individualize your stance to what feels best for your hips.

Do not push too hard when performing the stretching and mobility exercises in this protocol, especially the knee to opposite shoulder stretch and the hip flexion mobility movements. Pushing into a position of impingement typically causes more pain. Phases 2 and 3 focus on multiplanar hip and core strengthening, which is the most important part of rehabilitating this condition. For exercises that take you into hip flexion (the banded squat, split squat, hip flexor march, and hip thrust), go only as deep as you can without pain. Like the mobility exercises, if you push to the point of pain, you are likely to aggravate your hip joint.

## HOW DO I DETERMINE IF I HAVE A TRUE HIP IMPINGEMENT?

Bony growths are easy to miss, especially in people who are new to weightlifting. But if you feel a pinch in deep hip flexion positions, there may be something unusual about your hip anatomy. It doesn't necessarily mean you have an impingement with bony buildup on either side, because labral tears and some soft tissue irritations also can create that symptom.

What's more, a lot of people have a socket that is oriented differently. If you feel a pinch in deep hip flexion, even when your hip is neutral, there's probably something atypical about your anatomy. You don't want to push into it because doing so might cause a flare-up and make your pain worse. Instead, you may need to adjust your stance, experiment with different ranges of motion, or switch exercise variations to see if the issue is mechanical. If you still feel pain, then you might have a bony buildup, and you should consult with a doctor.

For an accurate diagnosis, an X-ray is typically required; that way, the doctor can see the bony changes and shave them off in surgery if you don't improve with rehab. Remember, if it's the hip flexor, it'll tend to hurt with an active contraction. With a labrum injury or hip impingement, you will have pain at end-range positions of the hip joint, especially those that combine flexion, adduction, and internal rotation.

# LABRAL TEAR

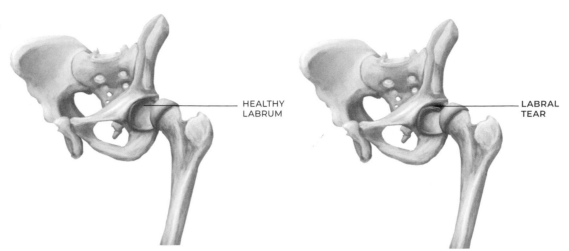

HEALTHY LABRUM

LABRAL TEAR

**DESCRIPTION:** The labrum of the hip is a fibrocartilaginous structure that forms a rim along the periphery of the joint socket and is designed to improve joint congruency and stability. Athletes who participate in dance, martial arts, hockey, golf, and other activities that take the hips into end-range positions are more likely to experience tears. It's not one movement at end range but rather the way the hips are stressed frequently (overuse or repetitive stress) or suddenly (a traumatic injury like a fall or blunt force).

Although labral tears can happen in the shoulder or hip, the hip experiences less instability because it has a deep socket. It's usually just pain in the groin or front hip area. Identifying a labral tear is tricky because hip pains can mimic one another. If your doctor suspects a tear, the issue is usually best diagnosed using an MRI with contrast.

However, you have to think of imaging as just one piece of the pain puzzle, and do not assume that the presence of a labral tear on an MRI is the cause of your pain. Research has shown that up to 54 percent of asymptomatic (pain-free) people have labral tears.[5]

**SIGNS AND SYMPTOMS:** Labral injuries typically produce sharp pain in the anterior (front) hip and groin regions that is provoked by moving the hip into a combination of flexion (knee to chest), adduction (moving the leg toward your midline), and internal rotation.

**AGGRAVATING FACTORS:** Prolonged sitting, stretches that place the hip in deep flexion, and exercises like squats and lunges that require the hip to move into end-range flexion.

**PROGNOSIS:** Many labral tears significantly improve within six to eight weeks when aggravating activities are modified and rehab exercises that strengthen the hip muscles in all planes of motion are implemented.

**TREATMENT STRATEGY:** Ease pain by resting and modifying movements that require deep hip flexion, such as adopting a wider, externally rotated stance for squats and deadlifts. Anti-inflammatory medication may be helpful in the acute pain phase. Labral tears are treated with rehab exercises that improve hip strength and stability. If your pain persists after you complete the exercise protocol, not counting any flare-ups, you may need arthroscopic surgery to repair the tear or remove a portion of your labrum.

Because hip impingements and labral tears produce similar symptoms and limitations, you approach the protocol in a similar way. While working through it, do not push into positions that cause your familiar hip pain. This usually comes up with deep hip flexion, so be careful with the knee to opposite shoulder stretch and the hip flexion mobility exercises in phase 1. The mobility exercises address commonly limited movements (flexion, internal and external rotation, and abduction) and include stretches targeting muscles that often tighten with joint mobility impairments. Phases 2 and 3 focus on multiplanar hip and core strengthening, which is important for rehabilitating a labral tear. However, for the exercises that require hip flexion (banded squat, split squat, hip flexor march, and hip thrust), go only as deep as you can without pain. Pushing deeper doesn't help and often makes pain worse.

# OSTEOARTHRITIS

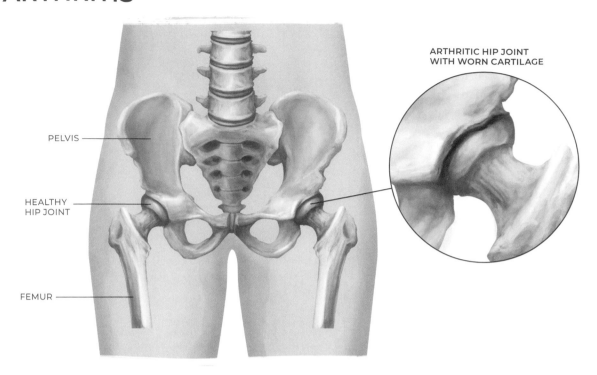

ARTHRITIC HIP JOINT
WITH WORN CARTILAGE

PELVIS

HEALTHY
HIP JOINT

FEMUR

**DESCRIPTION:** Osteoarthritis (OA) is the most common cause of hip pain in adults over 50.[6,7] The condition affects the structure (breakdown of cartilage) and function of the hip joint and is usually associated with mobility and strength deficits. OA is often associated with a loss of the cartilage that normally creates a small space between the ball and socket, changes in the underlying bone, and inflammation.[8] Physical therapy can alleviate pain and build hip strength, but it won't fix the cartilage. If the pain becomes severe enough to limit your functional activities, your doctor may recommend a hip replacement.

OA usually results from either an injury to the joint or factors that impair the joint's ability to heal.[6] If you are sedentary and/or overweight or you're repeatedly stressing the tissue beyond its capacity, your cartilage may become injured or may be unable to repair itself effectively.

What's more, arthritis is inflammatory, and so many things in life, from nutrition to sleep hygiene to stress levels, can affect inflammation.[6,7] It is important to review the factors that influence pain in Chapter 4 and manage the variables that are within your control to prevent and alleviate pain and optimize your physical health.

**SIGNS AND SYMPTOMS:** Like most hip issues, OA hurts mainly in the groin, although it also can hurt on the side of the hip. Individuals with hip OA typically experience morning joint stiffness that improves within an hour of awakening and limited mobility in at least two of the six hip movements (flexion, extension, abduction, adduction, internal rotation, and external rotation).

**AGGRAVATING FACTORS:** Pain typically occurs during weight-bearing tasks such as walking, stair climbing, squatting, twisting, and deep bending of the hip.

**PROGNOSIS:** While physical therapy cannot correct osteoarthritis, doing the rehab exercises can help slow its development by strengthening the surrounding muscles.

**TREATMENT STRATEGY:** Hip OA is primarily treated with physical therapy and exercise.[9-11] If the pain becomes severe and significantly compromises function (i.e., you can no longer participate in recreational activities or normal daily tasks), a total hip replacement is usually recommended.

OA typically limits joint mobility, so phase 1 of the protocol includes stretches for muscles that tend to tighten with joint range of motion impairments. Do not push into pain when performing the mobility exercises. Doing so would provide little benefit and can make your pain worse. Phases 2 and 3 focus on resistance training to improve hip strength. Research recommends resistance training for individuals with arthritis because it can improve function with daily tasks. Like the mobility exercises, if you feel joint pain, stop or modify the movement. It's OK to perform partial range of motion with these exercises. For instance, when you do exercises that require more hip range of motion (banded squat, split squat, hip flexor march, and hip thrust), you may reach a point where you feel pain. Going deeper wouldn't be helpful because it could flare up your pain and force you to take a few days off from exercise.

# GLUTEAL TENDINOPATHY AND TROCHANTERIC BURSITIS

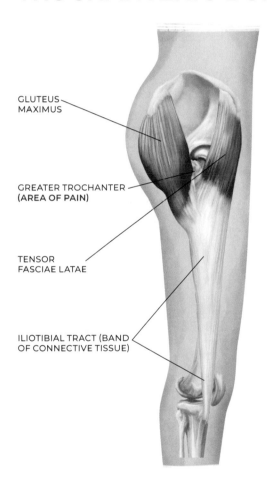

GLUTEUS MAXIMUS

GREATER TROCHANTER (AREA OF PAIN)

TENSOR FASCIAE LATAE

ILIOTIBIAL TRACT (BAND OF CONNECTIVE TISSUE)

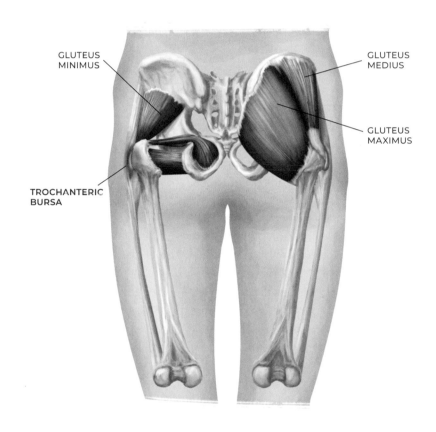

GLUTEUS MINIMUS

GLUTEUS MEDIUS

GLUTEUS MAXIMUS

TROCHANTERIC BURSA

**DESCRIPTION:** Bursas are fluid-filled sacs located in joints and under tendons that provide a thin cushion and reduce friction between the surfaces of tissues. When a bursa becomes irritated and inflamed, the condition is referred to as bursitis. You can get bursitis in many areas, such as the shoulder, knee, or hip.

Previously, pain on the outside of the hip, right on top of the bone, was always diagnosed as trochanteric bursitis because that bursa is right over the bone, on the outside of the femur. But your glute tendons also go over that bursa and attach to the bone. Many tendons do that. Now that this condition has been studied further, we know that pain on the outside of the hip is most often due to gluteal tendinopathy.[12,13]

Gluteal tendinopathy is associated with dysfunction of the gluteus medius and minimus muscles and their respective tendons as they attach on the greater trochanter on the side of the hip. Stress or an insufficiency in those tendons produces lateral hip pain. Either the tendons were stressed suddenly in a new way, or the volume of an existing activity (usually a sagittal plane activity) was increased too rapidly—for example, lots of running, walking, stair climbing, or hiking.

People tend to get tears in those tendons as they get older, and only 20 percent of cases are estimated to be true bursitis.[12] Regardless, the treatment strategy is the same.

**SIGNS AND SYMPTOMS:** Gluteal tendinopathy and trochanteric bursitis produce pain on the lateral hip over the greater trochanter that can range from a dull ache at rest to sharp pain. You can reproduce the pain by touching around the greater trochanter.

**AGGRAVATING FACTORS:** Pain typically occurs when applying pressure to the irritated tendons or bursa (such as sleeping on that side) or moving the hip into adduction (where one leg moves inward toward the other), which can happen during running and walking and when lying on the opposite side as the painful leg falls toward the other leg. When the leg falls inward, the tendons on the bone are compressed, and compression irritates a lot of tendon disorders. So, if you have trochanteric bursitis or gluteal tendinopathy on your right side, sleeping on that side is painful due to direct compression. Sleeping on your left side might also be painful because when your right leg is on top, it drops past your midline, which compresses the tendons on the greater trochanter. The same concept applies to an inward (valgus) twisting of the knee when squatting or sitting.

Pain is aggravated with deep flexion movements and positions, such as deep squats or sitting in a low chair. You would do better with a taller seat, keeping your thighs and femur bones coming straight out from the hip joint. If your legs come together, that position can irritate the area, too.

**PROGNOSIS:** Once you modify or eliminate aggravating positions and activities and implement a resistance training program that targets the gluteal tendons, the condition typically improves within four to 12 weeks.

**TREATMENT STRATEGY:** Both gluteal tendinopathy and trochanteric bursitis require modifying or eliminating aggravating activities and positions and doing rehab exercises designed to strengthen the gluteal muscles and tendons.[13-15] Applying heat to the side of the hip and sleeping on the non-painful side with a body pillow between your legs to limit hip adduction also can relieve pain.

Consider limiting dynamic valgus (inward knee movement) by controlling the alignment of your leg when performing squats and single-leg movements and then transferring that alignment to activities like hiking, running, and stair climbing. Much of this is accomplished by strengthening the gluteus medius and minimus muscles and then transferring that strength to functional tasks.

Phase 1 focuses on relieving pain and improving hip mobility. Most people with gluteal tendinopathy do not have significant hip mobility restrictions, so these exercises can reduce pain by adding gentle movement. Complete only the range of motion that you can do without pain. Also be careful with the knee to opposite shoulder stretch, which targets the glutes but also applies tensile stress to the gluteal tendons, which could cause pain. If it seems to aggravate your symptoms, I recommend removing it.

Phases 2 and 3 strengthen the hip muscles in multiple planes of movement with an emphasis on the hip abductors (gluteus medius and minimus). Research shows that strengthening these muscles and their respective tendons usually relieves pain associated with gluteal tendinopathy.[13-15] The banded hip abduction, single-leg bridge, and lateral squat walk exercises target these two muscles. That said, don't skip the squat and hip hinge exercises, because they require the gluteus medius and minimus to act as stabilizers of the hip joint and pelvis.

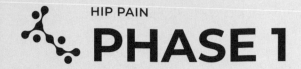

# HIP PAIN
# PHASE 1

**NOTE:** Because most of the conditions linked to this protocol affect the joint, which is deep, soft tissue mobilizations tend not to help much. Therefore, I have omitted them from the protocol to make rehab more efficient.

## GOOD FOR:

- Alleviating pain stemming from the hip, glutes, and groin
- Improving hip range of motion
- Warm-up for phase 2 and 3 exercises

## GUIDELINES:

- Perform every day
- Tools: stretch strap, balance pad, dowel
- Add phase 2 when you have no pain at rest and no more than mild pain (3/10) with the exercises

## STRETCHING EXERCISES:

- ▸ Do 3 reps with 30- to 60-second holds
- ▸ Perform in any order on both sides
- ▸ Don't stretch into pain

### knee to opposite shoulder

Lie on your back and bring one knee toward your chest. Interlock your fingers over your lower knee and upper shin. Keeping your low back flush with the floor, use your arms to pull your knee across your body toward your opposite shoulder.

### hamstring stretch with strap

Hook a strap around your foot. Keeping your leg completely relaxed, use your arms to pull your foot toward your head and hold it in place once you feel a moderate stretch.

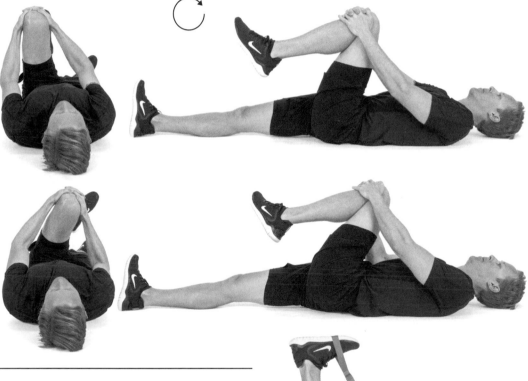

# hip flexor stretch

In a kneeling position, squeeze your abdominals and glutes to rotate your pelvis backward (posteriorly). Keeping your back neutral, shift your body forward slightly until you feel a stretch on the front of your hip and leg. To increase the intensity of the stretch, bend your knee and grab your ankle. You can also prop your foot on a bench or chair or position your shin flush against a wall.

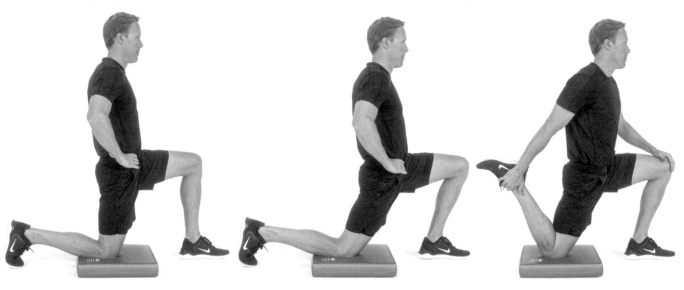

## MOBILITY EXERCISES:

▸ Do 3 sets of 10–15 reps

▸ Active range of motion (AROM)—move as far as you can without pain

▸ Perform in any order on both sides

▸ Pause at end range for 2–3 seconds

## hip external and internal rotation

Stand with your feet straight and positioned underneath your hips. Shift your weight onto one leg and lift your unweighted foot an inch or two off the floor, keeping your leg straight. To help maintain balance, place one hand against a wall or hold a dowel. Externally rotate your hip by turning your foot outward, then internally rotate your hip by turning your foot inward.

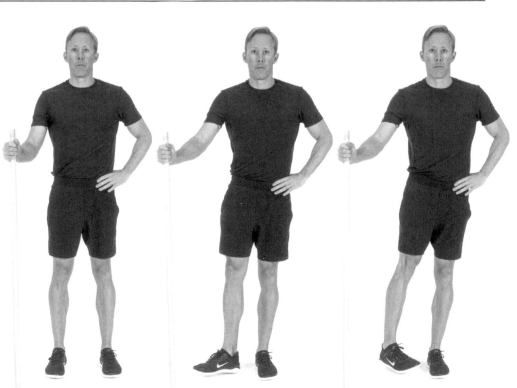

## hip abduction

As you shift your weight onto one leg, use your hip and glute muscles to raise your other leg out to the side of your body (abduction). Try not to lean excessively or rotate your foot; stay fairly upright and keep the toes of your moving foot facing forward.

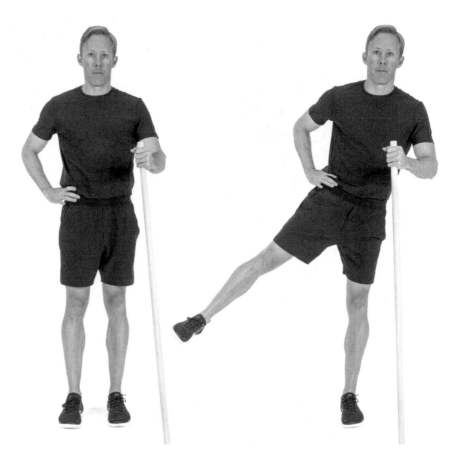

## hip flexion

Raise one knee as high as you can without assistance. As you reach end range, cup your hands around the front of your knee and gently pull it toward your chest. Stop if you hit a point where you feel pain.

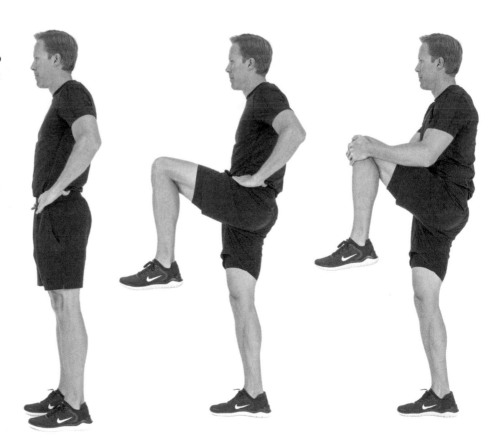

# PHASE 2

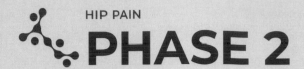

## GOOD FOR:

- Reducing hip pain
- Improving hip range of motion
- Early hip and glute strengthening
- Warm-up for phase 3

## GUIDELINES:

- Perform 3 or 4 days a week
- Do 3 sets of 10–15 reps unless otherwise noted
- Push sets to fatigue
- Tools: resistance loop, dumbbells

## bridge *(choose one)*

### bodyweight

Lie on your back with your knees bent and your feet flat on the floor. Push into the floor and lift your butt, fully extending your hips—a straight line runs from your shoulders to your knees. Squeeze your glutes as you reach full hip extension and pause in the top position for 1–2 seconds.

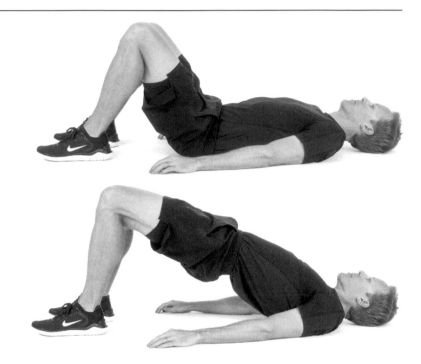

### banded

To increase glute activation and make the exercise more challenging, position a resistance loop just above your knees. Perform a bridge—drive your heels into the floor and extend your hips—while driving your knees out into the band. Maintain abduction resistance (knees out) throughout the entire range of the movement.

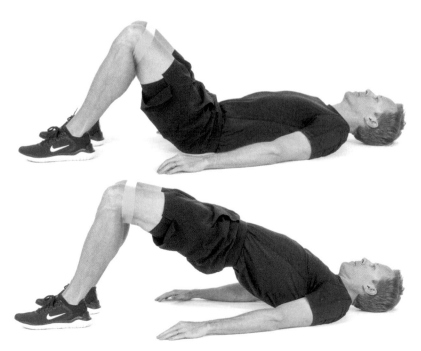

## side plank

Lie on your side, position your elbow underneath your shoulder to elevate your upper body, and stack your top leg over your bottom leg. Use your trunk and core muscles to lift your hips. Do 3 reps with 20- to 30-second holds.

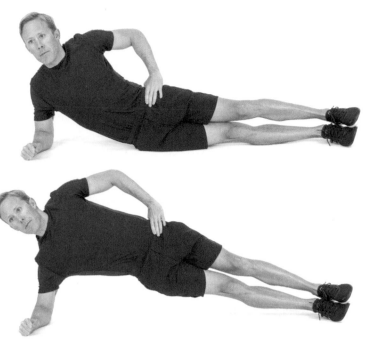

## banded hip abduction

With the resistance loop above your knees, shift your weight onto one leg, then raise your unweighted leg out to the side (abduction). Keep your foot pointed straight forward and try not to lean your upper body excessively. Place your hand against a wall or use a dowel to maintain balance.

## banded hip flexor march

Position the loop around your feet. Stand with your feet straight and aligned under your hips. Keeping your foot flexed (parallel to the floor), lift your knee to hip level or as far as you can without pain. You can place your hands on your hips or hold onto something sturdy to maintain balance.

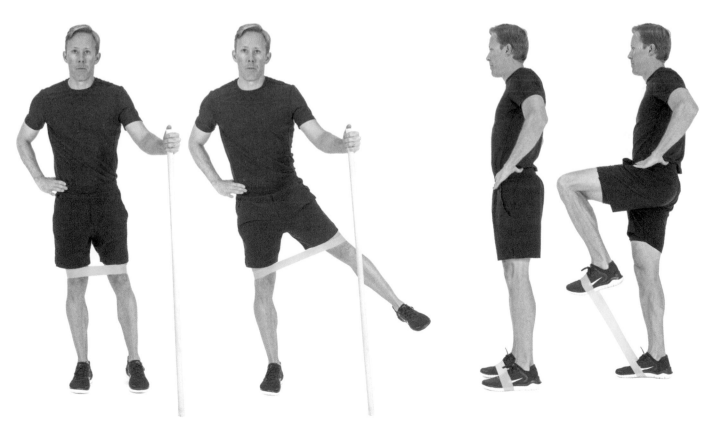

## banded squat

With the loop above your knees, stand with your feet roughly shoulder width apart. When it comes to foot flare, you can orient your feet straight or turn them out slightly—whichever feels better and allows you to reach the lowest depth without discomfort. To perform the movement, reach your hips back slightly and sit straight down. As you lower into the bottom position, drive your knees outward into the band, keep your spine neutral (not excessively arching or rounding), and keep your knees aligned over your toes. Lower as far as you can while maintaining good form.

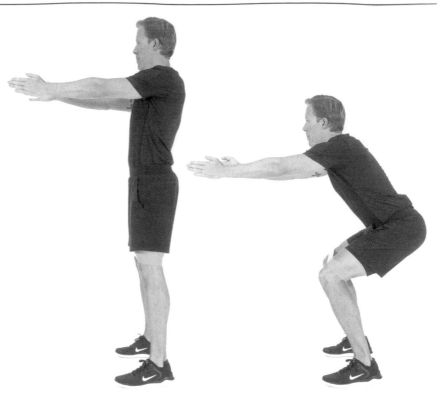

## split squat

Get into a split squat stance: torso upright, slight bend in your lead leg with your shin vertical, and back leg straight. Drop your hips straight down and lower your rear knee to the floor. Driving off the heel of your front foot and the ball of your rear foot, extend your knees and raise your body back into the start position. You can hold one dumbbell to challenge your trunk stability or two dumbbells to add load to the movement.

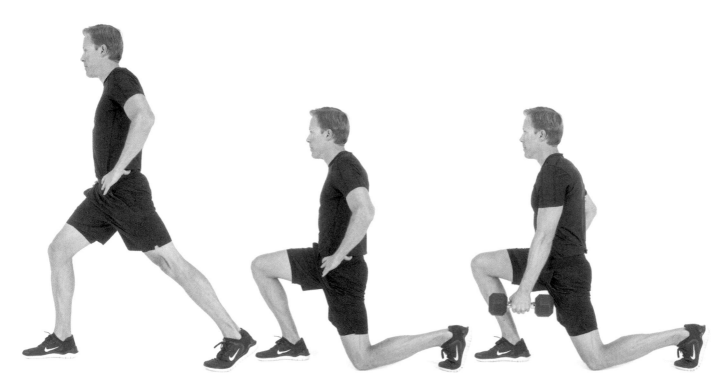

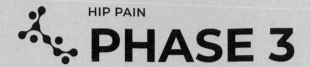

# PHASE 3

## GOOD FOR:

- Strengthening the hips, glutes, and legs
- Preventing hip pain and injury

## GUIDELINES:

- Perform 3 or 4 days a week
- Do 3 sets of 10–15 reps unless otherwise noted
- Push sets to fatigue
- Add load or reps to increase difficulty
- Tools: bench, resistance loop, dumbbell, plyo box

## kickback

Get into the quadruped position with your shoulders aligned over your wrists and hips over your knees. Keeping your knee bent to roughly 90 degrees, raise your foot toward the ceiling. Squeeze your glutes in the top position. Try to keep your back flat (core tight), get your thigh parallel to the floor, and reach full hip extension. Reduce the range of motion if you arch your back excessively. Place a resistance loop above your knees to make the exercise more challenging.

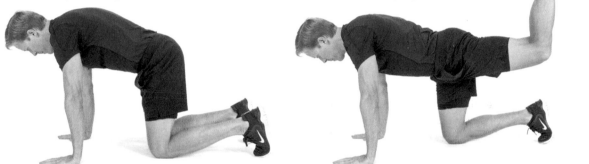

## single-leg hip extension *(choose one)*

## single-leg bridge

Get into the bridge start position and elevate one leg—you can either straighten it or keep it bent at about 90 degrees. Push into the floor and extend your hips. Focus on squeezing your glutes as you reach full hip extension, holding the contraction for 1–2 seconds. Add a resistance loop above your knees or do the single-leg hip thrust (page 342) to make the exercise more challenging.

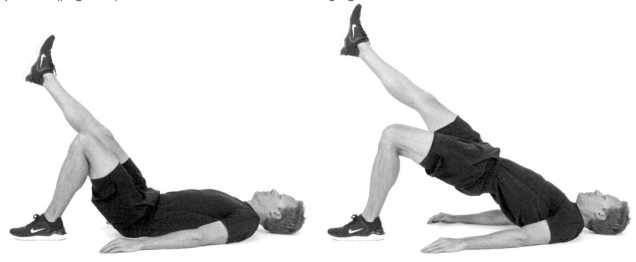

# single-leg hip thrust

Position your mid-back on the edge of a bench and lift one leg—you can either straighten it or keep it bent at about 90 degrees. Push into the floor and extend your hips. Focus on squeezing your glutes as you reach full hip extension, holding the contraction for 1–2 seconds.

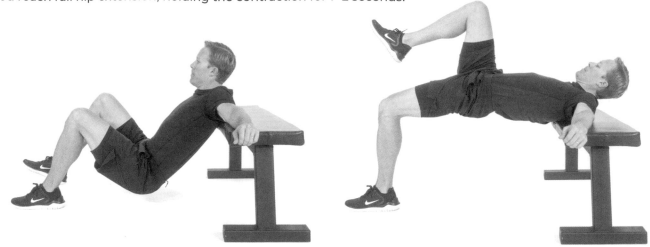

# lateral squat walk
## (choose one)

Wrap a resistance loop above your knees (harder) or ankles (easier). Position your feet shoulder width apart and bend your hips and knees slightly. Take a wide lateral step so there is a full stretch in the band. You can either walk along a line and then switch after a given number of steps or stay in one area by switching back and forth between legs. Choose a distance or rep range that is challenging—usually 15–20 steps in each direction. Don't pause between steps, and keep tension in the band during the entire movement.

**band above knees**

**band above ankles**

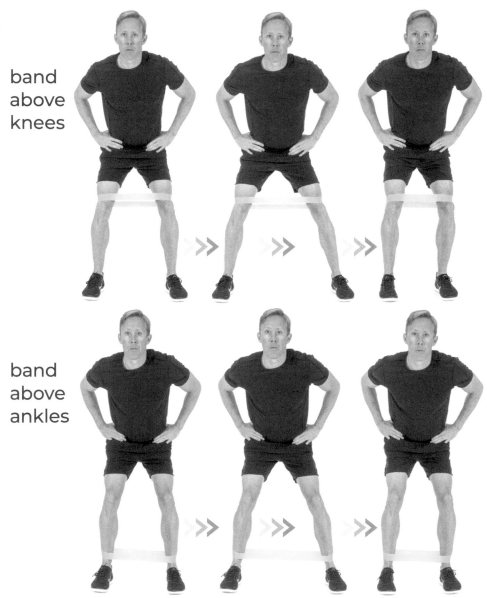

## sumo squat

Holding one end of a dumbbell in front of your body, position your feet outside shoulder width and turn your toes out to about 45 degrees. Keeping your torso upright and arms relaxed, sit your hips back and down, lowering the dumbbell to the floor. Push through your heels and extend your hips and knees simultaneously into the top position.

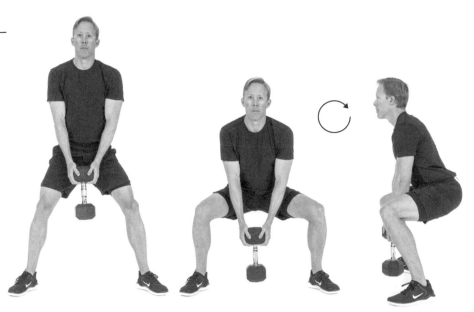

## bulgarian split squat

Stand about 2 feet in front of a bench. Reach back with one leg and place the ball of your foot on the bench. Keeping the majority of your weight over your front leg, lower your body slowly—sinking your hips down and back at an angle—until your front thigh is roughly parallel to the floor. Keep your back leg mostly relaxed during the exercise; don't push off the bench.

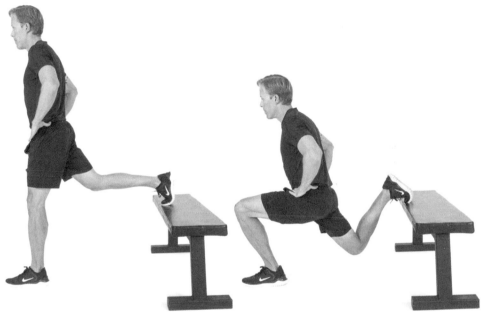

## step-up

Step onto a plyo box with your knee aligned over your foot. Without pushing off the floor, shift your weight onto your elevated leg, drive through your heel or mid-foot, and raise your torso and hips in one fluid motion. Progress this exercise by increasing the height of the box or holding a dumbbell.

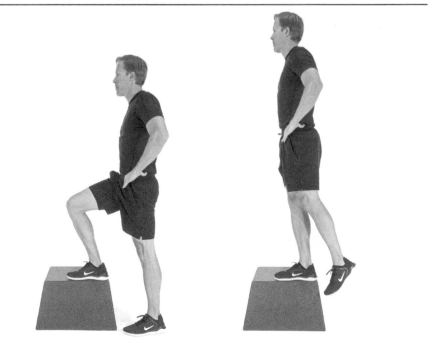

# NERVE PAIN

**Follow this program to treat:**

- Nerve pain radiating down the buttock, back of the thigh, and calf
- Piriformis syndrome (deep gluteal pain syndrome)
- Sciatica stemming from the pelvis

## PIRIFORMIS SYNDROME (DEEP GLUTEAL PAIN SYNDROME)

**DESCRIPTION:** The piriformis is a deep muscle underneath the glutes and part of a group of muscles called P-GO-GO-Q that includes the piriformis, obturator internus and externus, two gemelli muscles (minor and major), and the quadratus femoris. These six muscles form what is sometimes referred to as the "rotator cuff" of your hip because they share a similar function to the rotator cuff in your shoulder: they stabilize the hip joint and power rotation.

Piriformis syndrome creates discomfort in the buttock, hip, and leg. It can be subdivided into two categories:

- **PRIMARY PIRIFORMIS SYNDROME** is believed to result from anatomical variations of the sciatic nerve or the piriformis muscle. However, little evidence exists to support this type, and it is considered much less prevalent than was once thought.

- **SECONDARY PIRIFORMIS SYNDROME** results from a direct insult to the region, including trauma or issues that reduce blood flow (ischemia). Common insults include falls, hip-related surgery, pain-induced muscle guarding/spasm, and prolonged mechanical compression, like sitting on a wallet. Extreme hip extensor or hip rotator exercises (too many loaded squats and lunges) and overstretching the nerve (too much yoga or stretching) also can lead to this condition.

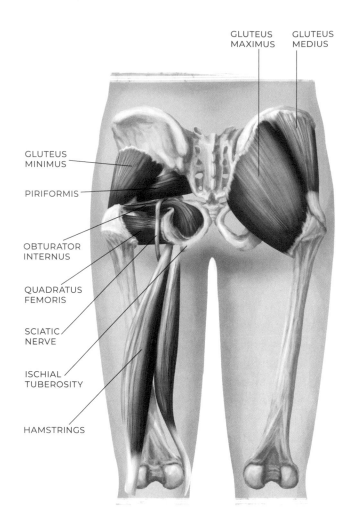

GLUTEUS MAXIMUS
GLUTEUS MEDIUS
GLUTEUS MINIMUS
PIRIFORMIS
OBTURATOR INTERNUS
QUADRATUS FEMORIS
SCIATIC NERVE
ISCHIAL TUBEROSITY
HAMSTRINGS

Piriformis syndrome is starting to be phased out as a diagnosis because the pain associated with this condition can be related to numerous muscles (glutes, P-GO-GO-Q, and hamstrings), not just the piriformis, which is a single structure. The more appropriate name—and the one becoming more common among practitioners—is deep gluteal pain syndrome because it captures the region instead of the exact muscle.[16] It is also sometimes interpreted as sciatica that comes from the pelvis or buttock rather than the low back because it mirrors sciatica symptoms.[17,18] Regardless of what you call it, if you have pain originating from your hip that refers down your thigh, this protocol will help.

**SIGNS AND SYMPTOMS:** Piriformis syndrome typically produces symptoms that are similar to sciatica—pain in the buttock, possibly with radiating nerve pain into the back of the thigh, calf, and foot. You will feel the pain deep in the hip socket or back pocket area. Some people just have a deep ache in their buttock, while others have numbness and tingling down their leg.

**AGGRAVATING FACTORS:** Putting pressure on the piriformis muscle and underlying sciatic nerve, such as with prolonged sitting or sitting on hard surfaces, typically aggravates symptoms.

Often, symptoms are triggered by a big workout or hard run followed by a long flight or car ride—basically, any prolonged seated position where you can't get up and move frequently. This probably has to do with delayed onset muscle soreness (DOMS) and the inflammatory process going on in the area. Many people seem to do worse if they sit after an intense exercise session versus only sitting. Another example is asymmetrical sitting, such as sitting on a wallet or an uneven hard surface.

When piriformis syndrome flares up, contracting the gluteal muscles may be painful. That's why activities like stair climbing can hurt; squeezing your glutes and activating those deep rotators of the hip compresses the nerve.

**PROGNOSIS:** Piriformis syndrome typically resolves within four to six weeks if you modify or eliminate aggravating factors. Rehab exercises designed to improve muscle and sciatic nerve health can help speed up the recovery process.

**TREATMENT STRATEGY:** Piriformis syndrome is primarily treated by applying heat to the buttock, stretching nearby muscles, taking muscle relaxants or anti-inflammatories, and doing rehab exercises.[19] In severe cases, a corticosteroid injection can reduce pain and inflammation.

For an acute flare-up or injury, phase 1 includes myofascial release and other techniques that relieve pain. The glute/piriformis mobilization can reduce muscle tension and pain, but do not push too hard; the sciatic nerve is right under the roller, and too much pressure can flare up symptoms. The hamstring mobilization helps reduce tension in the back of the leg, and the knee to opposite shoulder stretch is a favorite of many patients because it tends to reduce glute and hip rotator muscle tension and pain considerably. The lumbar rotation exercise works on mobility from the hips to the low back, where the sciatic nerve's branches originate. At the end of phase 1 is a sciatic nerve mobilization, which helps improve nerve mobility and oxygen and nutrient delivery to reduce pain, numbness, tingling, and other symptoms.

Phase 2 increases the challenge for many of the movements from phase 1. You progress from the sciatic nerve mobilization on your back in phase 1 to the slump mobilization in phase 2, which involves sitting with your back rounded. Do not push too hard into these stretches or you risk making your symptoms worse. Go to the point where you feel tension and stop. As your pain dissipates, your range of motion will improve, allowing you to increase the movement and position of the stretch. The lumbar rotation and glute/hip rotator stretches are also progressions from phase 1. Because your pain should be getting better, you want to challenge your mobility and flexibility further. Phase 2 wraps up with knee-banded bridges and clamshells, resistance exercises that start strengthening the glutes and deep hip rotators in a low-load fashion. You can do either exercise without a band if these movements cause pain.

Phase 3 focuses on more challenging resistance training exercises to strengthen your glutes, deep hip rotators, and low back muscles and should reduce the likelihood that piriformis syndrome will reoccur. The first three exercises work all three gluteal muscles, which help stabilize the hip and protect the underlying structures, including the sciatic nerve. The last two exercises, side plank and skydiver, strengthen the low back and core muscles, which is important because the sciatic nerve originates in the low back.

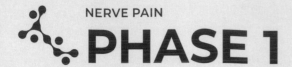

# NERVE PAIN
# PHASE 1

## GOOD FOR:

- Alleviating nerve pain and deep gluteal pain
- Reducing muscle stiffness
- Improving range of motion
- Warm-up for phase 2 and 3 exercises

## GUIDELINES:

- Perform every day
- Tools: foam roller, massage ball, stretch strap
- Add phase 2 when you have no pain at rest and no more than mild pain (3/10) with the exercises

## glute/piriformis mobilization

Sit on a foam roller and lean to one side, putting your weight over your glute muscles. Roll throughout the gluteal region: up, down, and side to side. To increase the pressure, stretch the muscles by crossing your leg over your opposite knee. Spend 1–2 minutes massaging the area, stopping on tender points for 10–20 seconds.

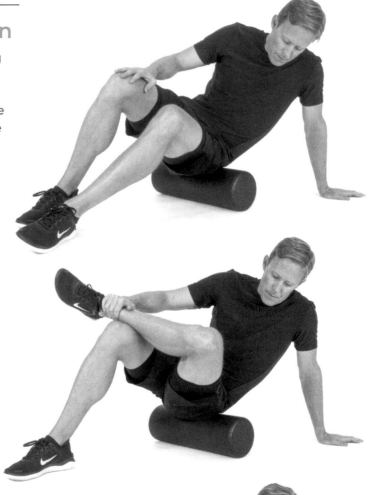

For more precise pressure, use a large or small massage ball.

**Skip this mobilization or add it to phase 2 if it creates more than mild pain.**

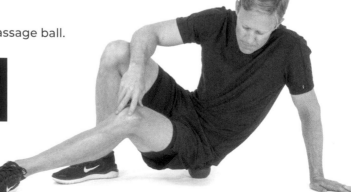

# hamstring mobilization

Sit on a bench or chair and place a massage ball under your hamstring muscles. Roll up and down the entire length of your hamstring. Flex and extend your knee to dynamically mobilize the muscles. Spend 1–2 minutes massaging the area, stopping on tender points for 10–20 seconds.

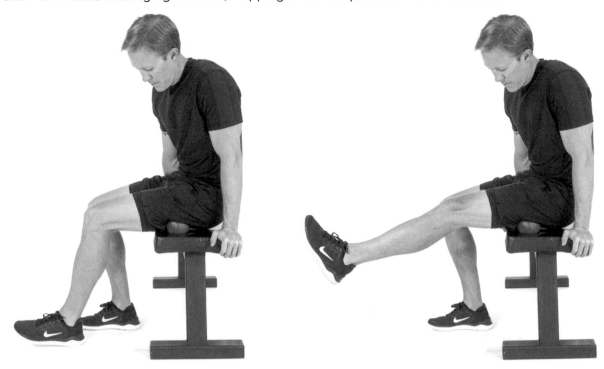

# knee to opposite shoulder

Lie on your back and bring one knee toward your chest. Interlock your fingers over your lower knee and upper shin. Keeping your low back flush with the floor, use your arms to pull your knee across your body toward your opposite shoulder. Do 3 reps on each side with 30- to 60-second holds. Don't stretch into pain.

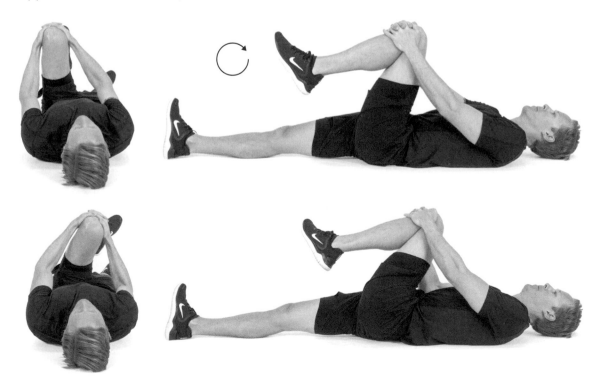

# MOBILITY EXERCISES:

▸ Do 3 sets of 10–15 reps

▸ Active range of motion (AROM)—move as far as you can without pain

▸ Pause at end range for 2–3 seconds

## lumbar rotation

Lie on your back with your knees bent and your feet on the floor. Rock your knees slowly from side to side, moving as far as you can without pain.

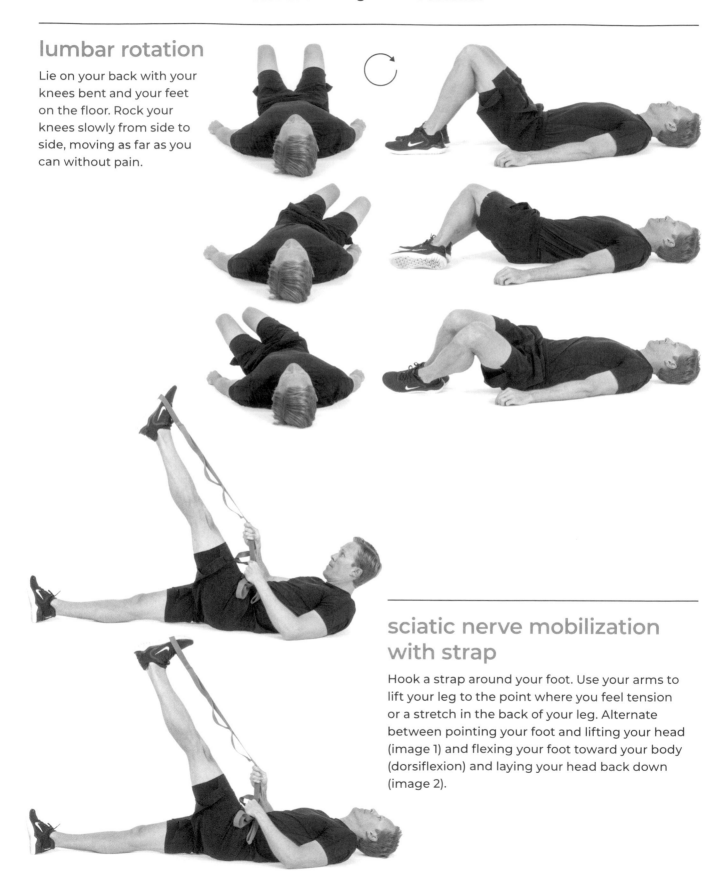

## sciatic nerve mobilization with strap

Hook a strap around your foot. Use your arms to lift your leg to the point where you feel tension or a stretch in the back of your leg. Alternate between pointing your foot and lifting your head (image 1) and flexing your foot toward your body (dorsiflexion) and laying your head back down (image 2).

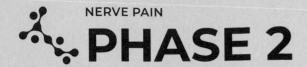

# NERVE PAIN
# PHASE 2

**GOOD FOR:**

- Reducing nerve sensitivity
- Improving hip range of motion
- Warm-up for phase 3 exercises

**GUIDELINES:**

- Perform every day
- Tools: resistance loop, bench
- Add phase 3 when you can do the exercises with no more than mild pain (3/10)

## MOBILITY EXERCISE:

- ▸ Do 3 sets of 10–15 reps
- ▸ Active range of motion (AROM)—move as far as you can without pain
- ▸ Pause at end range for 2–3 seconds

---

## slump sciatic nerve mobilization

Sit on a stool or table so that your feet are off the floor. Slouch your shoulders and round your back. Slowly straighten your knee until you feel tension or a stretch in the back of your leg. Alternate between pointing your foot and looking down and lifting your foot and extending your neck (looking forward).

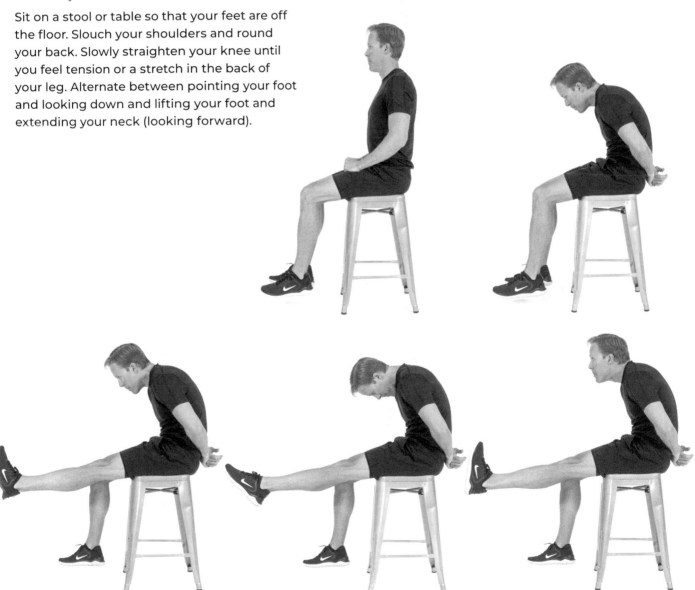

# STRETCHING EXERCISES:

- ▸ Do 3 reps with 30- to 60-second holds
- ▸ Perform in any order on both sides
- ▸ Don't stretch into pain

## lumbar rotation stretch

Lie on your back and bend your knee and hip to about 90 degrees. Reach across your body and cup your hand around the outside of your elevated knee. Keeping both shoulders on the floor, use your hand to pull your knee across your body and toward the floor. Rotate as far as your spine will comfortably allow.

## glute/hip rotator stretch
*(choose one)*

### seated figure-four stretch

Sit on a bench or chair, cross one leg over the opposite knee, and then hinge forward from the hips until you feel a stretch in your glute region.

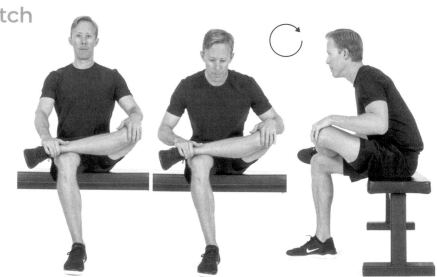

## supine figure-four stretch

Lie on your back with your legs bent and your feet on the floor. Cross one leg over the opposite knee. Reach one arm between your legs, the other arm around the outside of your leg, and then interlock your fingers around the front of your knee. Use your arms to pull your knee toward your chest.

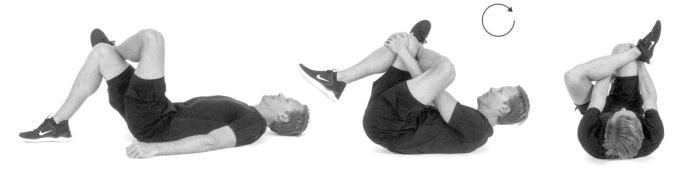

## pigeon stretch

Position one knee flush on the bench with your lower leg perpendicular to your body, then slide your rear foot back. Hinge forward from your waist until you feel a stretch in your glute region. If you feel pain in your knee or are unable to comfortably get into the start position, place a pillow under your knee or elevate one side of the bench (on the same side as your bent knee).

To increase the stretch, do this exercise on the floor.

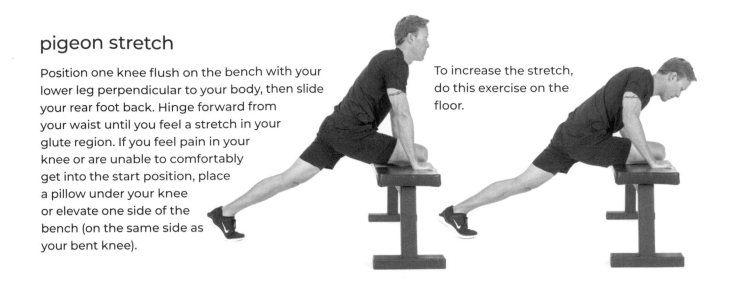

## RESISTANCE EXERCISES:

- ▸ Do 3 sets of 10–15 reps
- ▸ Push sets to fatigue
- ▸ Add reps to make the exercise more challenging

## bridge *(choose one)*

### banded frog bridge

Position a resistance loop above your knees. Bend your knees and position the insides of your feet together. Driving through the lateral edge of your heels and pushing your knees laterally into the band, extend your hips, squeezing your glutes as you reach full hip extension.

### banded bridge

Drive your heels into the floor and extend your hips. Maintain abduction resistance (knees out) throughout the entire range of the movement.

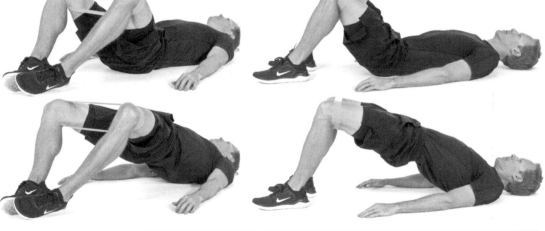

## clamshell

Lie on your side with your hips bent to about 45 degrees, your knees bent to about 90 degrees, and your feet and legs stacked. Lift your top knee as far as you can without rotating your spine.

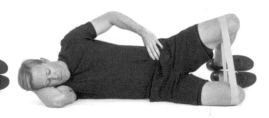

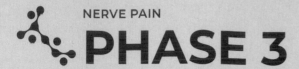

# PHASE 3

## GOOD FOR:

- Reducing nerve sensitivity and preventing future flare-ups
- Improving glute and hip strength

## GUIDELINES:

- Perform 3 or 4 days a week
- Do 3 sets of 10–15 reps unless otherwise noted
- Push sets to fatigue
- Tools: plyo box, resistance loop, dowel

## single-leg bridge

Get into the bridge start position and elevate one leg—you can either straighten it or keep it bent at about 90 degrees. Push into the floor and extend your hips. Focus on squeezing your glutes as you reach full hip extension, holding the contraction for 1–2 seconds. Add a resistance loop above your knees or do the single-leg hip thrust (page 342) to make the exercise more challenging.

## lateral step-up

Stand next to a plyo box. Step onto the box, positioning your entire foot on the box. Your feet should be roughly shoulder width apart. Shifting your weight onto your elevated leg, extend your hips and knee in one fluid motion. Don't push off the floor with your supporting leg. Increase the height of the box to make the exercise more challenging. The taller the box, the more you have to lean forward and at an angle over your elevated foot. You can extend your arms in front of you to counterbalance your weight.

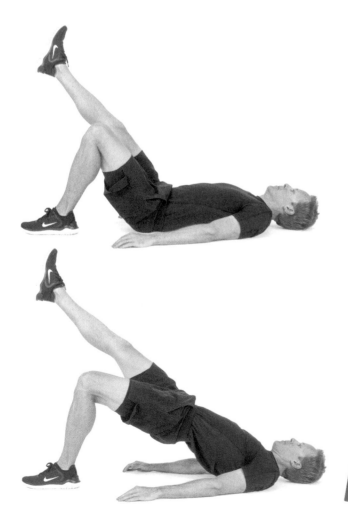

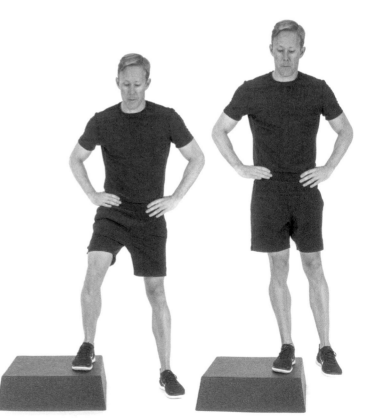

## banded hip abduction

Position a resistance loop above your knees. Shift your weight onto one leg, then raise the other leg out to the side (abduction). Keep your foot pointed straight forward and try not to lean your upper body excessively. Place your hand against a wall or use a dowel to maintain balance.

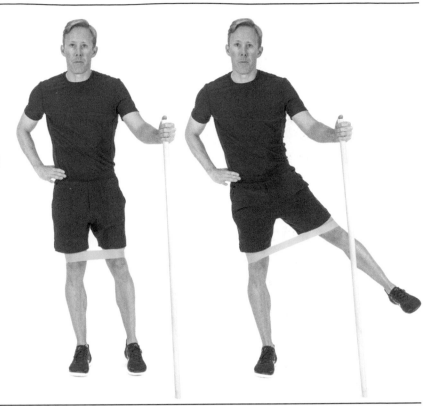

## skydiver

Lie on your stomach with your arms at your sides. Use your low back extensors to lift your lower and upper body segments off the floor. As you arch, squeeze your glutes and pull your shoulders back while maintaining a neutral neck position.

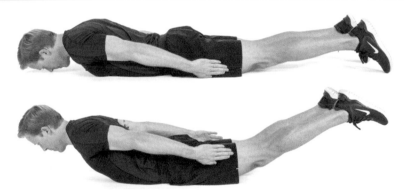

## side plank

Lie on your side, position your elbow underneath your shoulder to elevate your upper body, and stack your top leg over your bottom leg. Use your trunk and core muscles to lift your hips. Do 3 reps with 20- to 30-second holds.

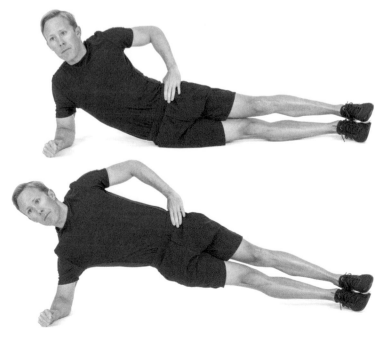

# HIP FLEXOR PAIN

**Follow this program to treat:**

- Pain on the front of the hip
- Hip flexor tendinopathy or strain
- Iliopsoas bursitis

## HIP FLEXOR STRAINS AND TENDINOPATHY

**DESCRIPTION:** The iliopsoas muscle is your major hip flexor (it pulls your thigh bone toward your chest) and is formed by the joining of three smaller muscles: the psoas major, psoas minor, and iliacus. These muscles blend together into one tendon deep in the stomach area and attach to a bony spot called the lesser trochanter on the inside of the femur.

Pain in this area is usually associated with hip flexion, such as in high-volume walking, running, hiking, or stair climbing. Any activity that involves a repetitious marching motion can affect the iliopsoas or hip flexor tendon.[20] Hip flexor strains are also common, either from repetitive stress, overstretching, or a quick, forceful contraction that tears the muscle or tendon.

**SIGNS AND SYMPTOMS:** Hip flexor tendon issues typically produce sharp pain in the front of the hip and groin region with activities that contract the muscles or place the joint in a position that compresses the tendon. You may feel a dull ache in the area following activities that irritate the tendon.

**AGGRAVATING FACTORS:** Activities that stress the iliopsoas tendon include those that require frequent hip flexion contractions, such as running and fast walking. Deep squats, lunges, or sitting in a low seat can compress the tendon and provoke symptoms.

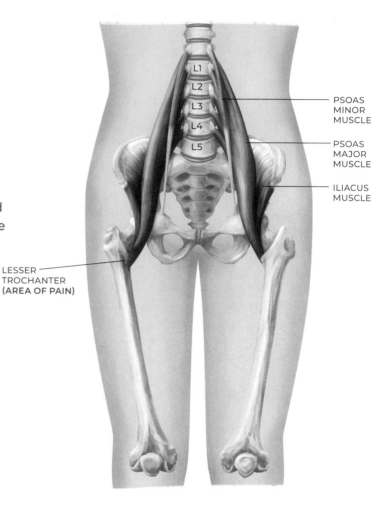

PSOAS MINOR MUSCLE

PSOAS MAJOR MUSCLE

ILIACUS MUSCLE

LESSER TROCHANTER (AREA OF PAIN)

### HOW DO I DISTINGUISH BETWEEN HIP FLEXOR TENDINOPATHY AND HIP IMPINGEMENT PAIN?

Hip flexor tendinopathy and hip impingement can create similar symptoms, but the hip flexors usually hurt when you're actively contracting them. You can do a self-assessment by trying to lift and hold up your leg while seated. If that effort causes pain, it's probably the hip flexor tendon and not an impingement.

**PROGNOSIS:** Once you modify or eliminate the aggravating activities and implement a rehab program designed to strengthen the hip flexor muscles, most cases resolve within six to 12 weeks.

**TREATMENT STRATEGY:** Hip flexor tendinopathy, strains, and bursitis are primarily treated with physical therapy aimed at calming the tissue and then strengthening the hip flexor muscles and tendon.[21] Anti-inflammatory medication and a steroid injection may be used to reduce acute pain.[22]

In phase 1 of the protocol, you start by mobilizing your quadriceps muscles. Because one of the quads (the rectus femoris) is a hip flexor, these muscles act as synergists with the iliopsoas muscles. Performing soft tissue mobilizations (massage) on the psoas and hip flexors can reduce pain and tightness for some people, but I didn't include these mobilizations because most evidence-based practitioners now believe that a deep structure like the iliopsoas group can't truly be massaged, as you would have to push past your abdominals and intestines to reach it. However, if you do find relief with hip flexor massage (usually done with a large ball), add it to your program.

Phase 1 also includes a hip flexor stretch, which can reduce general pain and tightness. However, if you have suffered a severe strain, such as from running or sprinting, perform this stretch gently or skip it altogether. Aggressive stretching can make muscle strains worse and is often contraindicated. Because the psoas muscle attaches to the low back, the lumbar rotation stretch targets this area and can reduce hip flexor–related pain. The last two exercises in phase 1 focus on hip flexion. First is a hip flexion mobility exercise that causes the hip flexors to contract strongly enough to lift the leg against gravity. If it is too painful, do it while lying on your back or perform only the range of motion that you can do standing without pain. Second is a hip flexor isometric, which starts strengthening the hip flexors in a controlled fashion. Apply only as much force with your arm as your muscles can tolerate. As they heal, you will be able to apply more resistance.

Phases 2 and 3 focus on resistance training, as the primary goal is to regain strength. All the exercises in phase 2 target the main action of the hip flexor muscles (hip flexion) except for the clamshell, which targets hip external rotation (your hip flexors assist with hip external rotation). Phase 3 makes the exercises from phase 2 more challenging. Once your injury has healed, practice the phase 2 and 3 exercises periodically to keep your hip flexors strong and prevent reinjury.

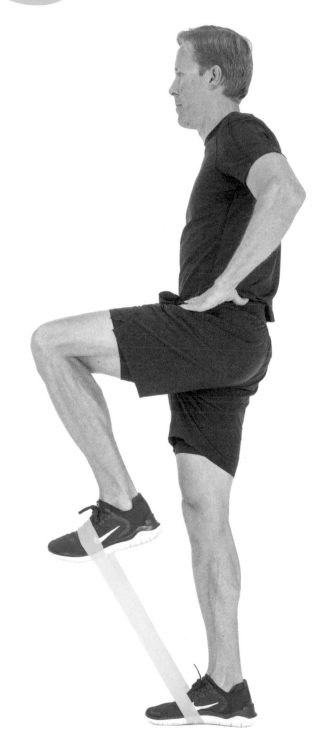

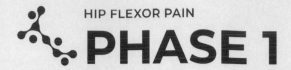

## HIP FLEXOR PAIN
# PHASE 1

### GOOD FOR:

- Alleviating pain on the front of the hip (hip flexor pain)
- Improving hip range of motion
- Warm-up for phase 2 and 3 exercises

### GUIDELINES:

- Perform every day
- Tools: foam roller, balance pad
- Add phase 2 when you have no pain at rest and no more than mild pain (3/10) with the exercises

---

## quad mobilization

Lie on your stomach with your weight supported on your forearms or hands and one leg positioned over a foam roller with your toes pointed toward the floor. Supporting your weight with your grounded foot and arms, roll up and down to mobilize the entire quadriceps muscles on the front of your thigh—from hip to knee. Spend 1–2 minutes on each leg. Stop on tender points for 10–20 seconds and straighten your knee to dynamically mobilize the muscles.

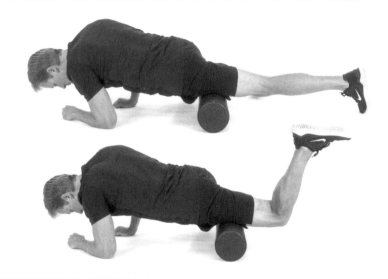

---

## hip flexor stretch

In a kneeling position, squeeze your abdominals and glutes to rotate your pelvis posteriorly. Keeping your back neutral, shift your body forward slightly until you feel a stretch on the front of your hip and leg. To increase the intensity of the stretch, bend your knee and grab your ankle. You can also prop your foot on a bench or chair or position your shin flush against a wall. Do 3 reps with 30- to 60-second holds. Remember, don't stretch into pain. Skip or be extra careful with this exercise if you have a strain or tendinopathy.

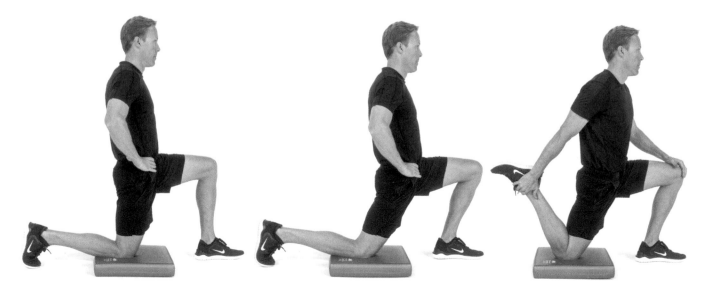

## lumbar rotation stretch

Lie on your back and bend your knee and hip to about 90 degrees. Reach across your body and cup your hand around the outside of your elevated knee. Keeping both shoulders on the floor, use your hand to pull your knee across your body and toward the floor. Rotate as far as your spine will comfortably allow. Perform 3 reps with 30- to 60-second holds.

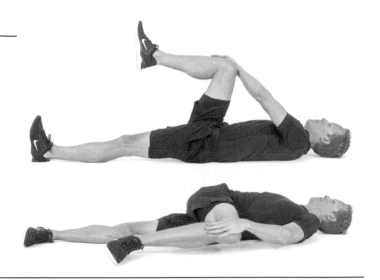

## hip flexion mobility

Stand with your feet straight and positioned underneath your hips. Raise your knee as high as you can without assistance. As you reach end range, cup your hands around the front of your knee and pull it toward your chest. Do 3 sets of 10–15 reps with active range of motion (move as far as you can without pain). Pause at end range for 2–3 seconds.

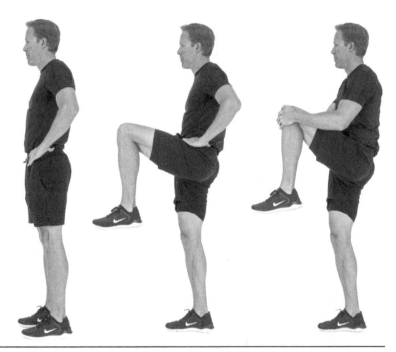

## hip flexor isometrics
### *(choose one)*

You can do this exercise standing or seated. For both variations, you want to bend your hip to about 90 degrees (knee at hip level). Place your palm on the top of your knee and press down. Using your hip flexor muscles, resist the downward pressure by driving your knee into your hand. Apply as much force as you can tolerate with no more than mild pain. Perform 4 or 5 reps on each leg with 30- to 45-second resisted holds.

standing          seated

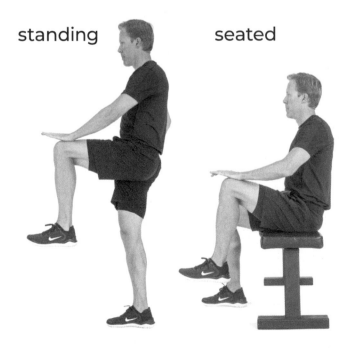

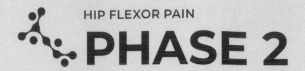

# PHASE 2

## GOOD FOR:

- Reducing hip pain
- Early hip flexor, abdominal, and glute strengthening
- Warm-up for phase 3

## GUIDELINES:

- Perform 3 or 4 days a week
- Do 3 sets of 10–15 reps unless otherwise noted
- Add reps or time to increase difficulty
- Tools: physio (exercise) ball, resistance loop

## front plank

Lie on your stomach, position your elbows underneath your shoulders with your forearms flush with the floor, spread your legs to about hip width, and get onto the balls of your feet. Lift your hips off the floor so that your back is flat. Try to get your hips on the same horizontal plane as your shoulders. Contract your abdominal muscles and squeeze your glutes to stabilize the position. Do 3 reps with 20- to 45-second holds.

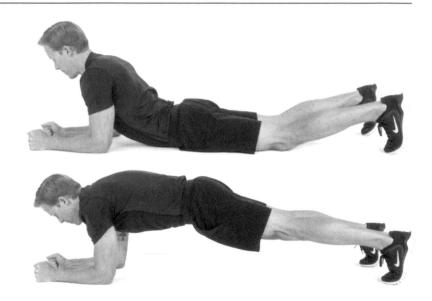

## supine straight-leg raise

Lie on your back with one leg bent, which will help keep you from arching through the low back. Keeping your knee locked, slowly raise your straight leg to just above your opposite knee, then lower it to the floor.

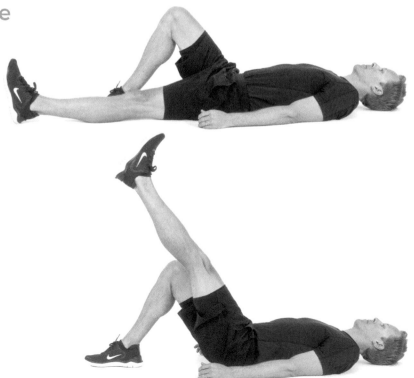

# abdominal curl with knees bent

Lie on your back with your knees bent and your hands by your sides. Reach your hands toward your feet and bend your waist and hips to sit up, bringing your chest to your knees. You can tuck your feet under a brace or overhang, such as a dumbbell handle or couch, or have a partner hold your feet.

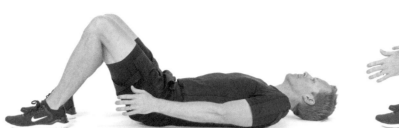

# abdominal draw-in

Get into the top of a push-up— shoulders aligned over wrists, back flat, glutes squeezed, and core tight—with your feet and shins positioned over a physio (exercise) ball. Keeping the weight of your legs on the ball, elevate your hips slightly and pull your knees toward your chest. Try not to let your shoulders travel over your hands.

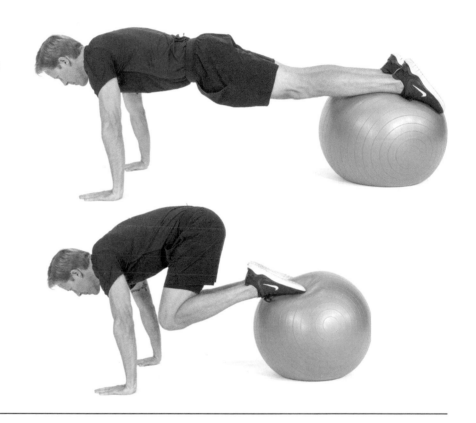

# clamshell

Place a resistance loop above your knees. Lie on your side with your hips bent to about 45 degrees, knees bent to about 90 degrees, and feet and legs stacked. Lift your top knee as far as you can without rotating your spine.

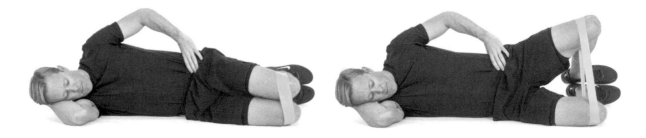

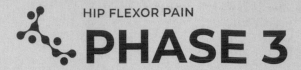

# PHASE 3

## GOOD FOR:

- Improving hip flexor and core strength
- Preventing hip flexor injuries

## GUIDELINES:

- Perform 3 or 4 days a week
- Do 3 sets of 10–15 reps unless otherwise noted
- Push sets to fatigue
- Add reps or time to increase difficulty
- Tool: resistance loop

## plank with leg lifts and arm reaches

Get into the plank position: elbows aligned under your shoulders, back flat, legs spread to about hip width, and up on the balls of your feet. Tighten your abdominals and squeeze your glutes to maintain the position. Then remove one limb from your base of support: raise one leg at a time, then extend one arm at a time. Try to complete 2–4 cycles per set.

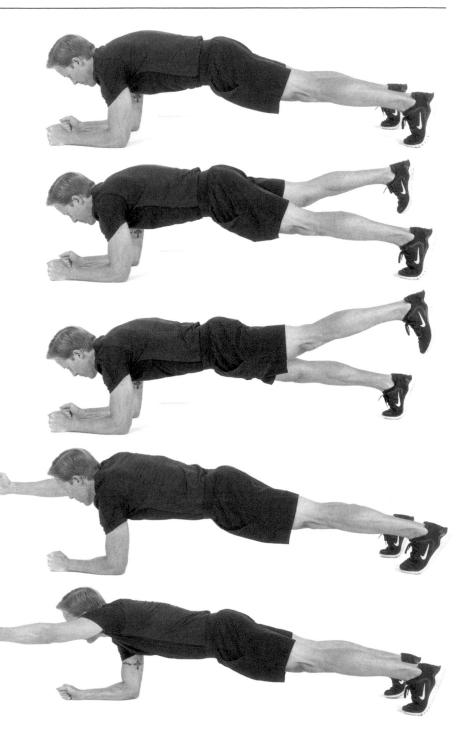

# banded hip flexor march

Position a resistance loop around your feet. Stand with your feet straight and aligned under your hips. Keeping your foot flexed (parallel to the floor), lift one knee to hip level or as far as you can without pain. You can place your hands on your hips or hold onto something sturdy to maintain balance.

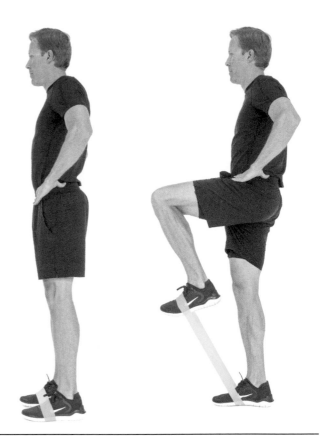

# abdominal curl with one knee bent

Lie on your back with one knee bent and your hands by your sides. Reach your hands toward your feet and bend your waist and hips to sit up, bringing your chest to your knee.

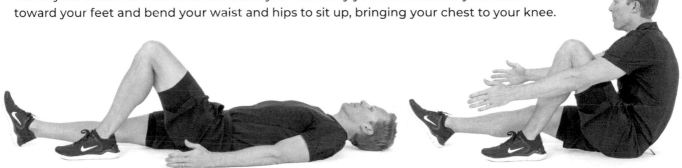

# seated straight-leg raise

Sit with one leg straight and the other leg bent so that your foot is flat on the floor. Keeping your knee extended, slowly raise your straight leg to just above your opposite knee, then lower it to the floor.

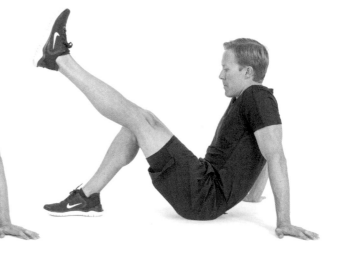

# HAMSTRING PAIN

**Follow this program to treat:**

- Pain stemming from the back of the thigh or sit bone
- Hamstring strain (pulled hamstring)
- Hamstring tendinopathy (buttock or sit bone pain when stretching and sitting)

## HAMSTRING STRAIN

**DESCRIPTION:** The hamstrings (biceps femoris, semitendinosus, and semimembranosus) are located on the back of the thigh and are responsible for extending (straightening) the hip and flexing (bending) the knee. Hamstring strains commonly occur when the muscles are contracting forcefully while lengthening (eccentric contraction), which is seen during the late swing phase of sprinting—the muscle group is maximally lengthened and working to decelerate hip flexion and knee extension to prepare for the foot to hit the ground—when the knee swings straight and the hamstring acts as a brake to slow knee extension before the foot hits.[23,24]

Hamstring strains can occur in the upper or lower part of the muscle. The main difference is that lower strains produce symptoms closer to the knee, while upper strains produce symptoms closer to the hip. In either case, the treatment strategy is similar.

**SIGNS AND SYMPTOMS:** Pain is typically located on the back of the thigh somewhere between where the hamstrings attach to the sit bone and the knee. You feel sharp pain when contracting the muscles and may feel a dull ache when not using the muscles. You may hear or feel a pop, which is the muscle fibers tearing.

**AGGRAVATING FACTORS:** Running and hip hinging movements like deadlifting and hamstring stretches can cause flare-ups and pain. Modify any movement that stretches or creates tension in the hamstring at end range in the early phases of recovery.

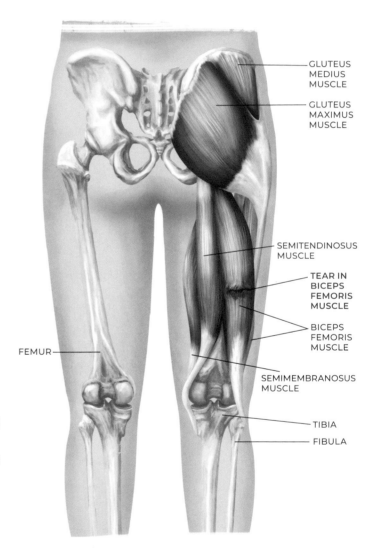

GLUTEUS MEDIUS MUSCLE

GLUTEUS MAXIMUS MUSCLE

SEMITENDINOSUS MUSCLE

TEAR IN BICEPS FEMORIS MUSCLE

BICEPS FEMORIS MUSCLE

FEMUR

SEMIMEMBRANOSUS MUSCLE

TIBIA

FIBULA

**PROGNOSIS:** Healing times vary based on the severity (grade I–III) and location of the injury. A strain of the muscle itself takes around three to six weeks to heal. An injury of the junction between the muscle and tendon (musculotendinous region) takes longer, averaging four to eight weeks. Injuries of the hamstring tendon (tears at musculotendinous junction or the area where muscle turns into tendon) are the slowest to heal and can take up to four months to improve fully.

**TREATMENT STRATEGY:** Hamstring strains require strengthening exercises that gradually load the injured muscle and/or tendon.[24] In severe cases where the muscle tears completely or pulls away from the bone (avulsion), surgery may be indicated.

Three major signs suggest a complete hamstring tear. The first is extreme bruising over the entire back of the thigh. If the muscles detach from the bone, you will also have a divot where the tendon pulled away and feel a gap where the muscles are not connected. Finally, you will have significant strength loss. This last symptom can be tricky because a painful injury that isn't a tear can cause weakness, too. But it's the combination that matters.

If you notice these symptoms, consult with a doctor. You will have options depending on your needs, functionality, injury severity, and so on. There's a lot of redundancy in the musculoskeletal system, so you may be able to get by without surgery. For almost every condition in this book (except a major trauma), it generally doesn't hurt to try the protocol first. If you're not getting better, then check with a medical professional so you can make an informed decision.

**1** The rehab protocol progressively challenges the hamstring muscles. Phase 1 starts with the heel slide. Use a strap or belt to assist with the movement, and then as your pain lessens and the injury heals, do the movement with your hamstrings without help from your arms. The toe-elevated bridge makes the traditional glute bridge more hamstring focused, but you can do a regular bridge with your feet flat on the floor if the toe-elevated variation creates pain. If you can do the double-leg toe-elevated bridge easily, I recommend progressing to the eccentric variation, where you go up on both legs but come down (eccentric contraction) on the injured side. This starts building strength, as muscles are naturally stronger with eccentric contractions than concentric contractions. You finish with the standing hamstring curl, which is another early strengthening and neuromuscular control exercise.

**2 3** Phases 2 and 3 progressively increase the challenge on the hamstring muscles, so do only the exercises that create mild or no pain. Pushing too hard can compromise the tissue and delay healing. The hamstrings are hip extensors and knee flexors, so all these exercises include one or both of those movements. After your strain has healed, you should incorporate the exercises in phases 2 and 3 into your leg training to reduce the likelihood of another strain. The Nordic exercise, for instance, is powerful for not only rehab, but also reducing the odds of a second strain.[25,26]

# PROXIMAL HAMSTRING TENDINOPATHY

**DESCRIPTION:** Proximal hamstring tendinopathy (PHT) is a relatively new diagnosis that describes pain where the hamstring tendon attaches to the ischial tuberosity (sit bone) on the back of the pelvis. It occurs when the hamstring tendon cannot meet the external demand being placed on it—your hips are in flexion, your knees are straight, and then you stretch your hamstrings—and is usually associated with repeatedly compressing against the ischial tuberosity (think of sitting on a hard surface or doing a hamstring stretch).[27]

**SIGNS AND SYMPTOMS:** PHT produces pain at the sit bone—right at the bottom of the buttock where the hamstrings attach and toward the inner groin region—and is reproduced when the hip is in flexion and the hamstrings are contracting or being stretched. Pain is typically sharp with activities that stress the tendon (quick movements, hamstring stretches), and the region aches at rest.

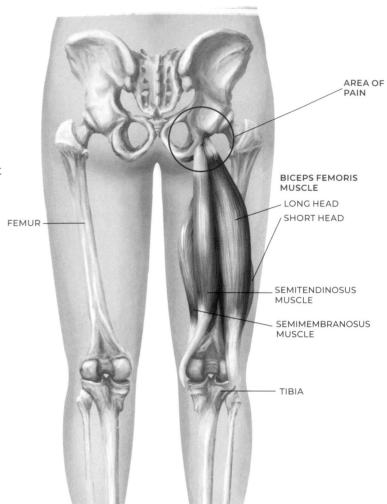

AREA OF PAIN

BICEPS FEMORIS MUSCLE

LONG HEAD

SHORT HEAD

FEMUR

SEMITENDINOSUS MUSCLE

SEMIMEMBRANOSUS MUSCLE

TIBIA

## HOW DO I DIFFERENTIATE BETWEEN AN UPPER HAMSTRING TENDINOPATHY AND AN UPPER HAMSTRING STRAIN (TEAR)?

Most people are not aware that tendinopathy can occur in the upper hamstring, so they assume they have a tear. Although pain symptoms for these two problems can be very similar, the location of the pain usually differs. Upper hamstring tendinopathy is typically brought on by uphill and long-distance running or by sprinting (much like strains) and is exacerbated by hamstring stretching and sitting, both of which compress the tendon against the ischial tuberosity. As a result, you typically feel pain where the tendon connects to the bone, right on the back of your pelvis near the sit bone. An upper hamstring strain, on the other hand, occurs when a forceful muscle contraction (think sprinting or stiff-leg deadlifts) creates a tear in the tissue, usually an inch or two below the tendon or toward the middle of the thigh. So you may feel or hear a pop, which is the muscle fibers tearing.

Because tendinopathy and partial muscle tears (strains) present with similar symptoms, differentiating them is only possible with an MRI. But in most cases, imaging is not necessary (unless you think you have a complete rupture or avulsion), as the rehab process is nearly identical.

**AGGRAVATING FACTORS:** Stretching the hamstrings, hip hinging movements (such as deadlifting), running uphill, sprinting, and similar activities often provoke this issue. You may need to temporarily halt stretching and limit prolonged sitting to desensitize the tendon and allow it to heal.

**PROGNOSIS:** This type of injury can take a long time to heal because it is easy to stress the area given how much time most of us spend sitting. But in most cases, PHT resolves within six to 12 weeks when you modify aggravating activities and work to strengthen the tendon. If you have frequent flare-ups, tendon issues can take up to four months to improve or fully heal.

**TREATMENT STRATEGY:** PHT is predominantly treated with physical therapy integrating resistance training exercises that gradually increase the strength and capacity of the hamstring tendon.[27,28] As with many issues that affect a tendon, stretching can make PHT worse. Stretching might be included in a preventative protocol, but it would compress an injured tendon and aggravate it in the acute stage. That's why the program doesn't include stretching exercises and instead focuses on loading and strengthening the tendon and muscles gradually.

Early in the protocol are lower-load exercises that don't allow the hip to move into much flexion, such as the toe-elevated bridge, standing hamstring curl, ball hamstring curl, and step-up. As you progress through the phases, you add exercises like the split squat, elevated hamstring bridge, skater squat, deadlift, and Nordic to gradually increase hamstring demand and hip flexion angles. The protocol limits hip flexion early on because this position (imagine the bottom of a deadlift or lunge) compresses the upper hamstring tendon against the sit bone on the pelvis. Adopting this position too early in the rehab process usually exacerbates the issue and delays healing. The key is to test each exercise; if you have mild or no pain, it is probably OK to add to your program. Once the issue has resolved, do the phase 2 and 3 exercises periodically to maintain hamstring muscle and tendon strength.

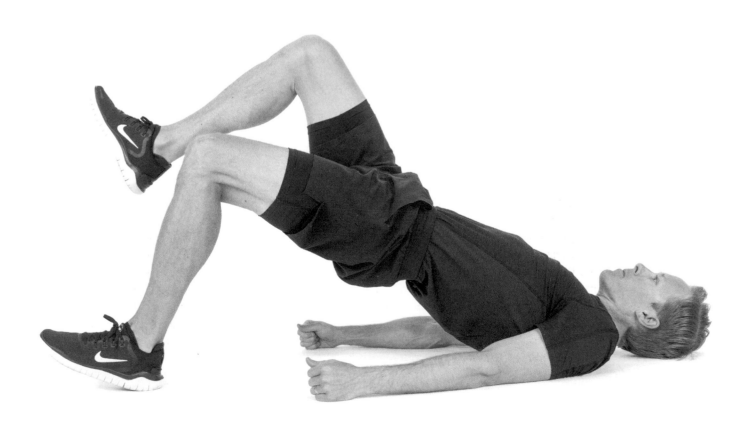

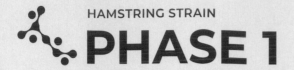

HAMSTRING STRAIN

# PHASE 1

## GOOD FOR:

- Alleviating hamstring pain
- Improving neuromuscular control
- Warm-up for phase 2 and 3 exercises

## GUIDELINES:

- Perform the heel slide and hamstring curl every day and the toe-elevated bridge 3 or 4 times a week
- Tool: stretch strap
- Add phase 2 when you have no pain at rest and no more than mild pain (3/10) with the exercises

---

## heel slide *(choose one)*

Hook a strap around your foot. Bend one knee and slide your heel toward your butt, pulling on the strap to assist with the movement. If you don't feel pain, perform the movement without the strap and go as far as you can with no more than mild pain. Do 3 sets of 10 reps.

### with strap

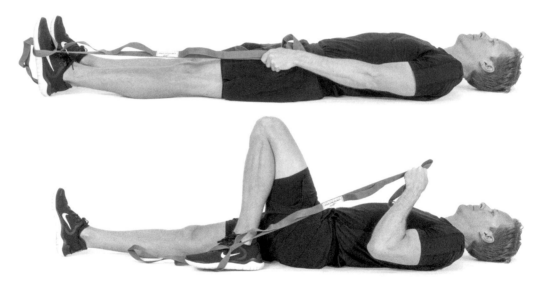

### without strap

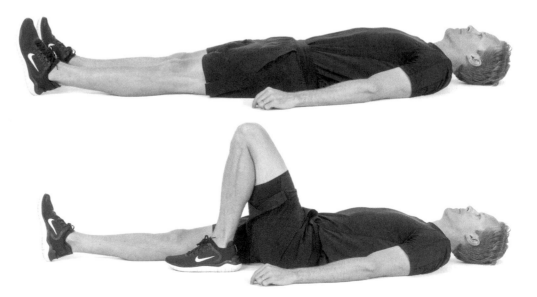

# toe-elevated bridge *(choose one)*

## double-leg

Bend your knees and elevate your toes. Drive through your heels and lift your butt, fully extending your hips. Squeeze your glutes as you reach full hip extension and pause in the top position for 1–2 seconds. Do 3 sets of 10 reps. If you can perform this exercise without pain, try the single-leg eccentric variation.

## single-leg eccentric

Perform the double-leg toe-elevated bridge. From the top position, lift one leg off the floor, then slowly lower your hips to do the eccentric (lowering) phase of the movement. Reclaim the double-leg start position and repeat the exercise—two legs up, one leg down.

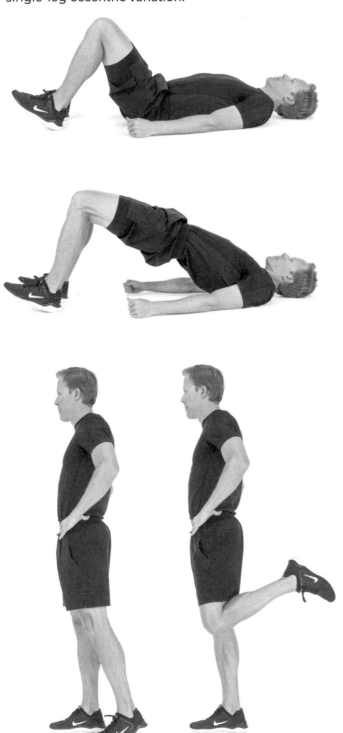

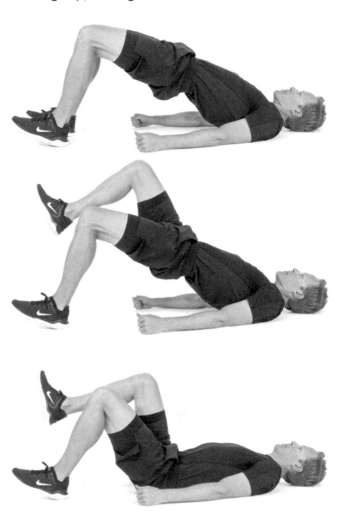

## standing hamstring curl

Shift your weight onto one leg, then curl the heel of your unweighted foot toward your butt. Keep your knee pointed toward the floor and your hips extended; don't bring your knee forward or bend your hips. Do 3 sets of 10–15 reps.

# PHASE 2

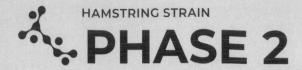

## GOOD FOR:

- Reducing hamstring pain
- Early hamstring strengthening
- Warm-up for phase 3 exercises

## GUIDELINES:

- Perform 3 or 4 days a week
- Do 3 sets of 10–15 reps
- Tools: physio (exercise) ball, plyo box
- Add phase 3 when you can do the exercises with no more than mild pain (3/10)

## kickback

Get into the quadruped position with your shoulders aligned over your wrists and hips over your knees. Keeping your knee bent to roughly 90 degrees, raise one foot toward the ceiling. Squeeze your glutes in the top position. Try to keep your back flat (core tight), get your thigh parallel to the floor, and reach full hip extension. Reduce the range of motion if you arch your back excessively. Place a resistance loop above your knees to make the exercise more challenging.

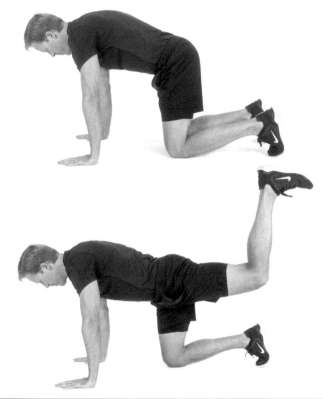

## toe-elevated hamstring bridge

Set up as if you were doing a toe-elevated bridge (page 366) but position your feet farther away from your body, with a roughly 45-degree bend in your knees. Lift one leg off the floor. To extend your hips, imagine pulling your heel toward your butt. Due to the angle of your leg, your foot will not move, but you will increase hamstring activation. If this version is too challenging or painful, you can perform the two-up, one-down variation: keep both heels on the floor into the top position, then lift one leg and perform a single-leg eccentric into the bottom position.

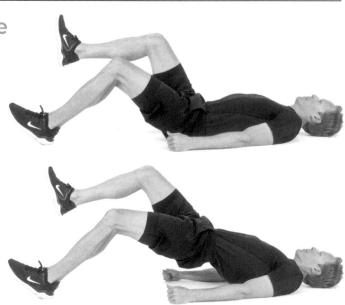

## ball hamstring curl

Lie on your back and center your feet on a physio (exercise) ball. Spread your arms slightly and keep them flush with the floor. Drive your heels into the ball and extend your hips. As you reach full hip extension, slowly curl your heels toward your butt.

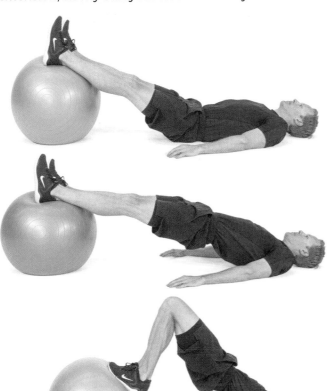

## step-up

Step on a plyo box with your knee aligned over your foot. Without pushing off the floor, shift your weight onto your elevated leg, drive through your heel or mid-foot, and raise your torso and hips in one fluid motion. Progress this exercise by increasing the height of the box or holding a dumbbell.

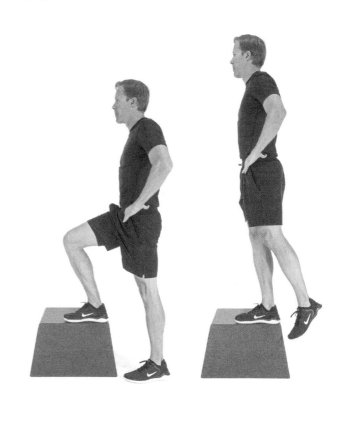

## split squat

Get into a split squat stance: torso upright, slight bend in your lead leg with your shin vertical, and back leg straight. Drop your hips straight down and lower your rear knee to the floor. Driving off the heel of your front foot and the ball of your rear foot, extend your knees and raise your body back to the start position. You can hold one dumbbell to challenge your trunk stability or two dumbbells to add load to the movement.

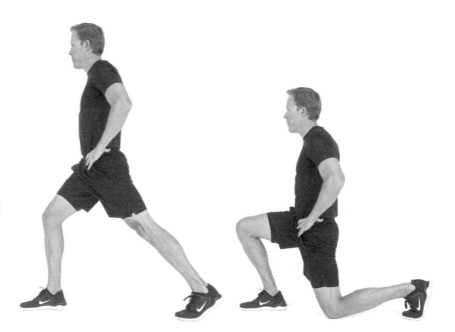

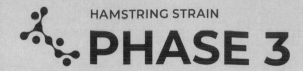

# PHASE 3

## GOOD FOR:

- Increasing hamstring strength
- Preventing hamstring pain and injury

## GUIDELINES:

- Perform 3 or 4 days a week
- Do 3 sets of 10–15 reps unless otherwise noted
- Push sets to fatigue
- Tools: bench, physio (exercise) ball, dumbbell, balance pad

## foot-elevated hamstring bridge

Lie on your back with your arms splayed out to your sides. Place your heel on the center of a bench with your knee bent just outside 90 degrees. Keeping your other leg off the bench and knee bent to about 90 degrees, drive your heel into the bench and raise your butt off the floor until you reach full hip extension. The goal is to get your knee, hip, and shoulder on the same diagonal line.

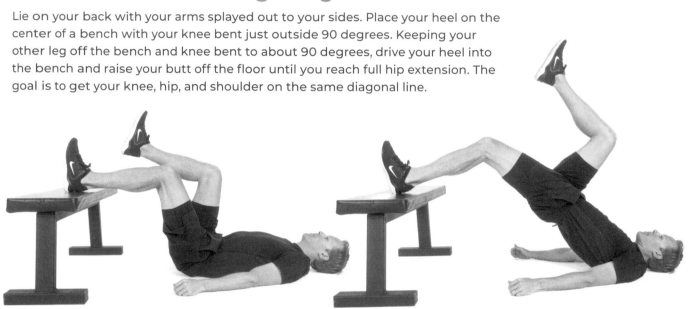

## skater squat

Stand on one leg with your unweighted knee bent and foot positioned behind your body. Keeping your torso and hips square, hinge forward from your hips, tilt your torso forward, and lower your unweighted knee toward the floor. Lower your knee to a pad to gauge distance. You can hold a light weight plate or dumbbells out in front of you to counterbalance your weight.

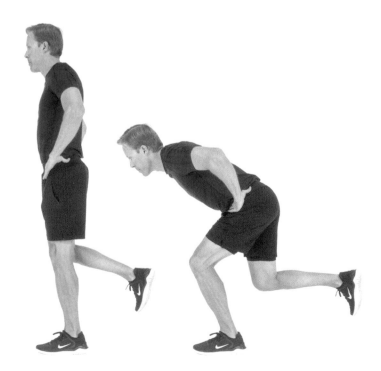

## single-leg hip thrust

Position your mid-back on the edge of the bench and lift one leg—you can either straighten it or keep it bent at about 90 degrees. Push into the floor and extend your hips. Focus on squeezing your glutes as you reach full hip extension, holding the contraction for 1–2 seconds.

## single-leg hamstring curl

Lie on your back and center your foot on a physio (exercise) ball, keeping your other leg off the ball and bent. Spread your arms slightly and keep them flush with the floor. Drive your heel into the ball and extend your hips. As you reach full hip extension, slowly curl your heel toward your butt.

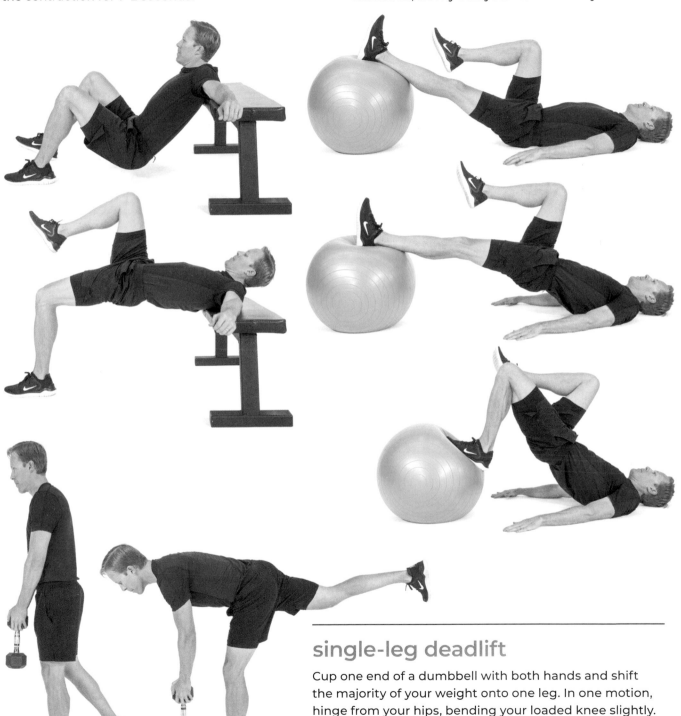

## single-leg deadlift

Cup one end of a dumbbell with both hands and shift the majority of your weight onto one leg. In one motion, hinge from your hips, bending your loaded knee slightly. As you lower your torso and the weight toward the floor, keep your back flat, grounded shin vertical, arms relaxed, and shoulders and hips square (try not to twist or rotate). Do 3 sets of 5–10 reps on each leg.

# nordic hamstring curl

Kneel on a pad and have a helper press on your heels, or use a leg curl machine to anchor your feet. If you're performing the partner-assisted variation, try to get the balls of your feet flush with the floor. Start in an upright posture with your hips fully extended and your knees bent to 90 degrees. Slowly lower your torso to the floor by extending your knees. As you do, curl your heels into the helper's hands to control the speed of your descent. You should only see movement at your knees. As you lower to the floor, use your arms to absorb the weight of your upper body while maintaining tension on your hamstrings. When you reach your breaking point, don't just fall; use your arms just enough to continue lowering with control. You should feel tension in your hamstrings during the entire eccentric phase of the movement. Push off the floor while continuing to curl your heels into the helper's hands. Use the momentum of your push combined with the power of your hamstrings to pull yourself back to the start position. Do 3 sets of 3–6 reps.

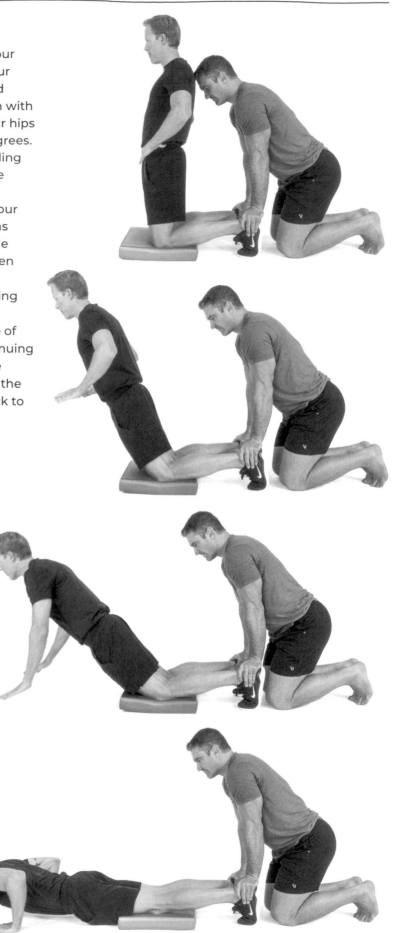

# GROIN STRAIN

**Follow this program to treat:**

- Pain on the inside of the hip and thigh
- Adductor strain (pulled groin)

**DESCRIPTION:** The hip adductors, or groin muscles, run along the inside of the thigh and are responsible for moving the hip joint from an abducted position to closer in line with the body (adduction) and stabilizing the lower extremities during activities such as standing, hopping, and propelling off one limb in a side-to-side fashion. Of the major groin muscles, adductor longus is thought to be the most commonly strained, but any of the adductors could be involved.

The most common site of injury is the musculotendinous junction (where muscle turns into tendon), as the tissue in this region is thought to be less elastic. Injuries to the adductor group are often associated with movements such as kicking, pivoting, skating, and sprinting and with sports such as hockey, gymnastics, soccer, martial arts, football, and track and field.[29,30]

**SIGNS AND SYMPTOMS:** A groin strain causes pain on the inside of the thigh that is usually felt closer to the groin rather than farther down the thigh. Pain is sharp when the muscles contract, and you may feel a dull ache when not using the muscles.

**AGGRAVATING FACTORS:** Because the groin muscles aid in hip extension and leg stabilization, pain is typically experienced with activities that require high degrees of hip stability (surfing, ice skating, running, hopping, etc.), along with stair climbing, standing from a seated position, and getting in and out of a car (especially a low one).

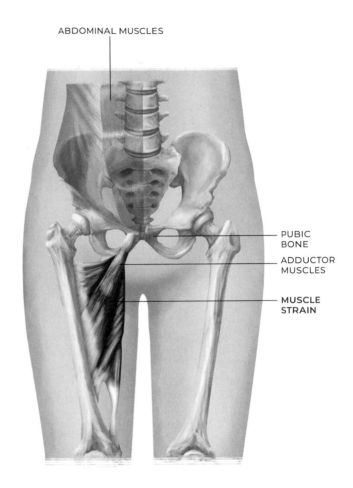

ABDOMINAL MUSCLES

PUBIC BONE

ADDUCTOR MUSCLES

MUSCLE STRAIN

## HOW DO I DIFFERENTIATE BETWEEN GROIN AND HAMSTRING STRAINS?

Determining whether you have an adductor strain or a strain of the upper hamstring can be tricky because they can create similar symptoms. You can use palpation (touch), the mechanism of injury, and the aggravating factors to make this determination.

If the pain is closer to your groin and the inside of your hip, the Groin Strain protocol on page 375 will probably be more effective. If the pain is more toward the back of your leg, you might try the Hamstring Pain protocol on page 366 first. But both protocols include exercises that will help.

**PROGNOSIS:** Healing times vary based on the severity (grade I–III) and location of the injury. Muscle strains take around three to six weeks to heal. An injury to the junction between the muscle and tendon (musculotendinous region) averages four to eight weeks. Injuries to the tendon are the slowest to heal and can take up to four months to improve fully.

**TREATMENT STRATEGY:** Adductor strains are treated with strengthening exercises that gradually load the injured muscle and/or tendon. Although stretching is sometimes useful for reducing pain, research shows that resistance training restores tissue integrity, reduces strain frequency, and helps prevent reinjury.[31,32]

In severe cases where the muscle tears completely or pulls away from the bone (avulsion), surgery may be indicated. Your adductors attach to your pubic bone, so if they tore, the consistency of that structure would break down, causing bleeding and bruising in the groin along with severe pain and weakness. These signs should prompt you to consult with a medical professional.

**1** Phase 1 focuses on reducing acute pain and includes basic hip mobility exercises (flexion, abduction, and adduction) and a bridge with an isometric adductor squeeze. Isometrics begin strengthening the injured muscles while adding force in a controlled fashion. Squeeze only as hard as you can without creating more than mild discomfort. Contracting the muscles too hard can worsen the injury and delay healing.

**2** The resistance training exercises in phase 2 gradually increase the demand on the adductor muscles. Side-lying adduction targets the adductors but only requires you to lift the weight of your leg. If this is too painful, do the other phase 2 exercises and revisit side-lying adduction in one or two weeks. If the side-lying raise is too easy, add an ankle weight. The offset side plank works the injured adductors when that leg is in the top position. Because the top leg is offset, the adductors push into the ground to help lift the pelvis. The single-leg bridge and chair squat focus on hip extension, which is important to address because some of the adductors assist the glutes with hip extension.

**3** The phase 3 exercises demand more of the adductors, helping you maximize the muscle group's strength and integrity. The wider stance of the sumo squat recruits the groin muscles. The split squat works on hip extension but is harder than the chair squat because the legs are separated. The lateral lunge and lateral step-up also work hip extension, but the movement of the hip away from the body (abduction) requires the adductors to contract to stabilize the hip joint and pull the body over the stance leg. The Copenhagen or adductor plank is the most challenging groin exercise but is one of the best for strengthening these muscles and reducing your chances of straining them again.[33,34] Start with the short lever option. If you can do it easily and without pain, move on to the long lever variation.

As with other types of strains, add the phase 2 and 3 exercises to your regular training program after your injury has healed to keep the muscles and tendon healthy.

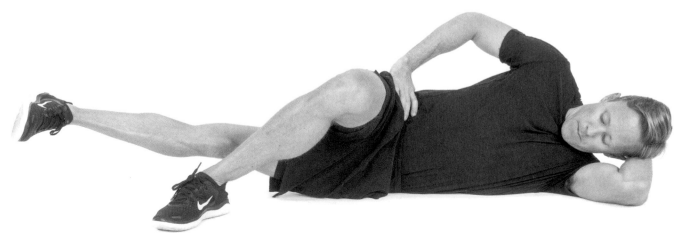

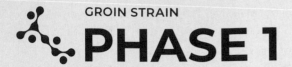

# GROIN STRAIN
# PHASE 1

### GOOD FOR:

- Alleviating groin pain
- Improving neuromuscular control
- Warm-up for phase 2 and 3 exercises

### GUIDELINES:

- Perform every day
- Do 3 sets of 10–15 reps
- Tools: dowel, sports ball
- Add phase 2 when you have no pain at rest and no more than mild pain (3/10) with the exercises

## hip flexion

Stand with your feet straight and positioned underneath your hips. Raise one knee as high as you can without assistance. As you reach end range, cup your hands around the front of your knee and pull it toward your chest. Pause at end range for 2–3 seconds.

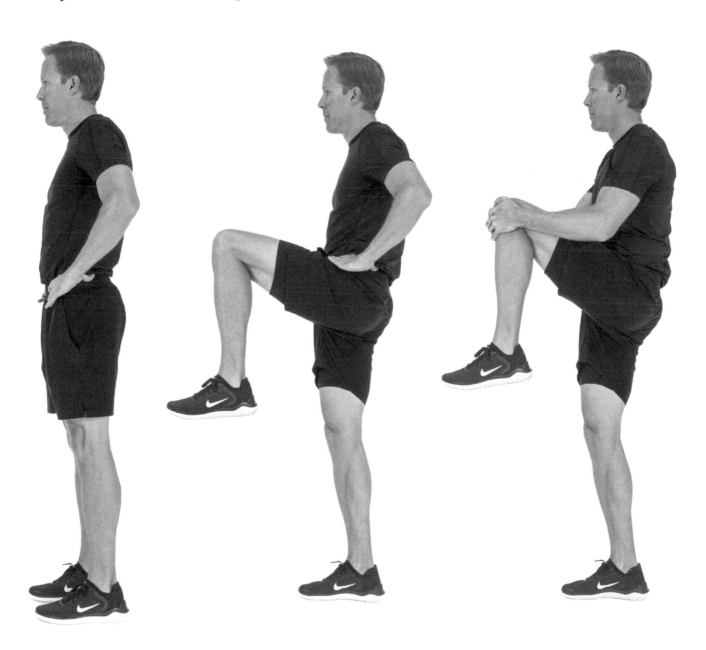

# hip abduction

Using a dowel for balance, shift your weight onto one leg, then use your hip and glute muscles to raise your unweighted leg to the side (abduction). Try not to lean excessively or rotate your foot. In other words, stay fairly upright and keep your moving foot facing forward.

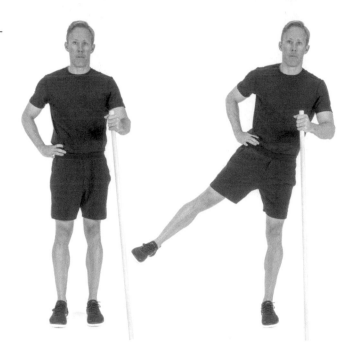

# hip adduction

Shift your weight onto one leg, then use your adductor muscles to move your unweighted leg across your body.

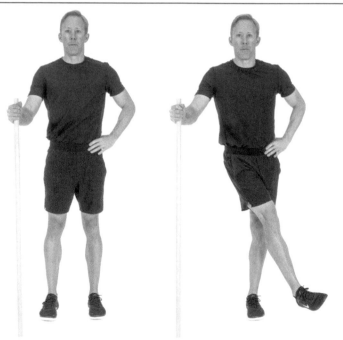

# bridge with adduction

Position a volleyball, soccer ball, or basketball between your knees. Perform a bridge—drive your heels into the floor and extend your hips—while squeezing your knees into the ball and contracting your glutes. Maintain pressure on the ball throughout the entire range of motion.

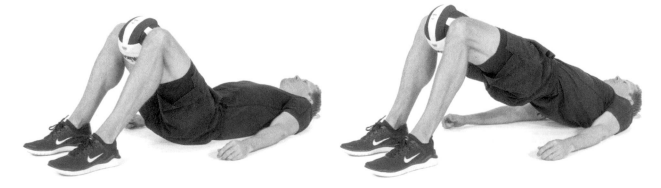

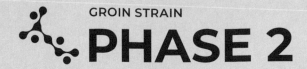

## GROIN STRAIN
# PHASE 2

**GOOD FOR:**

- Reducing groin pain
- Early adductor/groin strengthening
- Warm-up for phase 3 exercises

**GUIDELINES:**

- Perform 3 or 4 days a week
- Do 3 sets of 10–15 reps unless otherwise noted
- Add phase 3 when you can do the exercises with no more than mild pain (3/10)

---

## side-lying adduction

Lie on your side and cross your top leg over your bottom leg. Keeping your knee extended, lift your bottom foot straight up. Hold the top position for 1–2 seconds.

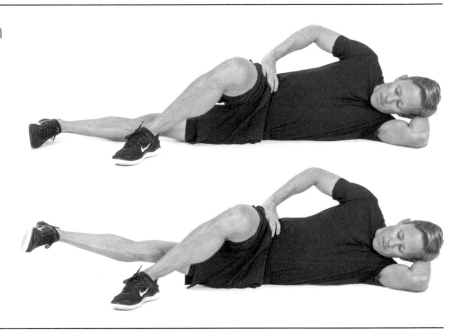

---

## side plank offset

Position your elbow underneath your shoulder to elevate your upper body and cross your top leg over your bottom leg. Driving your top leg into the floor, use your trunk and adductor muscles to lift your hips. Do 3 reps with 20- to 30-second holds.

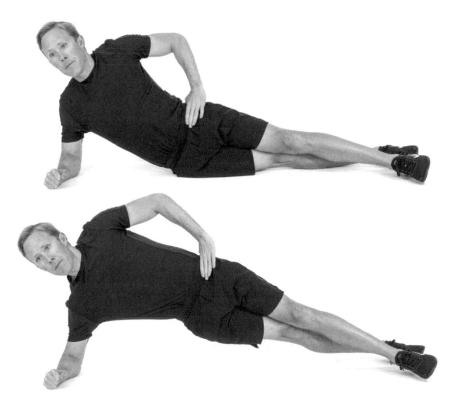

## single-leg bridge

Get into the bridge start position and elevate one leg—you can either straighten it or keep it bent at about 90 degrees. Push into the floor and extend your hips. Focus on squeezing your glutes as you reach full hip extension, holding the contraction for 1–2 seconds. Add a resistance loop above your knees or do a single-leg hip thrust (page 371) to make the exercise more challenging.

## chair squat

Stand in front of a chair or box with your feet roughly shoulder width apart. When it comes to foot flare, you can orient your feet straight or turn them out slightly—whichever feels better. To perform the movement, extend your arms in front of you to counterbalance your weight, reach your hips back slightly, and sit straight down. As you lower into the bottom position, keep your spine in the neutral zone (not excessively arching or rounding) and your knees aligned over your toes.

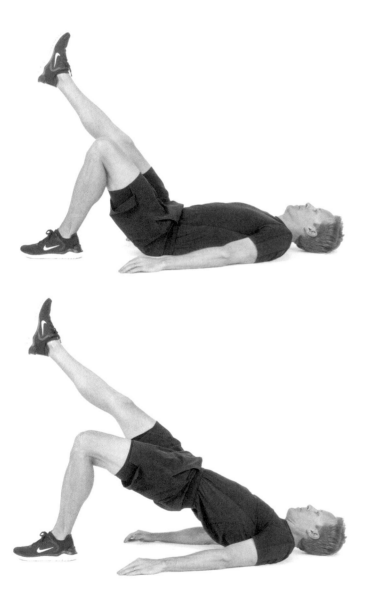

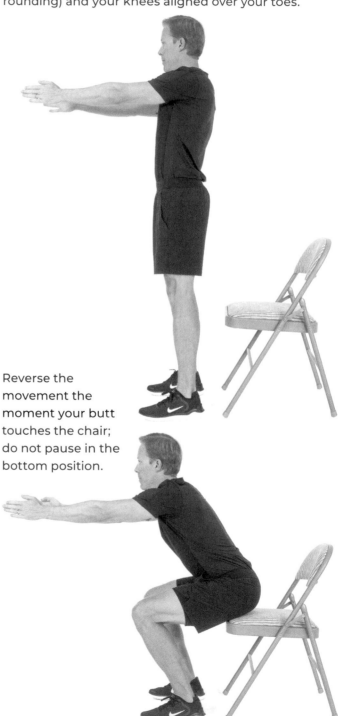

Reverse the movement the moment your butt touches the chair; do not pause in the bottom position.

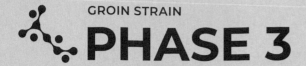
**GOOD FOR:**

- Increasing groin and lower body strength
- Preventing groin pain and injury

**GUIDELINES:**

- Perform 3 or 4 days a week
- Do 3 sets of 10–15 reps
- Push sets to fatigue
- Tools: dumbbell, plyo box, balance pad, bench

## sumo squat

Holding one end of a dumbbell in front of your body, position your feet outside shoulder width, and turn your toes out to about 45 degrees. Keeping your torso upright and arms relaxed, sit your hips back and down, lowering the dumbbell to the floor. Push through your heels and extend your hips and knees simultaneously into the top position.

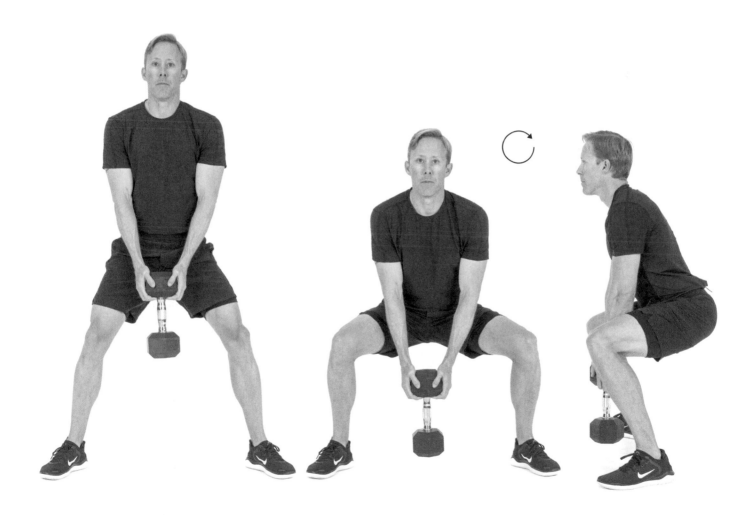

# split squat

Get into a split squat stance: torso upright, slight bend in your lead leg with your shin vertical, and back leg straight. Drop your hips straight down and lower your rear knee to the floor. Driving off the heel of your front foot and the ball of your rear foot, extend your knees and raise your body back to the start position. You can hold one dumbbell to challenge your trunk stability or two dumbbells to add load to the movement.

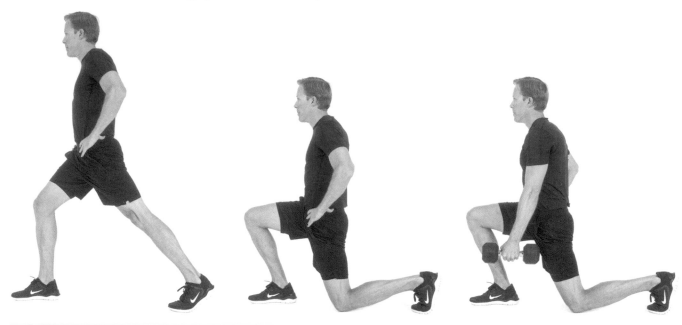

# lateral lunge

Stand with your feet positioned underneath your hips. Take a large lateral step so that your feet are positioned outside your shoulders. As your foot touches down, shift your weight over that foot, hinge from your hips, and tilt your torso forward slightly. Keeping your opposite leg straight and your hips and shoulders square, bend your knee and lower your hips. Keep your bent knee positioned over or just outside your foot; don't let it cave inward. You can extend your arms in front of you to counterbalance your weight. Push off your mid-foot while extending your hips and knee simultaneously, returning to the start position.

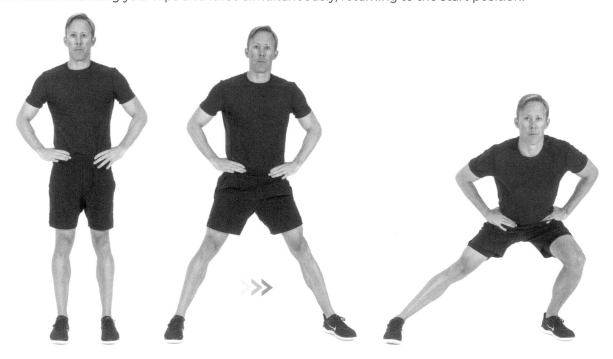

# lateral step-up

Stand next to a plyo box. Step onto the box, positioning your entire foot on the surface. Your feet should be roughly shoulder width apart. Shifting your weight onto your elevated leg, extend your hips and knee in one fluid motion. Don't push off the floor with your supporting leg. Increase the height of the box to make the exercise more challenging. The taller the box, the more you have to lean forward and at an angle over your elevated foot. You can extend your arms in front of you to counterbalance your weight.

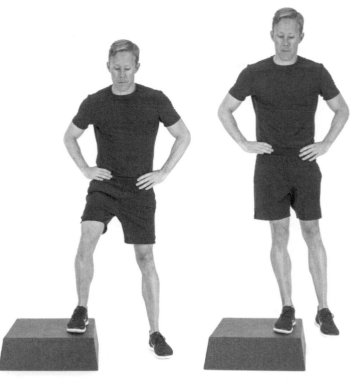

# adductor raise *(choose one)*

Try the short lever variation first, and if it's too easy, do the long lever variation. To set up for the short lever adductor raise, place a balance pad on a bench, then lie on your side and hook your top leg over the pad. Bend your knee slightly so that the inside of your shin is flush with the pad. Raise your bottom leg off the floor, then bring your bottom knee toward your top knee, using your adductor muscles to lift your hips. The long lever variation works the same muscles, but your top leg is straight and you drive your ankle and inside of your foot into the bench as you bring your legs together.

### short lever                    ### long lever

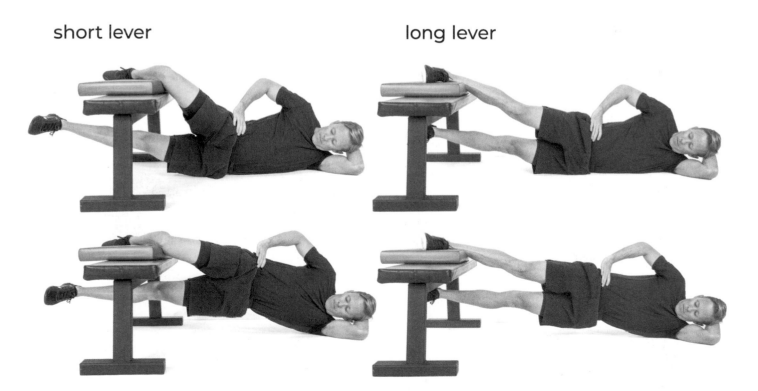

## CHAPTER 21

# KNEE
# PROTOCOLS

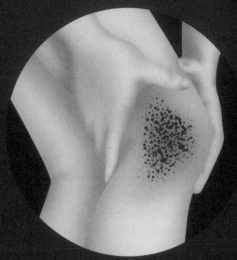

**KNEE PAIN**
(p. 383)

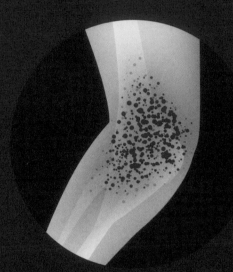

**KNEE INSTABILITY**
(p. 393)

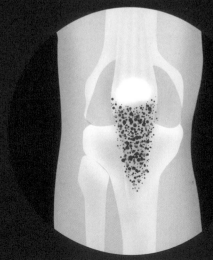

**PATELLAR TENDINOPATHY**
(p. 408)

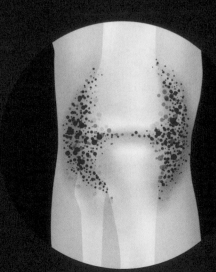

**OSTEOARTHRITIS**
(p. 418)

# KNEE PAIN

**Follow this program to treat:**

- General knee pain
- Patellofemoral joint pain (pain around the front of the knee or behind the kneecap)
- Iliotibial (IT) band syndrome (pain on the outside of the thigh just above the knee)

## PATELLOFEMORAL JOINT PAIN

**DESCRIPTION:** The patellofemoral joint is a synovial joint that involves an interaction between the kneecap (patella) and a groove on the femur. Essentially, the patella slides through the femoral groove as the knee moves through flexion and extension, which is why we used to think that kneecap pain was related to a tracking problem where the kneecap wasn't moving through the groove appropriately. While mechanical issues like poor patellar tracking contribute to pain in some cases, we now know that patellofemoral pain is more complicated and can be influenced by nonmechanical variables like our psychological and emotional states.[1]

Patellofemoral joint pain syndrome (PFPS) is a common condition that produces pain behind the kneecap.

Similar to patellar tendinopathy (see page 408), PFPS pain is typically brought on by activities that involve a lot of running (especially in heel strikers, who place more load on their quads and knees), jumping, and squatting. And although it's not inherently harmful, movements that require the knees to move forward over the toes (lunges, front squats, high-bar back squats, hiking downhill, walking down stairs, etc.) might amplify the condition because they compress the patellofemoral joint, placing extra stress on the area.

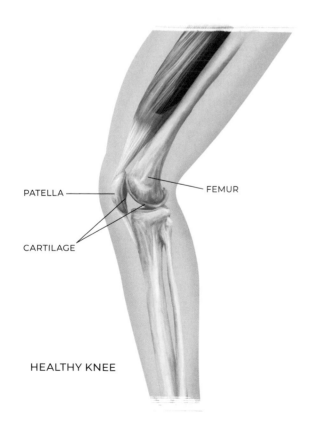

PATELLA

FEMUR

CARTILAGE

HEALTHY KNEE

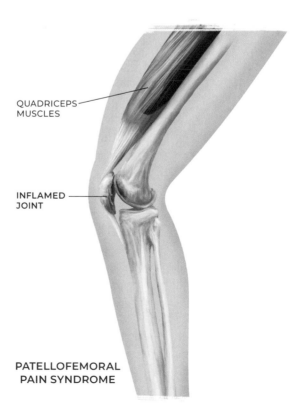

QUADRICEPS MUSCLES

INFLAMED JOINT

PATELLOFEMORAL PAIN SYNDROME

For most people, PFPS is a temporary irritation caused by overuse and inflammation. However, it can be associated with a gradual deterioration of cartilage (chondromalacia patellae) on the back of the kneecap. This is considered an arthritic condition. While a diagnosis of chondromalacia patellae might sound intimidating, you still treat it with the same exercises outlined in this protocol.

The best way to prevent arthritis—and the pain associated with PFPS—is to address aggravating factors, increase hip and knee strength, and avoid activities that place more load or volume on the joint than it is conditioned to handle.[2]

**SIGNS AND SYMPTOMS:** Pain is located behind the kneecap and is typically sharp. Because the pain stems from the joint behind the kneecap, touching the soft tissue in the region usually does not reproduce symptoms.

**AGGRAVATING FACTORS:** PFPS is aggravated with activities that compress and place increased stress on the joint, such as squatting, walking up and down stairs, sitting for long periods, running (especially in heel strikers), and cycling.

**PROGNOSIS:** PFPS typically improves within four to six weeks when aggravating activities are modified and rehab exercises that strengthen the hip and knee are implemented.

**TREATMENT STRATEGY:** PFPS is treated exclusively with physical therapy, which focuses on strengthening the kinetic chain (the joints and tissues that work together to assist the knee) and improving neuromuscular control with aggravating activities (running, squatting, etc.). The temporary use of orthotics for individuals with increased foot pronation and patellofemoral joint taping can be helpful in some cases.[2] Applying ice, taking anti-inflammatory medication, and refraining from aggravating activities all tend to reduce pain.

In phase 1, you use soft tissue mobilizations and stretches to reduce pain on the front of the knee. Mobilizing and stretching the muscles surrounding the knee (especially the quads) is thought to reduce pain by temporarily altering the stresses being applied to the joint and giving sensitive structures a break.

Because the phase 1 strategies typically create temporary changes in symptoms, you follow them with sensorimotor control and strengthening exercises in phases 2 and 3. One of the best first steps to combat patellofemoral pain is to strengthen your gluteal muscles, especially your abductors and external rotators. Strengthening these muscles and learning to control the hip joint and femur can reduce knee pain, as the femur makes up half of the hip joint and half of the knee joint. Because the hip is a ball-and-socket joint, poor control can increase stress on knee structures such as the patellofemoral joint. So, many of the exercises target these muscles (side-lying hip abduction, single-leg bridge, fire hydrant, and lateral squat walk).

After focusing on the hip, you add exercises that strengthen your knee muscles, especially your quads. However, high-volume and heavy quad training is associated with patellofemoral pain, so you start with exercises that limit the compressive loads applied to the joint. For instance, the lateral step-up, reverse lunge, split squat, and skater squat all strengthen the quads and glutes without putting high stress on the patellofemoral joint. While the knees-over-toes training concept has become popular recently, those types of exercises can make patellofemoral joint pain worse. When the knee moves past the toes, patellofemoral joint contact forces go up, which can create more pain if your knee isn't ready for it. These exercises aren't off-limits forever, but you want to start with the ones outlined in this program, and, once your symptoms have resolved, you can consider integrating more stressful quadriceps and patellofemoral joint exercises such as forward lunges, pistol squats, and front squats.

## SHOULD I BE WORRIED ABOUT CLICKING AND POPPING (CREPITUS) BEHIND MY KNEECAP?

In most cases, no. Healthy joints often make noise, and there is no research to suggest that noise indicates pathology will develop in the future.[3] If your knee makes a sound when you squat, that's usually your kneecap. If the clicking and popping—called crepitus—come with pain, it would be wise to look further into the issue. The rehab exercises included in this protocol will help build neuromuscular control (the connection between your nervous system and muscles) and strengthen your hips and knees, both of which can reduce crepitus and the pain associated with it.

# ILIOTIBIAL (IT) BAND SYNDROME

**DESCRIPTION:** The iliotibial (IT) band is a dense, fibrous band of connective tissue that runs along the lateral (outer) thigh from the hip to the knee. It is one of the primary causes of lateral knee pain in runners.[4]

Although several factors can contribute to IT band syndrome, such as anatomy, exercise volume, and mechanics, it's believed that repetitive compression of the fat pad and/or bursa under the IT band leads to inflammation and pain.[5,6] While the fat pad and bursa are designed to accommodate compressive forces, high-volume loading (such as high-mileage running) or loading that is unfamiliar (a new sport or activity) can spark an inflammatory response. The situation can be further amplified when a runner's foot lands with an inward (valgus) or outward (varus) deviation from neutral.

To prevent and treat this condition, it's important to look at three potential causes: mechanics (neuromuscular control), hip and knee strength, and training volume.

In most cases, you address a mechanical issue by strengthening the hip and knee using the exercises within this protocol, experimenting with new footwear that improves your form, and paying more attention to technique—squatting with your knees aligned over your feet or patterning a neutral knee landing, for example.

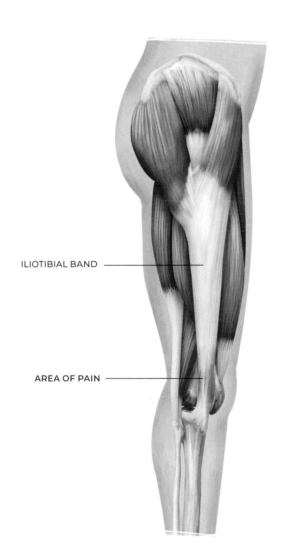

ILIOTIBIAL BAND

AREA OF PAIN

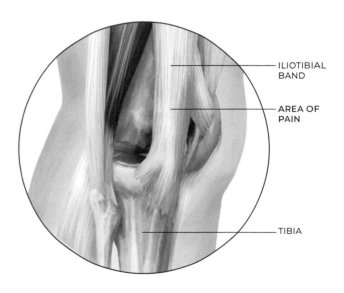

ILIOTIBIAL BAND

AREA OF PAIN

TIBIA

However, some people move their knee inward or outward away from neutral and have no knee issues. In these cases, their tissues have likely developed the capacity to handle the forces being placed on them, and they don't need to alter their movement patterns. If you do have pain and notice that your knee deviates from neutral, it's probably worth trying to change that tendency. Again, how you move is the tip of the iceberg when it comes to pain management and prevention.

The best strategies for preventing and treating most connective tissue conditions are strength training and program design (managing training volume). Even if it's a mechanical issue that you can't correct—which shouldn't be perceived as a negative or a dysfunction—you can still benefit from strengthening your hips and knees with exercise because it will improve the capacity of your tissues.

What's more, IT band syndrome is a connective tissue disorder, like patellar or Achilles tendinopathy, which means pain is usually caused by overuse—you did more than your tissues are conditioned to handle. Because this condition mainly affects runners, it's important to address the mileage you're putting on your body. Remember to increase volume gradually and give your tissues time to adapt. Combine intelligent program design with rehab exercises that target the IT band and the muscles to which it attaches, and you have a template for alleviating pain, moving better, and improving performance.

**SIGNS AND SYMPTOMS:** IT band syndrome typically produces sharp pain on the outside of the knee during activities like running. Some people also experience a popping or snapping sensation. IT band syndrome can sometimes hurt higher, such as at the hip, but it is most common in the knee.

**AGGRAVATING FACTORS:** High-volume running, running downhill or on uneven terrain, starting a new running program, and squatting are commonly associated with this type of pain.

**PROGNOSIS:** In most cases, IT band syndrome improves within four to six weeks when aggravating activities are modified and rehab exercises that strengthen the hip and knee are implemented.

**TREATMENT STRATEGY:** You treat IT band syndrome by managing the stress on the tissue, which means reducing running volume, temporarily running on flat surfaces, and potentially trying running shoes or orthotics that limit foot pronation and promote a more neutral knee alignment. It's also important to strengthen the gluteus medius and minimus and knee muscles and address neutral knee alignment mechanics during functional tasks.

**1** Addressing IT band syndrome is similar to addressing patellofemoral joint pain. Phase 1 mobilizes and stretches the quads and calf, which can reduce pain by temporarily altering the stresses applied to the lateral knee.

**2 3** Once your pain is under control, you use the exercises in phases 2 and 3 to improve hip and knee strength and movement control. The hip strengthening exercises, which include side-lying abduction, lateral squat walk, and fire hydrant, target the abductors (gluteus medius and minimus) and external rotators. These muscles help you control the hip joint and femur, which translates down the kinetic chain to better knee control. The lateral step-up, split squat, skater squat, reverse lunge, and other strengthening exercises combine quadriceps and gluteal strengthening movements, which again build tissue capacity and control. Focus on your movements and do not allow your knee to move in or out, which is associated with the development of IT band syndrome.

# PHASE 1

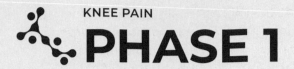

**GOOD FOR:**

- Alleviating knee pain
- Relieving muscle tension above and below the knee
- Warm-up for phase 2 and 3 exercises

**GUIDELINES:**

- Perform every day
- Tools: foam roller, slant board
- Add phase 2 when you have no pain at rest and no more than mild pain (3/10) with the exercises

## SOFT TISSUE MOBILIZATIONS:

- ▸ Spend 1–2 minutes on each area
- ▸ Perform in any order on both sides
- ▸ Stop on tender points for 10–20 seconds

### quad mobilization

Lie facedown with your weight supported on your forearms or hands and one leg positioned over a foam roller with your toes pointed toward the floor. Supporting your weight with your grounded foot and arms, roll up and down to mobilize the entire quadriceps muscles on the front of your thigh—from hip to knee. Bend and straighten your knee to dynamically mobilize the muscles and femoral nerve.

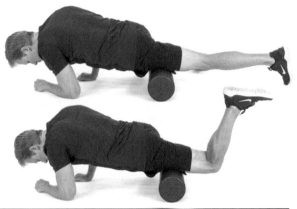

### lateral quad mobilization

The setup and execution are the same here: use your arms and grounded foot to control the pressure, roll up and down the entire thigh (from hip to knee), and stop on tender or stiff spots and bend and straighten your leg. But instead of mobilizing the front of your thigh, you target the lateral quadriceps along the outside of your leg.

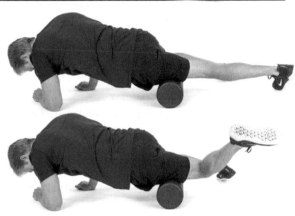

### calf mobilization

Sit on the floor with your calf positioned over a foam roller. Push off the floor with your hands and grounded foot—lifting your hips off the floor—to roll up and down your lower leg from ankle to knee.

Stop on any tender or stiff spots and move your foot (flex, extend, and rotate from side to side).

To increase the pressure, stack your other leg on top.

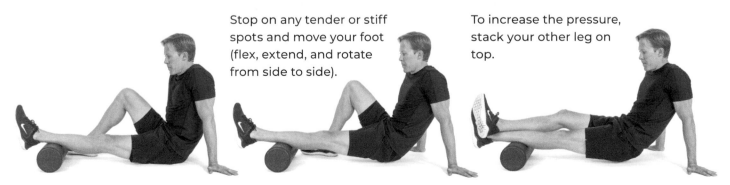

# STRETCHING EXERCISES:

## quad stretch
*(choose one)*

### standing

Grab your ankle and use your arm to bend your knee until you feel a stretch along the front of your thigh. Keep your posture upright and your knee vertical to maximize the stretch.

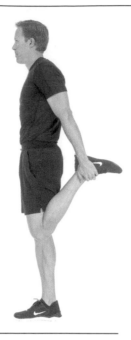

### side-lying

You can do the same stretch while lying on your side. Make sure your leg is in line with (not in front of) your body or pulled slightly back (hip extension) to maximize the stretch.

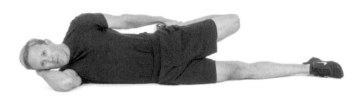

## side-bend stretch/ lateral flexion stretch

Cross one leg in front of the other. Reach up with the same-side arm. Without bending your spine forward or backward, lean away from your crossed leg until you feel a stretch along the side of your body.

## standing calf stretch

Stand with the ball of your foot on a slant board, incline, or elevated surface. Step your other foot in front of the leg you are stretching. You should feel a stretch through your calf and back of your ankle. To target your soleus muscle, sit your hips back, tilt your torso forward, and bend your knee.

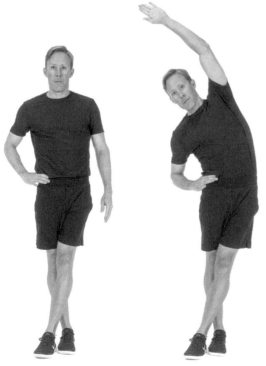

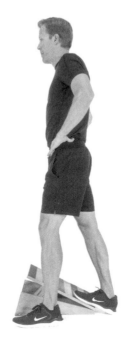

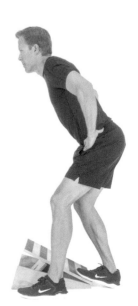

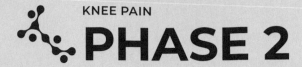

## KNEE PAIN
# PHASE 2

### GOOD FOR:

- Reducing knee pain
- Early knee and hip strengthening
- Warm-up for phase 3 exercises

### GUIDELINES:

- Perform 3 or 4 days a week
- Do 3 sets of 10–15 reps unless otherwise noted
- Tools: resistance loop, plyo box
- Add phase 3 when you can do the exercises with no more than mild pain (3/10)

## side-lying hip abduction

Lie on your side, rotate your hips toward the floor slightly, and internally rotate your top leg so that your big toe is angled toward the arch of your bottom foot. Lift your top leg at a backward angle. Keep your spine neutral and pause in the top position for 1–2 seconds. Reduce the range of motion if you start to arch your back excessively. Add a resistance loop above your knees to increase glute activation and make the exercise more challenging.

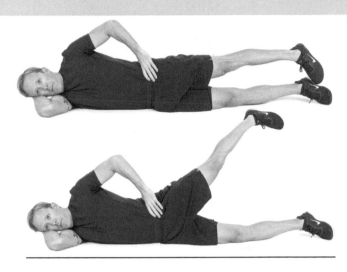

## single-leg bridge

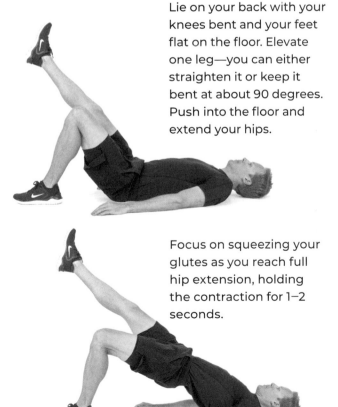

Lie on your back with your knees bent and your feet flat on the floor. Elevate one leg—you can either straighten it or keep it bent at about 90 degrees. Push into the floor and extend your hips.

Focus on squeezing your glutes as you reach full hip extension, holding the contraction for 1–2 seconds.

## lateral squat walk

Wrap a resistance loop above your ankles. Position your feet shoulder width apart and bend your hips and knees slightly. Take a wide lateral step so there is a full stretch in the band. You can either walk along a line and then switch after a given number of steps or stay in one area and switch back and forth between legs. Choose a distance or rep range that is challenging—usually 15–20 steps in each direction. Don't pause between steps, and keep tension in the band during the entire movement.

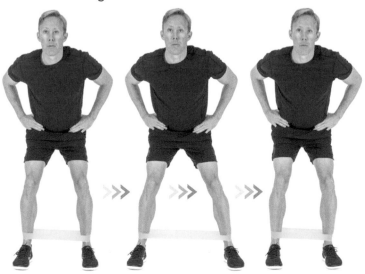

# banded squat

With the resistance loop above your knees, stand with your feet roughly shoulder width apart. When it comes to foot flare, you can orient your feet straight or turn them out slightly—whichever feels better and allows you to reach the lowest depth without discomfort. To perform the movement, reach your hips back slightly and sit straight down. As you lower into the bottom position, drive your knees outward into the band, keeping your spine in the neutral zone (not excessively arching or rounding) and your knees aligned over your toes. Lower as far as you can while maintaining good form.

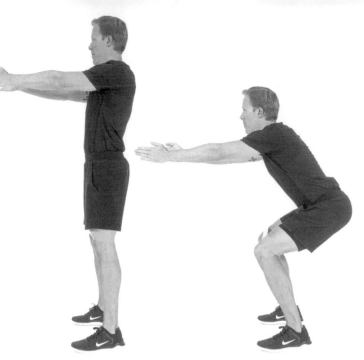

# lateral step-up

Stand next to a plyo box. Step onto the box, positioning your entire foot on the box. Your feet should be roughly shoulder width apart. Shifting your weight onto your elevated leg, extend your hips and knee in one fluid motion. Don't push off the floor with your supporting leg. Increase the height of the box to make the exercise more challenging. The taller the box, the more you have to lean forward and at an angle over your elevated foot. You can extend your arms in front of you to counterbalance your weight.

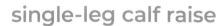

# single-leg calf raise

Stand with the ball of one foot on an elevated surface or step. Perform slow calf raises through the full range of motion. Your heel should drop slightly lower than your toes on the down phase.

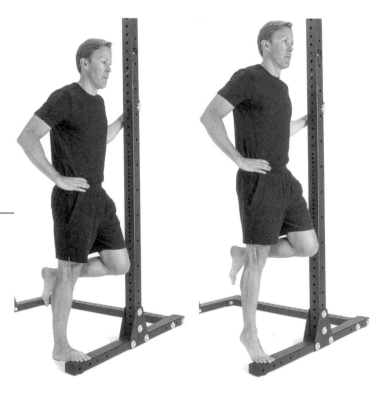

# PHASE 3

## GOOD FOR:

- Strengthening the knees, legs, and hips
- Preventing knee pain and injury

## GUIDELINES:

- Perform 3 or 4 days a week
- Do 3 sets of 10–15 reps
- Push sets to fatigue
- Tools: resistance loop, physio (exercise) ball, dumbbells, plyo box

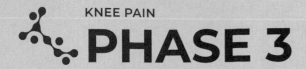

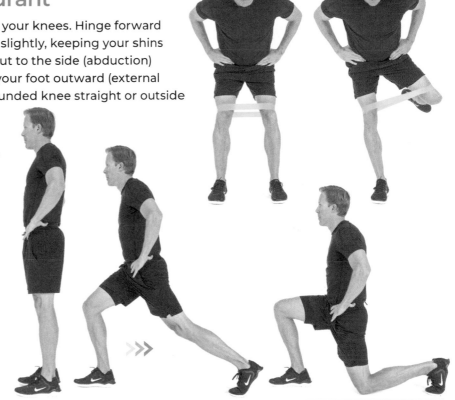

## standing banded hydrant

Position a resistance loop just above your knees. Hinge forward from your hips and bend your knees slightly, keeping your shins vertical. In one motion, lift your leg out to the side (abduction) and back (extension) while rotating your foot outward (external rotation). Focus on keeping your grounded knee straight or outside your foot; don't let it cave inward.

## reverse lunge

Stand with your legs together. Step back with one leg and slowly lower your knee to the floor, keeping your torso upright or leaning slightly forward. Your step back should be large enough that your front shin is approximately vertical. Keep the majority of your weight on your front leg and be careful not to slam your kneecap into the floor as you lower into the bottom position.

## ball hamstring curl

Lie on your back and center your feet on a physio (exercise) ball. Spread your arms slightly and keep them flush with the floor. Drive your heels into the ball and extend your hips. As you reach full hip extension, slowly curl your heels toward your butt.

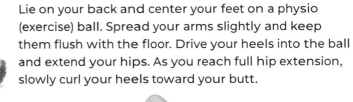

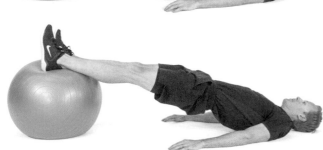

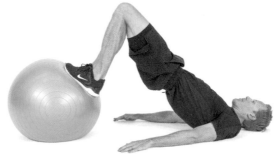

## split squat

Get into a split squat stance: torso upright, slight bend in your lead leg with your shin vertical, and back leg straight. Drop your hips straight down and lower your rear knee to the floor. Driving off the heel of your front foot and the ball of your rear foot (between your arch and your toes), extend your knees and raise your body back to the start position.

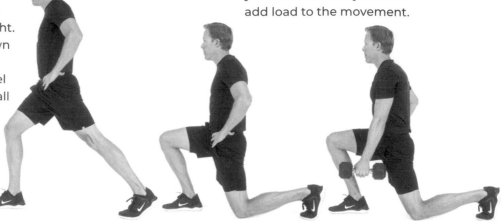

You can hold one dumbbell to challenge your trunk stability or two dumbbells to add load to the movement.

## skater squat

Stand on one leg with your unweighted knee bent and foot positioned behind your body. Keeping your torso and hips square, hinge forward from your hips, tilt your torso forward, and lower your unweighted knee toward the floor. Lower your knee to a pad to gauge distance. You can hold a light weight plate or dumbbells out in front of you to counterbalance your weight.

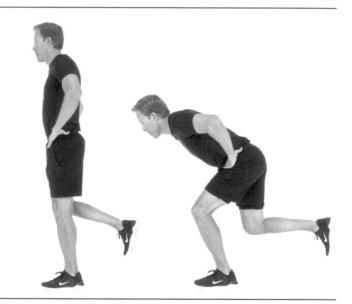

## lateral step-down

Stand next to a plyo box or small step. Perform a lateral step-up by placing your entire foot on the edge of the box and standing tall. Move your free leg forward slightly. Keeping your free leg straight, reach your heel toward the floor by slowly sitting back and bending your grounded knee. As soon as your heel contacts the floor, straighten your knee, extend your hips, and return to the start position. Keep your knee aligned over your foot; don't let it move in or out.

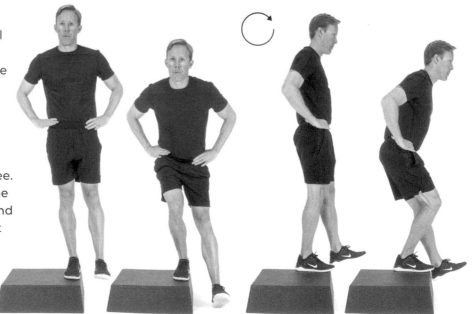

# KNEE INSTABILITY

**Follow this program to treat:**

- Knee that feels like it's going to give out or buckle
- Meniscus tear (limited knee range of motion with catching/locking, instability, and pain when standing and twisting on the injured leg)
- Ligament tear (ACL, PCL, MCL, LCL)
- Kneecap dislocation

## MENISCUS TEAR

**DESCRIPTION:** The menisci are C-shaped fibrocartilaginous structures that sit between the femur (thigh bone) and tibia (shin bone) and serve as the knee's primary shock absorbers. In addition to optimizing force transmission through the knee, they help stabilize the joint, with the medial meniscus acting as a secondary stabilizer of the anterior cruciate ligament (ACL). Meniscus tears can be degenerative or traumatic and typically involve twisting on a leg that is planted (imagine a soccer player planting and cutting to run across the field, for example). However, degenerative tears, which are more frequent in middle adulthood, can occur with simple activities that impart lower forces on the tissue, like twisting awkwardly when getting out of a car or playing a recreational sport such as tennis.

Many people have degenerative meniscus tears but don't experience pain or disruptions in functional ability.[7,8] In other cases, the symptoms are cyclical, like arthritis, which is why they are often associated with osteoarthritis of the knee. If you have frequent flare-ups and functional tasks become limited due to pain, your doctor might recommend surgery.

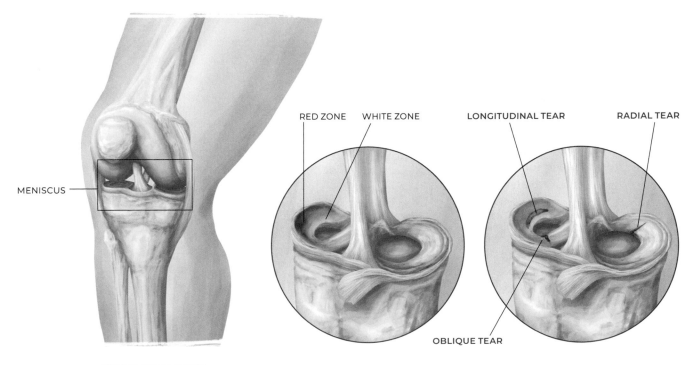

MENISCUS

RED ZONE    WHITE ZONE

LONGITUDINAL TEAR    RADIAL TEAR

OBLIQUE TEAR

RIGHT KNEE JOINT

## WHEN SHOULD I CONSIDER SURGERY?

Whether you should get surgery largely depends on your age, lifestyle, functional ability, pain symptoms, the grade of the injury, and where the tear is located. For instance, if you feel pain every time you squat and have mechanical symptoms such as locking—your knee catches or sticks when you try to bend it—then surgery is generally recommended. What's more, a younger athlete with a tear in the central part of the meniscus that's blocking knee motion—and interfering with your sport— is a good candidate for surgery because that area of the meniscus is unlikely to heal on its own. However, if you have a degenerative or less severe traumatic tear where you still have stability in your knee and full range of motion, you should focus on conservative treatment, including anti-inflammatory medication, physical therapy, and corticosteroid or hyaluronic injections.[9,10] Only if that fails, meaning your pain is reoccurring and function is limited beyond three months, should you explore surgical intervention.

**SIGNS AND SYMPTOMS:** Meniscus tears typically produce joint swelling (effusion) and sharp or aching pain when bending, straightening, or twisting. In more severe cases, people experience limited knee range of motion with catching/locking and instability or a feeling that the knee will give way or buckle. Many also report hearing or feeling a pop when the meniscus tears.

**AGGRAVATING FACTORS:** Standing on the affected leg and twisting or trying to move the knee through its full range of motion, such as when squatting, commonly reproduce pain. Prolonged sitting and standing may increase pain and swelling in the joint.

**PROGNOSIS:** Meniscus healing and recovery depends somewhat on your symptoms, the severity of the injury, and the location of the tear. The periphery (outer third) of the meniscus possesses a better blood supply and has a better chance of healing. The central two-thirds of the meniscus is not as well vascularized and may not heal well due to poor circulation. The bottom line is that not all meniscus tears are created equal. If the periphery of the meniscus is torn and you do not demonstrate instability or locking of the joint, symptoms often improve significantly within two to three months. If the tear is in the central two-thirds of the meniscus, rehab can improve pain and function, but you have a higher likelihood of needing surgical intervention to get the knee back to full function.

**TREATMENT STRATEGY:** Research suggests that most meniscus tears—specifically degenerative and less severe traumatic tears—should be addressed with rehab first.[11] Surgery should be reserved for younger individuals and athletes who have severe pain or tears that interfere with joint movement and function. In most cases, symptoms improve after six to 12 weeks of rehab when you modify or eliminate aggravating factors.

However, people often skip rehab and go straight to a doctor. The doctor orders an MRI—which shows a tear—and immediately recommends surgery. However, in most cases, surgery is not necessary. Are you active, and is the injury interfering with your functional tasks? Do you have a traumatic meniscus tear that limits function? Did you try 12 weeks of therapy, but pain and functional issues persist? If you answer "yes" to any of these questions, then surgery might be a good option.

The protocol does not include soft tissue mobilization or stretching techniques. These things are not off-limits, but you want to focus on restoring joint range of motion (as in the heel slide exercise) and then on boosting the strength and stability of the knee. Because the quadriceps muscles on the front of the thigh (knee extensors) are arguably the most important for knee joint stability, numerous exercises target this group, including the quad isometric, short arc quad, squats, knee

## WHAT ARE THE DIFFERENT TYPES OF SURGICAL INTERVENTIONS FOR MENISCUS INJURIES?

The most common type is meniscectomy, which is an arthroscopic surgery that involves cleaning up a tear. The tear could be getting between the tibia and femur and obstructing movement or causing pain, so the surgeon cleans that up without cutting you open or giving you stitches. With this procedure, you can put weight on the knee right away, and you're back to normal activity within a few weeks. A lot of people do well with meniscectomies, but because it is a lighter surgery, you may not be referred to a physical therapist, in which case this protocol can serve as your rehab after surgery. The major downside to the meniscectomy is that it has been shown to be associated with early development of knee osteoarthritis.[10-13] The surgeon cuts out part of the meniscus (the primary shock absorber of the knee), which means more force is transferred to the underlying cartilage, resulting in deterioration of that tissue.

Meniscus repair is a reconstructive surgery reserved for more severe traumatic tears. This procedure usually involves putting stitches in the part of the meniscus that has good blood flow, and you are on crutches for six weeks afterward. In this scenario, work with your assigned PT and follow the program that is designed for you. Once you finish with that protocol, you can either continue following it or use phase 3 of this protocol to maintain optimal strength and function.

extensions, and step-up. The glutes are important for controlling the femur, which makes up one half of the hip and knee joints, so the side-lying abduction, single-leg bridge, banded hydrant, and skater squat work those muscles. Additionally, I've included exercises like the ball hamstring curl and single-leg deadlift because the hamstrings, which are your primary knee flexors, also help stabilize the knee joint.

With the standing exercises, focus on sensorimotor control, which means moving slowly and thinking about the alignment of your leg so that your knee is not moving from side to side or in a jerky fashion. For instance, in the lateral step-down and clock exercises, take your time and pay attention to moving with precision. This type of training maximizes neuromuscular function and aids recovery.

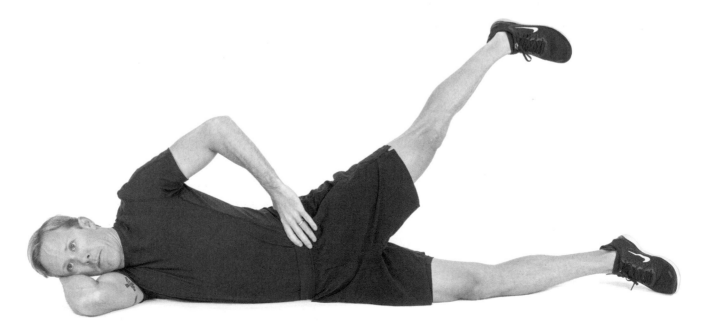

# LIGAMENT TEAR (ACL, PCL, MCL, LCL)

**DESCRIPTION:** Ligaments are connective tissues that hold bones together and keep joints stable. Two cruciate ligaments (anterior and posterior) are located in the center of the knee joint, and two collateral ligaments are located on the inside (medial) and outside (lateral) of the knee. Together, these ligaments help hold the femur (thigh bone) to the tibia and fibula (shin bones) and play a key role in maintaining joint stability. The anterior cruciate ligament (ACL) controls rotation and forward motion of the tibia. The posterior cruciate ligament (PCL) controls backward movement of the tibia. The medial collateral ligament (MCL) provides stability by resisting extreme inward or valgus motion. The lateral collateral ligament (LCL) provides stability by resisting extreme outward or varus motion.

These ligaments can be stretched or torn when the knee is forced to move in unnatural ways—usually extreme sideways, oblique, and/or rotational motions.

ACL and MCL tears tend to result from dynamic valgus knee movements. Imagine that the foot is planted and the knee caves inward (valgus) either from a hit or a twisting motion. As the knee caves, the tissue on the inside of the knee is stretched, which can tear or rupture the MCL. Add rotation, and that is how the ACL is typically injured.[14-16]

LCL tears usually happen due to varus stress, where the foot is planted and the knee bows outward, which stretches (and can rupture) the ligament on the outside of the knee. This scenario is less common and typically occurs during a football tackle or a traumatic impact to the joint.

The most common mechanism of injury for PCL tears is a fall on a bent knee. You often see these in athletes (football, rugby, basketball) who fall forward onto their knees or during car accidents when the knees hit the dashboard.

**SIGNS AND SYMPTOMS:** Knee ligament injuries typically produce joint swelling (effusion), pain, and, in many cases, a feeling of instability where the joint gives way or slips when weight is put on the leg. Individuals who suffer ligament tears usually report a popping sound at the time of injury and have difficulty moving the knee through its full range of motion.

Isolated MCL and LCL tears are often clearer because they're on the inside or outside of the knee and touching the area reproduces pain. With ACL and PCL tears, which are internal, pain often occurs on the back of the knee but can be diffuse and deep, making the injury difficult to pinpoint.

Feeling like you don't have control—feeling unstable, as if your leg might give out when you put weight on it—is a sign that is specific to ligament tears. It doesn't have to be a complicated or demanding movement—you might experience instability when standing on one leg, walking down stairs, or stepping out to catch yourself.

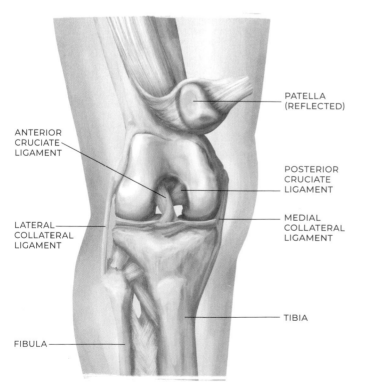

ANTERIOR CRUCIATE LIGAMENT

PATELLA (REFLECTED)

POSTERIOR CRUCIATE LIGAMENT

LATERAL COLLATERAL LIGAMENT

MEDIAL COLLATERAL LIGAMENT

TIBIA

FIBULA

## HOW MUCH INSTABILITY IS ACCEPTABLE?

Some degrees of instability are manageable, and some are not. The hallmark sign is whether you had a trauma involving a pop where it felt as though your knee gave way, and now you have not just pain but also a feeling that your knee is going to slip or come apart with certain positions and movements. This is more common with grade III tears, which often require surgery. With a grade I or II tear, you will have some tissue stability, meaning things still feel "attached" and you can typically control movement through a full range of motion (albeit with a little pain). These milder tears often don't require surgery and will heal with the appropriate treatment strategy and activity modifications.

**AGGRAVATING FACTORS:** Activities like standing on one leg (especially when twisting or pivoting), squatting, lunging, climbing stairs, running, and jumping are typically associated with pain and feelings of joint instability.

**PROGNOSIS:** Some ligament ruptures can be treated successfully with rehab that focuses on building muscle strength and improving neuromuscular control. After implementing these interventions, you should see significant changes within three to four months. If you continue to experience pain and episodes of instability, surgical reconstruction may be necessary.

**TREATMENT STRATEGY:** Isolated injuries of the LCL and MCL are predominantly treated with rehab exercises. How an ACL or PCL injury is treated depends on how it affects function.[17] Some people with ligament tears do not require surgery and can maintain joint stability by implementing strength and neuromuscular control exercises.[18] For others, the knee continues to give way, and they must undergo surgical ligament reconstruction to prevent further damage.

## WHEN SHOULD I SEEK MEDICAL ATTENTION?

If you have instability—for example, when you stand, your knee feels like it's going to slip apart or buckle—get it checked by a doctor to determine how much damage was done and whether surgery is recommended.

## HOW DO DOCTORS DETERMINE THE LOCATION AND GRADE OF THE INJURY?

Imaging such as an MRI is the best way to determine the location and grade of the injury. However, a clinician, orthopedic surgeon, or physical therapist might perform other common tests. For example, practitioners commonly use a stress test to differentiate between varus and valgus tears. To test for an MCL or LCL tear, the practitioner holds your lower leg and pushes your foot to either the inside or the outside. If it's torn, they will be able to separate the femur and tibia on either the inside or the outside. The bones will come apart and then snap back together.

For the ACL, there's a drawer test. The ACL keeps the tibia from sliding forward, so people who have ACL tears can see their tibia shift forward when they pull on it.

Both ligament and meniscus tears create pain and instability in the knee joint and affect passive subsystems (ligaments and cartilage), so rehab has many of the same objectives. In the beginning of rehab, you should focus on reducing any swelling that is present and restoring knee joint range of motion.[19] You can relieve pain and swelling by elevating the leg, applying a compression sleeve, and using ice and anti-inflammatory medication. After pain and swelling are under control and joint mobility is full, your attention should shift to maximizing muscle strength and joint stability via neuromuscular control exercises such as the squat, leg extension, step-up, lateral step-down, ball curl, and skater squat. When a passive subsystem element like a ligament is damaged, you must make up for this loss of stability with the active subsystem (muscles and nerves) through specific movements and exercises.

With all the standing exercises, focus on neuromuscular control by moving slowly and thinking about the alignment of your leg so that your knee does not move from side to side or in a jerky fashion. For example, in the lateral step-down and clock exercises, take your time and pay attention to moving with precision. This type of training maximizes neuromuscular function, aids recovery, and reduces future injury risk.

**NOTE:** This protocol is not intended for individuals who have undergone ligament reconstruction surgery. In that case, it is important to see a physical therapist who can evaluate your knee and guide you through the rehabilitation process, as this type of rehab is specialized and differs from person to person based on the severity of the injury and surgical intervention.

## SHOULD I GET SURGERY?

As with all surgical interventions, you must consider a myriad of factors before deciding whether to have surgery. What is the extent of the injury (for example, is more than one ligament torn)? Is it completely torn and unstable or partially torn and somewhat stable? How is the injury impacting your life? How long do you have to heal? And although you can regain stability by doing rehab, will you regain enough to function at the level you want? These are just a few of the types of questions you must ask yourself.

There are people with grade III tears who don't need surgery, and some of them are high-level athletes. That's why you need to base your decision on the kinds of tasks you need to be able to do, how stable you feel with those tasks, and how much time you can spend healing. Everyone's situation is different, and rehab for this type of injury can take time, even with surgery.

If you have an MCL or LCL tear, you can probably handle it with strengthening exercises. If you've torn your PCL or ACL, you might start with the strengthening, but if it isn't improving after a couple of months, reconstruction surgery might make sense. Or you may decide to get surgery right away because you have zero stability and you want to return to action as quickly as possible.

## WHAT TYPE OF SURGERY IS TYPICALLY PERFORMED, AND HOW LONG IS THE RECOVERY?

It depends—again—on the extent of the injury. For a torn ligament, reconstructive surgery is generally recommended. In this scenario, the surgeon takes some of your tissue, such as a piece of your patellar or semitendinosus (hamstring) tendon, and reconnects the ligament by anchoring it back on the bone.

Most athletes are advised not to return to sports for nine to 12 months after reconstructive surgery and rehab.[20] If they return sooner, the risk of reinjury is much higher—although, again, it depends on the grade of the tear and their function. If you don't have surgery, the timeline may be somewhat shorter, as surgery can come with deconditioning and other negative side effects, but you risk going through all the rehab, still having instability, and then deciding you need surgery anyway. It can be a tough choice for young athletes because they don't know if stability will return with just rehab.

# KNEECAP DISLOCATION

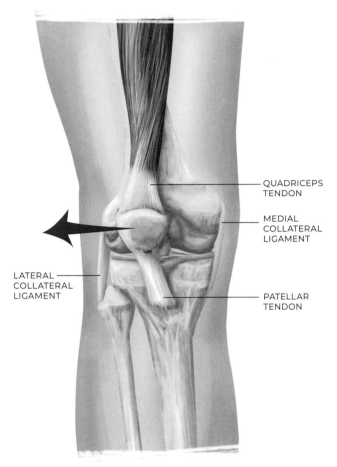

**PATELLA DISPLACED**

Labels on image:
- QUADRICEPS TENDON
- MEDIAL COLLATERAL LIGAMENT
- PATELLAR TENDON
- LATERAL COLLATERAL LIGAMENT

**DESCRIPTION:** The kneecap, or patella, slides through a groove in the femur (thigh bone) during movement, but certain injuries can force it out of this groove. Kneecap dislocations are fairly uncommon, occurring in only 2 to 3 percent of the population.[21] They're more often seen in adolescent female athletes and are typically associated with trauma or planting the foot and then suddenly changing direction, such as pivoting or landing hard on one leg. In most cases, the medial patellofemoral ligament is disrupted, which allows the patella to shift laterally from its normal resting position between the femoral condyles.

**SIGNS AND SYMPTOMS:** Kneecap dislocations typically produce an audible pop followed by intense, sharp pain. The knee swells, and bearing weight is usually difficult. After the joint moves back to its original position, dull, achy pain is often present.

**AGGRAVATING FACTORS:** Movements that stress the patellofemoral joint, such as pivoting, jumping, squatting, and running.

**PROGNOSIS:** For first-time kneecap dislocations, the prognosis is good, especially if you focus on glute and quadriceps strengthening.[22] You should feel significantly better after six to eight weeks of rehab. If you have dislocated the kneecap many times (chronic patellar instability), the prognosis becomes worse, and surgery is often required to prevent future dislocations.

**TREATMENT STRATEGY:** First-time dislocations should be managed with physical therapy, but re-dislocation rates following conservative care range from 15 to 44 percent.[21] When the cartilage or underlying bone is injured or dislocations recur, surgical intervention is often warranted to restabilize the joint.

In rehab, the knee is immobilized for six weeks with a cast or range of motion brace. Following this period of immobilization, you begin doing exercises designed to restore range of motion, improve motor control, and increase quad, hamstring, and hip strength.

Patellofemoral dislocations create joint instability, which is why I've lumped them in with meniscus and ligament tears. This protocol first walks you through regaining knee mobility and motor control in phase 1. Then it shifts to more challenging exercises in phases 2 and 3 that help build strength and neuromuscular control, which will ultimately result in improved knee stability.

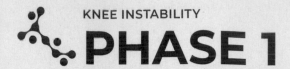

## KNEE INSTABILITY
# PHASE 1

### GOOD FOR:

- Alleviating knee pain
- Improving knee stability and neuromuscular control
- Warm-up for phase 2 and 3 exercises

### GUIDELINES:

- Perform every day
- Do 3 sets of 10–15 reps unless otherwise noted
- Tools: stretch strap, foam roller
- Add phase 2 when range of motion is greater than 90 degrees (see finish position in heel slide exercise)

---

## heel slide *(choose one)*

Hook a strap around your foot. Bend your knee and slide your heel toward your butt, pulling on the strap to assist with the movement. If you don't feel pain, perform the movement without the strap and go as far as you can with no more than mild pain.

### with strap

### without strap

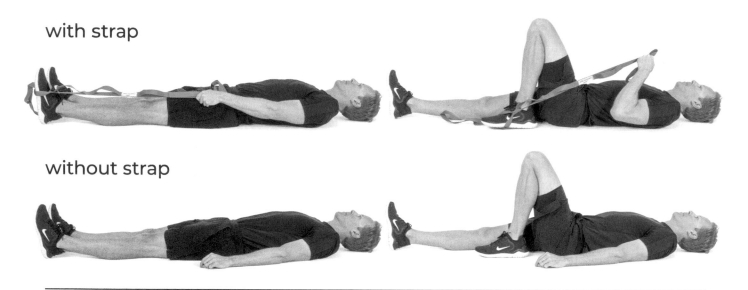

---

## quad isometrics

Sit with one leg straight. Squeeze your quadriceps muscles (think about straightening your knee as you engage your quads). As you squeeze, you should see your kneecap pull up slightly. Hold the contraction for 10 seconds and repeat 10 times.

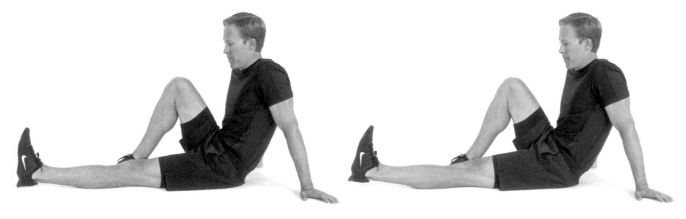

## short arc quad

Position a foam roller under your knee. Straighten your leg by squeezing your quadriceps. Focus your attention on the working muscles. Move slowly and with control. Hold the contraction for 1–2 seconds.

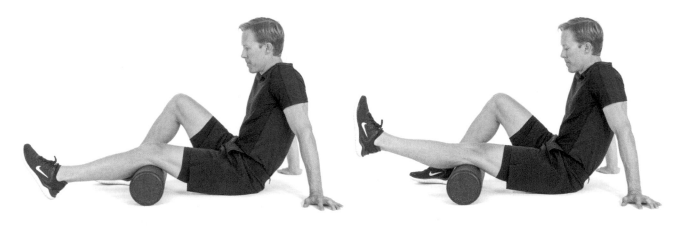

## supine straight-leg raise

Lie on your back with one leg bent, which will help keep you from arching through the low back. Keeping your knee locked, slowly raise your straight leg to just above your opposite knee, then lower it to the floor.

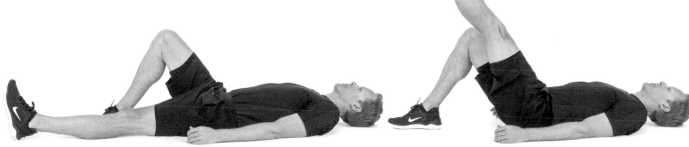

## side-lying hip abduction

Lie on your side, rotate your hips toward the floor slightly, and internally rotate your top leg so that your big toe is angled toward the arch of your bottom foot. Lift your top leg up and at a backward angle. Keep your spine neutral and pause in the top position for 1–2 seconds. Reduce the range of motion if you start to arch your back excessively. Add a resistance loop above your knees to increase glute activation and make the exercise more challenging.

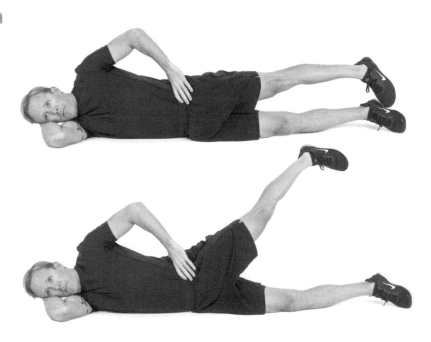

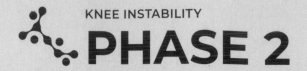

# PHASE 2

## GOOD FOR:

- Reducing knee pain
- Improving knee stability and neuromuscular control
- Early knee and hip strengthening
- Warm-up for phase 3 exercises

## GUIDELINES:

- Perform 3 or 4 days a week
- Do 3 sets of 10–15 reps unless otherwise noted
- Tools: resistance loop, physio (exercise) ball, plyo box, dumbbells
- Add phase 3 once you have full knee range of motion and can do the exercises without pain or instability

## banded squat

Place a resistance loop above your knees and stand with your feet roughly shoulder width apart. When it comes to foot flare, you can orient your feet straight or turn them out slightly—whichever feels better and allows you to reach the lowest depth without discomfort. To perform the movement, reach your hips back slightly and sit straight down. As you lower into the bottom position, drive your knees outward into the band, keeping your spine in the neutral zone (not excessively arching or rounding) and your knees aligned over your toes. Lower as far as you can while maintaining good form.

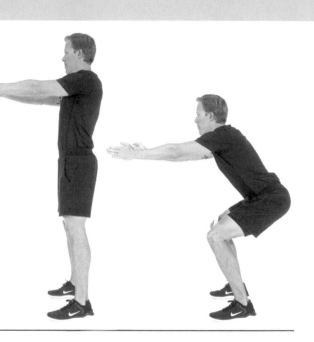

## knee extension

Sit on a bench or chair with your hips and knees bent to roughly 90 degrees. Slowly extend one knee by flexing your quadriceps muscles. Move with control and try to reach full knee extension with your leg straight. Hold the contraction for 1–2 seconds.

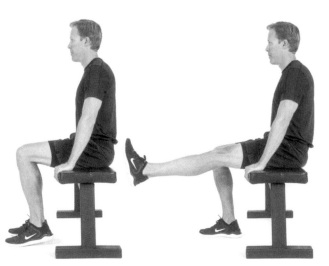

## single-leg bridge

Lie on your back with your knees bent and your feet flat on the floor.

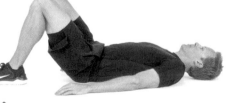

Elevate one leg—you can either straighten it or keep it bent at about 90 degrees. Push into the floor and extend your hips. Focus on squeezing your glutes as you reach full hip extension, holding the contraction for 1–2 seconds.

# ball hamstring curl

Lie on your back and center your feet on a physio (exercise) ball. Spread your arms slightly and keep them flush with the floor. Drive your heels into the ball and extend your hips. As you reach full hip extension, slowly curl your heels toward your butt.

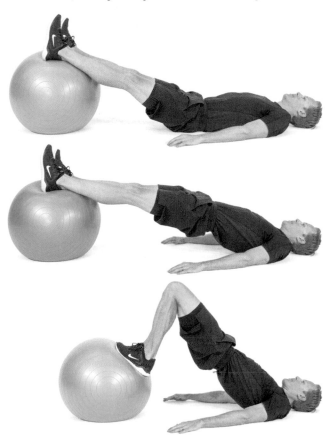

# split squat

Get into a split squat stance: torso upright, slight bend in your lead leg with your shin vertical, and back leg straight. Drop your hips straight down and lower your rear knee to the floor. Driving off the heel of your front foot and the ball of your rear foot, extend your knees and raise your body back to the start position. You can hold one dumbbell to challenge your trunk stability or two dumbbells to add load to the movement.

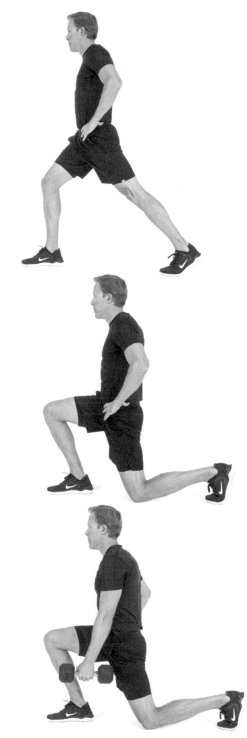

# step-up

Step on a plyo box with your knee aligned over your foot. Without pushing off the floor, shift your weight onto your elevated leg, drive through your heel or mid-foot, and raise your torso and hips in one fluid motion. Progress this exercise by increasing the height of the box or holding a dumbbell.

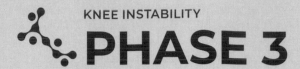

KNEE INSTABILITY

# PHASE 3

## GOOD FOR:

- Increasing knee and leg strength
- Preventing knee pain and injury

## GUIDELINES:

- Perform 3 or 4 days a week for 8–12 weeks, or until you have regained stability
- Do 3 sets of 10–15 reps unless otherwise noted
- Push sets to fatigue
- Tools: resistance loop, bench, dumbbell, plyo box

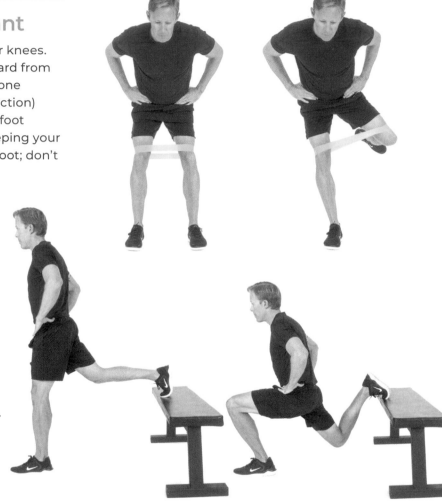

## standing banded hydrant

Position a resistance loop just above your knees. Bend your knees slightly and hinge forward from your hips, keeping your shins vertical. In one motion, lift your leg out to the side (abduction) and back (extension) while rotating your foot outward (external rotation). Focus on keeping your grounded knee straight or outside your foot; don't let it cave inward.

## bulgarian split squat

Stand about 2 feet in front of a bench. Reach back with one leg and place the ball of your foot on the bench. Keeping the majority of your weight over your front leg, lower your body slowly—sinking your hips down and back at an angle—until your front thigh is roughly parallel to the floor. Keep your back leg mostly relaxed; don't push off the bench.

## single-leg deadlift

Cup one end of a dumbbell with both hands and shift the majority of your weight onto one leg. In one motion, hinge from your hips and bend your loaded knee slightly. As you lower your torso and the weight toward the floor, keep your back flat, grounded shin vertical, arms relaxed, and shoulders and hips square (try not to twist or rotate). Do 3 sets of 5–10 reps on each leg.

# lateral step-down

Stand next to a plyo box or small step. Perform a lateral step-up by placing your entire foot on the edge of the box and standing tall. Move your free leg forward slightly. Keeping your free leg straight, reach your heel toward the floor by slowly sitting back and bending your grounded knee. As soon as your heel contacts the floor, straighten your knee, extend your hips, and return to the start position. Keep your knee aligned over your foot; don't let it move in or out.

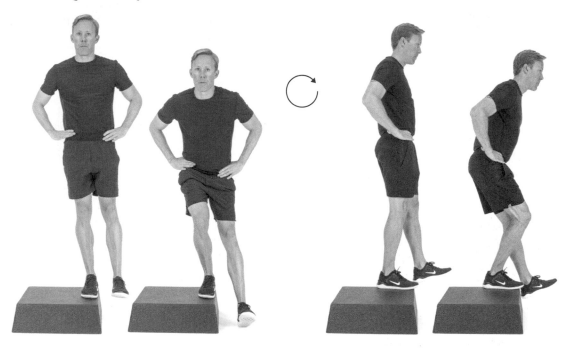

# clock

Stand with your feet positioned underneath your hips. Shift your weight onto one leg. Sink your hips back and bend your grounded knee, then reach out to the positions of an imaginary clock with the other leg. Start at 12 o'clock and work through each hour position—returning to the start position after every step—until you reach 6 o'clock. Each leg will work through one half of the clock, which counts as one rep.

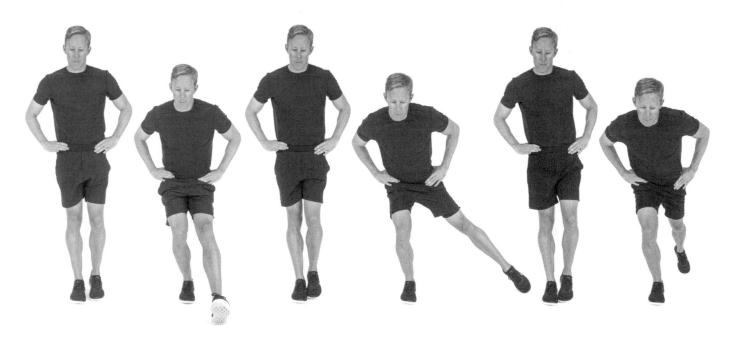

## skater squat

Stand on one leg with your unweighted knee bent and foot positioned behind your body. Keeping your torso and hips square, hinge forward from your hips, tilt your torso forward, and lower your unweighted knee toward the floor. Lower your knee to a pad to gauge distance. You can hold a light weight plate or dumbbells out in front of you to counterbalance your weight.

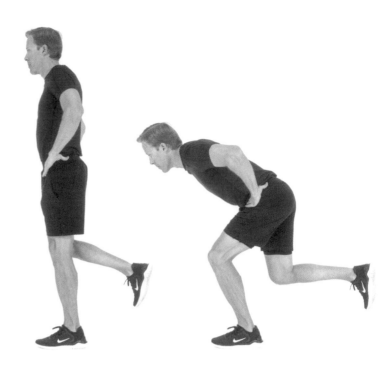

## single-leg hamstring curl

Lie on your back and center one foot on a physio (exercise) ball—keeping your other leg off the ball and bent. Spread your arms slightly and keep them flush with the floor. Drive your heel into the ball and extend your hips. As you reach full hip extension, slowly curl your heel toward your butt.

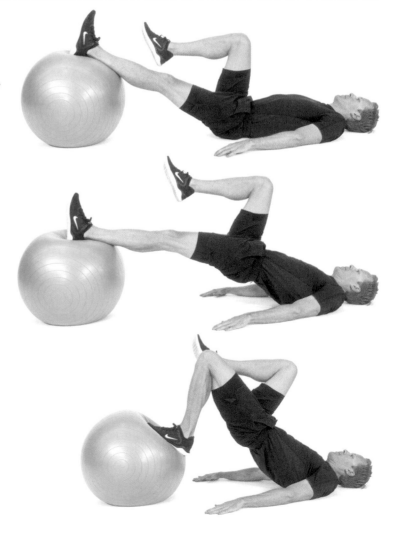

## tiptoe walk

You can perform this exercise with or without dumbbells. Try the bodyweight variation first, then add dumbbells if it's too easy. Start by getting into a half squat: hinge from your hips, tilt your torso forward, and bend your knees. Get onto the balls of your feet and take small steps. Keep your knees over your toes and your heels off the floor. Choose a distance or rep range that is challenging—usually 15–20 steps.

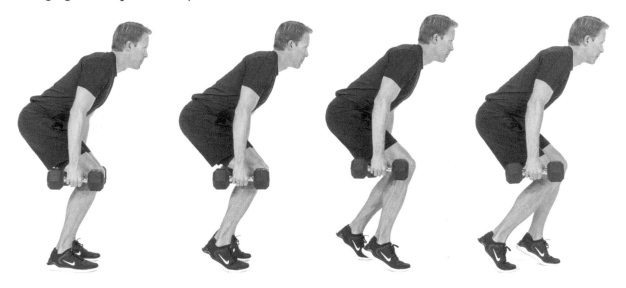

## bilateral jump to unilateral landing

Stand with your feet just inside shoulder width. Lower into a half squat and pull your elbows back. In one motion, extend your hips and knees, swing your arms forward, and jump vertically. While in the air, pull one leg back and prepare to land on one leg. Cushion your landing by bending your knee and hinging forward. Try to land with your knee aligned over your toes; don't let your knee or ankle collapse inward. Spread your arms to maintain balance. Do 3 sets of 6–12 reps (jumps).

**Only do this exercise if your knee stability is very high and you need to be able to perform jumping movements in daily life.**

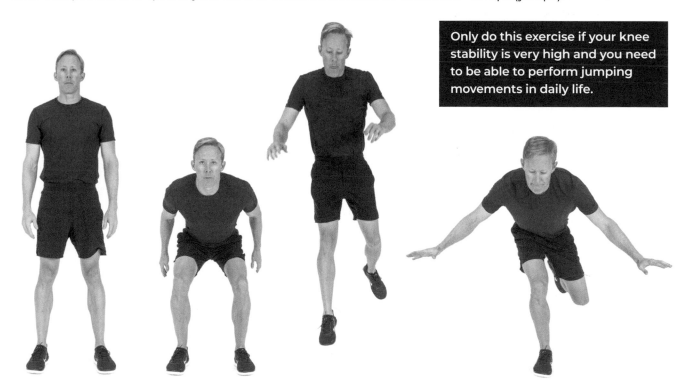

# PATELLAR TENDINOPATHY

**Follow this program to treat:**

- Jumper's knee
- Quadriceps tendinopathy
- Pain below or above the kneecap

DESCRIPTION: Patellar tendinopathy, or "jumper's knee," describes a condition in which the tendon that attaches the quadriceps muscles to the front of the shin becomes irritated—usually from doing a lot of jumping.

When you jump, your quadriceps contract forcefully, placing tension on the patellar tendon. As with most tendinopathies, pain manifests when your tissues are not conditioned to handle the load or volume of movement. That could mean doing something every day that builds up stress over time or doing more than you normally would in a short period.

Although jumping is a common cause of patellar tendinopathy, any activity that causes the quads to contract repeatedly—say, squatting, hiking downhill, or walking down stairs—can irritate the tendon, leading to an overuse or repetitive stress injury.

## DOES MOVING YOUR KNEES FORWARD OVER YOUR FEET CONTRIBUTE TO THIS PROBLEM?

Moving your knees forward over your toes is a common pattern when jumping, squatting, and lunging. While it can contribute to knee pain, it is not necessarily the cause. Again, it depends on how much stress you're putting on the tissue and what it's conditioned to handle. When your knees move over your toes, the eccentric load places constant tension on the patellar tendon because your quads must contract to slow and control the movement. But the movement is not inherently wrong or harmful. In fact, it's a requirement to maintain balance whenever you flex your hips while your torso remains upright, such as walking downhill or down stairs, vertical jumping, or upright squatting (high bar back squat or front squat). Do too much and the tendon can get irritated. If you're already in pain, recognize that the knees-over-toes movement pattern is a potential aggravating factor that may need to be modified in the beginning of rehab.

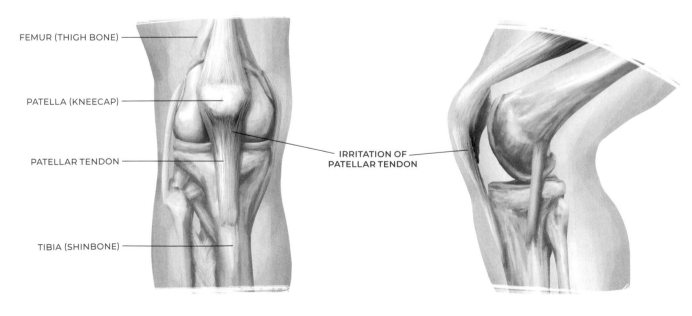

FEMUR (THIGH BONE)

PATELLA (KNEECAP)

PATELLAR TENDON

TIBIA (SHINBONE)

IRRITATION OF PATELLAR TENDON

**SIGNS AND SYMPTOMS:** Pain is typically sharp, and the knee may ache and throb at rest following aggravating activities. Patellar tendon pain usually occurs between the bottom point of the kneecap (inferior pole) and the spot where the tendon attaches to the front of the shin (tibial tuberosity) but can also be present above the kneecap.

**AGGRAVATING FACTORS:** Activities that require forceful contractions of the quadriceps, including jumping, squatting, lunging, climbing/descending stairs, hiking downhill, and running.

**PROGNOSIS:** Most cases resolve within eight to 12 weeks when you follow the rehab protocol and modify or temporarily eliminate aggravating activities.

**TREATMENT STRATEGY:** You treat patellar tendinopathy with exercises that improve tendon strength and capacity.[23,24] You may need to modify the volume and intensity of aggravating activities to give the tendon the opportunity to recover. Ease pain in the acute phase with a couple of days of rest and easy mobility work. You can use a patellar tendon strap, but this should be a very temporary strategy, as chronic use can lead to tendon deconditioning. A corticosteroid injection may reduce pain in more resistant cases, but because these medications weaken tendons, you should avoid them if possible.

Phase 1 of the protocol implements strategies to control acute pain. The soft tissue mobilization of the quadriceps can help since the patellar tendon attaches to those muscles. Most people with this issue do not have limited range of motion, so the heel slide is used as a general pain reducer. The knee extension isometric can reduce tendon pain when held for 30 to 45 seconds and begins to rebuild tendon strength and capacity. Phase 1 finishes with several hip/gluteal exercises to improve hip strength and promote knee health.

Phases 2 and 3 focus on hip and graded quadriceps/patellar tendon loading. Phase 2 includes lower-load quad exercises such as the isometric wall sit, front plank reach, tiptoe walk, and eccentric bench squat. Once isometric contractions have calmed tendon pain, you start eccentric contractions (where the muscle is contracting and lengthening at the same time). With a bench squat, this is the down part of the motion, so you do this phase of the movement on one leg only and do the concentric (up) portion with two legs. As you get stronger and your tendon can tolerate more loading, try performing the entire range of motion (down and up) on one leg. Phase 3 combines single-leg exercises that target the hip, hamstrings, and quads. The decline squat is one of the best for targeting the quads and patellar tendon. Phase 3 finishes with hopping movements, which help with the tendon's energy storage and release capacities. Non-athletes can omit these and focus on the other exercises in phases 2 and 3.

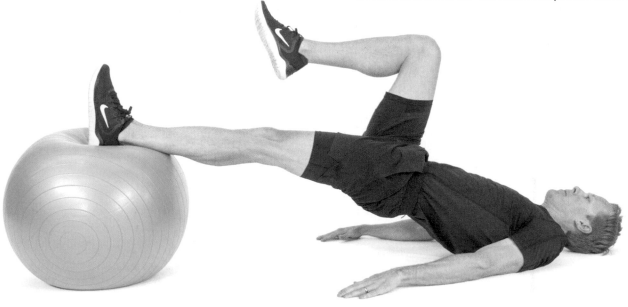

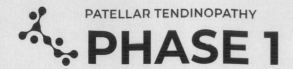

# PATELLAR TENDINOPATHY
# PHASE 1

## GOOD FOR:

- Alleviating knee pain
- Relieving muscle tension above and below the knee
- Warm-up for phase 2 and 3 exercises

## GUIDELINES:

- Perform every day, or every other day if tendon soreness increases
- Tools: foam roller, stretch strap
- Add phase 2 when you have no pain at rest and no more than mild pain (3/10) with the exercises

## quad mobilization

Lie on your stomach with your weight supported on your forearms or hands and one leg positioned over a foam roller. Supporting your weight with your grounded foot and arms, roll up and down to mobilize the entire quadriceps muscles on the front of your thigh, from hip to knee. Bend and straighten your knee to dynamically mobilize the muscles and femoral nerve. Spend 1–2 minutes on each leg.

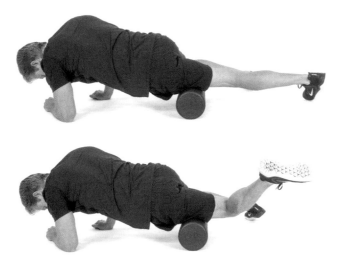

## lateral quad mobilization

The setup and execution are the same here: use your arms and grounded foot to control the pressure, roll up and down the entire thigh (from hip to knee), and stop on tender or stiff spots and bend and straighten your leg. But instead of mobilizing the front of your thigh, you target the lateral quadriceps along the outside of your leg. Spend 1–2 minutes on each leg.

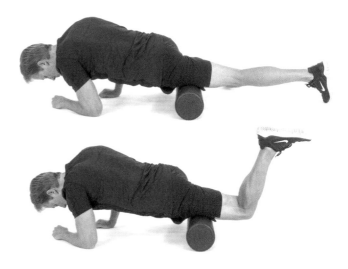

## heel slide *(choose one)*

Hook a strap around your foot. Bend your knee and slide your heel toward your butt, pulling on the strap to assist with the movement. If you don't feel pain, perform the movement without the strap and go as far as you can with no more than mild pain. Do 3 sets of 10 reps.

### with strap

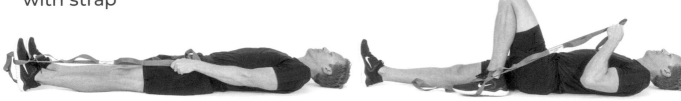

## without strap

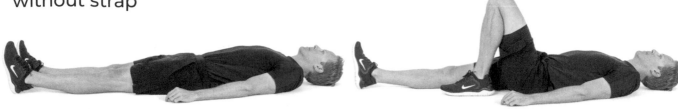

## knee extension isometrics

Sit on a bench or chair with your hips and knees bent to roughly 90 degrees. Slowly extend your knee by flexing your quadriceps muscles. Move with control and try to reach full knee extension with your leg straight. Perform 4 or 5 reps with 30- to 45-second contracted holds in the top position.

## side-lying hip abduction

Lie on your side, rotate your hips toward the floor slightly, and internally rotate your top leg so that your big toe is angled toward the arch of your bottom foot. Lift your top leg up and at a backward angle. Keep your spine neutral and pause in the top position for 1–2 seconds. Reduce the range of motion if you start to arch your back excessively. Add a resistance loop above your knees to increase glute activation and make the exercise more challenging.

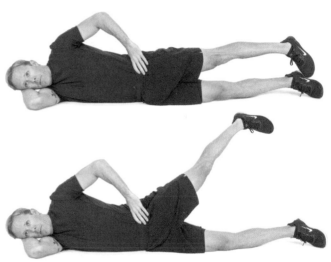

## single-leg bridge

Lie on your back with your knees bent and your feet flat on the floor. Elevate one leg—you can either straighten it or keep it bent at about 90 degrees.

Push into the floor and extend your hips. Focus on squeezing your glutes as you reach full hip extension, holding the contraction for 1–2 seconds.

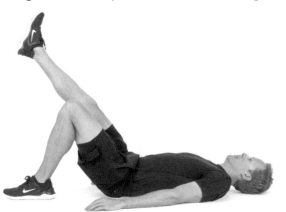

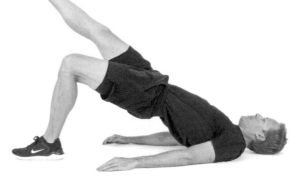

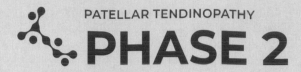

# PHASE 2

## GOOD FOR:

- Reducing knee pain
- Early knee and hip strengthening
- Warm-up for phase 3 exercises

## GUIDELINES:

- Perform 3 or 4 days a week
- Set, rep, and hold times for each exercise are covered in the captions
- Tools: resistance loop, dowel, dumbbells, physio (exercise) ball
- Skip any exercises that create pain and add them to phase 3
- Add phase 3 when you can do the exercises with no more than mild pain (3/10)

## banded hip abduction

Position a resistance loop above your knees. Shift your weight onto one leg, then raise your unweighted leg out to the side (abduction). Keep your foot pointed straight forward and try not to lean your upper body excessively. Place your hand against a wall or use a dowel to maintain balance. Do 3 sets of 10–15 reps.

## wall sit

With your back against a wall or rack, stand with your feet shoulder width apart and 1–2 feet from the wall. Slide down the wall into a squat. Keeping your knees over your toes, adjust your feet forward or backward to get your shins roughly vertical. When it comes to squat depth, find a position that is challenging—usually, that is thighs parallel to the floor—but doesn't create more than mild pain. Perform 4 or 5 reps with 30- to 45-second holds.

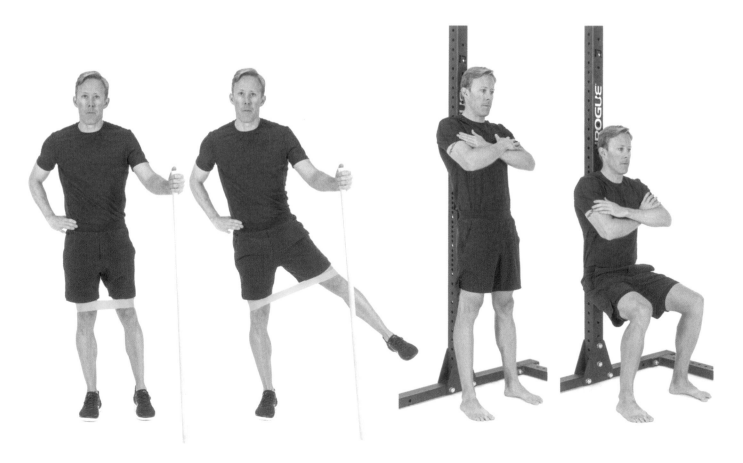

## plank with leg lifts and arm reaches

Get into the plank position: elbows aligned under your shoulders, back flat, legs spread to about hip width, and up on the balls of your feet. Tighten your abdominals and squeeze your glutes to maintain the position. Then remove one limb from your base of support: raise one leg at a time, then extend one arm at a time. Do 3 sets and complete 2–4 cycles per set.

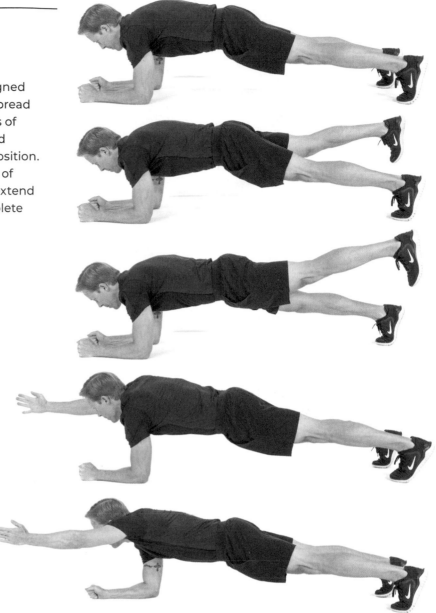

## tiptoe walk

You can perform this exercise with or without dumbbells. Try the bodyweight variation first, then add dumbbells if it's too easy. Start by getting into a half squat: hinge from your hips, tilt your torso forward, and bend your knees. Get onto the balls of your feet and take small steps. Keep your knees over your toes and your heels off the floor. Choose a distance or rep range that is challenging—usually 15–20 steps.

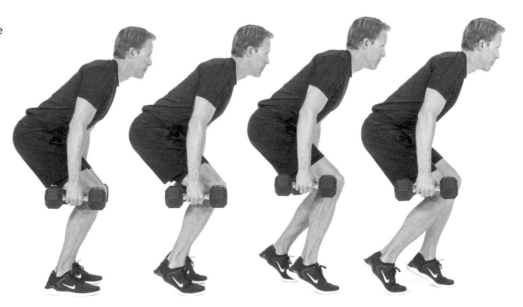

## single-leg eccentric bench squat

Stand with your back facing a bench or chair. Position your heels 6–12 inches from the bench and align your feet underneath your hips. Lift one leg out in front of your body. Slowly squat to the bench and sit down. Place your elevated foot on the floor next to your other foot and perform a bodyweight squat back into the standing position—one leg down, two legs up. To progress this exercise, keep your foot off the floor and perform the entire movement on one leg. Do 3 sets of 10–15 reps.

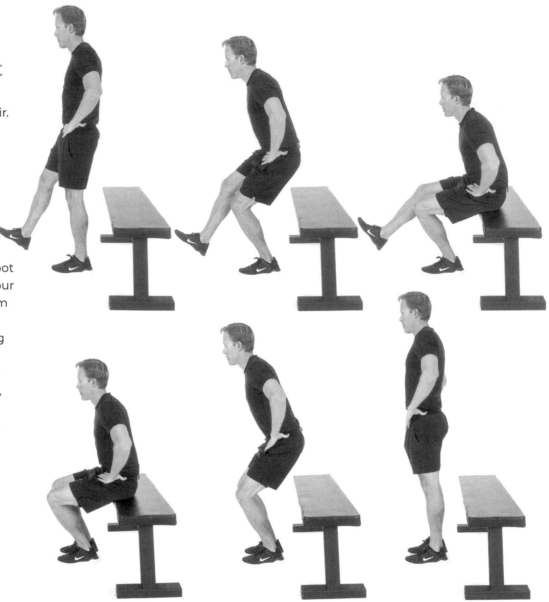

## ball hamstring curl

Lie on your back and center your feet on a physio (exercise) ball. Spread your arms slightly and keep them flush with the floor. Drive your heels into the ball and extend your hips. As you reach full hip extension, slowly curl your heels toward your butt. Do 3 sets of 10–15 reps.

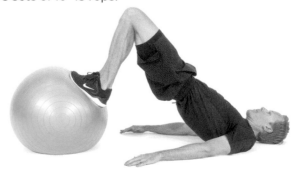

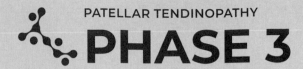

## PATELLAR TENDINOPATHY
# PHASE 3

**GOOD FOR:**

- Increasing knee and leg strength
- Preventing knee pain and injury

**GUIDELINES:**

- Perform 3 or 4 days a week
- Do 3 sets of 10–15 reps unless otherwise noted
- Push sets to fatigue
- Tools: resistance loop, plyo box, physio (exercise) ball, slant board

## standing banded hydrant

Position a resistance loop just above your knees. Hinge forward from your hips and bend your knees slightly, keeping your shins vertical. In one motion, lift your leg out to the side (abduction) and back (extension) while rotating your foot outward (external rotation). Focus on keeping your grounded knee straight or outside your foot; don't let it cave inward.

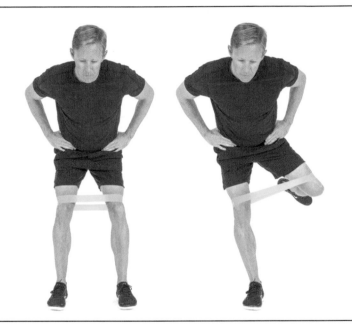

## step-up

Step on a plyo box with your knee aligned over your foot. Without pushing off the floor, shift your weight onto your elevated leg, drive through your heel or mid-foot, and raise your torso and hips in one fluid motion. Progress this exercise by increasing the height of the box or holding one dumbbell at your side to challenge your trunk stability or two dumbbells to increase the load.

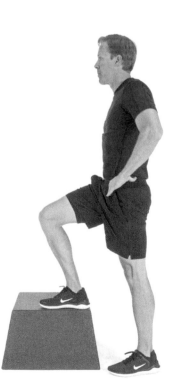
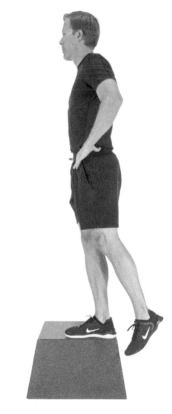

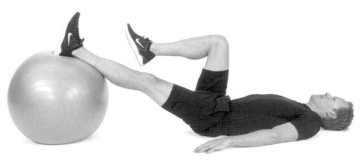

## single-leg hamstring curl

Lie on your back and center one foot on a physio (exercise) ball—keeping your other leg off the ball and bent. Spread your arms slightly and keep them flush with the floor. Drive your heel into the ball and extend your hips. As you reach full hip extension, slowly curl your heel toward your butt.

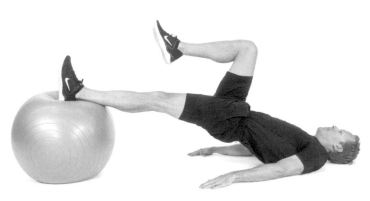

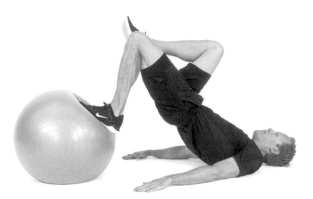

## decline single-leg eccentric squat

Stand on a slant board or squat wedge block with your heels above your toes and your feet underneath your hips. Lift one foot out in front of your body, then slowly lower into a squat—tilt your torso forward while maintaining a flat back and sit your hips down. Keep your knee aligned over your toes. Descend as far as you can while maintaining good form and balance. Place your elevated foot on the board next to your other foot and perform a bodyweight squat back to the standing position—one leg down, two legs up. To progress this exercise, increase the range of motion or keep your leg off the board and perform the entire movement on one leg.

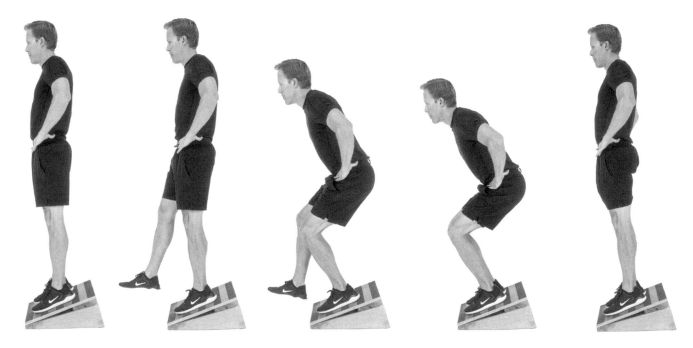

# bilateral jump to unilateral landing

Stand with your feet just inside shoulder width. Lower into a half squat and pull your elbows back. In one motion, extend your hips and knees, swing your arms forward, and jump vertically. While in the air, pull one leg back and prepare to land on one leg. Cushion your landing by bending your knee and hinging forward. Try to land with your knee aligned over your toes; don't let your knee or ankle collapse inward. Spread your arms to maintain balance. Do 3 sets of 6–12 reps (jumps).

> **Only do these exercises if your knee stability is very high and you need to be able to perform jumping movements in daily life.**

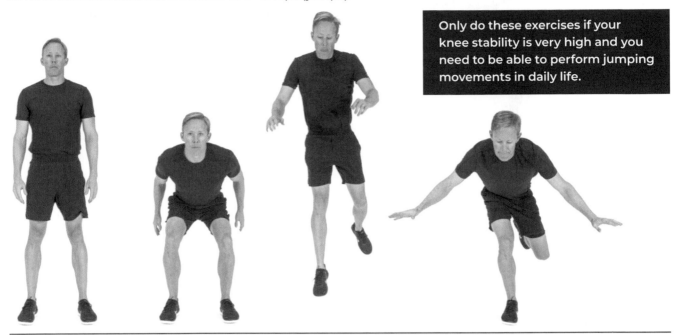

# skater jumps

Stand with your feet shoulder width apart. To generate momentum for the lateral jump, hinge forward from your hips and kick one leg back. As you do, rotate your shoulders toward your grounded leg. Think of an ice skater's stride—this is your start and finish position. Drive off the outside edge of your foot and extend your elevated leg laterally in the direction of the jump. As your foot leaves the floor, unwind your shoulders and bend your knee. Cushion the landing by reclaiming the start position on the opposite side—hinging from your hips, lowering into a single-leg (skater) squat, and rotating your shoulders toward your grounded leg. Immediately repeat the sequence, hopping rhythmically from side to side. Do 3 sets of 6–12 reps (jumps).

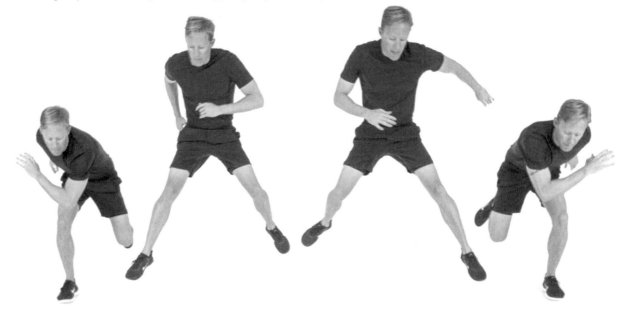

# OSTEOARTHRITIS

**Follow this program to treat:**

- Knee arthritis
- Pain inside the knee joint

**DESCRIPTION:** Osteoarthritis (OA) is a degenerative condition of the hyaline cartilage that usually affects the knee and hip joints. In the knee, the cartilage at the ends of the tibia and femur breaks down. Over time, it can deteriorate, creating bone-on-bone friction. At this stage, OA becomes a severe condition that limits your ability to complete daily tasks, and your doctor may recommend a knee replacement.

To avoid this outcome, it's imperative to listen to your body and address lifestyle factors that might be contributing to the problem.[25,26] Knee pain that increases in frequency and severity could be an early sign of arthritis. If you have a history of knee injuries, you are more susceptible to arthritis and must take special care to strengthen the surrounding tissues and modify your behavior.[27]

Remember, cartilage breaks down faster in people who are either very sedentary or very active, whereas moderate-dose activity protects it.[28] What's more, arthritis is an inflammatory condition that can accelerate the breakdown of cartilage. So, it's worth referencing Chapter 4 to see what behavior modifications you can make to reduce inflammation and slow the process—for example, get more sleep, clean up your diet, and reduce stress.

**SIGNS AND SYMPTOMS:** Osteoarthritis typically produces pain in the joint, swelling (effusion), joint stiffness, limited range of motion (flexion and extension), and difficulty with functional tasks such as standing, squatting, walking, and running.

**AGGRAVATING FACTORS:** Activities that require increased range of motion, such as squatting or getting in and out of a chair. Pain may increase when the joint is loaded, such as standing for extended periods, or after long walks.

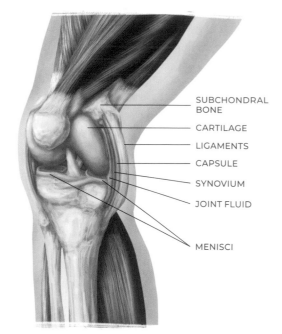

SUBCHONDRAL BONE
CARTILAGE
LIGAMENTS
CAPSULE
SYNOVIUM
JOINT FLUID
MENISCI

HEALTHY KNEE

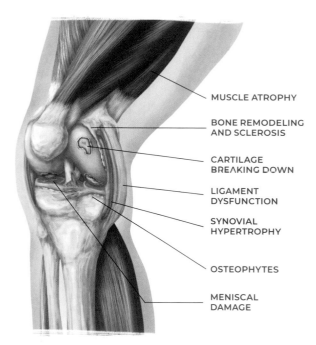

MUSCLE ATROPHY
BONE REMODELING AND SCLEROSIS
CARTILAGE BREAKING DOWN
LIGAMENT DYSFUNCTION
SYNOVIAL HYPERTROPHY
OSTEOPHYTES
MENISCAL DAMAGE

OSTEOARTHRITIC KNEE

**PROGNOSIS:** While rehab exercises will not reverse arthritic changes, improving range of motion and strengthening the muscles surrounding the knee joint can improve cartilage health and slow the progression. In some cases, you can manage pain and functional limitations with exercise alone.

TREATMENT STRATEGY: Physical therapy focuses on building knee and hip strength and implementing mobility exercises to maintain the joint range of motion needed for daily activities. Rest, anti-inflammatory medication, ice, and heat can reduce pain temporarily.

**1** Phase 1 is all about pain relief. You implement soft tissue mobilizations and stretches targeting the major muscle groups that directly influence the knee joint, such as the calf muscles, quadriceps, and hamstrings.

**2** Because many people with knee arthritis have limited knee flexion, extension, or both, phase 2 begins with passive and active mobility exercises. With the heel slide, you pull your leg in and then straighten it as far as you can without creating more than mild pain. You want to challenge the joint but not flare it up. Active mobility drills like the standing hamstring curl and knee extension teach your neuromuscular system to utilize the range of motion that you gain from the heel slide. The last three exercises in phase 2 strengthen the glute and calf muscles, which absorb shock and support the knee.

**3** The strength exercises in phase 3 are more challenging. If any of the single-leg options creates pain, stick with the double-leg version or one of the phase 2 variations. The strengthening exercises in phases 2 and 3 take off your knee and often reduce pain. As your muscles become stronger, they can accept more load, which means less force is transferred to sensitive joint structures.

## WHEN SHOULD I CONSIDER KNEE REPLACEMENT SURGERY?

When an X-ray shows bone-on-bone contact, pain becomes unmanageable, and function is severely limited, a total knee replacement is usually recommended.

## CAN I FOLLOW THE REHAB EXERCISE PROTOCOL IF I'M A CANDIDATE FOR SURGERY?

Research has shown that building strength before surgery can expedite your post-surgical recovery.[29] If you are planning to have a knee replacement, the exercises in this protocol can help. It's also critical to follow through with rehab after surgery. Because a total knee replacement is a serious surgery, you need to work with a physical therapist who can design a program specifically for you. Follow the program and see it all the way through. Once your time with the PT is over, you can either stick with the program they wrote or implement the rehab exercises in this protocol. The bottom line is that the work is not done once you finish with your PT. To maintain function and prevent pain, it's imperative to remain moderately active.

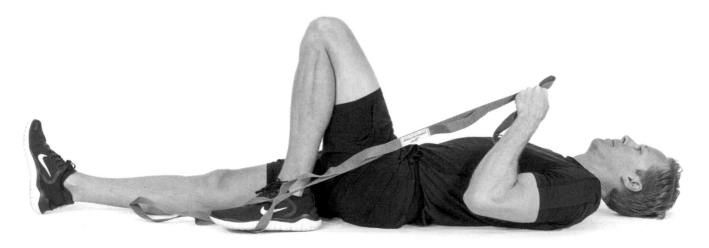

# PHASE 1

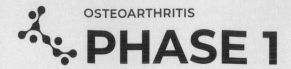

**GOOD FOR:**

- Alleviating knee pain
- Relieving muscle tension above and below the knee
- Warm-up for phase 2 and 3 exercises

**GUIDELINES:**

- Perform every day
- Tools: foam roller, massage ball, stretch strap, slant board
- Add phase 2 after 2 weeks

## SOFT TISSUE MOBILIZATIONS:

▸ Spend 1–2 minutes on each area

▸ Perform in any order on both sides

▸ Stop on tender points for 10–20 seconds

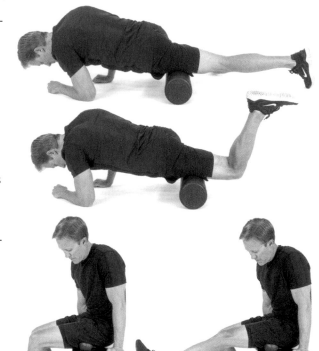

### quad mobilization

Lie on your stomach with your weight supported on your forearms or hands and one leg positioned over a foam roller with your toes pointed toward the floor. Supporting your weight with your grounded foot and arms, roll up and down to mobilize the entire quadriceps muscles on the front of your thigh—from hip to knee. Bend and straighten your knee to dynamically mobilize the muscles and femoral nerve.

### hamstring mobilization

Sit on a bench or chair and place a large or small massage ball under your hamstring muscles. Roll up and down the entire length of your hamstring. Flex and extend your knee to dynamically mobilize the muscles.

### calf mobilization

Sit on the floor with your calf positioned over a foam roller. Push off the floor with your hands and grounded foot—lifting your hips off the floor—to roll up and down your lower leg from ankle to knee.

Stop on any tender or stiff spots and move your foot (flex, extend, and rotate from side to side).

To increase the pressure, stack your other leg on top.

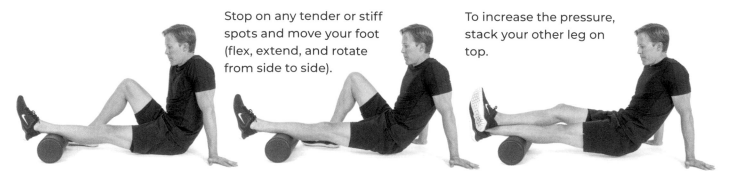

# STRETCHING EXERCISES:

▸ Do 3 reps with 30- to 60-second holds

▸ Perform in any order on both sides

▸ Don't stretch into pain

## quad stretch

*(choose one)*

### standing

Grab your ankle and use your arm to bend your knee until you feel a stretch along the front of your thigh. Keep your posture upright and your knee vertical to maximize the stretch.

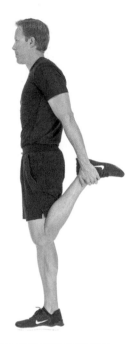

### side-lying

You can perform the same stretch while lying on your side. Make sure your leg is in line with (not in front of) your body or pulled slightly back (hip extension) to maximize the stretch.

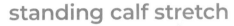

## hamstring stretch with strap

Lie on your back with a strap hooked around one foot. Keeping your leg completely relaxed, use your arms to pull your foot toward your head and hold it in place once you feel a moderate stretch.

## standing calf stretch

Stand with the front part of your foot on a slant board, incline, or elevated surface. Step your other foot in front of the leg you are stretching. You should feel a stretch through your calf and back of your ankle. To target your soleus muscle, sit your hips back, tilt your torso forward, and bend your knee.

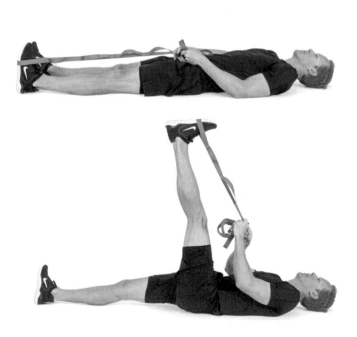

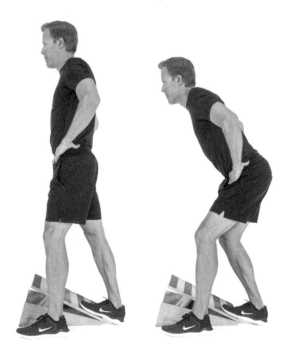

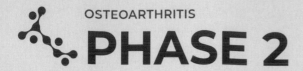

## OSTEOARTHRITIS
# PHASE 2

### GOOD FOR:

- Reducing knee pain
- Early knee and hip strengthening
- Warm-up for phase 3 exercises

### GUIDELINES:

- Perform 3 or 4 days a week
- Do 3 sets of 10–15 reps
- Tools: stretch strap, resistance loop
- Add phase 3 when you can do the exercises with no more than mild pain (3/10)

## heel slide *(choose one)*

Hook a strap around your foot. Bend your knee and slide your heel toward your butt, pulling on the strap to assist with the movement. If you don't feel pain, perform the movement without the strap and go as far as you can with no more than mild pain.

### with strap

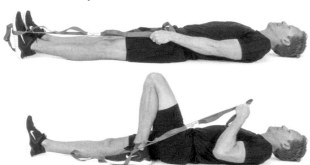

### without strap

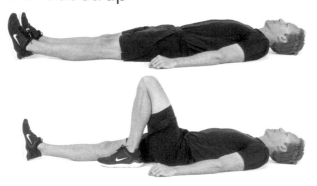

## standing hamstring curl

Shift your weight onto one leg, then curl the heel of your unweighted foot toward your butt. Keep your knee pointed toward the floor and your hips extended; don't bring your knee forward or bend your hips.

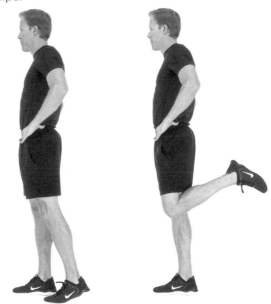

## knee extension

Sit on a bench or chair with your hips and knees bent to roughly 90 degrees. Slowly extend your knee by flexing your quadriceps muscles. Move with control and try to reach full knee extension with your leg straight. Hold the top position for 1–2 seconds.

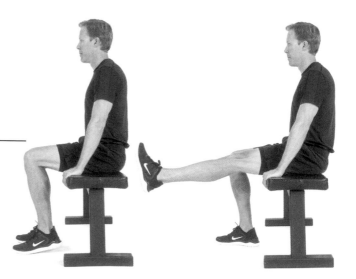

## lateral squat walk

Wrap a resistance loop above your knees. Position your feet shoulder width apart and bend your hips and knees slightly. Take a wide lateral step so there is a full stretch in the band. You can either walk along a line and then switch after a given number of steps or stay in one area and switch back and forth between legs. Choose a distance or rep range that is challenging—you feel your upper glutes burn—usually 15–20 steps in each direction. Don't pause between steps, and keep tension in the band during the entire movement.

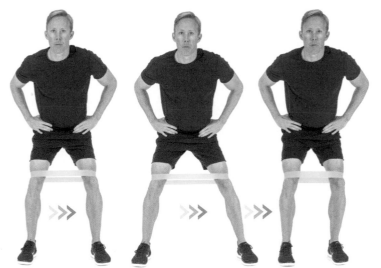

## chair squat

Stand in front of a chair or bench with your feet roughly shoulder width apart. When it comes to foot flare, you can orient your feet straight or turn them out slightly—whichever feels better. To perform the movement, extend your arms in front of you to counterbalance your weight, reach your hips back slightly, and sit straight down. As you lower into the bottom position, keep your spine in the neutral zone (not excessively arching or rounding) and your knees aligned over your toes. Reverse the movement the moment your butt touches the chair; do not pause in the bottom position.

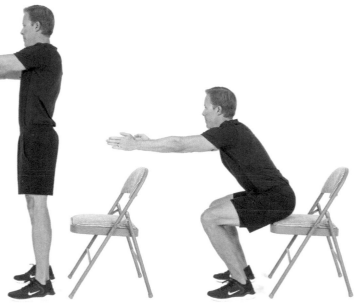

## double-leg calf raise

Stand with the balls of your feet on an elevated surface or step. Allow your heels to sink toward the floor. Perform slow calf raises through a full range of motion. Your heels should drop slightly lower than your toes on the down phase.

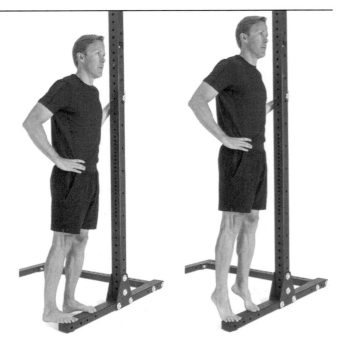

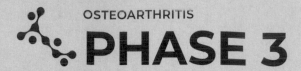

# PHASE 3

## GOOD FOR:

- Increasing knee and leg strength
- Improving functional mobility
- Preventing knee pain and injury

## GUIDELINES:

- Perform 3 or 4 days a week
- Do 3 sets of 10–15 reps
- Push sets to fatigue
- Tools: physio (exercise) ball, dumbbell, plyo box

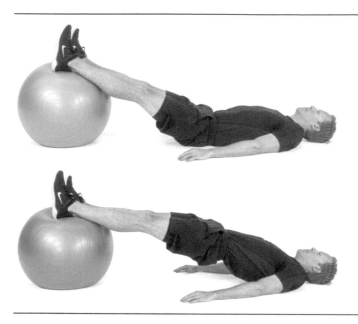

## ball hamstring curl

Lie on your back and center your feet on a physio (exercise) ball. Spread your arms slightly and keep them flush with the floor. Drive your heels into the ball and extend your hips. As you reach full hip extension, slowly curl your heels toward your butt.

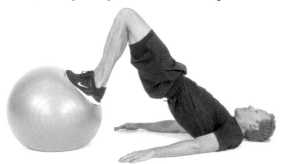

## bridge *(choose one)*

### double-leg

Lie on your back with your knees bent and your feet flat on the floor. Push into the floor and lift your butt, fully extending your hips—a straight line runs from your shoulders to your knees. Squeeze your glutes as you reach full hip extension and pause in the top position for 1–2 seconds.

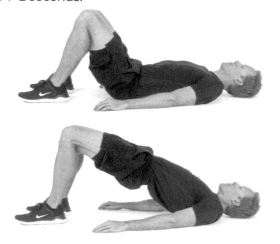

### single-leg

With your knees bent and your feet flat on the floor, elevate one leg—you can either straighten your raised leg or keep it bent at about 90 degrees. Push into the floor and extend your hips. Focus on squeezing your glutes as you reach full hip extension, holding the contraction for 1–2 seconds.

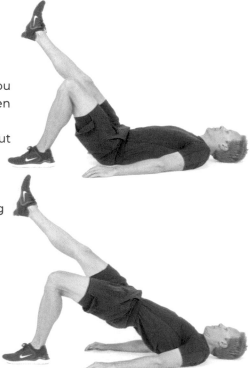

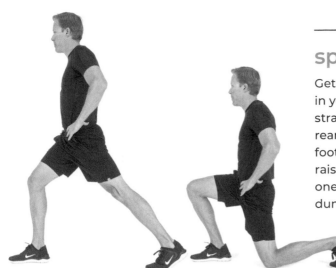

## split squat

Get into a split squat stance: torso upright, slight bend in your lead leg with your shin vertical, and back leg straight. Drop your hips straight down and lower your rear knee to the floor. Driving off the heel of your front foot and the ball of your rear foot, extend your knees and raise your body back to the start position. You can hold one dumbbell to challenge your trunk stability or two dumbbells to add load to the movement.

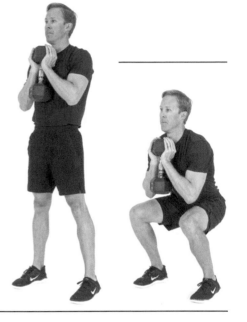

## goblet squat

Stand with your feet roughly shoulder width apart. When it comes to foot flare, you can orient your feet straight or turn them out slightly—whichever feels better and allows you to reach the lowest depth without discomfort. Cup one end of a dumbbell with both hands at the center of your chest. To perform the movement, reach your hips back slightly and sit straight down. As you lower into the bottom position, keep your spine in the neutral zone (not excessively arching or rounding), your knees aligned over your toes, and the weight close to your body. The goal is to keep your torso as upright as possible and lower as far as you can while maintaining good form.

## step-up

Step on a plyo box with your knee aligned over your foot. Without pushing off the floor, shift your weight onto your elevated leg, drive through your heel or mid-foot, and raise your torso and hips in one fluid motion. Progress this exercise by increasing the height of the box or holding a dumbbell.

## single-leg calf raise

Stand with the ball of one foot on an elevated surface or step. Perform slow calf raises through the full range of motion. Your heel should drop slightly lower than your toes on the down phase.

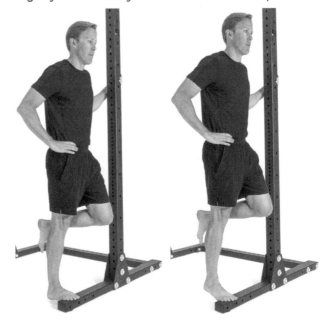

## CHAPTER 22

# ANKLE & FOOT
# PROTOCOLS

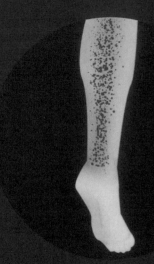

**CALF AND
ACHILLES PAIN**
(p. 427)

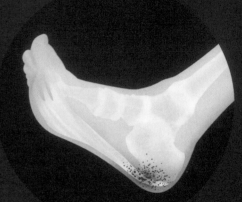

**PLANTAR
FASCIOPATHY
(FASCIITIS)**
(p. 436)

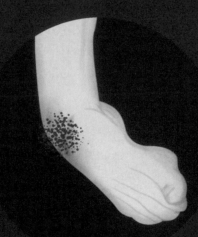

**ANKLE SPRAIN**
(p. 445)

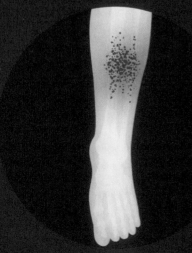

**SHIN SPLINTS**
(p. 454)

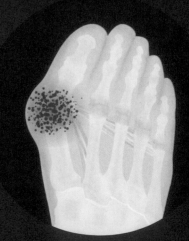

**BUNION**
(p. 463)

# CALF AND ACHILLES PAIN

**Follow this program to treat:**

- Achilles tendinopathy
- Achilles tear
- Calf strain

## ACHILLES TENDINOPATHY/ TEAR

**DESCRIPTION:** Achilles tendinopathy describes a condition in which the tendon that connects the calf muscles (gastrocnemius and soleus) to the heel bone (calcaneus) becomes irritated, resulting in pain, ankle stiffness, and difficulty plantarflexing (pointing the foot).

Think of your Achilles tendon as a spring that stores and releases energy. When you lift your heel to jump, land, or take a step—whether you are sprinting, jogging, or walking—your Achilles and calf muscles help propel your movement and then absorb the shock of your foot contacting the ground. More specifically, they slow the eccentric phase of the movement to soften the landing of your heel (spring stores energy). That energy can then be redirected into your next step or jump (spring releases energy).

Achilles tendinopathy generally stems from overuse but can come on rapidly if you are not warmed up or haven't built up your tissue to handle a high volume of jumping, sprinting, or running uphill. As with all pain symptoms, it's imperative to listen to your body's warnings that you may be vulnerable to serious injury. This is especially true for Achilles tendinopathy.

When the Achilles is in a weakened state, it is much more likely to rupture, and a full or partial tear often requires surgery. Interestingly, the Achilles is the strongest and thickest tendon in the human body, yet it is the one most commonly ruptured.[1,2] So, if you have pain in your lower leg, dial back the aggravating activities and start following the rehab protocol to strengthen your tissues. Doing so will not only alleviate pain and improve function but also help safeguard you from more severe injury.

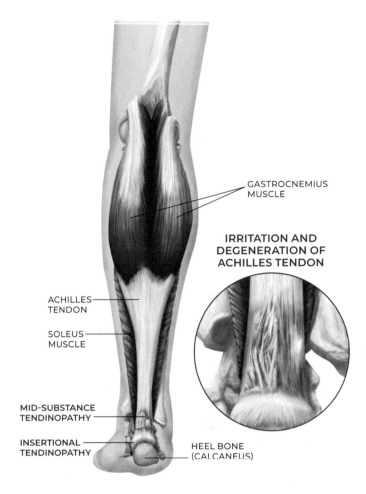

GASTROCNEMIUS MUSCLE

**IRRITATION AND DEGENERATION OF ACHILLES TENDON**

ACHILLES TENDON

SOLEUS MUSCLE

MID-SUBSTANCE TENDINOPATHY

INSERTIONAL TENDINOPATHY

HEEL BONE (CALCANEUS)

## HOW DO I DIFFERENTIATE BETWEEN A TENDINOPATHY AND A RUPTURE?

With a rupture, you typically hear or feel a pop, but there's an easy test called the Thompson's test that a friend can help you with. You lie on your stomach on a couch or table with your ankle hanging over the edge, and then your friend squeezes your calf muscle. If your Achilles tendon is attached, squeezing your calf muscle will make your foot point, as if your calf is contracting. If the Achilles is torn, your foot won't move when the calf is squeezed. In that case, surgery may be your only recourse. A medical professional can use imaging to determine if the tendon is partially or fully torn and whether surgery is necessary.

**SIGNS AND SYMPTOMS:** Achilles tendinopathy is divided into two categories based on the location of symptoms:

- Mid-substance tendinopathy causes pain several centimeters above the heel bone.

- Insertional tendinopathy causes pain on the back of the heel bone where the Achilles tendon attaches.

Pain can be sharp with activities that stress the tendon, and the area often aches at rest or after activity.

**AGGRAVATING FACTORS:** Walking, running, sprinting, jumping, climbing stairs, and any activity that involves lifting and lowering the heel.

**PROGNOSIS:** Achilles tendinopathy typically resolves within two to 12 weeks, depending on the severity of the problem and whether it is chronic, when you temporarily modify or halt aggravating activities and implement a tendon loading program.

**TREATMENT STRATEGY:** Treating Achilles tendinopathy involves modifying behaviors to allow the tendon to heal and gradually loading the tendon and calf muscles with resistance training exercises.[3,4]

If you have tendinopathy, you can use this protocol to start rehabbing your Achilles tendon. If you have a rupture, seek medical attention; you might need reconstructive surgery in which a surgeon uses either your own tissue or cadaver tissue to sew your Achilles back together, reattaching it to your heel bone. You may also be put in a boot that locks your ankle at 90 degrees to allow the tendon to heal, which is usually done for six weeks.

There is no stretching in this protocol because you shouldn't stretch an Achilles tendinopathy. A calf stretch, for example, might make the pain worse.

Phase 1 focuses on reducing pain. The calf and plantar mobilizations reduce muscle tension and tightness. The calf isometrics typically reduce Achilles tendon pain. The knee-straight calf raise targets the more superficial calf muscle (gastrocnemius), whereas the knee-bent version targets the deeper calf muscle (soleus), which research has shown to be important when rehabilitating the Achilles.[5] If your pain is acute and you cannot complete the double-leg calf raises, stick with the soft tissue mobilizations and calf isometrics and add the calf raises once your pain calms down.

In phase 2, you continue building calf and Achilles tendon strength with calf eccentrics. With Achilles tendinopathy, the up part of the calf raise is typically more painful, so you reduce the stress by going up on two legs. Then you shift your weight onto the painful leg and lower slowly into an eccentric contraction (the muscle fibers are contracting and lengthening). Again, you do knee-straight and knee-bent versions to target both calf muscles. Following these exercises is the band inversion, which targets muscles that assist the calf muscles, especially the tibialis posterior. Phase 2 ends with the split squat and ball hamstring curl, which target muscles farther up the kinetic chain that support the calf and Achilles tendon.

Phase 3 provides more challenging resistance exercises. You now complete the calf raises on one leg, as you must be able to do at least 20 to 25 single-leg calf raises (a measure of full strength) to return to full function, especially for sport-related activities.[6] The skater squat and forward lunge work muscles farther up the kinetic chain that support the calf complex. Last comes the tiptoe walk, which targets the calf muscles and ankle stabilizers, especially the soleus muscle.

# CALF STRAIN

**DESCRIPTION:** The gastrocnemius and soleus muscles run down the back of the lower leg and attach to the heel bone (calcaneus) via the Achilles tendon. These two calf muscles work together to move the ankle through plantarflexion (pointing the foot), absorb shock, and propel the body during activities like walking, running (especially in forefoot strikers), and jumping. When stressed suddenly with a forceful load—say you are running hill sprints and feel your calf spasm—chances are there is minor damage to the muscle fibers, and you strained your calf.

**SIGNS AND SYMPTOMS:** Strains typically produce sharp pain in the calf muscle region (not the Achilles tendon) when the muscles are in use and a dull ache at rest, especially in the early phases. For most people, pain occurs in the lower calf, where the muscle becomes tendon.

**AGGRAVATING FACTORS:** Walking, running, jumping, or standing on tiptoe.

**PROGNOSIS:** Healing times vary depending on the severity of the strain, but most strains heal within three to six weeks when you follow a rehab program.

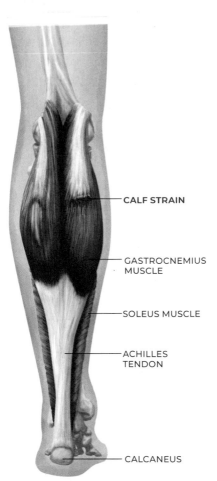

CALF STRAIN

GASTROCNEMIUS MUSCLE

SOLEUS MUSCLE

ACHILLES TENDON

CALCANEUS

## RED FLAG SYMPTOMS: SIGNS OF A BLOOD CLOT

If you have pain in your upper calf, it's vital to evaluate your symptoms and the mechanism of injury because calf strain pain can mimic signs of a blood clot.

A patient in my clinic came to me thinking she had strained her calf, but my evaluation revealed a couple of red flags. First, she didn't have a clear mechanism of injury. She hadn't hurt her calf while running or jumping; she just woke up with a swollen and tender lower leg. Second, her calf was warm to the touch. These are clear signs of a potential blood clot, so I sent her to her doctor, who performed a Doppler ultrasound and confirmed the diagnosis. It turned out that the clot was a side effect of her birth control medication.

As I've said, you need to pay close attention to the signs your body is sending you. Don't hesitate to seek medical attention if you have any doubt, especially when it comes to lower leg pain. If your lower leg is swollen, tender, or warm to the touch and there is no mechanism of injury—all red flag symptoms—seek medical attention immediately.

**TREATMENT STRATEGY:** Calf strains are treated almost exclusively with therapeutic exercises that gradually increase muscle strength and integrity.

Whether you have a calf strain or Achilles tendinopathy, you approach the protocol in nearly the same fashion. Phase 1 is all about reducing pain. With a strain, you may want to skip the calf mobilization, which could create more discomfort and delay healing. So, if your pain is in your calf muscles, you can gently test this exercise, but eliminate it if you experience more than mild discomfort. The plantar mobilization should reduce muscle tension and tightness. The calf isometrics begin to build strength and reduce stress on the healing muscle since there is no movement during the contraction. Following the isometrics, the knee-straight calf raise targets the more superficial calf muscle (gastrocnemius), whereas the knee-bent calf raise targets the deeper calf muscle (soleus). If your pain is acute and you cannot do the double-leg raises, do partial range of motion calf raises or stick with the isometrics until your injury has healed more, and then add the calf raises.

Phases 2 and 3 mirror the approach for Achilles tendinopathy (opposite).

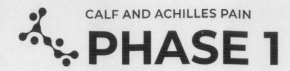

## CALF AND ACHILLES PAIN
# PHASE 1

### GOOD FOR:

- Alleviating calf and Achilles pain
- Relieving ankle and foot stiffness
- Warm-up for phase 2 and 3 exercises

### GUIDELINES:

- Perform every day
- Tools: foam roller, small massage ball
- Add phase 2 when you have no pain at rest and no more than mild pain (3/10) with the exercises

**Skip this exercise and add it to the next phase if you have a calf strain or you experience more than mild pain.**

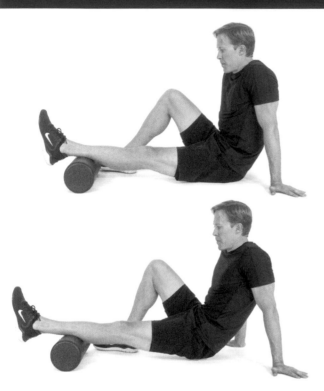

## calf mobilization

Sit on the floor with your calf positioned over a foam roller. Push off with your hands and grounded foot—lifting your hips off the floor—to roll up and down your lower leg from ankle to knee. Stop on any tender or stiff spots and move your foot (flex, extend, and rotate from side to side). Spend 1–2 minutes on each calf.

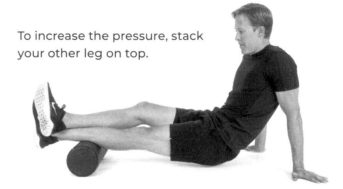

To increase the pressure, stack your other leg on top.

## plantar mobilization

Step on a small massage ball, positioning it under the arch of your foot. Roll from front to back and side to side across your plantar fascia, from the ball of your foot to the front of your heel. Flex and extend your toes to dynamically mobilize the plantar fascia and underlying muscles. Spend 1–2 minutes on each foot.

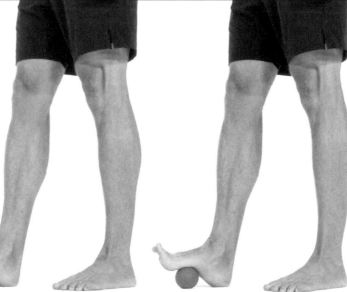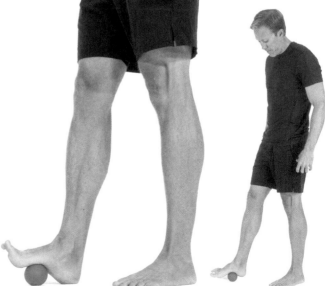

## double-leg calf raise (knees straight)

Stand with the balls of your feet on an elevated surface or step. Allow your heels to sink toward the floor. Perform slow calf raises through a full range of motion. Your heels should drop slightly lower than your toes on the down phase. Do 2 sets of 10–15 reps.

**If you have insertional Achilles tendinopathy, do this calf raise on the ground. Dropping the heel below the toes can make insertional tendinopathy worse.**

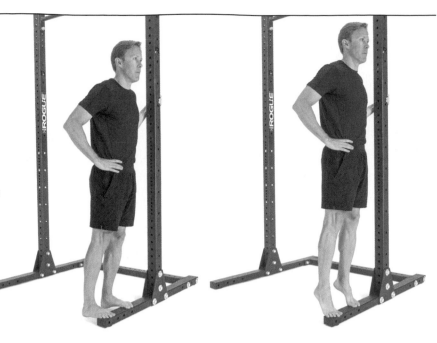

## double-leg calf raise (knees bent)

Hold onto a doorframe or rack. Sit your hips back and bend your knees into a half squat. Maintaining your knee angle, perform calf raises to target the soleus muscle. Do 3 sets of 10–15 reps.

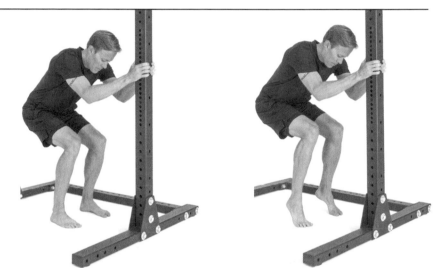

## single-leg calf isometrics

Stand with the balls of your feet on an elevated surface or step and perform a calf raise. At the top position, shift all your weight onto one leg—holding a single-leg calf raise. To stay balanced, grip something sturdy. Perform 4–5 reps with 30- to 45-second holds. Put your other foot down and lower into the start position on both legs.

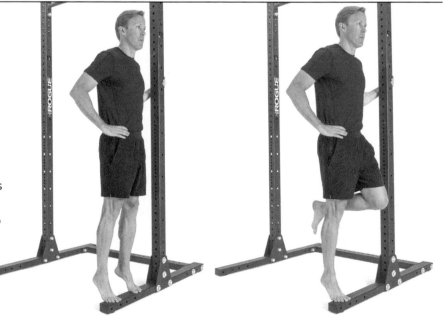

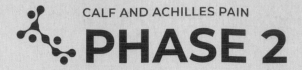

# PHASE 2

**GOOD FOR:**

- Reducing calf and Achilles pain
- Building early muscle and tendon strength
- Warm-up for phase 3 exercises

**GUIDELINES:**

- Perform 3 or 4 days a week
- Do 3 sets of 10–15 reps unless otherwise noted
- Tools: resistance band, dumbbell, physio (exercise) ball
- Add phase 3 when you can do the exercises with no more than mild pain (3/10)

## single-leg calf eccentrics (knee straight)

Stand with the balls of your feet on an elevated surface or step and perform a double-leg (bilateral) calf raise. At the top position, shift your weight onto one leg and do a single-leg (unilateral) eccentric into the start position. Then lift again with both legs and repeat—two up, one down. Do 2 sets of 15 reps.

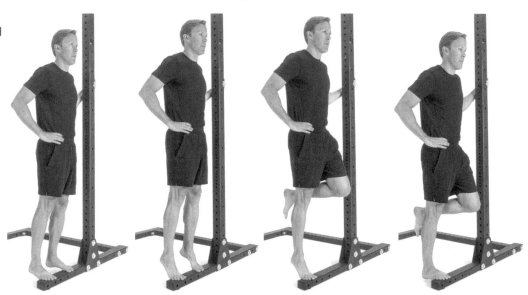

**If you have insertional Achilles tendinopathy, do this calf raise on the ground.**

## single-leg calf eccentrics (knee bent)

Hold onto a doorframe or rack. Sit your hips back, bend your knees, and lower into a half squat. Maintaining your knee angle, perform a double-leg calf raise. At the top position, shift your weight onto one leg and do a single-leg eccentric into the start position. Then lift again with both legs and repeat—two up, one down. Do 2 sets of 15 reps.

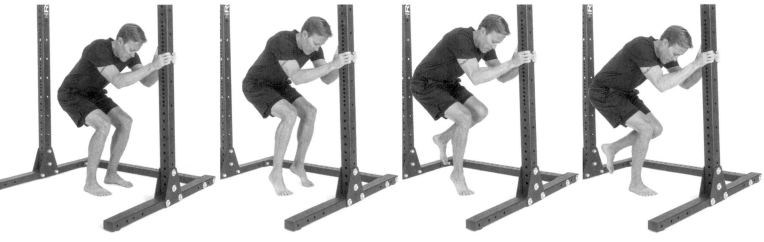

## band inversion

Tie a loop in a resistance band and wrap it around the top part of your foot. Apply tension to the band at an angle away from your body. Turn your ankle in (inversion) without moving the rest of your leg—your kneecap should point up the entire time. Move slowly and don't let the band snap your foot back to the start position.

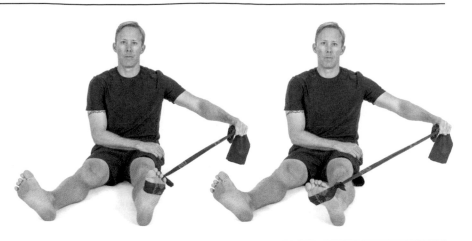
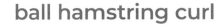

## split squat

Get into a split squat stance: torso upright, slight bend in your lead leg with your shin vertical, and back leg straight. Drop your hips straight down and lower your rear knee to the floor. Driving off the heel of your front foot and the ball of your rear foot, extend your knees and raise your body back to the start position.

You can hold one dumbbell to challenge your trunk stability or two dumbbells to add load to the movement.

## ball hamstring curl

Lie on your back and center your feet on a physio (exercise) ball. Spread your arms slightly and keep them flush with the floor. Drive your heels into the ball and extend your hips. As you reach full hip extension, slowly curl your heels toward your butt.

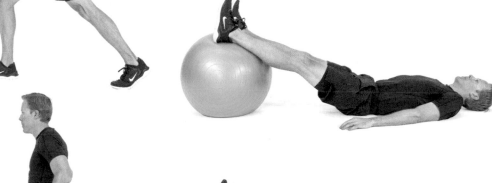
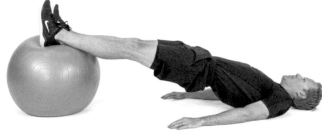
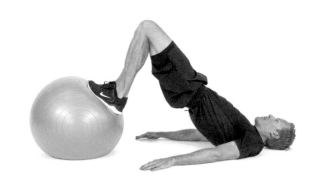

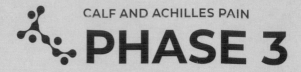

# PHASE 3

## GOOD FOR:

- Increasing Achilles, ankle, and calf strength
- Preventing ankle pain and injury

## GUIDELINES:

- Perform 3 or 4 days a week
- Do 3 sets of 10–15 reps unless otherwise noted
- Push sets to fatigue
- Tools: dumbbells

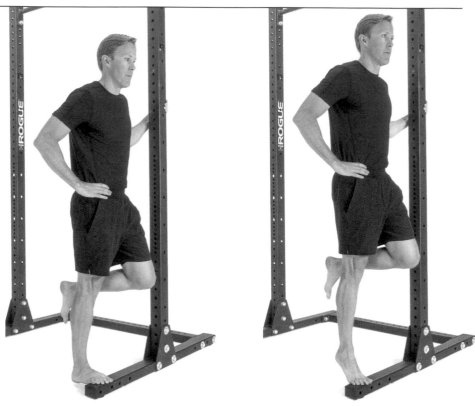

## single-leg calf raise (knee straight)

Stand with the ball of one foot on an elevated surface or step. Perform slow calf raises through a full range of motion. Your heel should drop slightly lower than your toes on the down phase.

> If you have insertional Achilles tendinopathy, start on level ground and progress to an elevated surface as your symptoms improve.

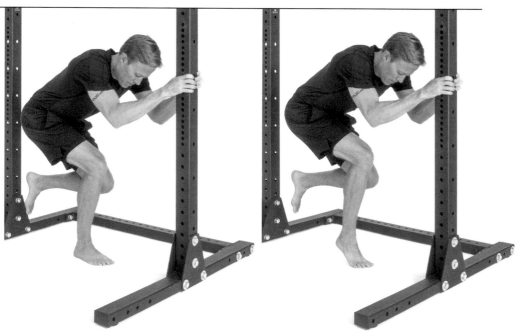

## single-leg calf raise (knee bent)

Hold onto a doorframe or rack. Sit your hips back, bend your knees, and lower into a half squat. Shift your weight onto one leg and perform single-leg calf raises. Maintain your knee and hip angle during the movement.

## skater squat

Stand on one leg with your unweighted knee bent and foot positioned behind your body. Keeping your torso and hips square, hinge forward from your hips, tilt your torso forward, and lower your unweighted knee toward the floor. Lower your knee to a pad to gauge distance. You can hold a light weight plate or dumbbells out in front of you to counterbalance your weight.

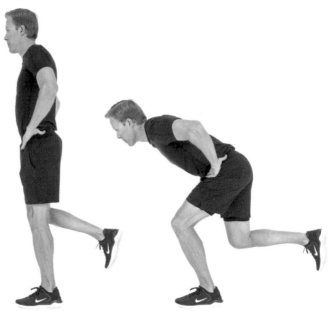

## forward lunge

Stand with your feet shoulder width apart. Take a big step forward and come up onto the ball of your rear foot. As your front foot makes contact, slowly lower your rear knee to the floor with control. You can keep your torso upright or tilt forward slightly. Shift your weight onto your lead leg, drive through your mid-foot, and stand upright. You can step into the start position or transition into your next forward step with the opposite leg. Do 10–15 steps with each leg.

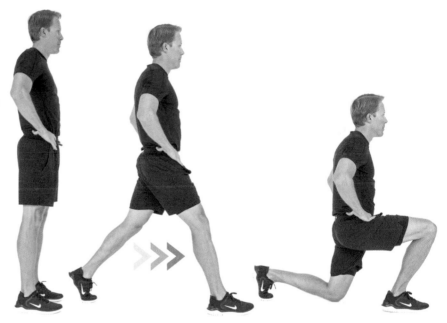

## tiptoe walk

You can perform this exercise with or without dumbbells. Try the bodyweight variation first, then add dumbbells if it's too easy. Start by getting into a half squat: hinge from your hips, tilt your torso forward, and bend your knees. Get onto the balls of your feet and take small steps. Keep your knees over your toes and your heels off the floor. Choose a distance or rep range that is challenging—usually 15–20 steps.

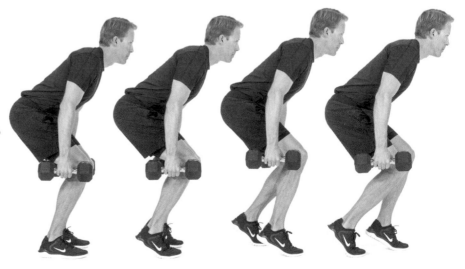

# PLANTAR FASCIOPATHY (FASCIITIS)

**Follow this program to treat:**

- Pain at the front of the heel on the sole of the foot
- Pain in the bottom of the foot

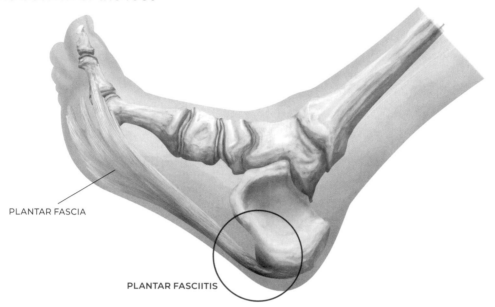

PLANTAR FASCIA

PLANTAR FASCIITIS

**DESCRIPTION:** Plantar fasciitis—or, as it is referred to in more recent research, plantar fasciopathy—is a disorder of the plantar fascia, which is a thick band that runs from your heel bone (calcaneus) up to the base of your toes. It is the most common cause of heel pain and occurs in both active and sedentary individuals.[7,8] The pain typically occurs at the front of the heel on the sole of the foot where the plantar fascia attaches to the heel bone. Plantar fasciopathy is more common in runners and overweight individuals and can be associated with other factors, such as arch height, lower body strength, and ankle and foot mobility.

The plantar fascia is a connective tissue, almost like a ligament. In addition to connecting two bones, it maintains the arch of your foot along with muscles and other ligaments. Arch height varies from person to person, but your plantar fascia helps maintain that position, and it stretches or shortens depending on whether your foot is pronating (collapsing inward) or supinating (rolling onto the outer edge).

Repeatedly straining the plantar fascia—say, from too much standing, walking, or running—can lead to plantar fasciitis, which is classified as a repetitive stress or overuse injury.

**SIGNS AND SYMPTOMS:** Pain is often sharp, especially upon standing first thing in the morning, returning to standing after being seated for long periods, or prolonged standing in place. It can also be a dull ache, usually around the front or inner side of the heel, or feel like a tender bruise on the bottom of the foot.

**AGGRAVATING FACTORS:** Standing or walking for long periods (especially barefoot or on hard surfaces), running, jumping, and adjusting to a new pair of shoes can worsen the problem.

**PROGNOSIS:** Most cases resolve within two to 12 weeks when you eliminate or modify aggravating factors and implement an appropriate rehab program, which includes loading (strength training) and stretching that targets the plantar fascia. However, some cases of plantar fasciopathy can last as long as 12 to 18 months.[9]

**TREATMENT STRATEGY:** Most cases are treated with physical therapy exercises, massage of the foot and lower leg, anti-inflammatory medication, night splints, and orthotics. Different shoes or orthotics often help not because they reposition the arch of the foot but because they change the load on the tissue, varying the source of stress. For resistant or chronic cases, steroid injections and extracorporeal shock wave therapy (sound waves that stimulate healing) can be used.

You might hear about tricks for changing your walking and running mechanics to prevent and alleviate pain, such as running with your feet straight or not letting your ankles collapse. While mechanical strategies may reduce pain in some cases, they're not a foolproof fix. For example, say you've had low arches your entire life. You went for a long run after taking some time off, and now you have pain in the bottom of your foot. Most likely, the cause of your pain is not your low arches because your body has adapted to them. In this scenario, training variables such as volume and intensity are what contributed to the issue.

If pain is a recurring problem, you need to address the speed, distance, and/or duration of your running regimen and make sure you're giving your body enough time to heal.

**1** Phase 1 of the rehab protocol aims to reduce pain with calf and plantar soft tissue mobilizations. Then you implement straight- and bent-knee plantar fascia calf stretches to eliminate pain and improve your stretch tolerance.[10] Changing your knee position alters how your calf muscles and plantar fascia are loaded, so experiment with both versions. I've included hamstring stretches in phase 1 because improving posterior chain flexibility and stretch tolerance farther up the leg can reduce pain in the calf and sole of the foot.

This is likely because the plantar nerves in the sole of the foot are branches of the tibial nerve in the calf, which is part of the sciatic nerve. Stretching the hamstring muscles also stretches the sciatic nerve, which may be why it often helps people with plantar fascia–related pain. The last exercise in phase 1 is the towel curl, which activates and strengthens the four layers of deep intrinsic muscles in the arch of the foot (muscles that support and stabilize the numerous joints in the foot).

**2** Phase 2 begins with straight- and bent-knee calf raises that target the gastrocnemius and soleus muscles. These exercises can reduce plantar fascia pain because the calf muscles and ankle joint have a direct biomechanical influence on the foot and plantar fascia.[11] The band inversion exercise works the tibialis posterior muscle, which aids in arch position and control. Improving tibialis posterior performance can take stress off the plantar fascia and intrinsic foot muscles. The doming exercise is similar to the towel curl in phase 1 and builds intrinsic foot muscle strength and control. Creating the neuromuscular pathways necessary to recruit these small muscles can take a while, so be patient and keep practicing. The last exercise in phase 2 is the kettlebell deadlift, which strengthens the hamstrings, glutes, and low back muscles and helps improve posterior chain flexibility (including the sciatic nerve) like the hamstring stretches in phase 1.

**3** Phase 3 focuses on increasing the load tolerance of the plantar fascia with knee-straight and knee-bent plantar fascia calf raises. These are similar to traditional calf raises except that the big toe is in dorsiflexion, which challenges the plantar fascia. The photos show me using a tool called the Fasciitis Fighter, which is specifically designed for this condition. If you don't have access to this tool, you can use a rolled-up towel instead. That said, if plantar fasciopathy is a common issue for you, then the Fasciitis Fighter is a good tool to have on hand.

The last three exercises target your glutes, hamstrings, and quads, which are major stabilizers of the upper kinetic chain. Improving strength and control at the hip and knee takes stress off the ankle and foot.

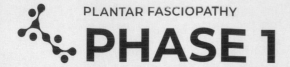

# PLANTAR FASCIOPATHY
# PHASE 1

## GOOD FOR:

- Alleviating pain in the bottom of the foot
- Relieving ankle and foot stiffness
- Warm-up for phase 2 and 3 exercises

## GUIDELINES:

- Perform every day
- Tools: foam roller, small massage ball, Fasciitis Fighter, stretch strap, towel
- Add phase 2 when you have no pain at rest and no more than mild pain (3/10) with the exercises

## SOFT TISSUE MOBILIZATIONS:

- ▸ Spend 1–2 minutes on each area
- ▸ Perform in any order on both sides
- ▸ Stop on tender points for 10–20 seconds

### calf mobilization

Sit on the floor with your calf positioned over a foam roller. Push off the floor with your hands and grounded foot—lifting your hips off the floor—to roll up and down your lower leg from ankle to knee. Stop on any tender or stiff spots and move your foot (flex, extend, and rotate from side to side).

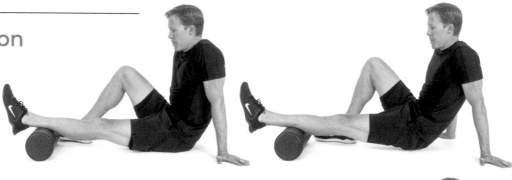

To increase the pressure, stack your other leg on top.

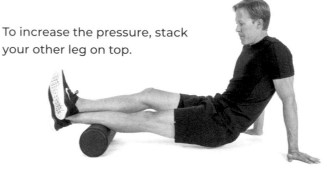

### plantar mobilization

Position a small massage ball under the arch of your foot. Roll front to back and side to side across your plantar fascia, from the ball of your foot to the front of your heel. Flex and extend your toes to dynamically mobilize the plantar fascia and underlying muscles.

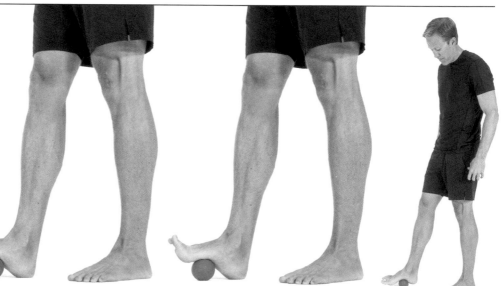

# STRETCHING EXERCISES:

▸ Do 3 reps with 30- to 60-second holds

▸ Perform in any order on both sides

▸ Don't stretch into pain

## plantar fascia calf stretch (knee straight)

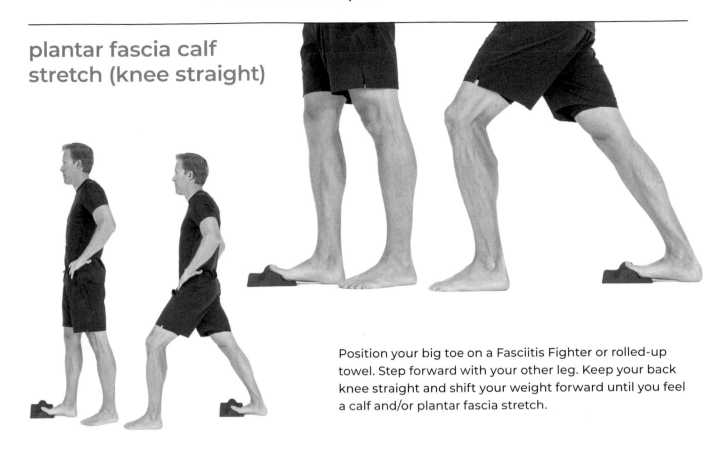

Position your big toe on a Fasciitis Fighter or rolled-up towel. Step forward with your other leg. Keep your back knee straight and shift your weight forward until you feel a calf and/or plantar fascia stretch.

## plantar fascia calf stretch (knee bent)

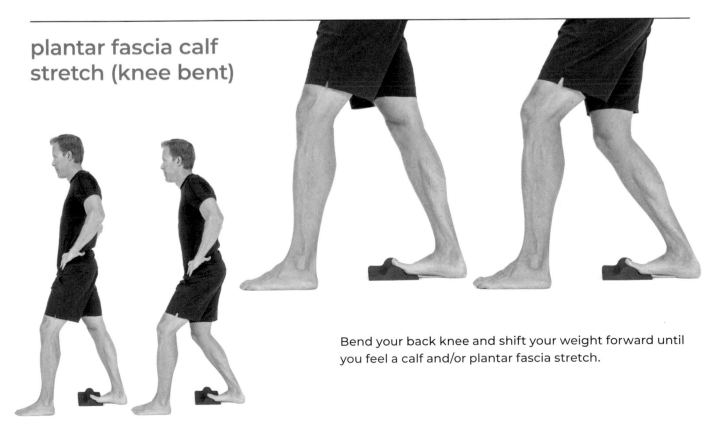

Bend your back knee and shift your weight forward until you feel a calf and/or plantar fascia stretch.

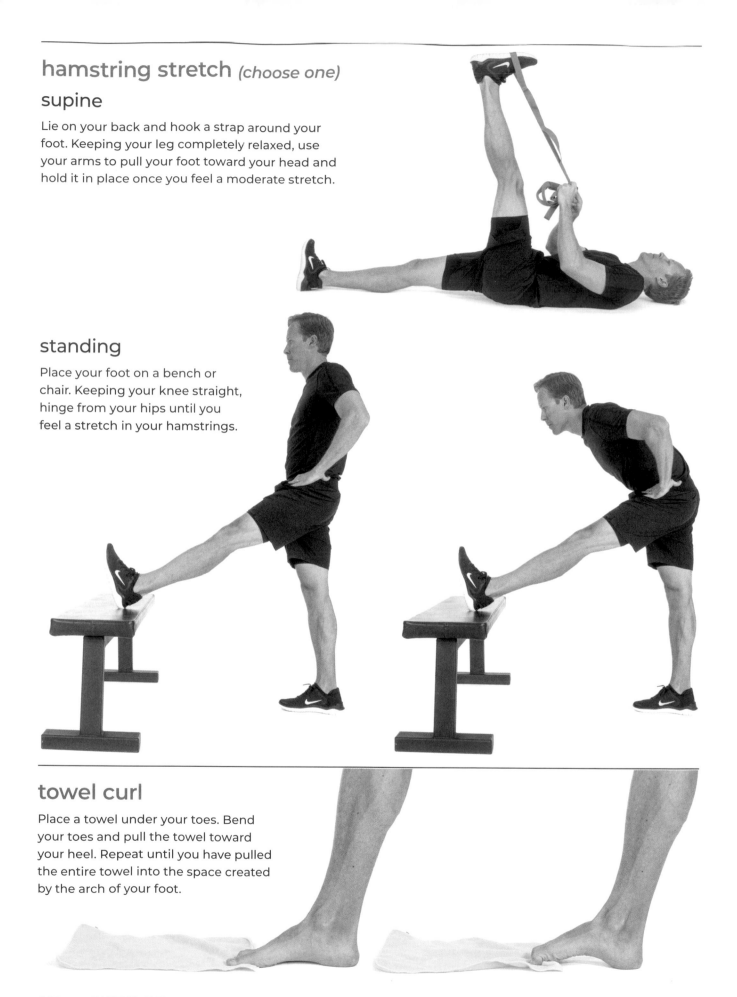

# hamstring stretch *(choose one)*

## supine

Lie on your back and hook a strap around your foot. Keeping your leg completely relaxed, use your arms to pull your foot toward your head and hold it in place once you feel a moderate stretch.

## standing

Place your foot on a bench or chair. Keeping your knee straight, hinge from your hips until you feel a stretch in your hamstrings.

# towel curl

Place a towel under your toes. Bend your toes and pull the towel toward your heel. Repeat until you have pulled the entire towel into the space created by the arch of your foot.

# PHASE 2

## GOOD FOR:

- Reducing ankle and foot pain
- Improving foot mobility and neuromuscular control
- Early ankle and foot strengthening
- Warm-up for phase 3 exercises

## GUIDELINES:

- Perform 3 or 4 days a week
- Do 3 sets of 10–15 reps unless otherwise noted
- Tools: resistance band, kettlebell or dumbbell
- Add phase 3 when you can do the exercises with no more than mild pain (3/10)

## double-leg calf raise (knees straight)

Stand with the balls of your feet on an elevated surface or step. Allow your heels to sink toward the floor. Perform slow calf raises through a full range of motion. Your heels should drop slightly lower than your toes on the down phase. Do 2 sets of 10–15 reps.

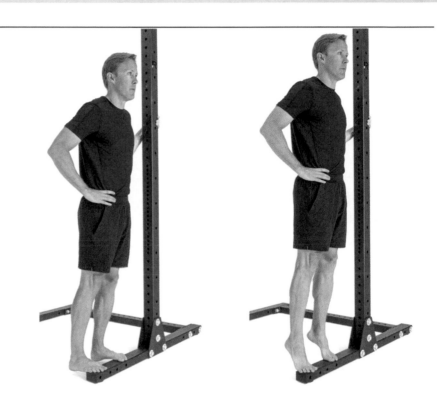

## double-leg calf raise (knees bent)

Hold onto a doorframe or rack. Sit your hips back and bend your knees into a half squat. Maintaining your knee angle, perform calf raises to target the soleus muscle. Do 2 sets of 10–15 reps.

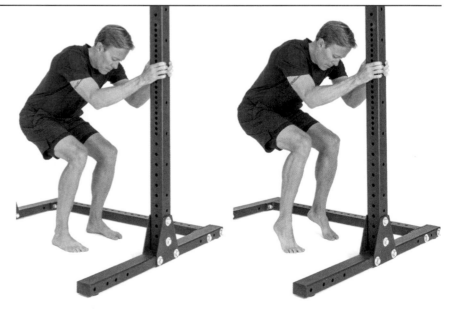

# band inversion

Tie a loop in a resistance band and wrap it around the top part of your foot. Apply tension to the band at an angle away from your body. Turn your ankle in (inversion) without moving the rest of your leg—your kneecap should point up the entire time. Move slowly and don't let the band snap your foot back to the start position.

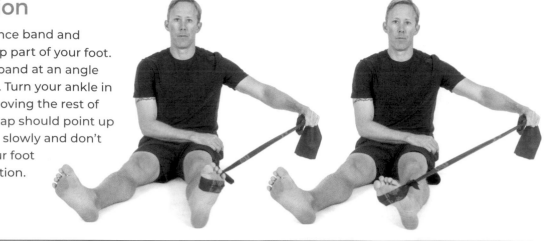

# doming

Standing with your feet staggered, squeeze the muscles in your front foot so that your arch lifts higher from the floor. Imagine trying to pull the ball of your big toe toward your heel so that your foot becomes shorter. Keep the ball of your big toe on the floor. To make the exercise easier, perform it while seated to take weight off your foot.

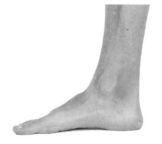
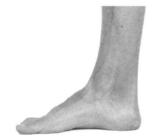
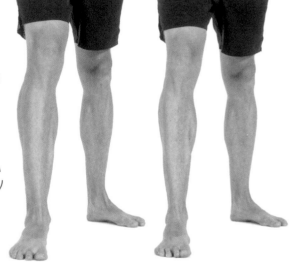

# kettlebell deadlift

Hold a kettlebell between your legs with your palms facing your body. Position your feet underneath your hips or just inside shoulder width. Keeping your back flat and arms relaxed, sit your hips back, bend your knees, and allow your torso to tilt forward—you should feel tension in your hips, hamstrings, and back. Keeping the kettlebell close to your body and your shins as vertical as possible, go as low as you can without rounding your back. To perform the upward movement, drive through your heels while extending your hips and knees. If you don't have a kettlebell, you can hold the top of a dumbbell or perform one of the variations on page 303.

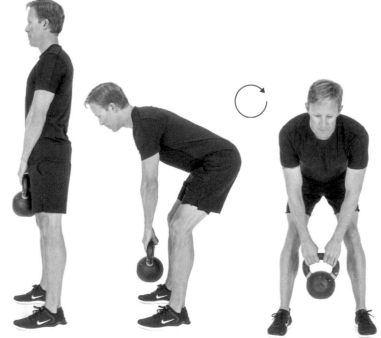

**GOOD FOR:**

- Increasing foot and ankle strength
- Preventing ankle and foot pain and injury

**GUIDELINES:**

- Perform 3 or 4 days a week
- Do 3 sets of 10–15 reps
- Push sets to fatigue
- Tools: Fasciitis Fighter, dowel, resistance loop, dumbbell

## plantar fascia calf raise (knee straight)

Stand inside a doorframe or hold something sturdy for balance and elevate your big toe on a Fasciitis Fighter or rolled-up towel. Perform single-leg calf raises with your knee straight to target the gastrocnemius (calf) muscle and plantar fascia.

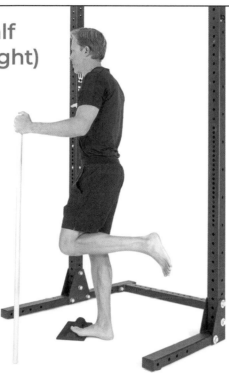 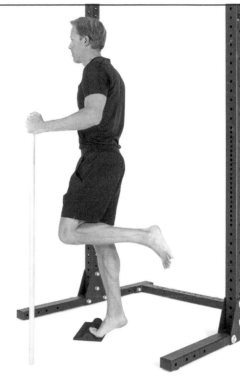

## plantar fascia calf raise (knee bent)

With your big toe elevated, lower into a half squat and perform single-leg calf raises with your knee bent to target the soleus muscle and plantar fascia.

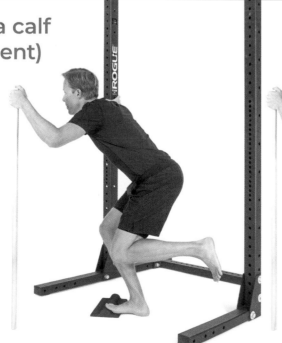 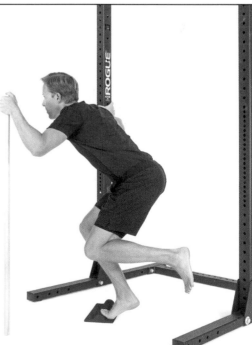

## banded hip abduction

Position a resistance loop above your knees. Shift your weight onto one leg, then raise your unweighted leg out to the side (abduction). Keep your foot pointed straight forward and try not to lean your upper body excessively. Place your hand against a wall or use a dowel to maintain balance.

## skater squat

Stand on one leg with your unweighted knee bent and foot positioned behind your body. Keeping your torso and hips square, hinge forward from your hips, tilt your torso forward, and lower your unweighted knee toward the floor. Lower your knee to a pad to gauge distance. You can hold a light weight plate or dumbbells out in front of you to counterbalance your weight.

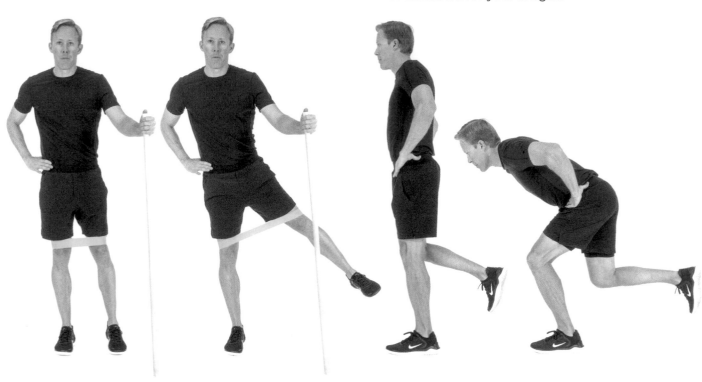

## single-leg deadlift

Cup one end of a dumbbell with both hands and shift the majority of your weight onto one leg. In one motion, hinge from your hips and bend your loaded knee slightly. As you lower your torso and the weight toward the floor, keep your back flat, grounded shin vertical, arms relaxed, and shoulders and hips square (try not to twist or rotate).

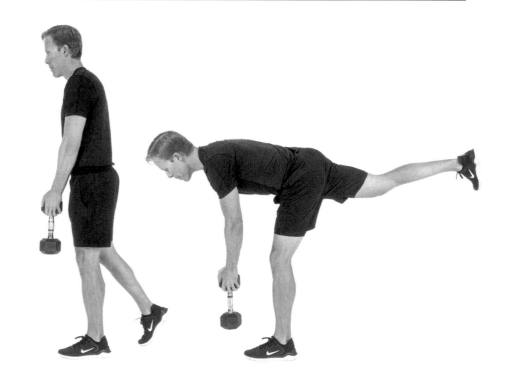

# ANKLE SPRAIN

**Follow this program to treat:**

- Ankle pain and instability

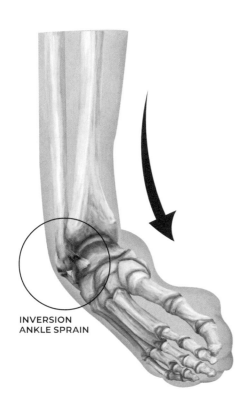

INVERSION
ANKLE SPRAIN

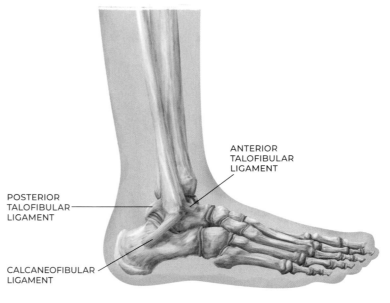

POSTERIOR
TALOFIBULAR
LIGAMENT

ANTERIOR
TALOFIBULAR
LIGAMENT

CALCANEOFIBULAR
LIGAMENT

**TEARS IN LATERAL COLLATERAL LIGAMENTS (LCL)**

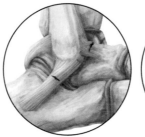

GRADE I

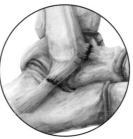

GRADE II

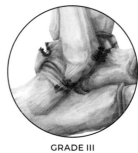

GRADE III

**DESCRIPTION:** Ankle sprains are common orthopedic injuries and can lead to long-term impairments, including pain, stiffness, and gait abnormalities in as many as 72 percent of individuals. Furthermore, nearly 80 percent of those who suffer a sprain are likely to experience reinjury.[12,13] Ankle sprains can be divided into two types—inversion (foot rolls in) and eversion (foot rolls out)—with inversion sprains accounting for more than three-quarters of cases.[14,15]

An inversion sprain damages ligaments on the outside of the ankle. You can tear one or all of the four ligaments located there. Imagine landing from a rebound in basketball and rolling your ankle; your foot's pointed and turns inward (plantarflexion plus inversion). It usually turns inward because the ligament on the inside is so strong that it's harder to turn out—that's why eversion sprains are less common.

With an ankle sprain, you typically feel a pop followed by sharp stabbing pain. Despite the pain, you should be able to bear some weight on the injured foot and take at least four steps immediately after the injury. If you can't put any weight on it, you likely have a fracture, and you should get an X-ray to determine the exact nature of your injury.

**SIGNS AND SYMPTOMS:** Sprains typically cause sharp pain on either the outside or the inside of the ankle when loading or moving the ankle and throbbing or aching at rest. Swelling and discoloration of the surrounding tissues can occur with more severe sprains.

**AGGRAVATING FACTORS:** Turning the foot in or out, walking or running on uneven surfaces, and other movements that stress the healing ligaments.

**PROGNOSIS:** Ankle sprains typically heal within four to 16 weeks depending on the severity and how quickly you implement an appropriate rehab program.

**TREATMENT STRATEGY:** Most sprains require a rehab program that focuses on regaining joint stability, strength, and neuromuscular control.[14] Resting and elevating the leg, along with wearing a compression garment, can reduce swelling and pain. If ligament damage is significant and the ankle feels unstable, surgical reconstruction may be necessary to restore function and stability.

The treatment strategy varies based on the grade of the sprain. For a substantial sprain with swelling and bruising up the leg, three to seven days of rest will allow you to protect the area, elevate the limb, and apply compression. You may be able to do ankle pumps (as in the plantarflexion-dorsiflexion mobility exercise) after a couple of days, which can help with blood flow and mobility during early recovery. The key is to let the injury calm down before starting the rest of the phase 1 exercises.

Phase 1 of the protocol focuses on reducing pain and improving active mobility via the calf mobilization and ankle mobility plantarflexion-dorsiflexion exercise. Limited ankle dorsiflexion is common after ankle sprains, so the standing dorsiflexion stretch comes next. With this movement, push only to the point where discomfort begins. The next two band exercises build strength in the sagittal (flexion-extension) plane of motion. You don't want to move into the frontal plane (inversion-eversion) early on, as these movements can stress the injured ligaments and delay healing.

As you begin phase 2, the exercise challenge increases. You now see ankle inversion and eversion with a band. Your ankle invertors and evertors run along the inside and outside of your lower leg and brace the ankle, so you want them to be strong before you return to tasks that challenge ankle stability. The kneeling dorsiflexion stretch is a more advanced version of the standing option from phase 1. Again, do not push into pain. Because the calf muscles help control and stabilize the joint, the double-leg calf raise builds calf strength without putting too much stress on the injured ankle. The last two exercises in phase 2, the standing banded hydrant and lateral step-down, involve balancing on one leg and strengthening the quad and glute muscles farther up the kinetic chain, which helps stabilize the hip and knee joints. Learning to control these joints can reduce the likelihood that your leg will move into a position that compromises your ankle.

Phase 3 progresses to single-leg calf raises because you want the ankle to support your full body weight so that you can complete sets of calf raises without pain. The knee-straight version targets the gastrocnemius muscle, which is closer to the surface, whereas the knee-bent version targets the deeper soleus muscle. The clock exercise improves dynamic balance and proprioception, which improves joint control and awareness and makes you less likely to sprain your ankle again. The tiptoe walk targets the calf muscles, especially the soleus, but performing it correctly requires ankle stability. Your ankle may want to twist, so move slowly and focus on controlling the joint. The last two exercises are mainly for athletes who wish to return to jumping and landing tasks. Even if you aren't an athlete, practicing small single-leg hops can teach you how to land and control your ankle in a more challenging fashion. Try to stick the landing without losing your balance.

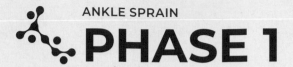

## ANKLE SPRAIN
# PHASE 1

### GOOD FOR:

- Alleviating ankle pain
- Reducing inflammation
- Improving mobility
- Warm-up for phase 2 and 3 exercises

### GUIDELINES:

- Perform every day
- Tools: foam roller, resistance band
- Add phase 2 when you have no pain at rest and no more than mild pain (3/10) with the exercises

## calf mobilization

Sit on the floor with your calf positioned over a foam roller. Push off the floor with your hands and grounded foot—lifting your hips off the floor—to roll up and down your lower leg from ankle to knee, spending 1–2 minutes on each leg. To increase the pressure, stack your other leg on top.

## ankle mobility plantarflexion-dorsiflexion

Sit on the floor or in a chair—any position where you can move your ankle freely. You can keep your knee straight or bend it. Move your toes toward your shin (dorsiflexion), then point your foot (plantarflexion). That counts as one rep. Do 3 sets of 15–20 reps with active range of motion—move as far as you can with no more than mild pain.

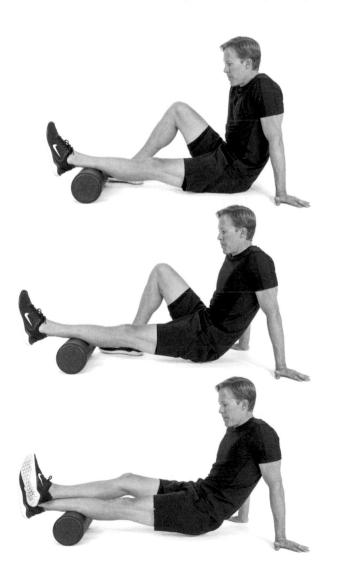

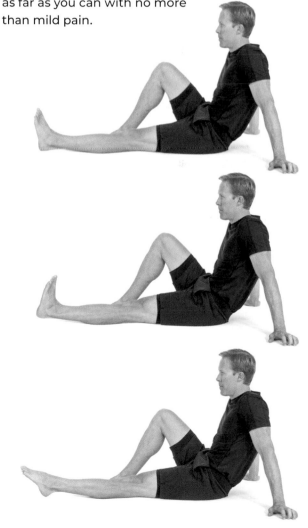

## standing dorsiflexion stretch

Stand in a staggered stance. Keep your back knee straight and feet flat on the floor. Shift your weight forward and lower your body by bending your knees, driving your rear knee forward over your toes until you feel a stretch in your calf/Achilles tendon. This stretch targets the ankle joint, so you may feel it on the front of your ankle. Perform 3 reps on each side with 30- to 60-second holds.

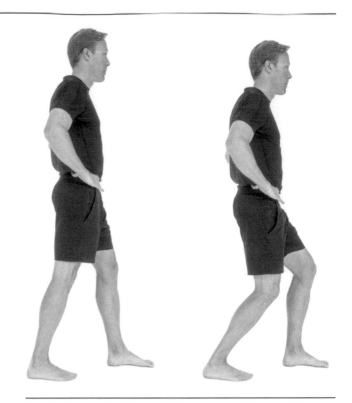

## band plantarflexion

Tie a loop in a resistance band, wrap it around the top part of your foot, and apply tension to the band with your arm. Extend your ankle as far as you can into plantarflexion with no more than mild pain. Slowly return to the start position. Do 3 sets of 10–15 reps.

## band dorsiflexion

With the band still looped around your foot, attach the other end to a fixed object or have a partner hold it to create tension. Pull your ankle as far as you can into dorsiflexion with no more than mild pain. Slowly return to the start position; don't let the band snap your ankle back down. Do 3 sets of 20 reps.

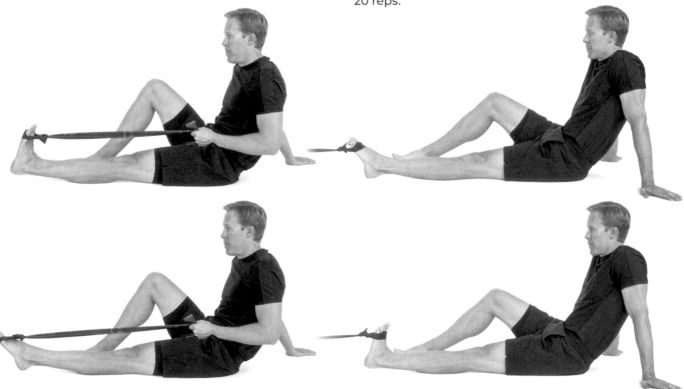

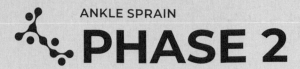

# PHASE 2

## GOOD FOR:

- Reducing ankle and foot pain
- Early ankle and foot strengthening
- Warm-up for phase 3 exercises

## GUIDELINES:

- Perform 3 or 4 days a week
- Tools: resistance band, resistance loop, plyo box
- Add phase 3 when you can do the exercises with no more than mild pain (3/10)

## band inversion

Tie a loop in a resistance band and wrap it around the top part of your foot. Apply tension to the band at an angle away from your body. Turn your ankle in (inversion) without moving the rest of your leg—your kneecap should point up the entire time. Move slowly and don't let the band snap your foot back to the start position. Do 3 sets of 15 reps.

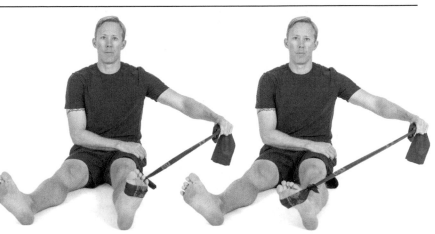

## band eversion

Apply tension to the band by pulling it around your other foot with your opposite-side arm. Start with your foot turned in (inversion), then turn your ankle out (eversion) without moving the rest of your leg—your kneecap should point up the entire time. Do 3 sets of 15 reps.

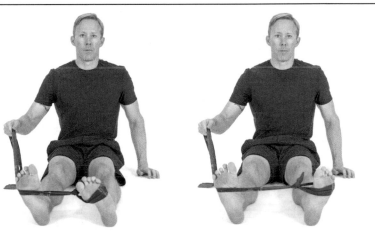

## kneeling dorsiflexion stretch

Kneel on the floor and get into the bottom of a split squat. Keeping your rear big toe flush with the floor, shift your weight forward so that your front ankle moves into dorsiflexion. Move as far as you can without pain. You should feel a stretch on the front of your ankle and/or the back side near your Achilles tendon. Perform 3 reps with 30- to 60-second holds. Don't stretch into pain.

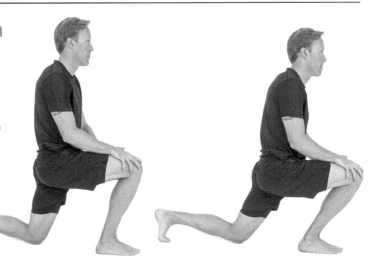

## double-leg calf raise

Stand with the balls of your feet on an elevated surface or step. Allow your heels to sink toward the floor. Perform slow calf raises through a full range of motion. Your heels should drop slightly lower than your toes on the down phase. Do 3 sets of 10–15 reps.

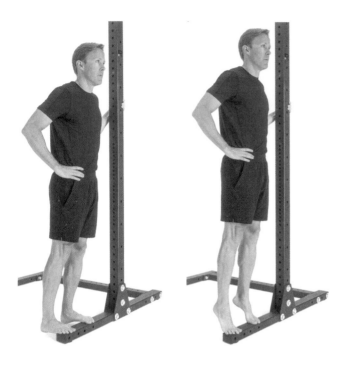

## standing banded hydrant

Position a resistance loop just above your knees. Hinge forward from your hips and bend your knees slightly, keeping your shins vertical. In one motion, lift your leg out to the side (abduction) and back (extension) while rotating your foot outward (external rotation). Focus on keeping your grounded knee straight; don't let it cave inward. Do 3 sets of 10–20 reps.

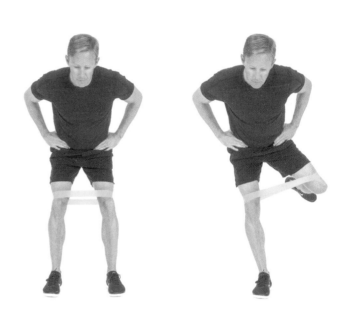

## lateral step-down

Stand next to a plyo box or small step. Perform a lateral step-up by placing your entire foot on the edge of the box and standing tall. Move your free leg forward slightly. Keeping that leg straight, reach your heel toward the floor by slowly sitting back and bending your grounded knee. As soon as your heel contacts the floor, straighten your knee, extend your hips, and return to the start position. Keep your knee aligned over your foot; don't let it move in or out. Do 3 sets of 10–15 reps.

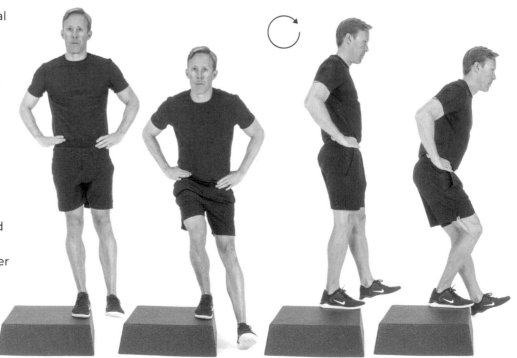

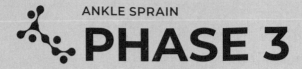

# PHASE 3

## GOOD FOR:

- Increasing ankle strength
- Improving stability and balance
- Preventing ankle pain and injury

## GUIDELINES:

- Perform 3 or 4 days a week
- Do 3 sets of 10–15 reps unless otherwise noted
- Push sets to fatigue
- Tools: dumbbells

## single-leg calf raise (knee straight)

Stand with the ball of one foot on an elevated surface or step. Perform slow calf raises through a full range of motion. Your heel should drop slightly lower than your toes on the down phase.

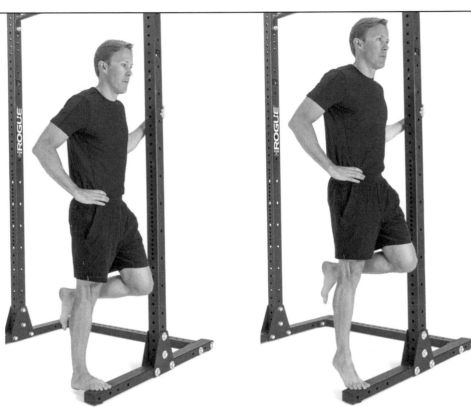

## single-leg calf raise (knee bent)

Hold onto a doorframe or rack, sit your hips back, bend your knees, and lower into a half squat. Shift your weight onto one leg and perform single-leg calf raises. Maintain your knee and hip angle during the movement.

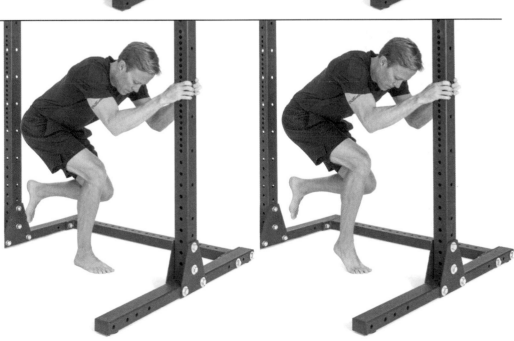

## clock

Stand with your feet positioned underneath your hips. Shift your weight onto one leg. Sink your hips back and bend your grounded knee, then reach out to the positions of an imaginary clock with the other leg. Start at 12 o'clock and work through each hour position—returning to the start position after every step—until you reach 6 o'clock. Each leg will work through one half of the clock.

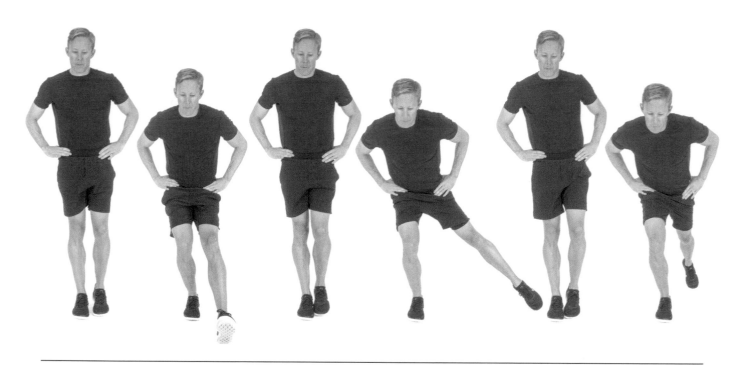

## tiptoe walk

You can perform this exercise with or without dumbbells. Try the bodyweight variation first, then add dumbbells if it's too easy. Start by getting into a half squat: hinge from your hips, tilt your torso forward, and bend your knees. Get onto the balls of your feet and take small steps. Keep your knees over your toes and your heels off the floor. Choose a distance or rep range that is challenging—usually 15–20 steps.

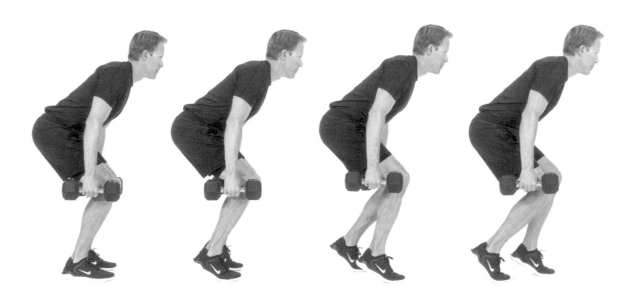

# single-leg hops

Stand on one leg and hop straight up. Land softly on the ball of your foot and allow your heel to come down with control. Jump only as high as feels comfortable and safe. Jumping too high without adequate control puts you at risk of suffering another sprain. Do 3 sets of 6–12 reps (hops).

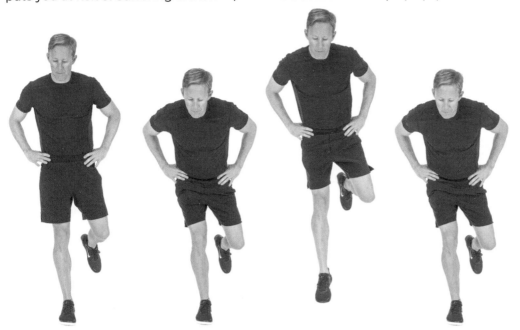

**Only do these exercises if your knee stability is very high and you need to be able to perform jumping movements in daily life.**

# skater jumps

Stand with your feet shoulder width apart. To generate momentum for the lateral jump, hinge forward from your hips and kick one leg back. As you do, rotate your shoulders toward your grounded leg. Think of an ice skater's stride—this is your start and finish position. Drive off the outside edge of your foot and extend your elevated leg laterally in the direction of the jump. As your foot leaves the floor, unwind your shoulders and bend your knee. Cushion the landing by reclaiming the start position on the opposite side—hinging from your hips, lowering into a single-leg (skater) squat, and rotating your shoulders toward your grounded leg. Immediately repeat the sequence, hopping from side to side rhythmically. Do 3 sets of 6–12 reps (jumps).

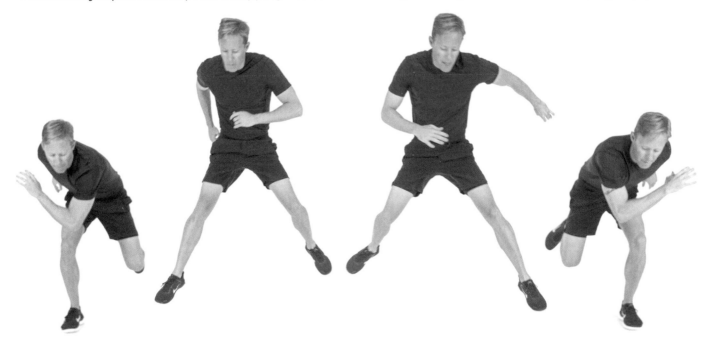

# SHIN SPLINTS
## (MEDIAL TIBIAL STRESS SYNDROME)

**Follow this program to treat:**

- Pain on the inside or outside of the shin
- Medial tibial stress syndrome

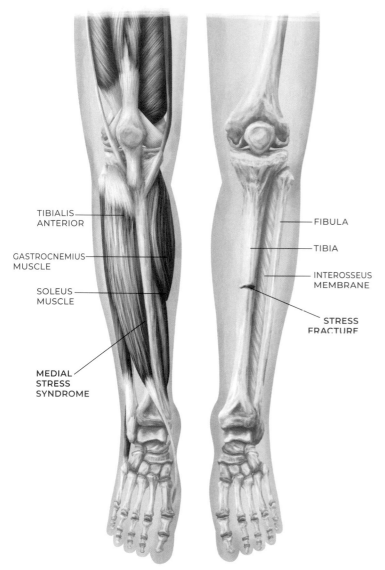

TIBIALIS ANTERIOR

GASTROCNEMIUS MUSCLE

SOLEUS MUSCLE

MEDIAL STRESS SYNDROME

FIBULA

TIBIA

INTEROSSEUS MEMBRANE

STRESS FRACTURE

**DESCRIPTION:** Medial tibial stress syndrome (MTSS), or shin splints, is a repetitive stress injury of the anteromedial shin region (inside of the lower leg). The most common running-related musculoskeletal injury, MTSS typically involves excessive loading of the tissues from which the body is unable to heal.[16] In most cases, shin splints develop because of an increase in training intensity, distance, or duration, but they can involve other variables, such as running on hard surfaces, wearing shoes with poor shock absorption, or engaging in a new activity—like going for a long walk on the beach.

A lot of issues with the bone or tendon create symptoms in similar areas, so they all get lumped together under the umbrella term MTSS. You can have shin splints on the inside, back, or front of the shinbone. You can also have anterior or posterior shin splints, which affect different muscular compartments.

Anterior shin splints have more to do with your ankle dorsiflexor muscles, especially the tibialis anterior, which lifts the front of your foot. They are more common in runners who heel-strike because the tibialis anterior muscle acts as a brake to lower the front of the foot after the heel strikes the ground. They also happen in people who do a lot of downhill hiking, where that muscle has to work over and over to lower the foot for the next step.

Posterior shin splints occur more often on the back side of the bone, in the posterior compartment with the calf and tibialis posterior muscles. The tibialis posterior works with your calf to point your foot and turn it inward. So, this type of shin splints is more common in forefoot strikers. People who go from wearing cushioned shoes to barefoot shoes or who run on hard or difficult surfaces (like sand) often develop posterior shin splints because they strike the ground with the ball of their foot, and the tibialis posterior and calf muscles have to work much harder to absorb shock.

**SIGNS AND SYMPTOMS:** Pain is typically felt in the front and inside of the shin region and is provoked when the area is stressed, such as during running or walking downhill. You may notice that touching the shinbone reproduces your pain. Symptoms can be sharp during activity, and the area may ache or throb afterward.

**AGGRAVATING FACTORS:** Walking, running, and jumping, which stress the shin region and surrounding muscles and connective tissue.

**PROGNOSIS:** Shin splints usually resolve with rest and rehab, but the time frame can vary based on the severity and your activity level. Most people recover within six to eight weeks once the area has been desensitized and they have modified their training to meet their current tissue capacity.

**TREATMENT STRATEGY:** Shin splints are typically managed with physical therapy and training program modifications. The rehab exercises focus on decreasing pain, building strength in the shin muscles, and gradually increasing running or jumping volume to give the sensitive tissues time to adapt. If your symptoms do not improve after six to eight weeks—assuming you have addressed aggravating factors and discounting potential flare-ups—you may want to consult with a doctor to rule out a stress fracture.

**1** Phase 1 of the protocol focuses on reducing pain and relieving tension in the anterior and posterior muscle compartments. The calf and tibialis posterior mobilizations are specific to posterior shin splints, whereas the tibialis anterior mobilization fits with anterior shin splints. It doesn't hurt to work all these muscle groups even if you have shin splints in only one location. Phase 1 also includes calf stretches because stretching your calves can help reduce pain associated with posterior shin splints. The knee-straight version targets the gastrocnemius muscle, and the knee-bent version targets the soleus muscle. There are also two tibialis anterior stretching options. Pick the one that creates a better stretch on the front of your shin.

**2** In phase 2, you use banded movements to start strengthening the muscles and tendons involved with shin splints. The band inversion exercise targets the tibialis posterior, and the band dorsiflexion exercise loads the tibialis anterior muscle and tendon. Because the tibialis posterior is in the posterior compartment with the calf muscles, I have included both calf raise variations in this phase: the knee-straight exercise biases the load toward the gastrocnemius, and the knee-bent exercise biases it toward the soleus. The skater squat strengthens the glutes and quads farther up the kinetic chain. These muscles are important shock absorbers and can take stress off the lower leg muscles.

**3** In phase 3, you continue to strengthen muscles located proximally in the kinetic chain. This is true except for the tiptoe walk, which targets the calf (and quads), especially the soleus, and can improve lower leg strength. The single-leg hops at the end place the most stress on the healing tissues, so do this exercise only when you can hop and land with little or no pain.

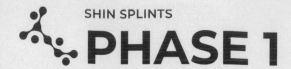

## SHIN SPLINTS
# PHASE 1

**GOOD FOR:**

- Alleviating shin splint pain
- Reducing muscle tension
- Improving flexibility
- Warm-up for phase 2 and 3 exercises

**GUIDELINES:**

- Perform every day
- Tools: foam roller, small massage ball, slant board
- Add phase 2 when you have no pain at rest and no more than mild pain (3/10) with the exercises

# SOFT TISSUE MOBILIZATIONS:

- ▸ Spend 1–2 minutes on each area
- ▸ Perform in any order on both sides
- ▸ Stop on tender points for 10–20 seconds

## calf mobilization

Sit on the floor with your calf positioned over a foam roller. Push off the floor with your hands and grounded foot—lifting your hips off the floor—to roll up and down your lower leg from ankle to knee. Stop on any tender or stiff spots and move your foot (flex, extend, and rotate from side to side). To increase the pressure, stack your other leg on top.

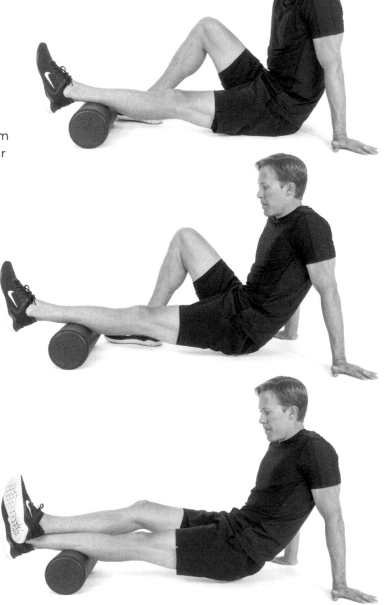

## tibialis anterior mobilization *(choose one)*

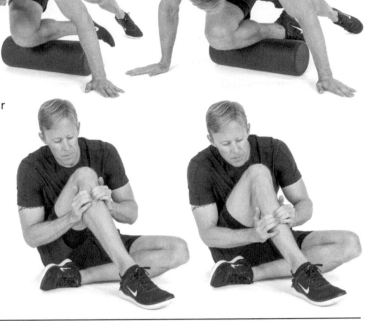

### with foam roller

Get into push-up position and place the meaty part of your shin (not the bone) on the foam roller. Roll up and down your lower leg, from knee to ankle. Apply pressure by sinking your hips down and getting your weight over your leg.

### manual variation

Sit with your leg bent (knee to chest) and apply pressure with your index and middle fingers to the muscles on the outside of your shin, from knee to ankle. Stop on tender points and flex and extend your ankle to further mobilize the muscle.

## tibialis posterior mobilization *(choose one)*

You can perform this mobilization using a small massage ball or your thumbs. Sit with your leg bent (knee to chest) and apply pressure to the muscles on the inside of your shin, from knee to ankle. Stop on tender points and flex and extend your ankle to further mobilize the muscle.

### with ball

### manual variation

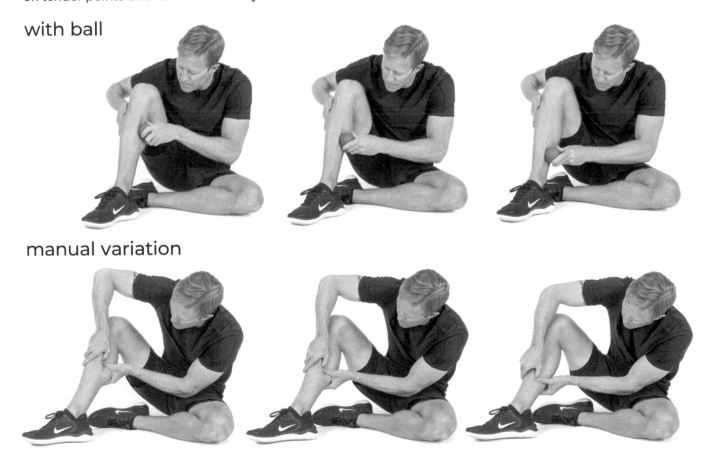

# STRETCHING EXERCISES:

- ▸ Do 3 reps with 30- to 60-second holds
- ▸ Perform in any order on both sides
- ▸ Don't stretch into pain

## pretibial stretch *(choose one)*

### double-leg

Start with the tops of your feet and shins flush on the floor. Keeping your knees on the floor, sit your hips toward your heels. Skip this exercise if you experience ankle pain. You can also try the single-leg variation for a more potent stretch.

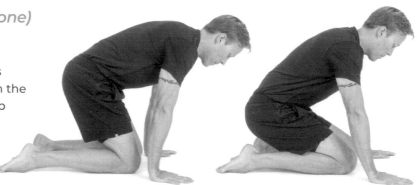

### single-leg

Sit with one foot on the floor and the other leg bent underneath your body, positioning your foot underneath your hips. Start with your foot and shin flush with the floor. Shift your weight toward your bent leg and use your arm to prop yourself up. Supporting your weight with your arm and leg, pull your knee toward your chest.

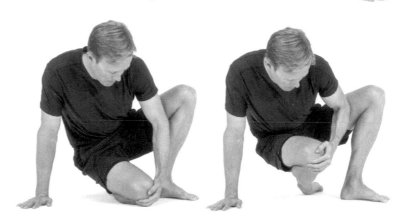

## standing calf stretch

Stand with the front part of your foot on a slant board, incline, or elevated surface. Step your other foot in front of the leg you are stretching. You should feel a stretch through your calf and the back of your ankle. To target your soleus muscle, sit your hips back, tilt your torso forward, and bend your knee.

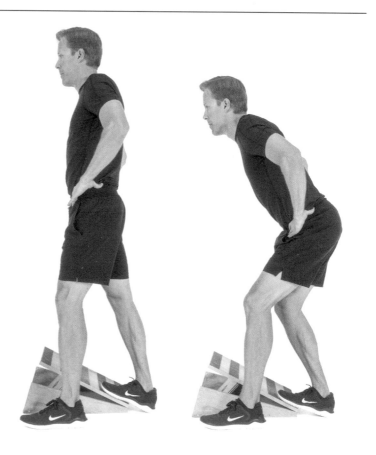

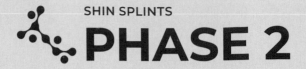

# PHASE 2

## GOOD FOR:

- Reducing shin splint pain
- Early ankle and shin strengthening
- Warm-up for phase 3 exercises

## GUIDELINES:

- Perform 3 or 4 days a week
- Do 3 sets of 10–15 reps
- Tool: resistance band
- Add phase 3 when you can do the exercises with no more than mild pain (3/10)

## band inversion

Tie a loop in a resistance band and wrap it around the top part of your foot. Apply tension to the band at an angle away from your body. Turn your ankle in (inversion) without moving the rest of your leg—your kneecap should point up the entire time. Move slowly and don't let the band snap your foot back when returning to the start position.

## band dorsiflexion

With the band still looped around your foot, attach the other end to a fixed object or have a partner hold it to create tension. Pull your ankle as far as you can into dorsiflexion with no more than mild pain. Slowly return to the start position; don't let the band snap your ankle back down.

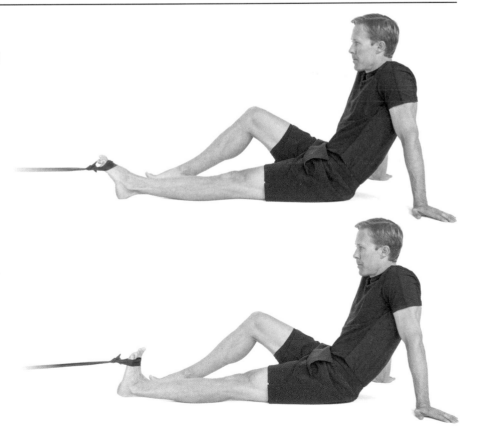

## single-leg calf raise (knee straight)

Stand with the ball of one foot on an elevated surface or step. Perform slow calf raises through the full range of motion. Your heel should drop slightly lower than your toes on the down phase.

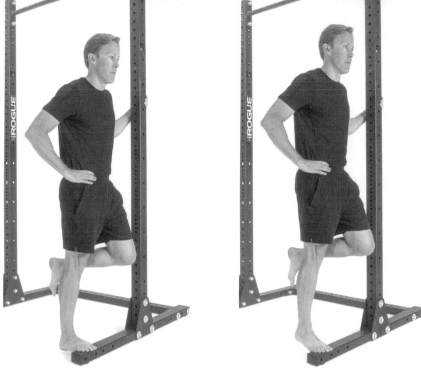

## single-leg calf raise (knee bent)

Hold onto a doorframe or rack, sit your hips back, bend your knees, and lower into a half squat. Shift your weight onto one leg and perform single-leg calf raises. Maintain your knee and hip angle during the movement.

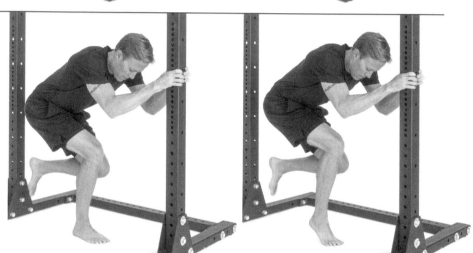

## skater squat

Stand on one leg with your unweighted knee bent and foot positioned behind your body. Keeping your torso and hips square, hinge forward from your hips, tilt your torso forward, and lower your unweighted knee toward the floor. Lower your knee to a pad to gauge distance. You can hold a light weight plate or dumbbells out in front of you to counterbalance your weight.

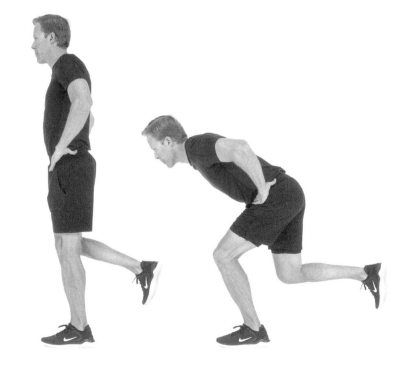

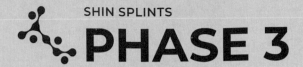

# PHASE 3

**GOOD FOR:**

- Increasing lower leg strength
- Preventing shin splint pain and injury

**GUIDELINES:**

- Perform 3 or 4 days a week
- Do 3 sets of 10–15 reps unless otherwise noted
- Push sets to fatigue
- Tools: dumbbells, plyo box

## tiptoe walk

You can perform this exercise with or without dumbbells. Try the bodyweight variation first, then add dumbbells if it's too easy. Start by getting into a half squat: hinge from your hips, tilt your torso forward, and bend your knees. Get onto the balls of your feet and take small steps. Keep your knees over your toes and your heels off the floor. Choose a distance or rep range that is challenging—usually 15–20 steps.

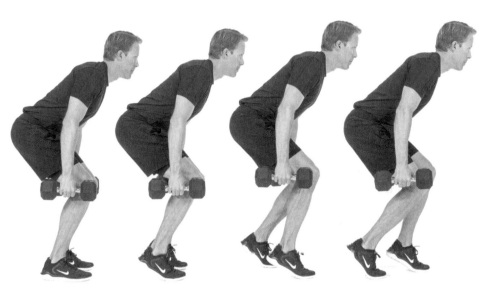

## goblet squat

Stand with your feet roughly shoulder width apart. When it comes to foot flare, you can orient your feet straight or turn them out slightly—whichever feels better and allows you to reach the lowest depth without discomfort. Cup a dumbbell with both hands at the center of your chest. To perform the movement, reach your hips back slightly and sit straight down. As you lower into the bottom position, keep your spine in the neutral zone (not excessively arching or rounding), your knees aligned over your toes, and the weight close to your body. The goal is to keep your torso as upright as possible and lower as far as you can while maintaining good form.

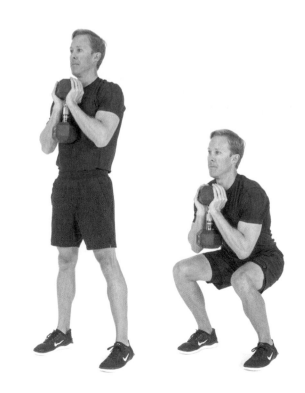

## step-up

Step on a plyo box with your knee aligned over your foot. Without pushing off the floor, shift your weight onto your elevated leg, drive through your heel or mid-foot, and raise your torso and hips in one fluid motion. Progress this exercise by increasing the height of the box or holding a dumbbell.

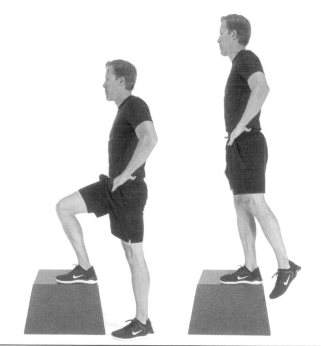

## forward lunge

Stand with your feet shoulder width apart. Take a big step forward and come up onto the ball of your rear foot. As your front foot makes contact, slowly lower your rear knee to the floor with control. You can keep your torso upright or tilt slightly forward. Shift your weight onto your lead leg, drive through your mid-foot, and stand upright. You can step into the start position or transition into your next forward step with the opposite leg. Do 10–15 steps with each leg.

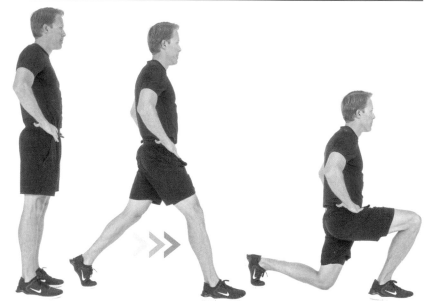

## single-leg hops

Stand on one leg and hop straight up. Land softly on the ball of your foot and allow your heel to come down with control. Jump only as high as feels comfortable and safe.

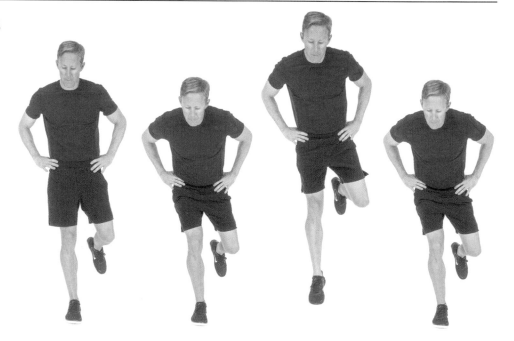

# BUNION

**Follow this program to treat:**

- Painful bump at the base of the big toe
- Big toe stiffness, swelling, and redness

**DESCRIPTION:** Hallux valgus (bunion) is a deformity in which the first metatarsal, or big toe, deviates medially toward the other toes, creating a bump at its base. This issue occurs more often in women than in men by a ratio of 2:1 to 4:1.[17] About 70 percent of bunion patients have a positive family history, suggesting that there is a genetic component to this condition.[18-20] Certain biomechanical characteristics of the ankle and foot (limited big toe and ankle dorsiflexion) as well as wearing high heels or shoes with a narrow toe box are also thought to contribute to the development of bunions. When ankle or big toe dorsiflexion is limited and mobility is restricted, people typically pronate their feet when walking. This extra pronation creates a shearing force on the big toe and pushes it toward the other toes, exacerbating the issue.

**SIGNS AND SYMPTOMS:** Bunions typically cause pain, stiffness, redness, and swelling in and around the joint at the base of the big toe (first metatarsophalangeal, or MTP).

**AGGRAVATING FACTORS:** Activities that stress the big toe, such as walking, running, and rising onto the toes, work the first MTP joint and can worsen bunion pain.

**PROGNOSIS:** Conservative interventions such as physical therapy and shoe modifications can reduce bunion pain significantly within four to six weeks. However, these interventions will not correct the alignment of the toe. If your pain is ongoing and function remains severely impaired, consider consulting with a podiatrist.

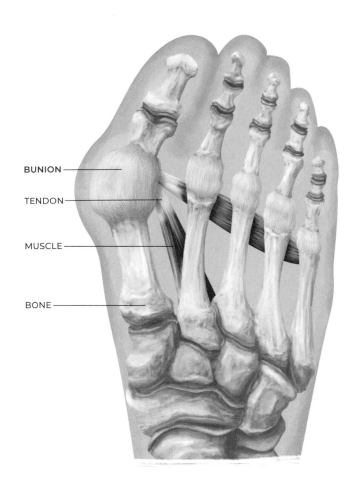

BUNION

TENDON

MUSCLE

BONE

## WILL THIS PROTOCOL WORK FOR HAMMERTOE, TAILOR'S BUNION, METATARSALGIA, MORTON'S NEUROMA, AND OTHER TOE CONDITIONS?

The rehab exercises and recommendations might benefit other toe conditions, but in my experience—and this might also be the case with a severe bunion—it's best to work with a podiatrist and a manual therapy specialist because these conditions are hard to treat with exercise alone. Also, you may need a special type of orthotic or a shoe modification, which should be made by an expert based on your individual needs.

**TREATMENT STRATEGY:** Nonoperative treatment usually includes choosing shoes with a wider toe box and doing mobilization and stretching exercises to reduce pain and improve the mobility of the big toe and ankle joint. Operative treatment involves surgical realignment of the big toe. Do not rush into surgery, however; many patients who undergo this procedure end up having considerable toe stiffness and functional limitations.

**1** In phase 1, you implement techniques to loosen muscles that have a direct biomechanical influence on your ankle, foot, and big toe. The calf and plantar mobilizations allow the ankle and big toe to move more easily through dorsiflexion, which is necessary for many functional tasks, including walking. The standing calf and plantar fascia stretches are the next step and again encourage dorsiflexion mobility. The big toe mobilization at the end of phase 1 involves using your hands to position the toe in a neutral alignment and then pull it down into plantarflexion and up into dorsiflexion. As mobility in your big toe joint improves, you will notice less pain with functional tasks. The big toe joint must have at least 60 degrees of dorsiflexion for you to walk normally.

**2** In phase 2, you continue moving your big toe and ankle into dorsiflexion with more aggressive stretches. Do not push into pain, especially with the big toe dorsiflexion stretch. The hamstring stretch helps improve posterior chain flexibility, which can influence the sole of the foot and the big toe. The three mobility exercises teach you how to better control your big toe and the arch of your foot. The big toe abduction exercise involves using your abductor muscles to pull your big toe to the side and away from the smaller toes into a more neutral alignment. It is quite challenging if you have never practiced it, so be patient and stick with it; your nervous system will figure it out. The big toe dorsiflexion exercise involves lifting your big toe as high as you can on your own and then using your hand to add more stretch at the top. The doming exercise, in which you lift the arch of your foot while keeping the ball of your big toe on the floor, improves the strength and control of the muscles in the arch. Imagine doing a crunch exercise with your arch muscles.

**3** Phase 3 is all about strengthening muscles farther up the kinetic chain that support and protect the big toe. The towel curl is similar to the doming exercise but focuses more on the toe flexor muscles. The band dorsiflexion and calf raise exercises target the ankle muscles, and the lateral step-down works the quads and glutes. Improving strength and control at the hip, knee, and ankle takes stress off sensitive toe structures, so these exercises can help optimize the health of the entire leg, including the big toe.

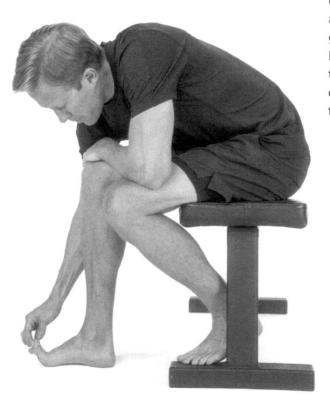

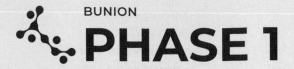

## BUNION
# PHASE 1

### GOOD FOR:

- Alleviating big toe and foot pain
- Reducing inflammation
- Improving mobility
- Warm-up for phase 2 and 3 exercises

### GUIDELINES:

- Perform every day
- Tools: foam roller, small massage ball, slant board
- Add phase 2 when you have no pain at rest and no more than mild pain (3/10) with the exercises

## SOFT TISSUE MOBILIZATIONS:

- ▸ Spend 1–2 minutes on each area
- ▸ Perform in any order on both sides
- ▸ Stop on tender points for 10–20 seconds

### calf mobilization

Sit on the floor with your calf positioned over a foam roller. Push off the floor with your hands and grounded foot—lifting your hips off the floor—to roll up and down your lower leg from ankle to knee. Stop on any tender or stiff spots and move your foot (flex, extend, and rotate from side to side).

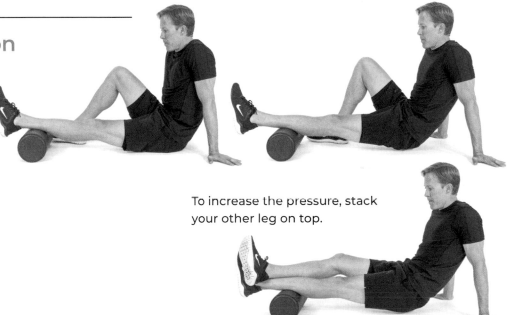

To increase the pressure, stack your other leg on top.

### plantar mobilization

Step on a small massage ball, positioning it under the arch of your foot. Roll from front to back and side to side across your plantar fascia, from the ball of your foot to the front of your heel. Flex and extend your toes to dynamically mobilize the plantar fascia and underlying muscles.

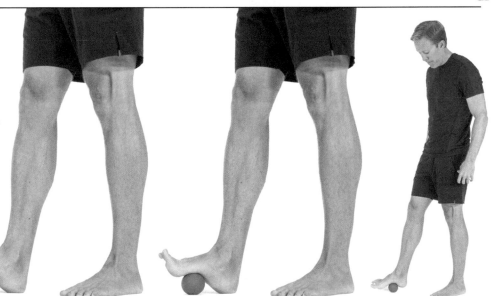

## standing calf stretch

Stand with the front part of your foot on a slant board, incline, or elevated surface. Step your other foot in front of the leg you are stretching. You should feel a stretch through your calf and back of your ankle. To target your soleus muscle, sit your hips back, tilt your torso forward, and bend your knee. Do 3 reps with 30- to 60-second holds. Don't stretch into pain.

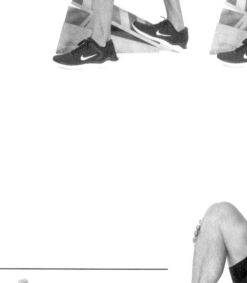

## plantar fascia stretch

In a seated position, bend your ankle into dorsiflexion (toes toward your shin). Push down on the back of your heel to hold the position. Grip the bottom of your big toe and pull it toward your shin, stretching the plantar fascia and big toe joint. Do 3 reps with 30- to 60-second holds. Don't stretch into pain.

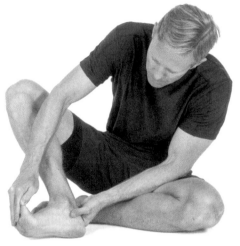

## big toe mobilization

Wrap your thumb and index finger around the base of your big toe, gripping the long bone (metatarsal) to stabilize the joint. Pinch-grip your big toe with your other hand and pull it into a neutral or straight alignment. Maintaining your grips, mobilize the toe up into dorsiflexion and down into plantarflexion. Do 3 sets of 10–15 reps, moving the toe as far as you can without pain and holding at end range for 2–3 seconds.

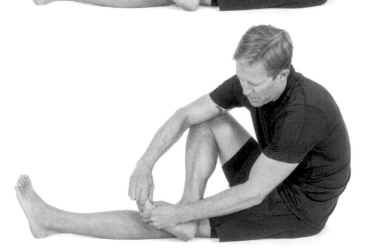

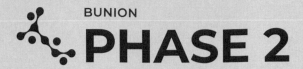

# BUNION
# PHASE 2

**GOOD FOR:**

- Reducing big toe and foot pain
- Improving mobility
- Warm-up for phase 3 exercises

**GUIDELINES:**

- Perform 3 or 4 days a week
- Tool: stretch strap
- Add phase 3 when you can do the exercises with no more than mild pain (3/10)

## STRETCHING EXERCISES:

▸ Do 3 reps with 30- to 60-second holds
▸ Perform in any order on both sides
▸ Don't stretch into pain

## big toe dorsiflexion stretch

Get into a staggered stance and shift your weight onto your lead leg. Keeping your rear big toe flush with the floor, bend your knee and lift your heel until you feel a moderate stretch. To increase the stretch, shift more weight onto your back leg and straighten your knee.

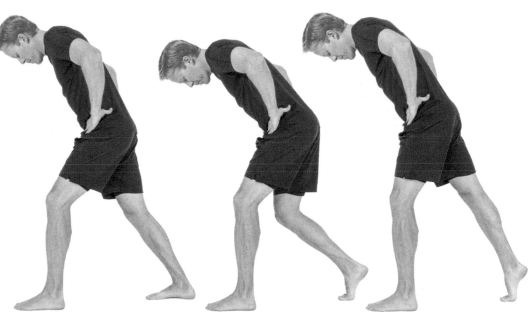

## kneeling dorsiflexion stretch

Kneel on the floor and get into the bottom of a split squat. Keeping your rear big toe flush with the floor, shift your weight forward so that your front ankle moves into dorsiflexion. Move as far as you can without pain. You should feel a stretch on the bottom of your foot, the front of your ankle, and/or the back side near your Achilles tendon.

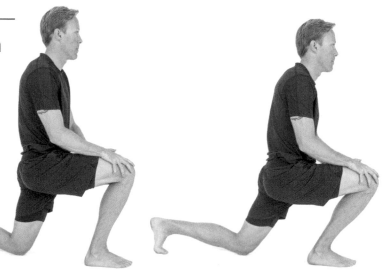

# hamstring stretch with strap

Lie on your back with a strap hooked around your foot. Keeping your leg completely relaxed, use your arms to pull your foot toward your head and hold it in place once you feel a moderate stretch.

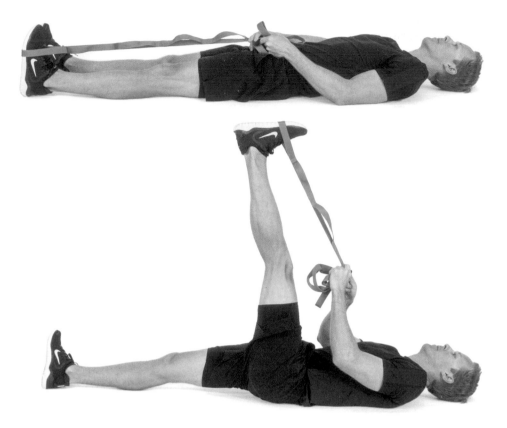

## MOBILITY EXERCISES:

- ▶ Do 3 sets of 10–15 reps
- ▶ Active range of motion (AROM)—move as far as you can without pain
- ▶ Pause at end range for 2–3 seconds

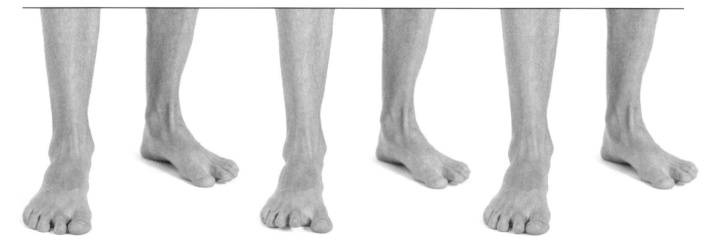

# big toe abduction

In a seated or standing position, lift your big toe and move it to the side away from the other toes. This teaches your toe abductor muscle how to pull the toe into a straighter alignment. The exercise is quite challenging and can take a fair bit of practice, so don't give up on it.

## big toe dorsiflexion

Lift your big toe toward your shin as far as you can without pain. When you hit end range, pinch-grip the end of your toe and pull it into a deeper stretch. Hold for 1–2 seconds, then release and return to the start position.

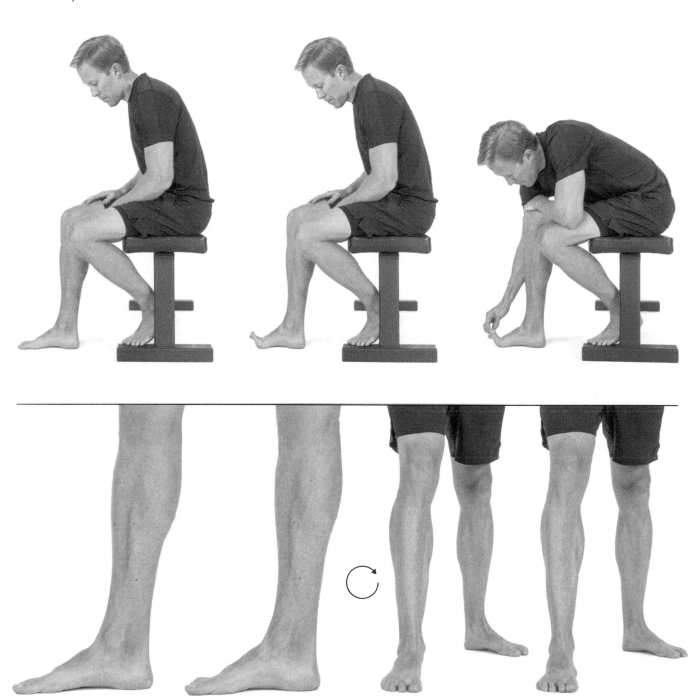

## doming

Standing with your feet staggered, squeeze the muscles in your front foot so that your arch lifts higher from the floor. Imagine trying to pull the ball of your big toe toward your heel so that your foot becomes shorter. Keep the ball of your big toe on the floor. To make the exercise easier, perform it while seated to take weight off your foot.

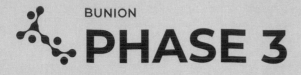

## BUNION
# PHASE 3

**GOOD FOR:**

- Increasing ankle, foot, and toe strength
- Preventing bunion pain and big toe injury

**GUIDELINES:**

- Perform 3 or 4 days a week
- Do 3 sets of 10–15 reps unless otherwise noted
- Push sets to fatigue
- Tools: towel, resistance band, plyo box

## towel curl

Place a towel under your toes. Bend your toes and pull the towel toward your heel. Repeat until you have pulled the entire towel into the space created by the arch of your foot.

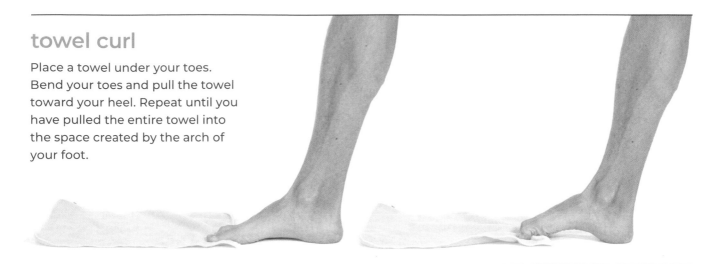

## band dorsiflexion

Tie a loop in a resistance band and wrap it around the top part of your foot. Attach the other end to a fixed object or have a partner hold it to create tension. Pull your ankle as far as you can into dorsiflexion with no more than mild pain. Slowly return to the start position; don't let the band snap your ankle back down. Do 3 sets of 20 reps.

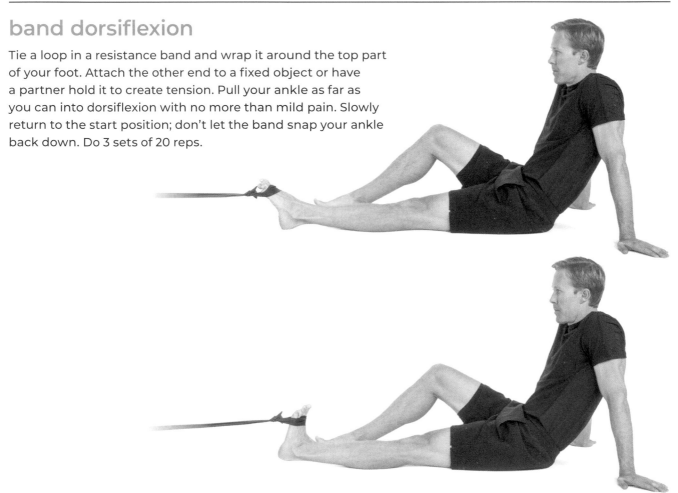

## double-leg calf raise (knees straight)

Stand with the balls of your feet on an elevated surface or step. Allow your heels to sink toward the floor. Perform slow calf raises through a full range of motion. Your heels should drop slightly lower than your toes on the down phase.

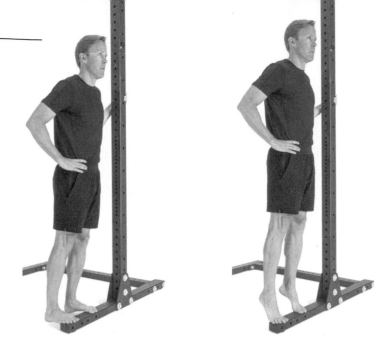

## double-leg calf raise (knees bent)

Hold onto a doorframe or rack. Sit your hips back and bend your knees into a half squat. Maintaining your knee angle, perform calf raises to target the soleus muscle.

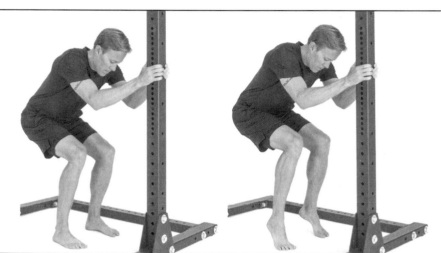

## lateral step-down

Stand next to a plyo box or small step. Perform a lateral step-up by placing your entire foot on the edge of the box and standing tall. Move your free leg forward slightly. Keeping your free leg straight, reach your heel toward the floor by slowly sitting back and bending your grounded knee. As soon as your heel contacts the floor, straighten your knee, extend your hips, and return to the start position. Keep your knee aligned over your foot; don't let it move in or out.

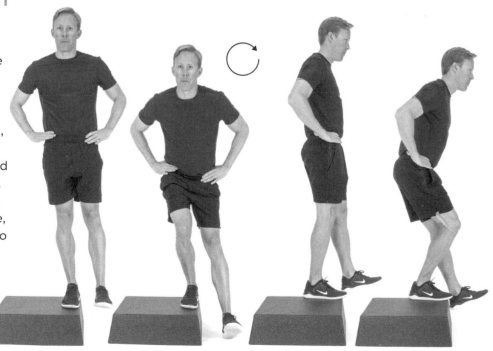

# REFERENCES

## Chapter 1

1. Malik NA. Revised definition of pain by International Association for the Study of Pain: concepts, challenges and compromises. *Anaesthesia, Pain & Intensive Care*. 2020;24(5).
2. Descartes, R. (1644). *L'Homme*.
3. Kuffler DP. Coping with phantom limb pain. *Mol Neurobiol*. 2018;55(1):70-84.
4. Stankevicius A, Wallwork SB, Summers SJ, Hordacre B, Stanton TR. Prevalence and incidence of phantom limb pain, phantom limb sensations and telescoping in amputees: a systematic rapid review. *Eur J Pain*. 2021;25(1):23-38.
5. Davis RW. Phantom sensation, phantom pain, and stump pain. *Arch Phys Med Rehabil*. 1993;74(1):79-91.
6. Jensen TS, Krebs B, Nielsen J, Rasmussen P. Immediate and long-term phantom limb pain in amputees: incidence, clinical characteristics and relationship to pre-amputation limb pain. *Pain*. 1985;21(3):267-278.
7. Moseley GL, Arntz A. The context of a noxious stimulus affects the pain it evokes. *Pain*. 2007;133(1-3):64-71.
8. Brinjikji W, Luetmer PH, Comstock B, et al. Systematic literature review of imaging features of spinal degeneration in asymptomatic populations. *AJNR Am J Neuroradiol*. 2015;36(4):811-816.
9. Sher JS, Uribe JW, Posada A, Murphy BJ, Zlatkin MB. Abnormal findings on magnetic resonance images of asymptomatic shoulders. *J Bone Joint Surg Am*. 1995;77(1):10-15.
10. Moosmayer S, Smith HJ, Tariq R, Larmo A. Prevalence and characteristics of asymptomatic tears of the rotator cuff: an ultrasonographic and clinical study. *J Bone Joint Surg Br*. 2009;91(2):196-200.
11. Milgrom C, Schaffler M, Gilbert S, van Holsbeeck M. Rotator-cuff changes in asymptomatic adults. The effect of age, hand dominance and gender. *J Bone Joint Surg Br*. 1995;77(2):296-298.
12. Horga LM, Hirschmann AC, Henckel J, et al. Prevalence of abnormal findings in 230 knees of asymptomatic adults using 3.0 T MRI. *Skeletal Radiol*. 2020;49(7):1099-1107.
13. Zanetti M, Pfirrmann CW, Schmid MR, Romero J, Seifert B, Hodler J. Patients with suspected meniscal tears: prevalence of abnormalities seen on MRI of 100 symptomatic and 100 contralateral asymptomatic knees. *AJR Am J Roentgenol*. 2003;181(3):635-641.
14. *The Times,* 17 Feb 2003, p. 5, London.
15. Melzack R. Pain and the neuromatrix in the brain. *J Dent Educ*. 2001;65(12):1378-1382.
16. Moseley GL. A pain neuromatrix approach to patients with chronic pain. *Man Ther*. 2003;8(3):130-140.
17. Lederman E. The fall of the postural-structural-biomechanical model in manual and physical therapies: exemplified by lower back pain. *J Bodyw Mov Ther*. 2011;15(2):131-138.
18. Engel GL. The need for a new medical model: a challenge for biomedicine. *Science*. 1977;196(4286):129-136.

## Chapter 2

1. Melzack R. Pain and the neuromatrix in the brain. *J Dent Educ*. 2001;65(12):1378-1382.
2. Moseley GL. A pain neuromatrix approach to patients with chronic pain. *Man Ther*. 2003;8(3):130-140.
3. Watson JA, Ryan CG, Cooper L, et al. Pain neuroscience education for adults with chronic musculoskeletal pain: a mixed-methods systematic review and meta-analysis. *J Pain*. 2019;20(10):1140.e1-1140.e22.
4. Louw A, Zimney K, Puentedura EJ, Diener I. The efficacy of pain neuroscience education on musculoskeletal pain: a systematic review of the literature. *Physiother Theory Pract*. 2016;32(5):332-355.
5. Moseley GL, Nicholas MK, Hodges PW. A randomized controlled trial of intensive neurophysiology education in chronic low back pain. *Clin J Pain*. 2004;20(5):324-330.
6. Meeus M, Nijs J, Van Oosterwijck J, Van Alsenoy V, Truijen S. Pain physiology education improves pain beliefs in patients with chronic fatigue syndrome compared with pacing and self-management education: a double-blind randomized controlled trial. *Arch Phys Med Rehabil*. 2010;91(8):1153-1159.
7. Clarke CL, Ryan CG, Martin DJ. Pain neurophysiology education for the management of individuals with chronic low back pain: systematic review and meta-analysis. *Man Ther*. 2011;16(6):544-549.
8. Louw A, Diener I, Butler DS, Puentedura EJ. The effect of neuroscience education on pain, disability, anxiety, and stress in chronic musculoskeletal pain. *Arch Phys Med Rehabil*. 2011;92(12):2041-2056.
9. Devor M. Sodium channels and mechanisms of neuropathic pain. *J Pain*. 2006;7(1 Suppl 1):S3-S12.
10. Devor M, Govrin-Lippmann R, Angelides K. Na+ channel immunolocalization in peripheral mammalian axons and changes following nerve injury and neuroma formation. *J Neurosci*. 1993;13(5):1976-1992.
11. Devor M. Response of nerves to injury in relation to neuropathic pain. In: McMahon S, Koltzenburg M. *Wall and Melzack's Textbook of Pain*. Philadelphia: Elsevier; 2013.
12. Flor H. The functional organization of the brain in chronic pain. *Prog Brain Res*. 2000;129:313-322.
13. Apkarian AV, Bushnell MC, Treede RD, Zubieta JK. Human brain mechanisms of pain perception and regulation in health and disease. *Eur J Pain*. 2005;9(4):463-484.
14. Tracey I, Mantyh PW. The cerebral signature for pain perception and its modulation. *Neuron*. 2007;55(3):377-391.
15. Doidge N. *The Brain That Changes Itself*. New York: Penguin Books; 2007.

## Chapter 3

1. Treede RD, Rief W, Barke A, et al. A classification of chronic pain for ICD-11. *Pain*. 2015;156(6):1003-1007.

2. Bonica JJ. *The Management of Pain*. Philadelphia: Lea & Febiger; 1953.
3. Merskey H, Bogduk N. *Classification of Chronic Pain*. 2nd ed. Seattle: IASP Press; 1994. p. 1.

## Chapter 4

1. Paller CJ, Campbell CM, Edwards RR, Dobs AS. Sex-based differences in pain perception and treatment. *Pain Med*. 2009;10(2):289-299.
2. Riley JL 3rd, Robinson ME, Wise EA, Myers CD, Fillingim RB. Sex differences in the perception of noxious experimental stimuli: a meta-analysis. *Pain*. 1998;74(2-3):181-187.
3. Assa T, Geva N, Zarkh Y, Defrin R. The type of sport matters: pain perception of endurance athletes versus strength athletes. *Eur J Pain*. 2019;23(4):686-696.
4. Peterson JA, Schubert DJ, Campbell J, Bemben MG, Black CD. Endogenous pain inhibitory function: endurance-trained athletes vs. active controls. *Pain Med*. 2019;20(9):1822-1830.
5. Tesarz J, Schuster AK, Hartmann M, Gerhardt A, Eich W. Pain perception in athletes compared to normally active controls: a systematic review with meta-analysis. *Pain*. 2012;153(6):1253-1262.
6. Geva N, Defrin R. Enhanced pain modulation among triathletes: a possible explanation for their exceptional capabilities. *Pain*. 2013;154(11):2317-2323.
7. Ohel I, Walfisch A, Shitenberg D, Sheiner E, Hallak M. A rise in pain threshold during labor: a prospective clinical trial. *Pain*. 2007;132 Suppl 1:S104-S108.
8. Berlit S, Lis S, Häfner K, et al. Changes in birth-related pain perception impact of neurobiological and psycho-social factors. *Arch Gynecol Obstet*. 2018;297(3):591-599.
9. Sluka KA, Frey-Law L, Hoeger Bement M. Exercise-induced pain and analgesia? Underlying mechanisms and clinical translation. *Pain*. 2018;159 Suppl 1(Suppl 1):S91-S97.
10. Landmark T, Romundstad P, Borchgrevink PC, Kaasa S, Dale O. Associations between recreational exercise and chronic pain in the general population: evidence from the HUNT 3 study. *Pain*. 2011;152(10):2241-2247.
11. Landmark T, Romundstad PR, Borchgrevink PC, Kaasa S, Dale O. Longitudinal associations between exercise and pain in the general population—the HUNT pain study. *PLoS One*. 2013;8(6):e65279. Published 2013 Jun 12.
12. Bobinski F, Ferreira TAA, Córdova MM, et al. Role of brainstem serotonin in analgesia produced by low-intensity exercise on neuropathic pain after sciatic nerve injury in mice. *Pain*. 2015;156(12):2595-2606.
13. Brito RG, Rasmussen LA, Sluka KA. Regular physical activity prevents development of chronic muscle pain through modulation of supraspinal opioid and serotonergic mechanisms. *Pain Rep*. 2017;2(5):e618. Published 2017 Aug 21.
14. Lima LV, DeSantana JM, Rasmussen LA, Sluka KA. Short-duration physical activity prevents the development of activity-induced hyperalgesia through opioid and serotoninergic mechanisms. *Pain*. 2017;158(9):1697-1710.
15. Naugle KM, Riley JL III. Self-reported physical activity predicts pain inhibitory and facilitatory function. *Med Sci Sports Exerc*. 2014;46(3):622-629.
16. Gong WY, Abdelhamid RE, Carvalho CS, Sluka KA. Resident macrophages in muscle contribute to development of hyperalgesia in a mouse model of noninflammatory muscle pain. *J Pain*. 2016;17(10):1081-1094.
17. Leung A, Gregory NS, Allen LH, Sluka KA. Regular physical activity prevents chronic pain by altering resident muscle macrophage phenotype and increasing interleukin-10 in mice. *Pain*. 2016;157(1):70-79.
18. Bobinski F, Teixeira JM, Sluka KA, Santos ARS. Interleukin-4 mediates the analgesia produced by low-intensity exercise in mice with neuropathic pain. *Pain*. 2018;159(3):437-450.
19. Grace PM, Fabisiak TJ, Green-Fulgham SM, et al. Prior voluntary wheel running attenuates neuropathic pain. *Pain*. 2016;157(9):2012-2023.
20. Belavy DL, Van Oosterwijck J, Clarkson M, et al. Pain sensitivity is reduced by exercise training: evidence from a systematic review and meta-analysis. *Neurosci Biobehav Rev*. 2021;120:100-108.
21. Grooten WJA, Boström C, Dedering Å, et al. Summarizing the effects of different exercise types in chronic low back pain—a systematic review of systematic reviews. *BMC Musculoskelet Disord*. 2022;23(1):801.
22. Bair MJ, Robinson RL, Katon W, Kroenke K. Depression and pain comorbidity: a literature review. *Arch Intern Med*. 2003;163(20):2433-2445.
23. IsHak WW, Wen RY, Naghdechi L, et al. Pain and depression: a systematic review. *Harv Rev Psychiatry*. 2018;26(6):352-363.
24. Lewis GN, Rice DA, McNair PJ, Kluger M. Predictors of persistent pain after total knee arthroplasty: a systematic review and meta-analysis. *Br J Anaesth*. 2015;114(4):551-561.
25. Doan L, Manders T, Wang J. Neuroplasticity underlying the comorbidity of pain and depression. *Neural Plast*. 2015;2015:504691.
26. Kroslak M, Murrell GAC. Surgical treatment of lateral epicondylitis: a prospective, randomized, double-blinded, placebo-controlled clinical trial. *Am J Sports Med*. 2018;46(5):1106-1113.
27. Moseley JB, O'Malley K, Petersen NJ, et al. A controlled trial of arthroscopic surgery for osteoarthritis of the knee. *N Engl J Med*. 2002;347(2):81-88.
28. Buchbinder R, Osborne RH, Ebeling PR, et al. A randomized trial of vertebroplasty for painful osteoporotic vertebral fractures. *N Engl J Med*. 2009;361(6):557-568.
29. Blasini M, Corsi N, Klinger R, Colloca L. Nocebo and pain: an overview of the psychoneurobiological mechanisms. *Pain Rep*. 2017;2(2):e585.
30. Manaï M, van Middendorp H, Veldhuijzen DS, Huizinga TWJ, Evers AWM. How to prevent, minimize, or extinguish nocebo effects in pain: a narrative review on mechanisms, predictors, and interventions. *Pain Rep*. 2019;4(3):e699. Published 2019 Jun 7.
31. Petersen GL, Finnerup NB, Colloca L, et al. The magnitude of nocebo effects in pain: a meta-analysis. *Pain*. 2014;155(8):1426-1434.
32. Hohenschurz-Schmidt D, Thomson OP, Rossettini G, et al. Avoiding nocebo and other undesirable effects in chiropractic, osteopathy and physiotherapy: an invitation to reflect. *Musculoskelet Sci Pract*. 2022;62:102677.

33. Hasenbring MI, Chehadi O, Titze C, Kreddig N. Fear and anxiety in the transition from acute to chronic pain: there is evidence for endurance besides avoidance. *Pain Manag.* 2014;4(5):363-374.

34. Leeuw M, Goossens ME, Linton SJ, Crombez G, Boersma K, Vlaeyen JW. The fear-avoidance model of musculoskeletal pain: current state of scientific evidence. *J Behav Med.* 2007;30(1):77-94.

35. Miller GE, Cohen S, Ritchey AK. Chronic psychological stress and the regulation of pro-inflammatory cytokines: a glucocorticoid-resistance model. *Health Psychol.* 2002;21(6):531-541.

36. Thacker MA, Clark AK, Marchand F, McMahon SB. Pathophysiology of peripheral neuropathic pain: immune cells and molecules. *Anesth Analg.* 2007;105(3):838-847.

37. Togo F, Natelson BH, Adler GK, et al. Plasma cytokine fluctuations over time in healthy controls and patients with fibromyalgia. *Exp Biol Med* (Maywood). 2009;234(2):232-240.

38. Van Looveren E, Bilterys T, Munneke W, et al. The association between sleep and chronic spinal pain: a systematic review from the last decade. *J Clin Med.* 2021;10(17):3836.

39. Hirshkowitz M, Whiton K, Albert SM, et al. National Sleep Foundation's updated sleep duration recommendations: final report. *Sleep Health.* 2015;1(4):233-243.

40. Short sleep duration among US adults. National Center for Chronic Disease Prevention and Health Promotion, Division of Population Health. Centers for Disease Control and Prevention. Updated September 12, 2022. Accessed December 31, 2022. https://www.cdc.gov/sleep/data_statistics.html.

41. Dragan S, Șerban MC, Damian G, Buleu F, Valcovici M, Christodorescu R. Dietary patterns and interventions to alleviate chronic pain. *Nutrients.* 2020;12(9):2510.

42. Bjørklund G, Aaseth J, Doșa MD, et al. Does diet play a role in reducing nociception related to inflammation and chronic pain? *Nutrition.* 2019;66:153-165.

43. Correa-Rodríguez M, Casas-Barragán A, González-Jiménez E, Schmidt-RioValle J, Molina F, Aguilar-Ferrándiz ME. Dietary inflammatory index scores are associated with pressure pain hypersensitivity in women with fibromyalgia. *Pain Med.* 2020;21(3):586-594.

44. Comee L, Taylor CA, Nahikian-Nelms M, Ganesan LP, Krok-Schoen JL. Dietary patterns and nutrient intake of individuals with rheumatoid arthritis and osteoarthritis in the United States. *Nutrition.* 2019;67-68:110533.

45. Atherton K, Wiles NJ, Lecky FE, et al. Predictors of persistent neck pain after whiplash injury. *Emerg Med J.* 2006;23(3):195-201.

46. Ritchie C, Ehrlich C, Sterling M. Living with ongoing whiplash associated disorders: a qualitative study of individual perceptions and experiences. *BMC Musculoskelet Disord.* 2017;18(1):531.

47. Buskila D. Genetics of chronic pain states. *Best Pract Res Clin Rheumatol.* 2007;21(3):535-547.

48. Clementi MA, Faraji P, Poppert Cordts K, et al. Parent factors are associated with pain and activity limitations in youth with acute musculoskeletal pain: a cohort study. *Clin J Pain.* 2019;35(3):222-228.

49. Walker SM. Long-term effects of neonatal pain. Semin Fetal *Neonatal Med.* 2019;24(4):101005.

50. Bates MS, Edwards TW, Anderson KO. Ethnocultural influences on variation in chronic pain perception. *Pain.* 1993;52(1):101-112.

51. Xygalatas D, Mitkidis P, Fischer R, et al. Extreme rituals promote prosociality. *Psychol Sci.* 2013;24(8):1602-1605.

52. Fischer R, Xygalatas D, Mitkidis P, et al. The fire-walker's high: affect and physiological responses in an extreme collective ritual. *PLoS One.* 2014;9(2):e88355. Published 2014 Feb 20.

53. Rabin BS. *Stress, Immune Function and Health: The Connection.* New York: Wiley Liss; 1999.

54. Lewis JS, Green A, Wright C. Subacromial impingement syndrome: the role of posture and muscle imbalance. *J Shoulder Elbow Surg.* 2005;14(4):385-392.

55. Lewis JS, Wright C, Green A. Subacromial impingement syndrome: the effect of changing posture on shoulder range of movement. *J Orthop Sports Phys Ther.* 2005;35(2):72-87.

56. Edmondston SJ, Chan HY, Ngai GC, et al. Postural neck pain: an investigation of habitual sitting posture, perception of "good" posture and cervicothoracic kinaesthesia. *Man Ther.* 2007;12(4):363-371.

57. Uvnas-Moberg K, Petersson M. Oxytocin, a mediator of anti-stress, well-being, social interaction, growth and healing. *Z Psychosom Med Psychother.* 2005;51(1):57-80.

## Chapter 5

1. Belavy DL, Van Oosterwijck J, Clarkson M, et al. Pain sensitivity is reduced by exercise training: Evidence from a systematic review and meta-analysis. *Neurosci Biobehav Rev.* 2021;120:100-108.

2. Vaegter HB, Jones MD. Exercise-induced hypoalgesia after acute and regular exercise: experimental and clinical manifestations and possible mechanisms in individuals with and without pain. *Pain Rep.* 2020;5(5):e823. Published 2020 Sep 23.

3. Sluka KA, Frey-Law L, Hoeger Bement M. Exercise-induced pain and analgesia? Underlying mechanisms and clinical translation. *Pain.* 2018;159 Suppl 1(Suppl 1):S91-S97.

4. Bishop MD, Torres-Cueco R, Gay CW, Lluch-Girbés E, Beneciuk JM, Bialosky JE. What effect can manual therapy have on a patient's pain experience? *Pain Manag.* 2015;5(6):455-464.

5. Bialosky JE, Bishop MD, Price DD, Robinson ME, George SZ. The mechanisms of manual therapy in the treatment of musculoskeletal pain: a comprehensive model. *Man Ther.* 2009;14(5):531-538.

6. Quintner JL, Bove GM, Cohen ML. A critical evaluation of the trigger point phenomenon. *Rheumatology* (Oxford). 2015;54(3):392-399.

7. Shah JP, Thaker N, Heimur J, Aredo JV, Sikdar S, Gerber L. Myofascial trigger points then and now: a historical and scientific perspective. *PM R.* 2015;7(7):746-761.

8. Tan L, Cicuttini FM, Fairley J, et al. Does aerobic exercise effect pain sensitisation in individuals with musculoskeletal pain? A systematic review. *BMC*

*Musculoskelet Disord.* 2022;23(1):113. Published 2022 Feb 3.

9. Tharmaratnam T, Civitarese RA, Tabobondung T, Tabobondung TA. Exercise becomes brain: sustained aerobic exercise enhances hippocampal neurogenesis. *J Physiol.* 2017;595(1):7-8.

10. Lima LV, Abner TSS, Sluka KA. Does exercise increase or decrease pain? Central mechanisms underlying these two phenomena. *J Physiol.* 2017;595(13):4141-4150.

11. Grooten WJA, Boström C, Dedering Å, et al. Summarizing the effects of different exercise types in chronic low back pain—a systematic review of systematic reviews. *BMC Musculoskelet Disord.* 2022;23(1):801.

12. Sluka KA, Frey-Law L, Hoeger Bement M. Exercise-induced pain and analgesia? Underlying mechanisms and clinical translation. *Pain.* 2018;159 Suppl 1(Suppl 1):S91-S97.

13. Støve MP, Hirata RP, Palsson TS. Muscle stretching—the potential role of endogenous pain inhibitory modulation on stretch tolerance. *Scand J Pain.* 2019;19(2):415-422.

14. Marshall PW, Cashman A, Cheema BS. A randomized controlled trial for the effect of passive stretching on measures of hamstring extensibility, passive stiffness, strength, and stretch tolerance. *J Sci Med Sport.* 2011;14(6):535-540.

15. Halbertsma JP, Göeken LN. Stretching exercises: effect on passive extensibility and stiffness in short hamstrings of healthy subjects. *Arch Phys Med Rehabil.* 1994;75(9):976-981.

16. Busch V, Magerl W, Kern U, Haas J, Hajak G, Eichhammer P. The effect of deep and slow breathing on pain perception, autonomic activity, and mood processing—an experimental study. *Pain Med.* 2012;13(2):215-228.

17. Jafari H, Gholamrezaei A, Franssen M, et al. Can slow deep breathing reduce pain? An experimental study exploring mechanisms. *J Pain.* 2020;21(9-10):1018-1030.

18. Hilton L, Hempel S, Ewing BA, et al. Mindfulness meditation for chronic pain: systematic review and meta-analysis. *Ann Behav Med.* 2017;51(2):199-213.

19. Cherkin DC, Sherman KJ, Balderson BH, et al. Effect of mindfulness-based stress reduction vs. cognitive behavioral therapy or usual care on back pain and functional limitations in adults with chronic low back pain: a randomized clinical trial. *JAMA.* 2016;315(12):1240-1249.

20. Usuba M, Akai M, Shirasaki Y, Miyakawa S. Experimental joint contracture correction with low torque—long duration repeated stretching. *Clin Orthop Relat Res.* 2007;456:70-78.

21. Flowers KR, LaStayo P. Effect of total end range time on improving passive range of motion. *J Hand Ther.* 1994;7(3):150-157.

22. Light KE, Nuzik S, Personius W, Barstrom A. Low-load prolonged stretch vs. high-load brief stretch in treating knee contractures. *Phys Ther.* 1984;64(3):330-333.

23. Slaven EJ, Goode AP, Coronado RA, Poole C, Hegedus EJ. The relative effectiveness of segment specific level and non-specific level spinal joint mobilization on pain and range of motion: results of a systematic review and meta-analysis. *J Man Manip Ther.* 2013;21(1):7-17.

24. Beattie PF, Arnot CF, Donley JW, Noda H, Bailey L. The immediate reduction in low back pain intensity following lumbar joint mobilization and prone press-ups is associated with increased diffusion of water in the L5-S1 intervertebral disc. *J Orthop Sports Phys Ther.* 2010;40(5):256-264.

25. Moss P, Sluka K, Wright A. The initial effects of knee joint mobilization on osteoarthritic hyperalgesia. *Man Ther.* 2007;12(2):109-118.

26. Conroy DE, Hayes KW. The effect of joint mobilization as a component of comprehensive treatment for primary shoulder impingement syndrome. *J Orthop Sports Phys Ther.* 1998;28(1):3-14.

27. Rio E, Kidgell D, Purdam C, et al. Isometric exercise induces analgesia and reduces inhibition in patellar tendinopathy. *Br J Sports Med.* 2015;49(19):1277-1283.

28. Malliaras P, Barton CJ, Reeves ND, Langberg H. Achilles and patellar tendinopathy loading programmes: a systematic review comparing clinical outcomes and identifying potential mechanisms for effectiveness. *Sports Med.* 2013;43(4):267-286.

29. Cardoso TB, Pizzari T, Kinsella R, Hope D, Cook JL. Current trends in tendinopathy management. *Best Pract Res Clin Rheumatol.* 2019;33(1):122-140.

30. Rio E, Kidgell D, Moseley GL, et al. Tendon neuroplastic training: changing the way we think about tendon rehabilitation: a narrative review. *Br J Sports Med.* 2016;50(4):209-215.

31. Turner MN, Hernandez DO, Cade W, Emerson CP, Reynolds JM, Best TM. The role of resistance training dosing on pain and physical function in individuals with knee osteoarthritis: a systematic review. *Sports Health.* 2020;12(2):200-206.

32. Ferreira RM, Torres RT, Duarte JA, Gonçalves RS. Non-pharmacological and non-surgical interventions for knee osteoarthritis: a systematic review and meta-analysis. *Acta Reumatol Port.* 2019;44(3):173-217.

## Chapter 6

1. Lauersen JB, Bertelsen DM, Andersen LB. The effectiveness of exercise interventions to prevent sports injuries: a systematic review and meta-analysis of randomised controlled trials. *Br J Sports Med.* 2014;48(11):871-877.

2. Raja SN, Carr DB, Cohen M, et al. The revised International Association for the Study of Pain definition of pain: concepts, challenges, and compromises. *Pain.* 2020;161(9):1976-1982.

3. Culvenor AG, Øiestad BE, Hart HF, Stefanik JJ, Guermazi A, Crossley KM. Prevalence of knee osteoarthritis features on magnetic resonance imaging in asymptomatic uninjured adults: a systematic review and meta-analysis. *Br J Sports Med.* 2019;53(20):1268-1278.

4. Frank JM, Harris JD, Erickson BJ, et al. Prevalence of femoroacetabular impingement imaging findings in asymptomatic volunteers: a systematic review. *Arthroscopy.* 2015;31(6):1199-1204.

5. Brinjikji W, Luetmer PH, Comstock B, et al. Systematic literature review of imaging features of spinal degeneration in asymptomatic populations. *AJNR Am J Neuroradiol.* 2015;36(4):811-816.

6. Wood KB, Garvey TA, Gundry C, Heithoff KB. Magnetic resonance imaging of the thoracic spine. Evaluation of asymptomatic individuals. *J Bone Joint Surg Am*. 1995;77(11):1631-1638.

7. Jerosch J, Castro WH, Assheuer J. Age-related magnetic resonance imaging morphology of the menisci in asymptomatic individuals. *Arch Orthop Trauma Surg*. 1996;115(3-4):199-202.

8. Schibany N, Zehetgruber H, Kainberger F, et al. Rotator cuff tears in asymptomatic individuals: a clinical and ultrasonographic screening study. *Eur J Radiol*. 2004;51(3):263-268.

9. Hall AM, Aubrey-Bassler K, Thorne B, Maher CG. Do not routinely offer imaging for uncomplicated low back pain. *BMJ*. 2021;372:n291.

10. Jacobs JC, Jarvik JG, Chou R, et al. Observational study of the downstream consequences of inappropriate MRI of the lumbar spine. *J Gen Intern Med*. 2020;35(12):3605-3612.

11. Webster BS, Bauer AZ, Choi Y, Cifuentes M, Pransky GS. Iatrogenic consequences of early magnetic resonance imaging in acute, work-related, disabling low back pain. *Spine* (Phila Pa 1976). 2013;38(22):1939-1946.

## Chapter 7

1. McCormick A, Charlton J, Fleming D. Assessing health needs in primary care. Morbidity study from general practice provides another source of information. *BMJ*. 1995;310(6993):1534.

2. Andarawis-Puri N, Flatow EL, Soslowsky LJ. Tendon basic science: development, repair, regeneration, and healing. *J Orthop Res*. 2015;33(6):780-784.

3. Alentorn-Geli E, Samuelsson K, Musahl V, Green CL, Bhandari M, Karlsson J. The association of recreational and competitive running with hip and knee osteoarthritis: a systematic review and meta-analysis. *J Orthop Sports Phys Ther*. 2017;47(6):373-390.

4. Lee DY, Park YJ, Kim HJ, et al. Arthroscopic meniscal surgery versus conservative management in patients aged 40 years and older: a meta-analysis. *Arch Orthop Trauma Surg*. 2018;138(12):1731-1739.

5. Giuffrida A, Di Bari A, Falzone E, et al. Conservative vs. surgical approach for degenerative meniscal injuries: a systematic review of clinical evidence. *Eur Rev Med Pharmacol Sci*. 2020;24(6):2874-2885.

## Chapter 8

1. Sørensen LT. Wound healing and infection in surgery: the pathophysiological impact of smoking, smoking cessation, and nicotine replacement therapy: a systematic review. *Ann Surg*. 2012;255(6):1069-1079.

2. Santiago-Torres J, Flanigan DC, Butler RB, Bishop JY. The effect of smoking on rotator cuff and glenoid labrum surgery: a systematic review. *Am J Sports Med*. 2015;43(3):745-751.

3. Kanneganti P, Harris JD, Brophy RH, Carey JL, Lattermann C, Flanigan DC. The effect of smoking on ligament and cartilage surgery in the knee: a systematic review. *Am J Sports Med*. 2012;40(12):2872-2878.

4. Novikov DA, Swensen SJ, Buza JA 3rd, Gidumal RH, Strauss EJ. The effect of smoking on ACL reconstruction: a systematic review. *Phys Sportsmed*. 2016;44(4):335-341.

5. Scolaro JA, Schenker ML, Yannascoli S, Baldwin K, Mehta S, Ahn J. Cigarette smoking increases complications following fracture: a systematic review. *J Bone Joint Surg Am*. 2014;96(8):674-681.

6. Steiner JL, Lang CH. Dysregulation of skeletal muscle protein metabolism by alcohol. *Am J Physiol Endocrinol Metab*. 2015;308(9):E699-E712.

7. Lang CH, Kimball SR, Frost RA, Vary TC. Alcohol myopathy: impairment of protein synthesis and translation initiation. *Int J Biochem Cell Biol*. 2001;33(5):457-473.

8. Alfredson H, Pietilä T, Jonsson P, Lorentzon R. Heavy-load eccentric calf muscle training for the treatment of chronic Achilles tendinosis. *Am J Sports Med*. 1998;26(3):360-366.

9. Ohberg L, Alfredson H. Effects on neovascularisation behind the good results with eccentric training in chronic mid-portion Achilles tendinosis? *Knee Surg Sports Traumatol Arthrosc*. 2004;12(5):465-470.

10. Shalabi A, Kristoffersen-Wilberg M, Svensson L, Aspelin P, Movin T. Eccentric training of the gastrocnemius-soleus complex in chronic Achilles tendinopathy results in decreased tendon volume and intratendinous signal as evaluated by MRI. *Am J Sports Med*. 2004;32(5):1286-1296.

11. Bahr R, Fossan B, Løken S, Engebretsen L. Surgical treatment compared with eccentric training for patellar tendinopathy (jumper's knee). A randomized, controlled trial. *J Bone Joint Surg Am*. 2006;88(8):1689-1698.

12. Cook JL, Purdam CR. Is tendon pathology a continuum? A pathology model to explain the clinical presentation of load-induced tendinopathy. *Br J Sports Med*. 2009;43(6):409-416.

13. Grafstein B. Role of slow axonal transport in nerve regeneration. *Acta Neuropathol*. 1971;5:144-152.

14. Hoffman PN, Lasek RJ. Axonal transport of the cytoskeleton in regenerating motor neurons: constancy and change. *Brain Res*. 1980;202(2):317-333.

## Chapter 9

1. McCrary JM, Ackermann BJ, Halaki M. A systematic review of the effects of upper body warm-up on performance and injury. *Br J Sports Med*. 2015;49(14):935-942.

2. Fradkin AJ, Zazryn TR, Smoliga JM. Effects of warming-up on physical performance: a systematic review with meta-analysis. *J Strength Cond Res*. 2010;24(1):140-148.

3. Herman K, Barton C, Malliaras P, Morrissey D. The effectiveness of neuromuscular warm-up strategies, that require no additional equipment, for preventing lower limb injuries during sports participation: a systematic review. *BMC Med*. 2012;10:75.

4. Gray SR, De Vito G, Nimmo MA, Farina D, Ferguson RA. Skeletal muscle ATP turnover and muscle fiber conduction velocity are elevated at higher muscle temperatures during maximal power output development in humans. *Am J Physiol Regul Integr Comp Physiol*. 2006;290(2):R376-R382.

5. Racinais S, Oksa J. Temperature and neuromuscular function. *Scand J Med Sci Sports*. 2010;20 Suppl 3:1-18.

6. Close R, Hoh JF. Influence of temperature on isometric contractions of rat skeletal muscles. *Nature.* 1968;217(5134):1179-1180.

7. Stewart D, Macaluso A, De Vito G. The effect of an active warm-up on surface EMG and muscle performance in healthy humans. *Eur J Appl Physiol.* 2003;89(6):509-513.

8. Pearce AJ, Rowe GS, Whyte DG. Neural conduction and excitability following a simple warm up. *J Sci Med Sport.* 2012;15(2):164-168.

9. Simic L, Sarabon N, Markovic G. Does pre-exercise static stretching inhibit maximal muscular performance? A meta-analytical review. *Scand J Med Sci Sports.* 2013;23(2):131-148.

10. Behm DG, Chaouachi A. A review of the acute effects of static and dynamic stretching on performance. *Eur J Appl Physiol.* 2011;111(11):2633-2651.

11. Fulton J, Wright K, Kelly M, et al. Injury risk is altered by previous injury: a systematic review of the literature and presentation of causative neuromuscular factors. *Int J Sports Phys Ther.* 2014;9(5):583-595.

12. Murphy DF, Connolly DA, Beynnon BD. Risk factors for lower extremity injury: a review of the literature. *Br J Sports Med.* 2003;37(1):13-29.

13. Hägglund M, Waldén M, Ekstrand J. Previous injury as a risk factor for injury in elite football: a prospective study over two consecutive seasons. *Br J Sports Med.* 2006;40(9):767-772.

14. Gaal BT, Knapik DM, Karns MR, Salata MJ, Voos JE. Contralateral anterior cruciate ligament injuries following index reconstruction in the pediatric athlete. *Curr Rev Musculoskelet Med.* 2020;13(4):409-415.

15. Swärd P, Kostogiannis I, Roos H. Risk factors for a contralateral anterior cruciate ligament injury. *Knee Surg Sports Traumatol Arthrosc.* 2010;18(3):277-291.

16. Arøen A, Helgø D, Granlund OG, Bahr R. Contralateral tendon rupture risk is increased in individuals with a previous Achilles tendon rupture. *Scand J Med Sci Sports.* 2004;14(1):30-33.

17. Milewski MD, Skaggs DL, Bishop GA, et al. Chronic lack of sleep is associated with increased sports injuries in adolescent athletes. *J Pediatr Orthop.* 2014;34(2):129-133.

18. Viegas F, Ocarino JM, Freitas LS, et al. The sleep as a predictor of musculoskeletal injuries in adolescent athletes. *Sleep Sci.* 2022;15(3):305-311.

19. Azboy O, Kaygisiz Z. Effects of sleep deprivation on cardiorespiratory functions of the runners and volleyball players during rest and exercise. *Acta Physiol Hung.* 2009;96(1):29-36.

20. McLean SG, Samorezov JE. Fatigue-induced ACL injury risk stems from a degradation in central control. *Med Sci Sports Exerc.* 2009;41(8):1661-1672.

21. Small K, McNaughton L, Greig M, Lovell R. The effects of multidirectional soccer-specific fatigue on markers of hamstring injury risk. *J Sci Med Sport.* 2010;13(1):120-125.

22. Kekelekis A, Nikolaidis PT, Moore IS, Rosemann T, Knechtle B. Risk factors for upper limb injury in tennis players: a systematic review. *Int J Environ Res Public Health.* 2020;17(8):2744.

23. Steele J, Bruce-Low S, Smith D, Osborne N, Thorkeldsen A. Can specific loading through exercise impart healing or regeneration of the intervertebral disc? *Spine J.* 2015;15(10):2117-2121.

24. Bohm S, Mersmann F, Arampatzis A. Human tendon adaptation in response to mechanical loading: a systematic review and meta-analysis of exercise intervention studies on healthy adults. *Sports Med Open.* 2015;1(1):7.

25. Grzelak P, Podgorski M, Stefanczyk L, Krochmalski M, Domzalski M. Hypertrophied cruciate ligament in high performance weightlifters observed in magnetic resonance imaging. *Int Orthop.* 2012;36(8):1715-1719.

26. O'Bryan SJ, Giuliano C, Woessner MN, et al. Progressive resistance training for concomitant increases in muscle strength and bone mineral density in older adults: a systematic review and meta-analysis. *Sports Med.* 2022;52(8):1939-1960.

27. Lauersen JB, Bertelsen DM, Andersen LB. The effectiveness of exercise interventions to prevent sports injuries: a systematic review and meta-analysis of randomised controlled trials. *Br J Sports Med.* 2014;48(11):871-877.

28. Papalia GF, Papalia R, Diaz Balzani LA, et al. The effects of physical exercise on balance and prevention of falls in older people: a systematic review and meta-analysis. *J Clin Med.* 2020;9(8):2595.

29. Wall BT, Morton JP, van Loon LJ. Strategies to maintain skeletal muscle mass in the injured athlete: nutritional considerations and exercise mimetics. *Eur J Sport Sci.* 2015;15(1):53-62.

30. Smith-Ryan AE, Hirsch KR, Saylor HE, Gould LM, Blue MNM. Nutritional considerations and strategies to facilitate injury recovery and rehabilitation. *J Athl Train.* 2020;55(9):918-930.

31. Tipton KD. Nutritional support for exercise-induced injuries. *Sports Med.* 2015;45 Suppl 1:S93-S104.

32. Kvist J, Silbernagel KG. Fear of movement and reinjury in sports medicine: relevance for rehabilitation and return to sport. *Phys Ther.* 2022;102(2):pzab272.

33. Mir B, Vivekanantha P, Dhillon S, et al. Fear of reinjury following primary anterior cruciate ligament reconstruction: a systematic review [published online ahead of print, 2022 Dec 23]. *Knee Surg Sports Traumatol Arthrosc.* 2022;10.1007/s00167-022-07296-6.

34. Hsu CJ, Meierbachtol A, George SZ, Chmielewski TL. Fear of reinjury in athletes. *Sports Health.* 2017;9(2):162-167.

35. Tagesson S, Kvist J. Greater fear of re-injury and increased tibial translation in patients who later sustain an ACL graft rupture or a contralateral ACL rupture: a pilot study. *J Sports Sci.* 2016;34(2):125-132.

36. Hartigan EH, Lynch AD, Logerstedt DS, Chmielewski TL, Snyder-Mackler L. Kinesiophobia after anterior cruciate ligament rupture and reconstruction: noncopers versus potential copers. *J Orthop Sports Phys Ther.* 2013;43(11):821-832.

37. Nuccio RP, Barnes KA, Carter JM, Baker LB. Fluid balance in team sport athletes and the effect of hypohydration on cognitive, technical, and physical performance. *Sports Med.* 2017;47(10):1951-1982.

38. Knapik JJ, Trone DW, Tchandja J, Jones BH. Injury-reduction effectiveness of prescribing running shoes on the basis of foot arch height: summary of military investigations. *J Orthop Sports Phys Ther.* 2014;44(10):805-812.

39. Knapik JJ, Trone DW, Swedler DI, et al. Injury reduction effectiveness of assigning running shoes based on plantar shape in Marine Corps basic training. *Am J Sports Med*. 2010;38(9):1759-1767.

40. Molloy JM. Factors Influencing running-related musculoskeletal injury risk among U.S. military recruits. *Mil Med*. 2016;181(6):512-523.

41. Ghosh N, Kolade OO, Shontz E, et al. Nonsteroidal anti-inflammatory drugs (NSAIDs) and their effect on musculoskeletal soft-tissue healing: a scoping review. *JBJS Rev*. 2019;7(12):e4.

42. Kapetanos G. The effect of the local corticosteroids on the healing and biomechanical properties of the partially injured tendon. *Clin Orthop Relat Res*. 1982;(163):170-179.

43. Wiggins ME, Fadale PD, Barrach H, Ehrlich MG, Walsh WR. Healing characteristics of a type I collagenous structure treated with corticosteroids. *Am J Sports Med*. 1994;22(2):279-288.

44. Hall MM, Finnoff JT, Smith J. Musculoskeletal complications of fluoroquinolones: guidelines and precautions for usage in the athletic population. *PM R*. 2011;3(2):132-142.

45. Khaliq Y, Zhanel GG. Musculoskeletal injury associated with fluoroquinolone antibiotics. *Clin Plast Surg*. 2005;32(4):495-vi.

## Chapter 11

1. American Physical Therapy Association. *Guide to Physical Therapist Practice*. Second Edition. American Physical Therapy Association. *Phys Ther*. 2001;81(1):9-746.

2. Sizer PS Jr, Brismée JM, Cook C. Medical screening for red flags in the diagnosis and management of musculoskeletal spine pain. *Pain Pract*. 2007;7(1):53-71.

3. Ramanayake RPJC, Basnayake BMTK. Evaluation of red flags minimizes missing serious diseases in primary care. *J Family Med Prim Care*. 2018;7(2):315-318.

4. Downie A, Williams CM, Henschke N, et al. Red flags to screen for malignancy and fracture in patients with low back pain: systematic review [published correction appears in *BMJ*. 2014;348:g7]. *BMJ*. 2013;347:f7095.

5. Henschke N, Maher CG, Refshauge KM. A systematic review identifies five "red flags" to screen for vertebral fracture in patients with low back pain. *J Clin Epidemiol*. 2008;61(2):110-118.

6. Ghosh N, Kolade OO, Shontz E, et al. Nonsteroidal anti-inflammatory drugs (NSAIDs) and their effect on musculoskeletal soft-tissue healing: a scoping review. *JBJS Rev*. 2019;7(12):e4.

## Chapter 12

1. Schoenfeld BJ, Vigotsky A, Contreras B, et al. Differential effects of attentional focus strategies during long-term resistance training. *Eur J Sport Sci*. 2018;18(5):705-712.

2. Calatayud J, Vinstrup J, Jakobsen MD, et al. Importance of mind-muscle connection during progressive resistance training. *Eur J Appl Physiol*. 2016;116(3):527-533.

3. Huygaerts S, Cos F, Cohen DD, et al. Mechanisms of hamstring strain injury: interactions between fatigue, muscle activation and function. *Sports* (Basel). 2020;8(5):65.

## Chapter 14

1. Minshull C, Gallacher P, Roberts S, Barnett A, Kuiper JH, Bailey A. Contralateral strength training attenuates muscle performance loss following anterior cruciate ligament (ACL) reconstruction: a randomised-controlled trial. *Eur J Appl Physiol*. 2021;121(12):3551-3559.

2. Green LA, Gabriel DA. The cross education of strength and skill following unilateral strength training in the upper and lower limbs. *J Neurophysiol*. 2018;120(2):468-479.

3. Frazer AK, Williams J, Spittle M, Kidgell DJ. Cross-education of muscular strength is facilitated by homeostatic plasticity. *Eur J Appl Physiol*. 2017;117(4):665-677.

4. Gabriel DA, Kamen G, Frost G. Neural adaptations to resistive exercise: mechanisms and recommendations for training practices. *Sports Med*. 2006;36(2):133-149.

5. Farthing JP, Borowsky R, Chilibeck PD, Binsted G, Sarty GE. Neuro-physiological adaptations associated with cross-education of strength. *Brain Topogr*. 2007;20(2):77-88.

6. Grande-Alonso M, Garrigos-Pedron M, Cuenca-Martinez F, et al. Influence of the generation of motor mental images on physiotherapy treatment in patients with chronic low back pain. *Pain Physician*. 2020;23(4):E399-E408.

7. Salik Sengul Y, Kaya N, Yalcinkaya G, Kirmizi M, Kalemci O. The effects of the addition of motor imagery to home exercises on pain, disability and psychosocial parameters in patients undergoing lumbar spinal surgery: a randomized controlled trial. *Explore* (NY). 2021;17(4):334-339.

8. Limakatso K, Madden VJ, Manie S, Parker R. The effectiveness of graded motor imagery for reducing phantom limb pain in amputees: a randomised controlled trial. *Physiotherapy*. 2020;109:65-74.

9. Louw A, Farrell K, Nielsen A, O'Malley M, Cox T, Puentedura EJ. Virtual McKenzie extension exercises for low back and leg pain: a prospective pilot exploratory case series [published online ahead of print, 2022 Jun 23]. *J Man Manip Ther*. 2022;1-7.

10. Louw A, Schmidt SG, Louw C, Puentedura EJ. Moving without moving: immediate management following lumbar spine surgery using a graded motor imagery approach: a case report. *Physiother Theory Pract*. 2015;31(7):509-517.

11. Moseley GL. Graded motor imagery is effective for long-standing complex regional pain syndrome: a randomised controlled trial. *Pain*. 2004;108(1-2):192-198.

12. Hughes L, Paton B, Rosenblatt B, Gissane C, Patterson SD. Blood flow restriction training in clinical musculoskeletal rehabilitation: a systematic review and meta-analysis. *Br J Sports Med*. 2017;51(13):1003-1011.

13. Karanasios S, Korakakis V, Moutzouri M, Xergia SA, Tsepis E, Gioftsos G. Low-load resistance training with blood flow restriction is effective for

managing lateral elbow tendinopathy: a randomized, sham-controlled trial. *J Orthop Sports Phys Ther.* 2022;52(12):803-825.

14. Kilgas MA, Lytle LLM, Drum SN, Elmer SJ. Exercise with blood flow restriction to improve quadriceps function long after ACL reconstruction. *Int J Sports Med.* 2019;40(10):650-656.

15. Hughes L, Rosenblatt B, Haddad F, et al. Comparing the effectiveness of blood flow restriction and traditional heavy load resistance training in the post-surgery rehabilitation of anterior cruciate ligament reconstruction patients: a UK National Health Service randomised controlled trial. *Sports Med.* 2019;49(11):1787-1805.

16. Ferraz RB, Gualano B, Rodrigues R, et al. Benefits of resistance training with blood flow restriction in knee osteoarthritis. *Med Sci Sports Exerc.* 2018;50(5):897-905.

17. Yildirim N, Filiz Ulusoy M, Bodur H. The effect of heat application on pain, stiffness, physical function and quality of life in patients with knee osteoarthritis. *J Clin Nurs.* 2010;19(7-8):1113-1120.

18. Michlovitz S, Hun L, Erasala GN, Hengehold DA, Weingand KW. Continuous low-level heat wrap therapy is effective for treating wrist pain. *Arch Phys Med Rehabil.* 2004;85(9):1409-1416.

19. French SD, Cameron M, Walker BF, Reggars JW, Esterman AJ. Superficial heat or cold for low back pain. *Cochrane Database Syst Rev.* 2006;2006(1):CD004750. Published 2006 Jan 25.

20. Nadler SF, Steiner DJ, Erasala GN, et al. Continuous low-level heat wrap therapy provides more efficacy than Ibuprofen and acetaminophen for acute low back pain. *Spine* (Phila Pa 1976). 2002;27(10):1012-1017.

21. Rodrigues P, Trajano GS, Stewart IB, Minett GM. Potential role of passively increased muscle temperature on contractile function. *Eur J Appl Physiol.* 2022;122(10):2153-2162.

22. Petrofsky J, Berk L, Bains G, et al. Moist heat or dry heat for delayed onset muscle soreness. *J Clin Med Res.* 2013;5(6):416-425.

23. Selsby JT, Rother S, Tsuda S, Pracash O, Quindry J, Dodd SL. Intermittent hyperthermia enhances skeletal muscle regrowth and attenuates oxidative damage following reloading. *J Appl Physiol* (1985). 2007;102(4):1702-1707.

24. Naito H, Powers SK, Demirel HA, Sugiura T, Dodd SL, Aoki J. Heat stress attenuates skeletal muscle atrophy in hindlimb-unweighted rats. *J Appl Physiol* (1985). 2000;88(1):359-363.

25. Hafen PS, Abbott K, Bowden J, Lopiano R, Hancock CR, Hyldahl RD. Daily heat treatment maintains mitochondrial function and attenuates atrophy in human skeletal muscle subjected to immobilization. *J Appl Physiol* (1985). 2019;127(1):47-57.

26. Selsby JT, Dodd SL. Heat treatment reduces oxidative stress and protects muscle mass during immobilization. *Am J Physiol Regul Integr Comp Physiol.* 2005;289(1):R134-R139.

27. Laukkanen JA, Laukkanen T, Kunutsor SK. Cardiovascular and other health benefits of sauna bathing: a review of the evidence. *Mayo Clin Proc.* 2018;93(8):1111-1121.

28. Laukkanen T, Khan H, Zaccardi F, Laukkanen JA. Association between sauna bathing and fatal cardiovascular and all-cause mortality events. *JAMA Intern Med.* 2015;175(4):542-548.

29. Laukkanen JA, Laukkanen T. Sauna bathing and systemic inflammation. *Eur J Epidemiol.* 2018;33(3):351-353.

30. Kunutsor SK, Laukkanen T, Laukkanen JA. Longitudinal associations of sauna bathing with inflammation and oxidative stress: the KIHD prospective cohort study. *Ann Med.* 2018;50(5):437-442.

31. Wu LC, Weng PW, Chen CH, Huang YY, Tsuang YH, Chiang CJ. Literature review and meta-analysis of transcutaneous electrical nerve stimulation in treating chronic back pain. *Reg Anesth Pain Med.* 2018;43(4):425-433.

32. Resende L, Merriwether E, Rampazo ÉP, et al. Meta-analysis of transcutaneous electrical nerve stimulation for relief of spinal pain. *Eur J Pain.* 2018;22(4):663-678.

33. Oosterhof J, Samwel HJ, de Boo TM, Wilder-Smith OH, Oostendorp RA, Crul BJ. Predicting outcome of TENS in chronic pain: a prospective, randomized, placebo controlled trial. *Pain.* 2008;136(1-2):11-20.

34. Hauger AV, Reiman MP, Bjordal JM, Sheets C, Ledbetter L, Goode AP. Neuromuscular electrical stimulation is effective in strengthening the quadriceps muscle after anterior cruciate ligament surgery. *Knee Surg Sports Traumatol Arthrosc.* 2018;26(2):399-410.

35. Stevens-Lapsley JE, Balter JE, Wolfe P, Eckhoff DG, Kohrt WM. Early neuromuscular electrical stimulation to improve quadriceps muscle strength after total knee arthroplasty: a randomized controlled trial. *Phys Ther.* 2012;92(2):210-226.

36. Fitzgerald GK, Piva SR, Irrgang JJ. A modified neuromuscular electrical stimulation protocol for quadriceps strength training following anterior cruciate ligament reconstruction. *J Orthop Sports Phys Ther.* 2003;33(9):492-501.

37. Brown F, Gissane C, Howatson G, van Someren K, Pedlar C, Hill J. Compression garments and recovery from exercise: a meta-analysis. *Sports Med.* 2017;47(11):2245-2267.

38. Marqués-Jiménez D, Calleja-González J, Arratibel I, Delextrat A, Terrados N. Are compression garments effective for the recovery of exercise-induced muscle damage? A systematic review with meta-analysis. *Physiol Behav.* 2016;153:133-148.

39. Hill J, Howatson G, van Someren K, Leeder J, Pedlar C. Compression garments and recovery from exercise-induced muscle damage: a meta-analysis. *Br J Sports Med.* 2014;48(18):1340-1346.

40. Dubois B, Esculier JF. Soft-tissue injuries simply need PEACE and LOVE. *Br J Sports Med.* 2020;54(2):72-73.

41. Moffet HH. Sham acupuncture may be as efficacious as true acupuncture: a systematic review of clinical trials. *J Altern Complement Med.* 2009;15(3):213-216.

42. Kong JT, Puetz C, Tian L, et al. Effect of electroacupuncture vs sham treatment on change in pain severity among adults with chronic low back pain: a randomized clinical trial [published correction appears in *JAMA Netw Open.* 2022 Apr 1;5(4):e229687]. *JAMA Netw Open.* 2020;3(10):e2022787. Published 2020 Oct 1.

43. Mu J, Furlan AD, Lam WY, Hsu MY, Ning Z, Lao L. Acupuncture for chronic nonspecific low back pain. *Cochrane Database Syst Rev*. 2020;12(12):CD013814. Published 2020 Dec 11.

44. Farag AM, Malacarne A, Pagni SE, Maloney GE. The effectiveness of acupuncture in the management of persistent regional myofascial head and neck pain: a systematic review and meta-analysis. *Complement Ther Med*. 2020;49:102297.

45. Su X, Qian H, Chen B, et al. Acupuncture for acute low back pain: a systematic review and meta-analysis. *Ann Palliat Med*. 2021;10(4):3924-3936.

46. Tu JF, Yang JW, Shi GX, et al. Efficacy of intensive acupuncture versus sham acupuncture in knee osteoarthritis: a randomized controlled trial. *Arthritis Rheumatol*. 2021;73(3):448-458.

47. Gattie E, Cleland JA, Pandya J, Snodgrass S. Dry needling adds no benefit to the treatment of neck pain: a sham-controlled randomized clinical trial with 1-year follow-up. *J Orthop Sports Phys Ther*. 2021;51(1):37-45.

48. Sánchez-Infante J, Navarro-Santana MJ, Bravo-Sánchez A, Jiménez-Díaz F, Abián-Vicén J. Is dry needling applied by physical therapists effective for pain in musculoskeletal conditions? A systematic review and meta-analysis. *Phys Ther*. 2021;101(3):pzab070.

49. Liu L, Huang QM, Liu QG, et al. Effectiveness of dry needling for myofascial trigger points associated with neck and shoulder pain: a systematic review and meta-analysis. *Arch Phys Med Rehabil*. 2015;96(5):944-955.

50. Callaghan MJ, McKie S, Richardson P, Oldham JA. Effects of patellar taping on brain activity during knee joint proprioception tests using functional magnetic resonance imaging. *Phys Ther*. 2012;92(6):821-830.

51. Aguilar-Ferrándiz ME, Castro-Sánchez AM, Matarán-Peñarrocha GA, Guisado-Barrilao R, García-Ríos MC, Moreno-Lorenzo C. A randomized controlled trial of a mixed kinesio taping-compression technique on venous symptoms, pain, peripheral venous flow, clinical severity and overall health status in postmenopausal women with chronic venous insufficiency. *Clin Rehabil*. 2014;28(1):69-81.

52. Logan CA, Bhashyam AR, Tisosky AJ, et al. Systematic review of the effect of taping techniques on patellofemoral pain syndrome. *Sports Health*. 2017;9(5):456-461.

53. Cheatham SW, Lee M, Cain M, Baker R. The efficacy of instrument assisted soft tissue mobilization: a systematic review. *J Can Chiropr Assoc*. 2016;60(3):200-211.

54. Ikeda N, Otsuka S, Kawanishi Y, Kawakami Y. Effects of instrument-assisted soft tissue mobilization on musculoskeletal properties [published correction appears in *Med Sci Sports Exerc*. 2020 Feb;52(2):524]. *Med Sci Sports Exerc*. 2019;51(10):2166-2172.

55. Gunn LJ, Stewart JC, Morgan B, et al. Instrument-assisted soft tissue mobilization and proprioceptive neuromuscular facilitation techniques improve hamstring flexibility better than static stretching alone: a randomized clinical trial. *J Man Manip Ther*. 2019;27(1):15-23.

56. Kawashima M, Kawanishi N, Tominaga T, et al. Icing after eccentric contraction-induced muscle damage perturbs the disappearance of necrotic muscle fibers and phenotypic dynamics of macrophages in mice. *J Appl Physiol* (1985). 2021;130(5):1410-1420.

57. Singh DP, Barani Lonbani Z, Woodruff MA, Parker TJ, Steck R, Peake JM. Effects of topical icing on inflammation, angiogenesis, revascularization, and myofiber regeneration in skeletal muscle following contusion injury. *Front Physiol*. 2017;8:93.

58. Raynor MC, Pietrobon R, Guller U, Higgins LD. Cryotherapy after ACL reconstruction: a meta-analysis. *J Knee Surg*. 2005;18(2):123-129.

59. Barber FA, McGuire DA, Click S. Continuous-flow cold therapy for outpatient anterior cruciate ligament reconstruction. *Arthroscopy*. 1998;14(2):130-135.

60. Merrick MA, Rankin JM, Andres FA, Hinman CL. A preliminary examination of cryotherapy and secondary injury in skeletal muscle. *Med Sci Sports Exerc*. 1999;31(11):1516-1521.

61. Scott A, Khan KM, Roberts CR, Cook JL, Duronio V. What do we mean by the term "inflammation"? A contemporary basic science update for sports medicine. *Br J Sports Med*. 2004;38(3):372-380.

62. Mawhinney C, Low DA, Jones H, Green DJ, Costello JT, Gregson W. Cold water mediates greater reductions in limb blood flow than whole body cryotherapy. *Med Sci Sports Exerc*. 2017;49(6):1252-1260.

63. Wilson LJ, Cockburn E, Paice K, et al. Recovery following a marathon: a comparison of cold water immersion, whole body cryotherapy and a placebo control. *Eur J Appl Physiol*. 2018;118(1):153-163.

64. Crystal NJ, Townson DH, Cook SB, LaRoche DP. Effect of cryotherapy on muscle recovery and inflammation following a bout of damaging exercise. *Eur J Appl Physiol*. 2013;113(10):2577-2586.

65. Ghosh N, Kolade OO, Shontz E, et al. Nonsteroidal anti-inflammatory drugs (NSAIDs) and their effect on musculoskeletal soft-tissue healing: a scoping review. *JBJS Rev*. 2019;7(12):e4.

66. Kristensen DM, Desdoits-Lethimonier C, Mackey AL, et al. Ibuprofen alters human testicular physiology to produce a state of compensated hypogonadism [published correction appears in *Proc Natl Acad Sci USA*. 2018 Apr 16]. *Proc Natl Acad Sci USA*. 2018;115(4):E715-E724.

67. Bittermann A, Gao S, Rezvani S, et al. Oral ibuprofen interferes with cellular healing responses in a murine model of Achilles tendinopathy. *J Musculoskelet Disord Treat*. 2018;4(2):049.

68. Hammerman M, Blomgran P, Ramstedt S, Aspenberg P. COX-2 inhibition impairs mechanical stimulation of early tendon healing in rats by reducing the response to microdamage. *J Appl Physiol* (1985). 2015;119(5):534-540.

69. Connizzo BK, Yannascoli SM, Tucker JJ, et al. The detrimental effects of systemic ibuprofen delivery on tendon healing are time-dependent. *Clin Orthop Relat Res*. 2014;472(8):2433-2439.

70. Wang W, Shi M, Zhou C, et al. Effectiveness of corticosteroid injections in adhesive capsulitis of shoulder: a meta-analysis. *Medicine* (Baltimore). 2017;96(28):e7529.

71. Kapetanos G. The effect of the local corticosteroids on the healing and biomechanical properties of the partially injured tendon. *Clin Orthop Relat Res*. 1982;(163):170-179.

72. Wiggins ME, Fadale PD, Barrach H, Ehrlich MG, Walsh WR. Healing characteristics of a type I collagenous structure treated with corticosteroids. *Am J Sports Med.* 1994;22(2):279-288.

73. Wang CJ. Extracorporeal shockwave therapy in musculoskeletal disorders. *J Orthop Surg Res.* 2012;7:11.

74. Lou J, Wang S, Liu S, Xing G. Effectiveness of extracorporeal shock wave therapy without local anesthesia in patients with recalcitrant plantar fasciitis: a meta-analysis of randomized controlled trials. *Am J Phys Med Rehabil.* 2017;96(8):529-534.

75. Cacchio A, Rompe JD, Furia JP, Susi P, Santilli V, De Paulis F. Shockwave therapy for the treatment of chronic proximal hamstring tendinopathy in professional athletes. *Am J Sports Med.* 2011;39(1):146-153.

76. van Leeuwen MT, Zwerver J, van den Akker-Scheek I. Extracorporeal shockwave therapy for patellar tendinopathy: a review of the literature. *Br J Sports Med.* 2009;43(3):163-168.

77. Staples MP, Forbes A, Ptasznik R, Gordon J, Buchbinder R. A randomized controlled trial of extracorporeal shock wave therapy for lateral epicondylitis (tennis elbow). *J Rheumatol.* 2008;35(10):2038-2046.

78. Belk JW, Kraeutler MJ, Houck DA, Goodrich JA, Dragoo JL, McCarty EC. Platelet-rich plasma versus hyaluronic acid for knee osteoarthritis: a systematic review and meta-analysis of randomized controlled trials. *Am J Sports Med.* 2021;49(1):249-260.

79. Kim CH, Park YB, Lee JS, Jung HS. Platelet-rich plasma injection vs. operative treatment for lateral elbow tendinosis: a systematic review and meta-analysis. *J Shoulder Elbow Surg.* 2022;31(2):428-436.

80. Chen X, Jones IA, Park C, Vangsness CT Jr. The efficacy of platelet-rich plasma on tendon and ligament healing: a systematic review and meta-analysis with bias assessment. *Am J Sports Med.* 2018;46(8):2020-2032.

81. Chahla J, Cinque ME, Piuzzi NS, et al. A call for standardization in platelet-rich plasma preparation protocols and composition reporting: a systematic review of the clinical orthopaedic literature. *J Bone Joint Surg Am.* 2017;99(20):1769-1779.

82. McIntyre JA, Jones IA, Han B, Vangsness CT Jr. Intra-articular mesenchymal stem cell therapy for the human joint: a systematic review. *Am J Sports Med.* 2018;46(14):3550-3563.

83. Chahla J, Piuzzi NS, Mitchell JJ, et al. Intra-articular cellular therapy for osteoarthritis and focal cartilage defects of the knee: a systematic review of the literature and study quality analysis. *J Bone Joint Surg Am.* 2016;98(18):1511-1521.

84. Chang CH, Tsai WC, Hsu YH, Pang JH. Pentadecapeptide BPC 157 enhances the growth hormone receptor expression in tendon fibroblasts. *Molecules.* 2014;19(11):19066-19077.

85. Krivic A, Majerovic M, Jelic I, Seiwerth S, Sikiric P. Modulation of early functional recovery of Achilles tendon to bone unit after transection by BPC 157 and methylprednisolone. *Inflamm Res.* 2008;57(5):205-210.

86. Staresinic M, Sebecic B, Patrlj L, et al. Gastric pentadecapeptide BPC 157 accelerates healing of transected rat Achilles tendon and in vitro stimulates tendocytes growth. *J Orthop Res.* 2003;21(6):976-983.

87. Ebadi S, Henschke N, Forogh B, et al. Therapeutic ultrasound for chronic low back pain. *Cochrane Database Syst Rev.* 2020;7(7):CD009169. Published 2020 Jul 5.

88. Desmeules F, Boudreault J, Roy JS, Dionne C, Frémont P, MacDermid JC. The efficacy of therapeutic ultrasound for rotator cuff tendinopathy: a systematic review and meta-analysis. *Phys Ther Sport.* 2015;16(3):276-284.

89. van den Bekerom MP, van der Windt DA, Ter Riet G, van der Heijden GJ, Bouter LM. Therapeutic ultrasound for acute ankle sprains. *Cochrane Database Syst Rev.* 2011;2011(6):CD001250. Published 2011 Jun 15.

90. Robertson VJ, Baker KG. A review of therapeutic ultrasound: effectiveness studies. *Phys Ther.* 2001;81(7):1339-1350.

91. Baker KG, Robertson VJ, Duck FA. A review of therapeutic ultrasound: biophysical effects. *Phys Ther.* 2001;81(7):1351-1358.

92. van der Windt DAWM, van der Heijden GJMG, van den Berg SGM, Ter Riet G, de Winter AF, Bouter LM. Ultrasound therapy for musculoskeletal disorders: a systematic review. *Pain.* 1999;81(3):257-271.

93. Almeida Silva HJ, Barbosa GM, Scattone Silva R, et al. Dry cupping therapy is not superior to sham cupping to improve clinical outcomes in people with non-specific chronic low back pain: a randomised trial. *J Physiother.* 2021;67(2):132-139.

94. Lauche R, Spitzer J, Schwahn B, et al. Efficacy of cupping therapy in patients with the fibromyalgia syndrome-a randomised placebo controlled trial. *Sci Rep.* 2016;6:37316.

95. Daly S, Thorpe M, Rockswold S, et al. Hyperbaric oxygen therapy in the treatment of acute severe traumatic brain injury: a systematic review. *J Neurotrauma.* 2018;35(4):623-629.

96. Deng Z, Chen W, Jin J, Zhao J, Xu H. The neuroprotection effect of oxygen therapy: a systematic review and meta-analysis. *Niger J Clin Pract.* 2018;21(4):401-416.

97. Kranke P, Bennett MH, Martyn-St James M, Schnabel A, Debus SE, Weibel S. Hyperbaric oxygen therapy for chronic wounds. *Cochrane Database Syst Rev.* 2015;2015(6):CD004123. Published 2015 Jun 24.

98. Bennett MH, Feldmeier J, Hampson NB, Smee R, Milross C. Hyperbaric oxygen therapy for late radiation tissue injury. *Cochrane Database Syst Rev.* 2016;4(4):CD005005. Published 2016 Apr 28.

99. Ince B, Ismayilzada M, Arslan A, Dadaci M. Does hyperbaric oxygen therapy facilitate peripheral nerve recovery in upper extremity injuries? A prospective study of 74 patients. *Eur J Trauma Emerg Surg.* 2022;48(5):3997-4003.

100. Millar IL, Lind FG, Jansson KÅ, et al. Hyperbaric oxygen for lower limb trauma (HOLLT): an international multi-centre randomised clinical trial. *Diving Hyperb Med.* 2022;52(3):164-174.

101. Webster AL, Syrotuik DG, Bell GJ, Jones RL, Hanstock CC. Effects of hyperbaric oxygen on recovery from exercise-induced muscle damage in humans. *Clin J Sport Med.* 2002;12(3):139-150.

102. Babul S, Rhodes EC, Taunton JE, Lepawsky M. Effects of intermittent exposure to hyperbaric oxygen for the treatment of an acute soft tissue injury. *Clin J Sport Med.* 2003;13(3):138-147.

## Chapter 15

1. Childs JD, Cleland JA, Elliott JM, et al. Neck pain: clinical practice guidelines linked to the international classification of functioning, disability, and health from the orthopedic section of the American Physical Therapy Association [published correction appears in *J Orthop Sports Phys Ther.* 2009 Apr;39(4):297]. *J Orthop Sports Phys Ther.* 2008;38(9):A1-A34.

2. Côté P, Cassidy DJ, Carroll LJ, Kristman V. The annual incidence and course of neck pain in the general population: a population-based cohort study. *Pain.* 2004;112(3):267-273.

3. Borghouts JAJ, Koes BW, Bouter LM. The clinical course and prognostic factors of non-specific neck pain: a systematic review. *Pain.* 1998;77(1):1-13.

4. Kazeminasab S, Nejadghaderi SA, Amiri P, et al. Neck pain: global epidemiology, trends and risk factors. *BMC Musculoskelet Disord.* 2022;23(1):26.

5. Andersen LL, Saervoll CA, Mortensen OS, Poulsen OM, Hannerz H, Zebis MK. Effectiveness of small daily amounts of progressive resistance training for frequent neck/shoulder pain: randomised controlled trial. *Pain.* 2011;152(2):440-446.

6. Andersen LL, Kjaer M, Søgaard K, Hansen L, Kryger AI, Sjøgaard G. Effect of two contrasting types of physical exercise on chronic neck muscle pain. *Arthritis Rheum.* 2008;59(1):84-91.

7. Hidalgo B, Hall T, Bossert J, Dugeny A, Cagnie B, Pitance L. The efficacy of manual therapy and exercise for treating non-specific neck pain: a systematic review. *J Back Musculoskelet Rehabil.* 2017;30(6):1149-1169.

8. Brinjikji W, Luetmer PH, Comstock B, et al. Systematic literature review of imaging features of spinal degeneration in asymptomatic populations. *AJNR Am J Neuroradiol.* 2015;36(4):811-816.

9. Gore DR. Roentgenographic findings in the cervical spine in asymptomatic persons: a ten-year follow-up. *Spine* (Phila Pa 1976). 2001;26(22):2463-2466.

10. Basson A, Olivier B, Ellis R, Coppieters M, Stewart A, Mudzi W. The effectiveness of neural mobilization for neuromusculoskeletal conditions: a systematic review and meta-analysis. *J Orthop Sports Phys Ther.* 2017;47(9):593-615.

11. Silveira A, Gadotti IC, Armijo-Olivo S, Biasotto-Gonzalez DA, Magee D. Jaw dysfunction is associated with neck disability and muscle tenderness in subjects with and without chronic temporomandibular disorders. *Biomed Res Int.* 2015;2015:512792.

12. Kraus S. Temporomandibular disorders, head and orofacial pain: cervical spine considerations. *Dent Clin North Am.* 2007;51(1):161-vii.

## Chapter 16

1. Zhao J, Luo M, Liang G, et al. Risk factors for supraspinatus tears: a meta-analysis of observational studies. *Orthop J Sports Med.* 2021;9(10):23259671211042826.

2. Yamamoto A, Takagishi K, Osawa T, et al. Prevalence and risk factors of a rotator cuff tear in the general population. *J Shoulder Elbow Surg.* 2010;19(1):116-120.

3. Matthewson G, Beach CJ, Nelson AA, et al. Partial thickness rotator cuff tears: current concepts. *Adv Orthop.* 2015;2015:458786.

4. Tsuchiya S, Davison EM, Rashid MS, et al. Determining the rate of full-thickness progression in partial-thickness rotator cuff tears: a systematic review. *J Shoulder Elbow Surg.* 2021;30(2):449-455.

5. Kim HM, Dahiya N, Teefey SA, Keener JD, Galatz LM, Yamaguchi K. Relationship of tear size and location to fatty degeneration of the rotator cuff. *J Bone Joint Surg Am.* 2010;92(4):829-839.

6. Eajazi A, Kussman S, LeBedis C, et al. Rotator cuff tear arthropathy: pathophysiology, imaging characteristics, and treatment options. *AJR Am J Roentgenol.* 2015;205(5):W502-W511.

7. Diercks R, Bron C, Dorrestijn O, et al. Guideline for diagnosis and treatment of subacromial pain syndrome: a multidisciplinary review by the Dutch Orthopaedic Association. *Acta Orthop.* 2014;85(3):314-322.

8. Pieters L, Lewis J, Kuppens K, et al. An update of systematic reviews examining the effectiveness of conservative physical therapy interventions for subacromial shoulder pain. *J Orthop Sports Phys Ther.* 2020;50(3):131-141.

9. Haik MN, Alburquerque-Sendín F, Moreira RF, Pires ED, Camargo PR. Effectiveness of physical therapy treatment of clearly defined subacromial pain: a systematic review of randomised controlled trials. *Br J Sports Med.* 2016;50(18):1124-1134.

10. Guerrero P, Busconi B, Deangelis N, Powers G. Congenital instability of the shoulder joint: assessment and treatment options. *J Orthop Sports Phys Ther.* 2009;39(2):124-134.

11. Misamore GW, Sallay PI, Didelot W. A longitudinal study of patients with multidirectional instability of the shoulder with seven- to ten-year follow-up. *J Shoulder Elbow Surg.* 2005;14(5):466-470.

12. Burkhead WZ Jr, Rockwood CA Jr. Treatment of instability of the shoulder with an exercise program. *J Bone Joint Surg Am.* 1992;74(6):890-896.

13. de la Serna D, Navarro-Ledesma S, Alayón F, López E, Pruimboom L. A comprehensive view of frozen shoulder: a mystery syndrome. *Front Med* (Lausanne). 2021;8:663703.

14. Favejee MM, Huisstede BM, Koes BW. Frozen shoulder: the effectiveness of conservative and surgical interventions—systematic review. *Br J Sports Med.* 2011;45(1):49-56.

15. Challoumas D, Biddle M, McLean M, Millar NL. Comparison of treatments for frozen shoulder: a systematic review and meta-analysis. *JAMA Netw Open.* 2020;3(12):e2029581. Published 2020 Dec 1.

16. Dempsey AL, Mills T, Karsch RM, Branch TP. Maximizing total end range time is safe and effective for the conservative treatment of frozen shoulder patients. *Am J Phys Med Rehabil.* 2011;90(9):738-745.

17. Wilk KE, Hooks TR. The painful long head of the biceps brachii: nonoperative treatment approaches. *Clin Sports Med.* 2016;35(1):75-92.

18. Nho SJ, Strauss EJ, Lenart BA, et al. Long head of the biceps tendinopathy: diagnosis and management. *J Am Acad Orthop Surg.* 2010;18(11):645-656.

19. Cardoso TB, Pizzari T, Kinsella R, Hope D, Cook JL. Current trends in tendinopathy management. *Best Pract Res Clin Rheumatol.* 2019;33(1):122-140.

## Chapter 17

1. Lenoir H, Mares O, Carlier Y. Management of lateral epicondylitis. *Orthop Traumatol Surg Res.* 2019;105(8S):S241-S246.
2. Kim YJ, Wood SM, Yoon AP, Howard JC, Yang LY, Chung KC. Efficacy of nonoperative treatments for lateral epicondylitis: a systematic review and meta-analysis. *Plast Reconstr Surg.* 2021;147(1):112-125.
3. Landesa-Piñeiro L, Leirós-Rodríguez R. Physiotherapy treatment of lateral epicondylitis: a systematic review. *J Back Musculoskelet Rehabil.* 2022;35(3):463-477.
4. Cullinane FL, Boocock MG, Trevelyan FC. Is eccentric exercise an effective treatment for lateral epicondylitis? A systematic review. *Clin Rehabil.* 2014;28(1):3-19.
5. Amin NH, Kumar NS, Schickendantz MS. Medial epicondylitis: evaluation and management. *J Am Acad Orthop Surg.* 2015;23(6):348-355.
6. Cardoso TB, Pizzari T, Kinsella R, Hope D, Cook JL. Current trends in tendinopathy management. *Best Pract Res Clin Rheumatol.* 2019;33(1):122-140.
7. Andres BM, Murrell GA. Treatment of tendinopathy: what works, what does not, and what is on the horizon. *Clin Orthop Relat Res.* 2008;466(7):1539-1554.
8. Casadei K, Kiel J, Freidl M. Triceps tendon injuries. *Curr Sports Med Rep.* 2020;19(9):367-372.

## Chapter 18

1. Atroshi I, Gummesson C, Johnsson R, Ornstein E, Ranstam J, Rosén I. Prevalence of carpal tunnel syndrome in a general population. *JAMA.* 1999;282(2):153-158.
2. Ferry S, Pritchard T, Keenan J, Croft P, Silman AJ. Estimating the prevalence of delayed median nerve conduction in the general population. *Br J Rheumatol.* 1998;37(6):630-635.
3. Yoshii Y, Zhao C, Amadio PC. Recent advances in ultrasound diagnosis of carpal tunnel syndrome. *Diagnostics* (Basel). 2020;10(8):596.
4. Harris-Adamson C, Eisen EA, Kapellusch J, et al. Biomechanical risk factors for carpal tunnel syndrome: a pooled study of 2474 workers. *Occup Environ Med.* 2015;72(1):33-41.
5. Meng S, Reissig LF, Beikircher R, Tzou CH, Grisold W, Weninger WJ. Longitudinal gliding of the median nerve in the carpal tunnel: ultrasound cadaveric evaluation of conventional and novel concepts of nerve mobilization. *Arch Phys Med Rehabil.* 2015;96(12):2207-2213.

## Chapter 19

1. Deyo RA, Weinstein JN. Low back pain. *N Engl J Med.* 2001;344(5):363-370.
2. Gianola S, Bargeri S, Del Castillo G, et al. Effectiveness of treatments for acute and subacute mechanical non-specific low back pain: a systematic review with network meta-analysis. *Br J Sports Med.* 2022;56(1):41-50.
3. Almeida M, Saragiotto B, Richards B, Maher CG. Primary care management of non-specific low back pain: key messages from recent clinical guidelines. *Med J Aust.* 2018;208(6):272-275.
4. Saragiotto BT, Maher CG, Yamato TP, et al. Motor control exercise for nonspecific low back pain: a Cochrane review. *Spine* (Phila Pa 1976). 2016;41(16):1284-1295.
5. Quentin C, Bagheri R, Ugbolue UC, et al. Effect of home exercise training in patients with nonspecific low-back pain: a systematic review and meta-analysis. *Int J Environ Res Public Health.* 2021;18(16):8430.
6. Seyedhoseinpoor T, Taghipour M, Dadgoo M, et al. Alteration of lumbar muscle morphology and composition in relation to low back pain: a systematic review and meta-analysis. *Spine J.* 2022;22(4):660-676.
7. Goubert D, Oosterwijck JV, Meeus M, Danneels L. Structural changes of lumbar muscles in non-specific low back pain: a systematic review. *Pain Physician.* 2016;19(7):E985-E1000.
8. O'Sullivan K, O'Keeffe M, Forster BB, Qamar SR, van der Westhuizen A, O'Sullivan PB. Managing low back pain in active adolescents. *Best Pract Res Clin Rheumatol.* 2019;33(1):102-121.
9. Warner WC Jr, de Mendonça RGM. Adolescent spondylolysis: management and return to play. *Instr Course Lect.* 2017;66:409-413.
10. Gagnet P, Kern K, Andrews K, Elgafy H, Ebraheim N. Spondylolysis and spondylolisthesis: a review of the literature. *J Orthop.* 2018;15(2):404-407.
11. Donaldson LD. Spondylolysis in elite junior-level ice hockey players. *Sports Health.* 2014;6(4):356-359.
12. Kalichman L, Hunter DJ. Diagnosis and conservative management of degenerative lumbar spondylolisthesis. *Eur Spine J.* 2008;17(3):327-335.
13. Vibert BT, Sliva CD, Herkowitz HN. Treatment of instability and spondylolisthesis: surgical versus nonsurgical treatment. *Clin Orthop Relat Res.* 2006;443:222-227.
14. Bernard TN Jr, Kirkaldy-Willis WH. Recognizing specific characteristics of nonspecific low back pain. *Clin Orthop Relat Res.* 1987;(217):266-280.
15. Hansen HC, McKenzie-Brown AM, Cohen SP, Swicegood JR, Colson JD, Manchikanti L. Sacroiliac joint interventions: a systematic review. *Pain Physician.* 2007;10(1):165-184.
16. Al-Subahi M, Alayat M, Alshehri MA, et al. The effectiveness of physiotherapy interventions for sacroiliac joint dysfunction: a systematic review. *J Phys Ther Sci.* 2017;29(9):1689-1694.
17. Koes BW, van Tulder MW, Peul WC. Diagnosis and treatment of sciatica. *BMJ.* 2007;334(7607):1313-1317.
18. Parreira P, Maher CG, Steffens D, Hancock MJ, Ferreira ML. Risk factors for low back pain and sciatica: an umbrella review. *Spine J.* 2018;18(9):1715-1721.
19. Vanti C, Panizzolo A, Turone L, et al. Effectiveness of mechanical traction for lumbar radiculopathy: a systematic review and meta-analysis. *Phys Ther.* 2021;101(3):pzaa231.
20. Brinjikji W, Luetmer PH, Comstock B, et al. Systematic literature review of imaging features of spinal degeneration in asymptomatic populations. *AJNR Am J Neuroradiol.* 2015;36(4):811-816.
21. Brinjikji W, Diehn FE, Jarvik JG, et al. MRI findings of disc degeneration are more prevalent in adults with low back pain than in asymptomatic controls: a systematic review and meta-analysis. *AJNR Am J Neuroradiol.* 2015;36(12):2394-2399.

22. Zhong M, Liu JT, Jiang H, et al. Incidence of spontaneous resorption of lumbar disc herniation: a meta-analysis. *Pain Physician*. 2017;20(1):E45-E52.

23. Videman T, Battié MC, Gibbons LE, Maravilla K, Manninen H, Kaprio J. Associations between back pain history and lumbar MRI findings. *Spine* (Phila Pa 1976). 2003;28(6):582-588.

24. Hahne AJ, Ford JJ, McMeeken JM. Conservative management of lumbar disc herniation with associated radiculopathy: a systematic review. *Spine* (Phila Pa 1976). 2010;35(11):E488-E504.

25. Katz JN, Harris MB. Clinical practice. Lumbar spinal stenosis. *N Engl J Med*. 2008;358(8):818-825.

26. Lurie J, Tomkins-Lane C. Management of lumbar spinal stenosis. *BMJ*. 2016;352:h6234.

27. Wood KB, Blair JM, Aepple DM, et al. The natural history of asymptomatic thoracic disc herniations. *Spine* (Phila Pa 1976). 1997;22(5):525-530.

28. Gundersen A, Borgstrom H, McInnis KC. Trunk injuries in athletes. *Curr Sports Med Rep*. 2021;20(3):150-156.

29. Foley CM, Sugimoto D, Mooney DP, Meehan WP 3rd, Stracciolini A. Diagnosis and treatment of slipping rib syndrome. *Clin J Sport Med*. 2019;29(1):18-23.

30. Proulx AM, Zryd TW. Costochondritis: diagnosis and treatment. *Am Fam Physician*. 2009;80(6):617-620.

# Chapter 20

1. Griffin DR, Dickenson EJ, O'Donnell J, et al. The Warwick Agreement on femoroacetabular impingement syndrome (FAI syndrome): an international consensus statement. *Br J Sports Med*. 2016;50(19):1169-1176.

2. Hoit G, Whelan DB, Dwyer T, Ajrawat P, Chahal J. Physiotherapy as an initial treatment option for femoroacetabular impingement: a systematic review of the literature and meta-analysis of 5 randomized controlled trials. *Am J Sports Med*. 2020;48(8):2042-2050.

3. Wall PD, Fernandez M, Griffin DR, Foster NE. Nonoperative treatment for femoroacetabular impingement: a systematic review of the literature. *PM R*. 2013;5(5):418-426.

4. Zhu Y, Su P, Xu T, Zhang L, Fu W. Conservative therapy versus arthroscopic surgery of femoroacetabular impingement syndrome (FAI): a systematic review and meta-analysis. *J Orthop Surg Res*. 2022;17(1):296. Published 2022 Jun 3.

5. Heerey JJ, Kemp JL, Mosler AB, et al. What is the prevalence of imaging-defined intra-articular hip pathologies in people with and without pain? A systematic review and meta-analysis. *Br J Sports Med*. 2018;52(9):581-593.

6. Johnson VL, Hunter DJ. The epidemiology of osteoarthritis. *Best Pract Res Clin Rheumatol*. 2014;28(1):5-15.

7. Litwic A, Edwards MH, Dennison EM, Cooper C. Epidemiology and burden of osteoarthritis. *Br Med Bull*. 2013;105:185-199.

8. National Clinical Guideline Centre (UK). *Osteoarthritis: Care and Management in Adults*. London: National Institute for Health and Care Excellence (UK); February 2014.

9. Zampogna B, Papalia R, Papalia GF, et al. The role of physical activity as conservative treatment for hip and knee osteoarthritis in older people: a systematic review and meta-analysis. *J Clin Med*. 2020;9(4):1167. Published 2020 Apr 18.

10. Gay C, Chabaud A, Guilley E, Coudeyre E. Educating patients about the benefits of physical activity and exercise for their hip and knee osteoarthritis. Systematic literature review. *Ann Phys Rehabil Med*. 2016;59(3):174-183.

11. Wellsandt E, Golightly Y. Exercise in the management of knee and hip osteoarthritis. *Curr Opin Rheumatol*. 2018;30(2):151-159.

12. Long SS, Surrey DE, Nazarian LN. Sonography of greater trochanteric pain syndrome and the rarity of primary bursitis. *AJR Am J Roentgenol*. 2013;201(5):1083-1086.

13. Reid D. The management of greater trochanteric pain syndrome: a systematic literature review. *J Orthop*. 2016;13(1):15-28.

14. Pianka MA, Serino J, DeFroda SF, Bodendorfer BM. Greater trochanteric pain syndrome: evaluation and management of a wide spectrum of pathology. *SAGE Open Med*. 2021;9:20503121211022582. Published 2021 Jun 3.

15. Torres A, Fernández-Fairen M, Sueiro-Fernández J. Greater trochanteric pain syndrome and gluteus medius and minimus tendinosis: nonsurgical treatment. *Pain Manag*. 2018;8(1):45-55.

16. Park JW, Lee YK, Lee YJ, Shin S, Kang Y, Koo KH. Deep gluteal syndrome as a cause of posterior hip pain and sciatica-like pain. *Bone Joint J*. 2020;102-B(5):556-567.

17. Kizaki K, Uchida S, Shanmugaraj A, et al. Deep gluteal syndrome is defined as a non-discogenic sciatic nerve disorder with entrapment in the deep gluteal space: a systematic review. *Knee Surg Sports Traumatol Arthrosc*. 2020;28(10):3354-3364.

18. Hopayian K, Heathcote J. Deep gluteal syndrome: an overlooked cause of sciatica. *Br J Gen Pract*. 2019;69(687):485-486.

19. Vij N, Kiernan H, Bisht R, et al. Surgical and non-surgical treatment options for piriformis syndrome: a literature review. *Anesth Pain Med*. 2021;11(1):e112825. Published 2021 Feb 2.

20. Hölmich P. Long-standing groin pain in sportspeople falls into three primary patterns, a "clinical entity" approach: a prospective study of 207 patients. *Br J Sports Med*. 2007;41(4):247-252.

21. Rauseo C. The rehabilitation of a runner with iliopsoas tendinopathy using an eccentric-biased exercise—a case report. *Int J Sports Phys Ther*. 2017;12(7):1150-1162.

22. Blankenbaker DG, De Smet AA, Keene JS. Sonography of the iliopsoas tendon and injection of the iliopsoas bursa for diagnosis and management of the painful snapping hip. *Skeletal Radiol*. 2006;35(8):565-571.

23. Carlson C. The natural history and management of hamstring injuries. *Curr Rev Musculoskelet Med*. 2008;1(2):120-123.

24. Biz C, Nicoletti P, Baldin G, Bragazzi NL, Crimì A, Ruggieri P. Hamstring strain injury (HSI) prevention in professional and semi-professional football teams: a systematic review and meta-analysis. *Int J Environ Res Public Health*. 2021;18(16):8272.

25. Arnason A, Andersen TE, Holme I, Engebretsen L, Bahr R. Prevention of hamstring strains in elite

soccer: an intervention study. *Scand J Med Sci Sports*. 2008;18(1):40-48.

26. Bahr R, Thorborg K, Ekstrand J. Evidence-based hamstring injury prevention is not adopted by the majority of Champions League or Norwegian Premier League football teams: the Nordic hamstring survey. *Br J Sports Med*. 2015;49(22):1466-1471.

27. Goom TS, Malliaras P, Reiman MP, Purdam CR. Proximal hamstring tendinopathy: clinical aspects of assessment and management. *J Orthop Sports Phys Ther*. 2016;46(6):483-493.

28. Beatty NR, Félix I, Hettler J, Moley PJ, Wyss JF. Rehabilitation and prevention of proximal hamstring tendinopathy. *Curr Sports Med Rep*. 2017;16(3):162-171.

29. Kerbel YE, Smith CM, Prodromo JP, Nzeogu MI, Mulcahey MK. Epidemiology of hip and groin injuries in collegiate athletes in the United States. *Orthop J Sports Med*. 2018;6(5):2325967118771676. Published 2018 May 11.

30. Maffey L, Emery C. What are the risk factors for groin strain injury in sport? A systematic review of the literature. *Sports Med*. 2007;37(10):881-894.

31. Hölmich P, Larsen K, Krogsgaard K, Gluud C. Exercise program for prevention of groin pain in football players: a cluster-randomized trial. *Scand J Med Sci Sports*. 2010;20(6):814-821.

32. Tyler TF, Nicholas SJ, Campbell RJ, Donellan S, McHugh MP. The effectiveness of a preseason exercise program to prevent adductor muscle strains in professional ice hockey players. *Am J Sports Med*. 2002;30(5):680-683.

33. Schaber M, Guiser Z, Brauer L, et al. The neuromuscular effects of the Copenhagen adductor exercise: a systematic review. *Int J Sports Phys Ther*. 2021;16(5):1210-1221.

34. Harøy J, Clarsen B, Wiger EG, et al. The Adductor Strengthening Programme prevents groin problems among male football players: a cluster-randomised controlled trial. *Br J Sports Med*. 2019;53(3):150-157.

## Chapter 21

1. McClinton SM, Cobian DG, Heiderscheit BC. Physical therapist management of anterior knee pain. *Curr Rev Musculoskelet Med*. 2020;13(6):776-787.

2. Willy RW, Hoglund LT, Barton CJ, et al. Patellofemoral pain. *J Orthop Sports Phys Ther*. 2019;49(9):CPG1-CPG95.

3. Robertson CJ, Hurley M, Jones F. People's beliefs about the meaning of crepitus in patellofemoral pain and the impact of these beliefs on their behaviour: a qualitative study. *Musculoskelet Sci Pract*. 2017;28:59-64.

4. Aderem J, Louw QA. Biomechanical risk factors associated with iliotibial band syndrome in runners: a systematic review. *BMC Musculoskelet Disord*. 2015;16:356.

5. Hutchinson LA, Lichtwark GA, Willy RW, Kelly LA. The iliotibial band: a complex structure with versatile functions. *Sports Med*. 2022;52(5):995-1008.

6. Fairclough J, Hayashi K, Toumi H, et al. The functional anatomy of the iliotibial band during flexion and extension of the knee: implications for understanding iliotibial band syndrome. *J Anat*. 2006;208(3):309-316.

7. Horga LM, Hirschmann AC, Henckel J, et al. Prevalence of abnormal findings in 230 knees of asymptomatic adults using 3.0 T MRI. *Skeletal Radiol*. 2020;49(7):1099-1107.

8. Englund M, Guermazi A, Gale D, et al. Incidental meniscal findings on knee MRI in middle-aged and elderly persons. *N Engl J Med*. 2008;359(11):1108-1115.

9. Wells ME, Scanaliato JP, Dunn JC, Garcia EJ. Meniscal injuries: mechanism and classification. *Sports Med Arthrosc Rev*. 2021;29(3):154-157.

10. Beaufils P, Pujol N. Management of traumatic meniscal tear and degenerative meniscal lesions. Save the meniscus. *Orthop Traumatol Surg Res*. 2017;103(8S):S237-S244.

11. Chirichella PS, Jow S, Iacono S, Wey HE, Malanga GA. Treatment of knee meniscus pathology: rehabilitation, surgery, and orthobiologics. *PM R*. 2019;11(3):292-308.

12. Feeley BT, Lau BC. Biomechanics and clinical outcomes of partial meniscectomy. *J Am Acad Orthop Surg*. 2018;26(24):853-863.

13. Drobnič M, Ercin E, Gamelas J, et al. Treatment options for the symptomatic post-meniscectomy knee. *Knee Surg Sports Traumatol Arthrosc*. 2019;27(6):1817-1824.

14. Hewett TE, Myer GD, Ford KR, Paterno MV, Quatman CE. Mechanisms, prediction, and prevention of ACL injuries: cut risk with three sharpened and validated tools. *J Orthop Res*. 2016;34(11):1843-1855.

15. Kobayashi H, Kanamura T, Koshida S, et al. Mechanisms of the anterior cruciate ligament injury in sports activities: a twenty-year clinical research of 1,700 athletes. *J Sports Sci Med*. 2010;9(4):669-675. Published 2010 Dec 1.

16. Boden BP, Sheehan FT, Torg JS, Hewett TE. Noncontact anterior cruciate ligament injuries: mechanisms and risk factors. *J Am Acad Orthop Surg*. 2010;18(9):520-527.

17. van Melick N, van Cingel RE, Brooijmans F, et al. Evidence-based clinical practice update: practice guidelines for anterior cruciate ligament rehabilitation based on a systematic review and multidisciplinary consensus. *Br J Sports Med*. 2016;50(24):1506-1515.

18. Kaplan Y. Identifying individuals with an anterior cruciate ligament-deficient knee as copers and noncopers: a narrative literature review. *J Orthop Sports Phys Ther*. 2011;41(10):758-766.

19. Eitzen I, Moksnes H, Snyder-Mackler L, Risberg MA. A progressive 5-week exercise therapy program leads to significant improvement in knee function early after anterior cruciate ligament injury. *J Orthop Sports Phys Ther*. 2010;40(11):705-721.

20. Grindem H, Snyder-Mackler L, Moksnes H, Engebretsen L, Risberg MA. Simple decision rules can reduce reinjury risk by 84% after ACL reconstruction: the Delaware-Oslo ACL cohort study. *Br J Sports Med*. 2016;50(13):804-808.

21. Smith TO, Song F, Donell ST, Hing CB. Operative versus non-operative management of patellar dislocation. A meta-analysis. *Knee Surg Sports Traumatol Arthrosc*. 2011;19(6):988-998.

22. Smith TO, Chester R, Cross J, Hunt N, Clark A, Donell ST. Rehabilitation following first-time patellar dislocation: a randomised controlled trial of purported vastus

medialis obliquus muscle versus general quadriceps strengthening exercises. *Knee.* 2015;22(4):313-320.

23. Challoumas D, Pedret C, Biddle M, et al. Management of patellar tendinopathy: a systematic review and network meta-analysis of randomised studies. *BMJ Open Sport Exerc Med.* 2021;7(4):e001110. Published 2021 Nov 29.

24. Malliaras P, Cook J, Purdam C, Rio E. Patellar tendinopathy: clinical diagnosis, load management, and advice for challenging case presentations. *J Orthop Sports Phys Ther.* 2015;45(11):887-898.

25. Allen KD, Golightly YM. State of the evidence. *Curr Opin Rheumatol.* 2015;27(3):276-283.

26. Litwic A, Edwards MH, Dennison EM, Cooper C. Epidemiology and burden of osteoarthritis. *Br Med Bull.* 2013;105:185-199.

27. Palazzo C, Nguyen C, Lefevre-Colau MM, Rannou F, Poiraudeau S. Risk factors and burden of osteoarthritis. *Ann Phys Rehabil Med.* 2016;59(3):134-138.

28. Alentorn-Geli E, Samuelsson K, Musahl V, Green CL, Bhandari M, Karlsson J. The association of recreational and competitive running with hip and knee osteoarthritis: a systematic review and meta-analysis. *J Orthop Sports Phys Ther.* 2017;47(6):373-390.

29. Calatayud J, Casaña J, Ezzatvar Y, Jakobsen MD, Sundstrup E, Andersen LL. High-intensity preoperative training improves physical and functional recovery in the early post-operative periods after total knee arthroplasty: a randomized controlled trial. *Knee Surg Sports Traumatol Arthrosc.* 2017;25(9):2864-2872.

## Chapter 22

1. Myhrvold SB, Brouwer EF, Andresen TKM, et al. Nonoperative or surgical treatment of acute Achilles' tendon rupture. *N Engl J Med.* 2022;386(15):1409-1420.

2. Järvinen TA, Kannus P, Maffulli N, Khan KM. Achilles tendon disorders: etiology and epidemiology. *Foot Ankle Clin.* 2005;10(2):255-266.

3. von Rickenbach KJ, Borgstrom H, Tenforde A, Borg-Stein J, McInnis KC. Achilles tendinopathy: evaluation, rehabilitation, and prevention. *Curr Sports Med Rep.* 2021;20(6):327-334.

4. Zhi X, Liu X, Han J, et al. Nonoperative treatment of insertional Achilles tendinopathy: a systematic review. *J Orthop Surg Res.* 2021;16(1):233.

5. O'Neill S, Barry S, Watson P. Plantarflexor strength and endurance deficits associated with mid-portion Achilles tendinopathy: the role of soleus. *Phys Ther Sport.* 2019;37:69-76.

6. Hébert-Losier K, Wessman C, Alricsson M, Svantesson U. Updated reliability and normative values for the standing heel-rise test in healthy adults. *Physiotherapy.* 2017;103(4):446-452.

7. Rhim HC, Kwon J, Park J, Borg-Stein J, Tenforde AS. A systematic review of systematic reviews on the epidemiology, evaluation, and treatment of plantar fasciitis. *Life* (Basel). 2021;11(12):1287.

8. Albers IS, Zwerver J, Diercks RL, Dekker JH, Van den Akker-Scheek I. Incidence and prevalence of lower extremity tendinopathy in a Dutch general practice population: a cross sectional study. *BMC Musculoskelet Disord.* 2016;17:16.

9. Morrissey D, Cotchett M, Said J'Bari A, et al. Management of plantar heel pain: a best practice guide informed by a systematic review, expert clinical reasoning and patient values. *Br J Sports Med.* 2021;55(19):1106-1118.

10. Rompe JD, Cacchio A, Weil L Jr, et al. Plantar fascia-specific stretching versus radial shock-wave therapy as initial treatment of plantar fasciopathy. *J Bone Joint Surg Am.* 2010;92(15):2514-2522.

11. Rathleff MS, Mølgaard CM, Fredberg U, et al. High-load strength training improves outcome in patients with plantar fasciitis: a randomized controlled trial with 12-month follow-up. *Scand J Med Sci Sports.* 2015;25(3):e292-e300.

12. Herzog MM, Kerr ZY, Marshall SW, Wikstrom EA. Epidemiology of ankle sprains and chronic ankle instability. *J Athl Train.* 2019;54(6):603-610.

13. Doherty C, Bleakley C, Delahunt E, Holden S. Treatment and prevention of acute and recurrent ankle sprain: an overview of systematic reviews with meta-analysis. *Br J Sports Med.* 2017;51(2):113-125.

14. Vuurberg G, Hoorntje A, Wink LM, et al. Diagnosis, treatment and prevention of ankle sprains: update of an evidence-based clinical guideline. *Br J Sports Med.* 2018;52(15):956.

15. Kobayashi T, Tanaka M, Shida M. Intrinsic risk factors of lateral ankle sprain: a systematic review and meta-analysis. *Sports Health.* 2016;8(2):190-193.

16. Menéndez C, Batalla L, Prieto A, Rodríguez MÁ, Crespo I, Olmedillas H. Medial tibial stress syndrome in novice and recreational runners: a systematic review. *Int J Environ Res Public Health.* 2020;17(20):7457.

17. Nix S, Smith M, Vicenzino B. Prevalence of hallux valgus in the general population: a systematic review and meta-analysis. *J Foot Ankle Res.* 2010;3:21.

18. Nguyen US, Hillstrom HJ, Li W, et al. Factors associated with hallux valgus in a population-based study of older women and men: the MOBILIZE Boston Study. *Osteoarthritis Cartilage.* 2010;18(1):41-46.

19. Arbeeva L, Yau M, Mitchell BD, et al. Genome-wide meta-analysis identified novel variant associated with hallux valgus in Caucasians. *J Foot Ankle Res.* 2020;13(1):11.

20. Hannan MT, Menz HB, Jordan JM, Cupples LA, Cheng CH, Hsu YH. High heritability of hallux valgus and lesser toe deformities in adult men and women. *Arthritis Care Res* (Hoboken). 2013;65(9):1515-1521.

# INDEX

## A

Achilles pain, rehab exercise protocol for, 427–435

Achilles tendinopathy/tear
overview, 427–428
rehab exercise protocol for, 430–435

ACL (anterior cruciate ligament), 70

ACL tear. *See* ligament tear (knee)

active assisted range of motion (AAROM), 53

active range of motion (AROM), 53

active strategies, in physical therapy, 47

acupuncture, 137

acute pain, chronic pain compared with, 27

aerobic exercise, for pain relief, 50

afferent input, 17

afferent (ascending) pathways, for pain, 22–23

age, as a red flag symptom, 111

aggravating factors, in rehab exercise protocols, 110

alcohol consumption, healing time and, 79

alternative in-person treatments, as a treatment option, 6

anatomy, as a factor influencing pain, 43–44

ankle sprain
overview, 445–446
rehab exercise protocol for, 447–453

ankles
ankle sprain, 445–453
ligament grades of injury, 71
rehab exercise protocols for, 426–471

anterior cruciate ligament (ACL), 70

anterior longitudinal ligament sprain, 75

anti-inflammatory cytokines, 36

anti-inflammatory medication, 140

anxiety, as a mental variable influencing injury, 96

ascending (afferent) pathways, for pain, 22–23

## B

back nerve pain, rehab exercise protocol for, 304–316

back pain (low back), rehab exercise protocol for, 281–303

back pain (mid-back and rib cage), rehab exercise protocol for, 304–327

"bad" movements, 37

balance pad, 130

balance/proprioception, as a physical variable influencing injury, 94

beliefs, as a mental variable influencing injury, 96

bench, 127

BFR (blood flow restriction), 134–135

biceps tendinopathy
overview, 224–225
rehab exercise protocol for, 226–233

biomechanics
as a factor influencing pain, 36–38
as a training variable influencing injury, 89

biopsychosocial (BPS) model, 14–15

bladder dysfunction, as a red flag symptom, 111

blood clots, 429

blood flow, sensing, 19

blood flow restriction (BFR), 134–135

body area map, 117

bone
about, 77
typical healing time frame for fractures of, 85

BPS (biopsychosocial) model, 14–15

braces, 142

brain, relationship with pain, 14–15

bunions
overview, 463–464
rehab exercise protocol for, 465–471

## C

calf pain, rehab exercise protocol for, 427–435

calf strain
overview, 429
rehab exercise protocol for, 430–435

CAMs. *See* complementary and alternative medicine (CAM) interventions

cancer history, as a red flag symptom, 111

carpal tunnel syndrome
overview, 30, 76, 271–273
rehab exercise protocol for, 274–279

Cartesian model of pain, 11

cartilage injuries
traumatic and degenerative, 73–75
typical healing time frame for, 83–84